Organ Specific Drug Delivery and Targeting to the Lungs

Organ Specific Drug Delivery and Targeting to the Lungs provides up to date information on the multidisciplinary field of particle engineering and drug delivery to the lungs, including advancements of nanotechnology. The text presents a unique, pragmatic focus with case studies that help translate scientific understanding to practical implementation. In addition to highlighting the successful case studies, it also offers practical advice on watchouts, limitations, and 'bookend' boundaries involved in the stages of testing and development.

Additional features include:

- An account of particle engineering, discovery, biology, development, and delivery in relation to the advancements of nanotechnology, unlike any previous book.
- Bringing together the leading experts and researchers in the field to critically assess and discuss various topics influencing drug delivery.
- Highlighting the interplay of different scientific disciplines and the balance of requirements that are critical to molecules and product design.

With a strategic focus on what matters during new product development, this book provides a guide to understanding and navigating new drug discovery and development for lung targets.

Organ-Specific Drug Delivery and Targeting

Series Editors

Ajit S. Narang, Ph.D.

Department of Pharmaceutical Sciences

ORIC Pharmaceuticals, Inc, South San Francisco, CA 94080, USA

&

Ram I. Mahato, Ph.D.

Department of Pharmaceutical Sciences, University of Nebraska Medical Center

Omaha, NE 68198, USA

The editors are leading experts in the field and will co-edit this brand new series on Organ-specific Drug Delivery and Targeting. In particular, the following organs will be featured: Lung, Liver, Brain, Kidney, Pancreas, GI and Eye. The vision is to provide a unique coverage of drug delivery to various organs through this series of volumes. Such a timely collection is sorely needed as the pharmaceutical industry is now in the midst of prioritizing research and development of COVID-19 related diagnostics, treatments, health technologies and vaccines, as well as looking at the potential of existing treatments.

Organ Specific Drug Delivery and Targeting to the Lungs
Edited by Ajit S. Narang, Ram I. Mahato

Organ Specific Drug Delivery and Targeting to the Lungs

Edited by
Ajit S. Narang, Ph.D.
Department of Pharmaceutical Sciences
ORIC Pharmaceuticals, Inc, South San Francisco, USA
&

Ram I. Mahato, Ph.D.
Department of Pharmaceutical Sciences, University of
Nebraska Medical Center
Omaha, USA

CRC Press
Taylor & Francis Group
Boca Raton London New York

CRC Press is an imprint of the
Taylor & Francis Group, an **informa** business

First edition published 2023
by CRC Press
6000 Broken Sound Parkway NW, Suite 300, Boca Raton, FL 33487-2742

and by CRC Press
4 Park Square, Milton Park, Abingdon, Oxon, OX14 4RN

CRC Press is an imprint of Taylor & Francis Group, LLC

Library of Congress Cataloging-in-Publication Data

Names: Narang, Ajit S., editor. | Mahato, Ram I., editor.
Title: Organ specific drug delivery and targeting to the lungs / edited by
Ajit S. Narang, Ph.D. (Department of Pharmaceutical Sciences, ORIC
Pharmaceuticals, Inc, South San Francisco, CA, USA) & Ram I. Mahato,
Ph.D. (Department of Pharmaceutical Sciences, University of Nebraska
Medical Center, Omaha, NE, USA).
Description: Boca Raton : CRC Press, 2023. | Includes bibliographical
references.
Identifiers: LCCN 2022015645 (print) | LCCN 2022015646 (ebook) | ISBN
9781032010397 (hardback) | ISBN 9781032022529 (paperback) | ISBN
9781003182566 (ebook)
Subjects: LCSH: Drugs--Dosage forms. | Drug targeting. | Respiratory
organs--Diseases--Treatment. | Nanomedicine.
Classification: LCC RS200 .O74 2023 (print) | LCC RS200 (ebook) | DDC
615.1--dc23/eng/20220625
LC record available at https://lccn.loc.gov/2022015645
LC ebook record available at https://lccn.loc.gov/2022015646

ISBN: 9781032010397 (hbk)
ISBN: 9781032022529 (pbk)
ISBN: 9781003182566 (ebk)

DOI: 10.1201/9781003182566

Typeset in Times
by Deanta Global Publishing Services, Chennai, India

To my mom, Gurdip Kaur, the silent warrior.

Ajit S. Narang

To the late Professor Sung Wan Kim of the University of Utah for his contribution and encouragement to young scientists.
To my late father-in law Professor Ram Mohan Mahto, who set higher goals of educating and igniting the young minds of Nepal.

Ram I. Mahato

Contents

Preface

The recent COVID-19 outbreak brought to the forefront the vulnerability and the potential of the inhalation route of access to systemic circulation. Drug delivery to and through the lungs has been recognized and practiced for long, including systemic delivery of nicotine by smoking and the lungs being the target organ for certain ailments such as asthma, chronic obstructive pulmonary disease (COPD), and tuberculosis. Nonetheless, the complexity of drug delivery to and absorption in/through the lungs belies the apparent simplicity of breathing in the desired medication. Consequently, drug development for lung delivery entails extraordinary uncertainty and risk from the relative lack of translational models, predictive in vitro and preclinical methods, and standardization of approaches – so much so that most discovery programs do not consider lung delivery as an enabler.

The objective of this book is to highlight key elements of this uncertainty and risk, with an emphasis on recent progress and strategies being adopted by the industry and academia to circumvent or overcome those technical risks.

The historical context of the inhalation route of drug administration is discussed in detail by Ruzycki et al. in Chapter 1. To establish a better correlation between in vitro and in vivo results, in Chapter 2 Bhattarai et al. discuss in vitro assessment of drug release, dissolution, and absorption in the lung. "Lung-on-a-chip" and other organoid models are richly discussed in Chapter 3 by Malik et al. In Chapter 4, Pan et al. discuss how interaction between inhalable nanomedicines and pulmonary surfactant can affect drug deposition, therapeutic efficacy, and toxicity. In Chapters 5 and 6, the effects of particle engineering and architectonics for pulmonary drug delivery are discussed by Karde and Heng, and Kawakami, respectively. In Chapter 7, Chang and Chan discuss engineered particles. In Chapter 8, Abdelaziz et al. discuss the recent advances in inhalable nanomedicine for lung cancer therapy. In Chapter 9, Moon et al. discuss the process and importance of thin film freeze-drying to generate versatile particles for inhalation drug delivery. There is an in-depth discussion on nanoparticles for delivery to the lung in Chapter 10 by Montanheiro et al. In Chapters 11 and 12, surface modification and spray drying of particles for inhalation are discussed by Bajaj et al. and Kumar et al., respectively. The use of inhalable phospholipid particles for targeted drug delivery to the lung is discussed in Chapter 13 by Eedara et al. Nebulizers are discussed in Chapter 14 by Berlinski. In Chapter 15, Xin et al. discuss protein and peptide delivery to the lung by inhalation. Chapter 16 is the last chapter of this book by Ramesh and Munshi, who discuss the use of extracellular vesicles called exosomes for drug delivery for the treatment of lung cancer.

Taken together, this book makes an attempt to highlight and address the key areas of drug development that have created bottlenecks to the wider utilization of the inhalation route of drug delivery. There are rapid advances in pulmonary drug delivery by inhalations and systemic administration. This book brings together several leading experts to critically assess and discuss various topics influencing drug delivery to the lung such that academics, industrial scientists, and graduate students can easily learn different facets of pulmonary drug delivery. This will further enable the reader to understand how particle size, shape, and surface modifications and devices affect drug deposition to the lung and therapeutic efficacy in more comprehensive manner.

Acknowledgments

We would like to thank all our contributors and the editorial staff at CRC Press for their time and effort in bringing this volume together.

We also thank our employers for supporting the pursuit of excellence in the emergent sciences as well as their investment in new drug development and delivery, and of the supporting sciences.

Ajit S. Narang and Ram I. Mahato

About the Authors

Ajit S. Narang works for the Department of Pharmaceutical Sciences at ORIC Pharmaceuticals, Inc., in south San Francisco, CA. His primary expertise is in oral drug delivery. He holds over 20 years of pharmaceutical industry experience in drug development. Prior to ORIC, Ajit also worked for Genentech, Inc.; Bristol-Myers Squibb, Co.; Ranbaxy Research Labs (currently a subsidiary of Daiichi Sankyo, Japan); and Morton Grove Pharmaceuticals (currently, Wockhardt USA). He holds an undergraduate pharmacy degree from the University of Delhi, India and graduate degrees in pharmaceutical sciences from the Banaras Hindu University, India, and the University of Tennessee Health Science Center (UTHSC) in Memphis, TN. He currently serves as the Chair of Biopharmaceutics Technical Committee of the Product Quality Research Institute. His current research interests focus on new drug discovery research. He has been credited with several publications, patents, and books throughout his career, and has contributed to the development of several clinical and marketed drug products.

Ram I. Mahato is Professor and Chairman of the Department of Pharmaceutical Sciences, University of Nebraska Medical Center, Omaha, NE. He was a professor at the University of Tennessee Health Science Center, Research Assistant Professor at the University of Utah, Senior Scientist at GeneMedicine, Inc., and postdoctoral fellow at the University of Southern California in Los Angeles, Washington University in St. Louis, and Kyoto University, Japan. He received a PhD in drug delivery from the University of Strathclyde, Great Britain, and a BS from China Pharmaceutical University, Nanjing. He has published 166 peer reviewed papers, 24 book chapters, holds three US patents, and has edited/written nine books and eleven journal issues (total Google citations = 13,060 and h-Index = 67). He is an associate editor of the Journal of Neuroimmune Pharmacology and was a feature editor of the Pharmaceutical Research (2006–2013). He is a CRS and AAPS Fellow. He applies sound principles in pharmaceutical sciences in the context of the latest advances in life and material sciences to solve challenging drug delivery problems in therapeutics. His areas of research include delivery and targeting of small molecules, miRNA and genes using novel polymeric and lipid carriers for treating cancer, liver fibrosis, and diabetes.

List of Contributors

Adnan A. Bekhit
Cancer Nanotechnology Research
    Laboratory (CNRL)
Faculty of Pharmacy
Alexandria University
Alexandria, Egypt
and
Department of Pharmaceutical Chemistry
Faculty of Pharmacy
Alexandria University
Alexandria, Egypt

Ahmed O. Elzoghby
Cancer Nanotechnology Research
    Laboratory (CNRL)
Faculty of Pharmacy
Alexandria University
Alexandria, Egypt
and
Department of Industrial Pharmacy
Faculty of Pharmacy
Alexandria University, Egypt
and
Division of Engineering in Medicine
Department of Medicine
Brigham and Women's Hospital
Harvard Medical School
Boston, Massachusetts

Ajit S. Narang
ORIC Pharmaceuticals
San Francisco, California

Amer S. Alali
Department of Pharmaceutics
College of Pharmacy
Prince Sattam Bin Abdulaziz University
Al-Kharj, Saudi Arabia

Andrew R. Martin
Department of Mechanical Engineering
University of Alberta
Edmonton, Alberta, Canada

Anupama Munshi
Department of Radiation Oncology
University of Oklahoma Health Sciences
    Center
Oklahoma City, Oklahoma
and
Stephenson Cancer Center
University of Oklahoma Health Sciences
    Center
Oklahoma City, Oklahoma

Ariel Berlinski
Pulmonary and Sleep Division
Department of Pediatrics
University of Arkansas for Medical
    Sciences
and
Pediatric Aerosol Research Laboratory at
    Arkansas Children's Research Institute
Little Rock, Arkansas

Basanth Babu Eedara
Center for Translational Science
Florida International University
Port St. Lucie, Florida

Charan Singh
Department of Pharmaceutics
ISF College of Pharmacy
Affiliated to IK Gujral Punjab Technical
    University Jalandhar
Kapurthala, Punjab, India

Chaeho Moon
Division of Molecular
  Pharmaceutics and Drug
  Delivery
College of Pharmacy
University of Texas at Austin
Austin, Texas

Chuanbin Wu
School of Pharmaceutical
  Sciences
Sun Yat-sen University
Guangzhou, China

Conor A. Ruzycki
Department of Mechanical
  Engineering
University of Alberta
Edmonton, Alberta, Canada

David Encinas-Basurto
Skaggs Pharmaceutical Sciences
  Center
University of Arizona
College of Pharmacy
Tucson, Arizona

David Oupicky
Center for Drug Delivery and
  Nanomedicine
Department of Pharmaceutical
  Sciences
University of Nebraska Medical
  Center
Omaha, Nebraska

Deepak Chitkara
Department of Pharmacy
Birla Institute of Technology and Science
  (BITS) Pilani
Vidya Vihar Campus
Pilani, Rajasthan, India

Don Hayes Jr
Division of Pulmonary Medicine
Cincinnati Children's Hospital Medical
  Center
Cincinnati, Ohio
and
Division of Pulmonary, Critical Care, and
  Sleep Medicine
University of Cincinnati
  Medical Center
Cincinnati, Ohio
and
Department of Pediatrics and Internal
  Medicine
University of Cincinnati College of
  Medicine
Cincinnati, Ohio

Gilmar Patrocínio Thim
Laboratory of Plasma and Processes
  (LPP)
Technological Institute of
  Aeronautics (ITA)
São José dos Campos, Brazil

Hadeer M.Abdelaziz
Cancer Nanotechnology Research
  Laboratory (CNRL)
Faculty of Pharmacy
Alexandria University
Alexandria, Egypt
and
Department of Pharmaceutics
Faculty of Pharmacy
Damanhur University
Damanhur, Egypt

Hak-Kim Chan
Advanced Drug Delivery Group
Sydney Pharmacy School
The University of Sydney
Sydney, Australia

Heidi M. Mansour
FIU Center for Translational Science
and
Robert Stempel College of Public Health
  & Social Work
Department of Environmental Health
  Sciences
and
Herbert Wertheim College of Medicine
Department of Cell Biology &
  Pharmacology
FIU Center for Translational Science
Port St. Lucie, Florida

Jerry Y.Y. Heng
Department of Chemical
  Engineering
Imperial College London
London, United Kingdom

Kadria A. Elkhodairy
Cancer Nanotechnology Research
  Laboratory (CNRL)
Faculty of Pharmacy
Alexandria University
Alexandria, Egypt
and
Department of Industrial Pharmacy
Faculty of Pharmacy
Alexandria University
Alexandria, Egypt

Karla Faquine Rodrigues
Laboratory of Plasma and Processes
  (LPP)
Technological Institute of Aeronautics
  (ITA)
São José dos Campos, Brazil

Kohsaku Kawakami
Medical Soft Matter Group
National Institute for Materials Science
Tsukuba, Ibaraki, Japan

Mohamed Teleb
Cancer Nanotechnology Research
  Laboratory (CNRL)
Faculty of Pharmacy
Alexandria University
Alexandria, Egypt
and
Department of Pharmaceutical Chemistry
Faculty of Pharmacy
Alexandria University
Alexandria, Egypt

Muhammad H. Malik
Department of Pharmacological and
  Pharmaceutical Sciences
College of Pharmacy
University of Houston
Houston, Texas

Sherine N.Khattab
Cancer Nanotechnology Research
  Laboratory (CNRL)
Faculty of Pharmacy
Alexandria University
Alexandria, Egypt
and
Department of Chemistry
Faculty of Science
Alexandria University
Alexandria, Egypt

Neha Kumari
Center for Drug Delivery and
  Nanomedicine
Department of Pharmaceutical Sciences
University of Nebraska Medical Center
Omaha, Nebraska

Qiyue Wang
Department of Pharmaceutical Sciences
University of Nebraska Medical Center
Omaha, Nebraska
and
School of Pharmaceutical Science
Nanjing Tech University
Nanjing, China

Rachel Yoon Kyung Chang
S341, Pharmacy and Bank Building A15
University of Sydney
Sydney, Australia

Raissa Monteiro Pereira
Laboratory of Plasma and Processes
(LPP)
Technological Institute of Aeronautics
(ITA)
São José dos Campos, Brazil

Rajagopal Ramesh
Department of Pathology
University of Oklahoma Health Sciences
Center
Oklahoma City, Oklahoma
and
Stephenson Cancer Center
University of Oklahoma Health Sciences
Center
Oklahoma City, Oklahoma

Raj Kumar
Center for Drug Delivery and
Nanomedicine
Department of Pharmaceutical Sciences
University of Nebraska Medical Center
Omaha, Nebraska

Rajan S. Bhattarai
Department of Pharmaceutical
Sciences
University of Nebraska Medical Center
Omaha, Nebraska

Ram I Mahato
Department of Pharmaceutical Sciences
University of Nebraska Medical Center
Omaha, Nebraska

Renata Guimarães Ribas
Laboratory of Plasma and Processes (LPP
Technological Institute of Aeronautics
(ITA)
São José dos Campos, Brazil

Robert O. Williams III
Division of Molecular Pharmaceutics and
Drug Delivery
College of Pharmacy
University of Texas at Austin
Austin, Texas

Sawittree Sahakijpijarn
TFF Pharmaceuticals, Inc.
Austin, Texas

Shalaleh Masoumi
Department of Pharmacological and
Pharmaceutical Sciences
College of Pharmacy
University of Houston
Houston, Texas

Tania Bajaj
Department of Pharmaceutics
ISF College of Pharmacy
affiliated to IK Gujral Punjab Technical
University Jalandhar
Kapurthala, Punjab, India
and
IK Gujral Punjab Technical University,
Jalandhar
Kapurthala, Punjab, India

Thaís Larissa do Amaral Montanheiro
Laboratory of Plasma and Processes (LPP)
Technological Institute of Aeronautics (ITA)
São José dos Campos, Brazil

Urvashi Anwekar
Department of Pharmacy
Birla Institute of Technology and Science
(BITS) Pilani
Vidya Vihar Campus
Pilani, Rajasthan, India

Vanessa Modelski Schatkoski
Laboratory of Plasma and Processes (LPP)
Technological Institute of Aeronautics
(ITA)
São José dos Campos, Brazil

Vikram Karde
Department of Chemical Engineering
Imperial College London
London, United Kingdom

Virender Kumar
Department of Pharmaceutical
    Sciences
University of Nebraska Medical Center
Omaha, Nebraska

Vishav Prabhjot Kaur
Department of Pharmaceutics
ISF College of Pharmacy
affiliated to IK Gujral Punjab Technical
    University, Jalandhar
Kapurthala, Punjab, India

Warren H. Finlay
Department of Mechanical Engineering
University of Alberta
Edmonton, Alberta, Canada

Xiaofei Xin
Department of Pharmaceutical Sciences
University of Nebraska Medical Center
Omaha, Nebraska
and
School of Pharmacy
China Pharmaceutical University
Nanjing, China

Xinli Liu
Department of Pharmacological and
    Pharmaceutical Sciences
College of Pharmacy
University of Houston
Houston, Texas

Xue Zhou
Department of Pharmacological and
    Pharmaceutical Sciences
College of Pharmacy
University of Houston
Houston, Texas

SECTION I

In-Vitro and
Ex-Vivo Methods

Estimating Clinically Relevant Measures of Inhaled Pharmaceutical Aerosol Performance with Advanced In Vitro and In Silico Methods

1

Conor A. Ruzycki, Warren H. Finlay,
Andrew R. Martin

DOI: 10.1201/9781003182566-2

Contents

1.1 INTRODUCTION

Inhaled pharmaceutical aerosols, having proved useful in the treatment of disease, are now a mainstay of modern medicine. The direct delivery of medication to the respiratory tract offers a number of advantages as a route of drug administration, including rapid onset of action, reduced systemic dosing for drugs targeting respiratory tract disease, and ease of use for patients. Consequently, therapeutic aerosols are routinely prescribed in the treatment of respiratory tract diseases and disorders, among them asthma, chronic obstructive pulmonary disease (COPD), and cystic fibrosis. Common inhaled therapies include corticosteroids, anticholinergic agents, and beta-agonists in the standard treatment of asthma and COPD[1-3]; antibiotics for managing lung infections that frequently occur in patients who suffer from cystic fibrosis, undergo prolonged mechanical ventilation, or experience lengthy stays in intensive care[4,5]; and mucoactive agents such as hypertonic saline to increase mucociliary clearance in patients with chronic lung disease.[6] For these therapies, whose goal is the treatment of disease locally within the lungs, the aerosol route allows for targeted delivery to the site of intended action, achieving local therapeutic doses while bypassing large systemic doses—a major advantage over other routes of administration.

There also exists a largely untapped potential for pharmaceutical aerosols in systemic drug delivery, for example, inhaled insulin for the treatment of diabetes,[7] antipsychotic[8] and anti-migraine[9,10] medications, and levodopa for treating Parkinson's disease.[11] Systemic delivery of macromolecules via the respiratory tract has been shown to yield higher bioavailability than other non-invasive delivery routes, which may help reduce the total dose required for efficacious treatment, while the large surface area provided by the alveolar airways allows for the rapid uptake of small molecules.[12] Formulations comprising dry powders for inhalation can remain stable for years when stored at room temperatures, making these an ideal vehicle for drug delivery in regions where access to refrigeration is limited.[13] Stable dry powder formulations of anti-tubercular therapies may thus prove extremely useful in treating tuberculosis in the developing world.[14]

Such advantages of inhaled pharmaceutical aerosols are countered somewhat by a number of factors that can reduce treatment success with these medications. For one, the drug must enter the airways to reach the site of intended action. Modern delivery devices typically lose a significant fraction of the nominal drug dose to deposition in the extrathoracic airways before it reaches the lungs, a process that can lead to deleterious side effects and reduced treatment efficacy.[15,16] Extrathoracic deposition, being subject-specific and variable,[17,18] can also cause a high degree of variability in the total dose delivered to the lungs, and complicates titration to efficacious minimal doses in patients with chronic conditions.[19] In addition to inflammation and associated immune responses, chronic lung diseases often cause pathophysiological and histological alterations in the airways that increase in severity with disease progression.[20] The site of intended action for some inhaled medications may therefore become a moving target as the disease advances.

An additional consideration with inhaled aerosols is the reliance of treatment efficacy on patient adherence to correct administration techniques. A large proportion of patients demonstrate improper technique when self-administering with inhalers, leading to jeopardized device performance and reduced treatment efficacy.[21] Noting the wide range of inhaler designs on the market, Laube et al.[22] provided a number of specific device recommendations for practitioners working with different patient groups to alleviate issues related to improper technique. And while pharmacist intervention can certainly improve inhalation technique and treatment outcomes,[23,24] the requirement of proper patient technique for treatment efficacy remains a key consideration.

With both local and systemic delivery of inhaled therapeutics, the deposition of aerosol particles in the airways of the respiratory tract is critical in determining the effective dose. The respiratory tract can be broadly classified into three regions: the extrathoracic region, which comprises the mouth, nose, and throat airways; the conducting region of the tracheobronchial airways; and the alveolar region, which facilitates gas exchange over the large surface area provided by hundreds of millions of alveoli. For local delivery, certain drugs may provide a more therapeutic effect when delivered to specific portions of the respiratory tract, as in the case of the proximal conducting airways for beta-agonists[25] or the more peripheral small airways for anti-inflammatories.[20,26] For systemic delivery, general consensus places the ideal location of deposition as the alveolar (gas-exchange) region, where the thin barrier between the alveolar lumen and surrounding capillaries facilitates rapid uptake and increased bioavailability compared to other administration routes.[12] With either form of delivery, deposition in the extrathoracic region for many inhaled pharmaceutical aerosols is often considered lost or wasted, as this dose is either swallowed (later undergoing first-pass metabolism) or expectorated.

1.1.1 Clinically Relevant Measures

Measures of inhaled pharmaceutical aerosol performance *in vivo* typically rely on clinical trials with quantifiable endpoints. Along with the classic endpoints of morbidity and mortality from large-scale clinical trials, quantifiable test metrics for use in evaluating inhaled pharmaceutical aerosol performance are invaluable. One of the most commonly used metrics in characterizing lung disease and treatment efficacy is the forced expiratory volume in one second (FEV1).[27] Measured via spirometry, the FEV1 sees widespread use in the characterization and treatment of asthma,[28] cystic fibrosis,[29] and COPD.[30] Correlations between the FEV1 and *in vitro* measures of pharmaceutical aerosol performance would thus be useful in optimizing therapies, and while the exact relation between dose and efficacy depends on numerous factors,[31] some basic inferences can be made for certain drug classes based on the literature.

Numerous dose-ranging studies have demonstrated relationships between the total administered dose and improvements in FEV1, reinforcing the logical notion that the amount of drug delivered to the lungs is related to treatment efficacy. Such relationships have been clinically demonstrated with both corticosteroids[32–35] and bronchodilators,[36–38] and the opposite effect (i.e., reductions in FEV1) are observed with challenge aerosols like methacholine.[39]

For some drugs, deposition in specific regions of the lungs may be more determinate of treatment efficacy than the total administered dose. Usmani, Biddiscombe, and Barnes[25] demonstrated *in vivo* that regional deposition was a larger determinant of the effect of albuterol on improvements to FEV1 for asthmatic patients than the total lung dose. 30 µg doses of albuterol delivered via large 6 µm mass median aerodynamic diameter particles (posited to deposit predominantly in the proximal airways) achieved greater improvements in FEV1 than 200 µg doses delivered via pressurized metered dose inhaler plus spacer, while equivalent 30 µg doses delivered via smaller 1.5 µm and 3.0 µm aerosols that demonstrated higher total lung doses than the 6.0 µm aerosol and more distal deposition showed reduced treatment efficacy. The authors surmised that since airway smooth muscle is predominately located in the conducting airways, and that the β2-agonist albuterol acts on this tissue to induce bronchodilation, treatment efficacy was increased by preferentially targeting deposition in this region.[25]

With inhaled corticosteroids, recent focus has shifted towards increasing deposition in the more peripheral regions of the lungs to treat small airway (<2 mm diameter) inflammation.[40] In a recent study on extra-fine beclomethasone dipropionate delivered via pressurized metered dose inhaler, Montanaro et al.[34] found the improvement in FEV1 in asthmatics plateaued at a nominal dose of 200 µg, with 400 µg showing increased adverse events at no additional clinical benefit. These results support the analysis of Beasley et al.,[41] who note that the traditional definition of a "low" dose of inhaled corticosteroids (100 to 250 µg of fluticasone propionate or equivalent for adults) actually captures 80 to 90% of the maximum achievable clinical effect for moderate to severe asthma. However, because these doses are the nominal doses metered by devices (not the actual doses depositing in the lungs or portions therein), the influence of regional deposition on clinical effect of corticosteroids is not well-established.

Regional targeting may also be of benefit with inhaled antibiotics. Ramsey et al.[42] demonstrated that inhaled tobramycin improved the FEV1 and decreased the need for hospitalizations of cystic fibrosis patients with *Pseudomonas aeruginosa* infections. Administration of high (300 mg) doses of tobramycin were performed using a jet nebulizer emitting relatively large droplets (4 µm), with the aim of preferentially targeting infection in the airways while limiting systemic absorption via the alveolar region. A companion study by Geller et al.[43] evaluated the pharmacokinetics and bioavailability of tobramycin, demonstrating that the majority of patients achieved sufficiently high concentrations of tobramycin in sputum to treat infection, with low systemic availability via the inhalation route (11.7%) helping to limit potential toxic systemic side effects that would otherwise be associated with such high doses. Inhaled antibiotics, in general, aim to provide the highest concentration of active drug at the site of infection while avoiding systemic toxicity.[44]

Common among the above examples is the notion that the quantification of the dose of drug delivered to the lungs, and even to specific regions of the lung, can aide in understanding treatment efficacy and the parameters that influence clinical outcomes. Beyond basic measures of total or regional dose, models allowing for the characterization of disposition are also useful in predicting drug concentrations in airway surface liquid, free vs. bound drug in specific tissues, and in characterizing systemic exposure. With novel treatments in development for various classes of therapeutics, the availability of *in vitro* and *in silico* methods that can accurately inform these fundamental characterizations of therapeutic agents are of interest in optimizing the drug development process.

1.1.2 Pharmacopeial Measures of Inhaler Performance

Methods for predicting where the aerosol generated by a particular inhaler and/or with a particular formulation will deposit within the respiratory tract are invaluable in characterizing existing treatments and creating new ones. Standard practice for examining and describing device and formulation performance follows the recommendations of compendial organizations such as the United States Pharmacopeia[45,46] and the European Pharmacopoeia,[47] or the guidance of regulatory bodies such as the United

States Food and Drug Administration[48] and European Medicines Agency.[49] These recommendations, which can vary depending on whether the device in question is a dry powder inhaler (DPI), pressurized metered dose inhaler (pMDI), soft mist inhaler (SMI), or nebulizer, aim at ensuring that manufactured devices on the market adhere to quality control metrics such as consistency and accuracy in delivered dose.[50] Less focus is placed on predicting *in vivo* performance. The delivered dose uniformity test, for example, provides no information concerning how much drug reaches the site of intended action, or the fate of the drug following deposition.

Fundamentally, this scarcity of information may hamper the development of new products, as the goalposts used in the early stages of inhaler and formulation design (delivered dose, basic aerodynamic particle size distribution groupings) are only tangentially related to *in vivo* deposition and disposition. Given such limitations, the development of new test methods that are more predictive of *in vivo* performance is an attractive prospect. Such methods may help streamline the development process for novel treatments by providing additional information on device and formulation performance in preclinical phases of drug development—well in advance of expensive clinical trials and associated ethical issues—while also providing quality control measures more applicable to health outcomes.

1.1.3 Defining Test Systems

Test systems for inhaled pharmaceutical aerosols can be broadly classified into several categories, including *in vitro* methods, *in silico* computational models, *ex vivo* experiments, and animal models. The present chapter focuses on *in vitro* methods for estimating extrathoracic and thoracic deposition together with aspects of *in silico* computational modeling, including algebraic deposition correlations, one-dimensional lung deposition models, and pharmacokinetic models of disposition following deposition (wherein some aspects of dissolution and absorption are discussed). Other categories of test systems, such as advanced *in vitro* and *ex vivo* dissolution and translocation testing,[51,52] three-dimensional lung deposition modeling,[53] and animal models[54] are not described in detail.

1.2 *IN VITRO* METHODS

In vitro methods are experimental methods performed in a laboratory setting under controlled conditions. With inhaled pharmaceutical aerosols, such methods allow for the in-depth examination of a multitude of parameters for device and formulation performance. A basic *in vitro* experiment to examine deposition may consist of an inhaler, extrathoracic geometry, and filter connected in a series to an inhalation source, shown schematically in Figure 1.1. As aerosol is emitted from the inhaler, some particles or droplets will impact on and deposit along the interior surfaces of the extrathoracic geometry, while others will continue downstream to be captured in the filter. In the

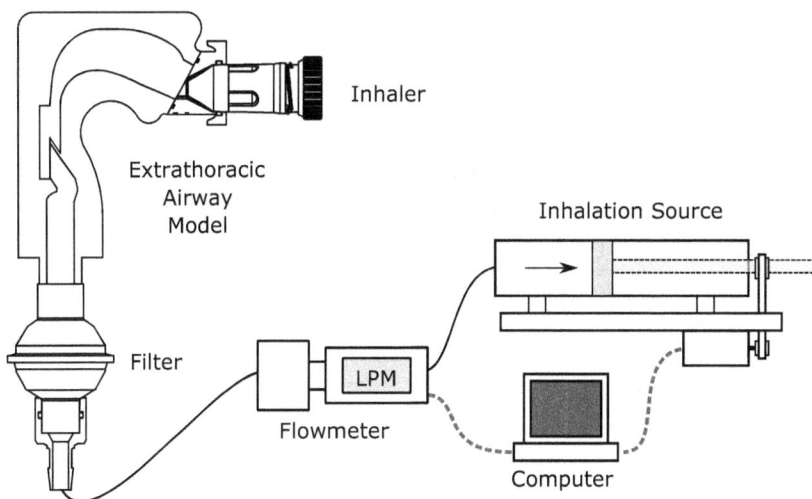

FIGURE 1.1   Schematic of a typical *in vitro* experiment for determining extra thoracic and total lung deposition from a dry powder inhaler. Adapted with permission from Ruzycki, Martin, and Finlay[89].

absence of a large exhaled dose, the dose depositing on this filter provides an estimate of the total dose delivered to the lungs, while the dose depositing in the extrathoracic geometry provides an estimate of oropharyngeal deposition.[17,55,56] Additional information can be gained by replacing the filter with a sizing instrument, such as a cascade impactor, from which the initial particle size distribution entering the thoracic airways can be inferred.[57,58]

The development of *in vitro* correlations capable of accurately predicting *in vivo* deposition has long been a topic of particular interest in the pharmaceutical industry,[59] leading to a number of recent advances that may improve the predictive capabilities of benchtop experiments. There are several factors to consider in the design of predictive *in vitro* methods, broadly summarized into categories of (i) airway geometry, (ii) inhalation maneuver, (iii) hygroscopic behavior, and (iv) real-world use.

1.2.1 Airway Geometry

Given the importance of extrathoracic deposition in determining the total dose delivered to the lungs, the design of *in vitro* geometries capable of replicating extrathoracic deposition is an obvious starting point in improving the clinical relevance of *in vitro* tests. The United States Pharmacopeia Induction Port (USP-IP)[45] is a commonly used geometry for interfacing with inhalers *in vitro* and consists of a simple design (two constant diameter tubes joined with a 90° elbow) allowing for ease of manufacture. Unfortunately, this simple design fails to replicate the complex fluid-dynamical interactions that occur within the extrathoracic airways and as a result consistently underestimates extrathoracic deposition of pharmaceutical aerosols in adults.[60–62]

TABLE 1.1   Examples of extrathoracic airway geometries for *in vitro* testing

GEOMETRY	TYPE	AGE GROUP	AIRWAY
Oropharyngeal Consortium (OPC) Models (Burnell et al.[67])	Realistic	Adults	Oral
Virginia Commonwealth University (VCU) Models (Delvadia, Longest, and Byron[69])	Semi-realistic	Adults	Oral
Sophia Anatomical Infant Nose-Throat (SAINT) Model (Janssens et al.[77])	Realistic	Infants (~9 months)	Nasal
Premature Infant Nose Throat (PrINT) Model (Minocchieri et al.[81])	Realistic	Premature infants (32-week gestational age)	Nasal
Alberta Idealized Throat (Stapleton et al.[82])	Idealized	Adults	Oral
Alberta Idealized Child Throat (Golshahi and Finlay[91])	Idealized	Children (school age, 6 to 14 years)	Oral
Idealized Infant Nasal Model (Javaheri, Golshahi, and Finlay[94])	Idealized	Infants (3–18 months)	Nasal
Idealized Neonatal Nasal Model (Tavernini et al.[95])	Idealized	Neonatal infants (0–3 months)	Nasal
Alberta Idealized Nasal Inlet (Kiaee et al.[97])	Idealized	Adults	Nasal

A natural progression from the USP-IP is the use of geometries that more accurately replicate the complex nature of the extrathoracic airways. Modern examples of this approach generally fall into one of two camps: the use of realistic (or semi-realistic) geometries that aim to directly replicate anatomical structures or the use of idealized geometries that mimic important anatomical features to capture the function of the airways. In either case, advances in medical imaging over the past few decades have proven extremely useful in the development of such geometries, which were previously obtainable only through airway casts on human cadavers.[63]

Several examples of both realistic and idealized extrathoracic airway geometries for *in vitro* tests can be found in the literature. For drug delivery to the lungs, the relevant extrathoracic airway is age-dependent: infants are obligate nose breathers, while older children and adults typically self-administer aerosols via the mouth. Thus, for treatments targeting delivery to the lungs, extrathoracic geometries for infants have focused on the nasal extrathoracic airways, while extrathoracic geometries for children and adults have focused on the oral extrathoracic airways. Table 1.1 and the following sections summarize some of the extrathoracic geometries that have been described in the literature for use *in vitro*.

1.2.1.1 Realistic and semi-realistic extrathoracic geometries

Drawing on a series of studies on human oropharyngeal airspaces using magnetic resonance imaging,[64–66] Burnell et al.[67] presented a set of three realistic extrathoracic airway models designed to predict low, median, and high oropharyngeal deposition in healthy adults using nebulizers, pMDIs, and DPIs. These three upper airway models were isolated from a large set of 80 MRI scans of 20 adult patients inhaling from four separate mouthpieces and were based on a statistical analysis of 11 dimensional variables and series of *in vitro* measurements using a DPI, pMDI, and nebulizer. Referred to as the Oropharyngeal Consortium (OPC) models, these geometries have been used to confirm the idea that the dose escaping deposition in an extrathoracic airway model is predictive of the total lung dose when the exhaled dose is negligible.[68]

Delvadia, Longest, and Byron[69] described a semi-realistic upper airway model spanning from the mouth and throat into the upper bronchi of the third airway generation. The mouth-throat model was adapted from Xi and Longest's[70] reconstruction of a fully realistic geometry using elliptical cross sections of equal hydraulic diameter and flow area, while the upper airways from the trachea to the third generation were based on morphological data from the literature.[71,72] The geometry, with a mouth-throat volume of 61.6 cm^3 and tracheobronchial dimensions corresponding to a lung volume of 3.5 L, was presented as a "medium-sized" geometry for the general adult population. Additional "small" and "large" geometries were created by a scaling procedure aimed at capturing the variations in airway sizes observed in adults. For the mouth-throat, scaling factors were obtained by adding and subtracting a volume of 37.8 cm^3 (corresponding to two times the standard deviation of the average mouth-throat volume reported by Burnell et al.[67]) to and from the original 65 cm^3 volume of Xi and Longest's[70] geometry, and then taking the cube root of the volume ratios. In effect, this approach created an isotropic scaling along each dimension of 1.165 for the large geometry and 0.748 for the small geometry. Here, Delvadia, Longest, and Byron[69] presumed that the "small" and "large" geometries generated via isometric scaling of the "medium" geometry would capture the 95th percentiles of physical dimensions observed in an adult population and hypothesized that these would translate into estimates of the median and variability of lung deposition when used *in vitro* to examine deposition from pharmaceutical inhalers. This approach does not account for geometric dissimilarity in extrathoracic geometries *in vivo*, however, (see discussion later in this chapter based on Ruzycki et al.[18]), and it is therefore unclear if these geometries provide rigorous estimates of variability in real populations. The geometries described by Delvadia, Longest, and Byron[69] are together referred to as the Virginia Commonwealth University (VCU) models, and a number of studies have used the VCU models, or portions thereof, to examine factors such as insertion angle,[73] the effects of realistic inhalation maneuvers on DPI performance,[74,75] and relative performance in comparisons with other throat models.[57,76]

Janssens et al.[77] presented the Sophia Anatomical Infant Nose-Throat (SAINT) model, a realistic nasopharyngeal geometry created from a computed tomography (CT) scan of a nine-month-old Caucasian female infant. The model, which included portions of the infant's face, provides a realistic interface for aerosol administration via facemasks and spacers. Janssens et al.[77] used the SAINT model to examine initial thoracic particle sizes and total lung doses of a budesonide pMDI delivered with a spacer and facemask using realistic inhalations. Deposition within the SAINT model itself was not directly measured, as the polymer resin of the model interfered with high performance liquid chromatographs (HPLCs) for the selected solvent, ethanol. The SAINT model has seen use in a number of studies on aerosol administration to infants, including investigations on high flow nebulization,[78] active dry powder inhalers,[79] and facemask seal leaks.[80]

Minocchieri et al.[81] developed a realistic nasopharyngeal airway model of a premature newborn from MRI scans of a healthy male with a gestational age of 32 weeks to address the absence of such a model in the literature. The authors noted somewhat limited scan resolution due to long acquisition times and coarse voxel sizes provided by MRI as compared to CT imaging, which was not used because of ethical issues concerning radiation exposure for preterm infants. A physical model including the face was rapid prototyped using a photopolymer, with post-build CT scans of the physical model confirming that the printing process adequately replicated the airways. Minocchieri et al.[81] then used a facemask to deliver a nebulized budesonide solution through the model at various inspiratory flow rates, measuring the total lung dose and particle sizes escaping deposition with a Next Generation Impactor. As with the study by Janssens et al.,[77] solvent interactions with the plastic extrathoracic airway geometry interfered with HPLC measurements, preventing the direct determination of deposition within the model itself.

1.2.1.2 Idealized extrathoracic geometries

The first idealized throat model for aerosol deposition measurements was developed by Stapleton et al.[82] using data from CT scans, MRI scans, observations of living subjects, and archival literature on extrathoracic airway dimensions in adults. The development of this geometry, called the Alberta Idealized Throat, was motivated in part by the desire to remove the bias of a particular individual's airway from studies using limited numbers of realistic airway replicas. Comprised of simplified analogues of important anatomical features including the pharynx, epiglottis, and larynx, the Alberta Idealized Throat can be reliably manufactured to tight tolerances with existing technologies while still capturing the function of the extrathoracic airways. Having been shown to predict the average deposition expected for various pharmaceutical aerosols in adult populations,[57,61,62,83] the Alberta Idealized Throat has seen extensive use following its commercialization through Copley Scientific. Recent examples include in vitro examinations of inhaler performance at altitude,[58,84] evaluation of novel inhaler designs and formulations,[83,85,86] and performance comparisons of various devices.[87–90] Ruzycki, Martin, and Finlay[89] recently demonstrated that the insertion angle used with high-momentum pMDIs and certain DPIs with large particle sizes or high mouthpiece exit velocities can significantly influence in vitro measurements obtained with the AIT. Their observations suggest that stronger correlations between in vitro measurements and in vivo scintigraphy data with inhalers demonstrating these characteristics are obtained with the AIT when the inhaler mouthpiece is aligned with the transverse plane, rather than directed towards the back of the oral cavity: such effects may explain disparities in in vitro–in vivo correlations reported by different authors (see e.g., Wei et al.[57]).

Golshahi and Finlay[91] found that an isometric scaling down of the Alberta Idealized Throat by a factor of 0.62 yielded a throat model that captures average extrathoracic deposition in school-age children. This particular scale factor was selected so that the characteristic diameter (equal to the throat volume divided by surface area) of the scaled model matched the average characteristic diameter measured in nine realistic airway models of children ages 6 to 14 that had been used to examine deposition in an earlier study.[92] Ruzycki et al.[93] then showed that this geometry, named the Alberta Idealized Child Throat, successfully replicated in vivo deposition of therapeutic aerosols from both pMDIs and DPIs in school-age children.

Javaheri, Golshahi, and Finlay[94] developed an idealized nasopharyngeal airway using CT scans from ten infants aged 3 to 18 months. Cross sections of airway scans were used to develop idealized cross sections that were then joined using two-dimensional splines to create the general form of the idealized model, incorporating such important airway features as the meatus, turbinates, nasal valve, and septum. This model was then scaled such that its hydraulic diameter (i.e., four times the volume divided by the airway surface area) matched the average hydraulic diameter measured in the ten infant airways. *In vitro* measurements suggested that deposition in this idealized geometry closely matched the trends in deposition observed in the ten realistic airway models, although Tavernini et al.[95] demonstrated that an additional isotropic scaling of 0.8 on this geometry yielded a geometry more predictive of the average deposition across the entire 3- to 18-month age range. An additional isotropic scale factor of 0.75 on this version of the geometry (i.e., a total isotropic scaling of 0.6 on the Javaheri, Golshahi, and Finlay[94] geometry) provided an idealized geometry representative of deposition in neonates with an average age of one month. At present, a lack of suitable *in vivo* deposition data in infants or neonates has prevented the full validation of either the idealized infant nasal geometry or the idealized neonate nasal geometry. Nevertheless, both may prove useful in guiding studies on aerosol administration to very young patients, a topic for which *in vitro* methods are particularly useful owing to ethical concerns.

Recent interest in intranasal drug delivery[96] has motivated the development of the Alberta Idealized Nasal Inlet,[97,98] representative of adult nasal extrathoracic airways. Kiaee et al.[97] developed the geometry via a sophisticated computational approach wherein airway geometries of ten subjects (obtained via computed tomography) were decomposed into cross sections that served as a basis for a heuristic and iterative development of an idealized model. Average numerical deposition of spray droplets in regions of interest including the vestibule, valve, anterior and posterior turbinates, olfactory mucosa, and nasopharynx observed in an earlier computational study[99] was used as a basis for iterating the design of the geometry. Chen et al.[98] demonstrated good *in vitro* agreement between deposition in this idealized model and the average deposition measured across five realistic nasal airway geometries, as well with *in vivo* data from the literature. Together these results suggest that the Alberta Idealized Nasal Inlet may serve as a useful platform for quantifying *in vitro* regional nasal-extrathoracic deposition for nasal sprays.

1.2.1.3 In vitro *measures of thoracic deposition*

The basic measurement of *in vitro* thoracic deposition is the total lung dose, typically measured by placing a high efficiency filter downstream of an extrathoracic geometry to capture any dose that would penetrate into the lungs. Such a procedure cannot differentiate between the dose that would deposit in the lungs and the dose that might be exhaled, but for many DPIs and pMDIs for which a long breath hold is advised during administration the exhaled dose is negligible.[100]

More in-depth characterization of thoracic deposition *in vitro* is complicated by the intricate anatomy of these airways: the fractal bifurcating nature of sequential airway generations with varying and continually decreasing dimensions quickly renders attempts to replicate such a complex geometry with a physical prototype untenable.

While a full *in vitro* model of the airways is not possible, partial upper-airway models consisting of the first few conducting airway generations and bifurcations have been described.[101-103] Such models have proven useful in exploratory research and in the development of empirical correlations[104] but are not widely used in practice.

An alternative is to combine the practice of particle size characterization via cascade impactors with extrathoracic deposition measurements using realistic or idealized mouth-throat geometries. Rather than simply providing a measure of the total lung dose as provided by a filter, the use of a cascade impactor downstream of a mouth-throat geometry allows for the estimation of the particle size distribution entering the thoracic airways.[67,75] These data can in turn be used as input in regional deposition models[58,90,105,106] to gather and elucidate more information on thoracic deposition than is provided by traditional *in vitro* measures such as the mass median aerodynamic diameter or fine particle dose.

The use of filters designed to mimic regional deposition is a promising development that may allow for the more direct estimation of broad trends in regional deposition without requiring numerical modeling and cascade impactor measurements. The physics of deposition in the human airways via impaction, sedimentation, and diffusion is in many ways analogous to that of deposition in filters, and in theory a properly designed filter should be able to replicate *in vivo* deposition of inhaled pharmaceutical aerosols in, for example, the tracheobronchial region. Tavernini et al.[107] described the development of such a filter capable of replicating numerical predictions of tracheobronchial deposition for various physiologically relevant inhalation profiles. Recent proof-of-concept tests have demonstrated good agreement between the *in vitro* tracheobronchial filter for four commercially available DPIs and *in vitro* NGI measurements plus *in silico* predictions of regional deposition.[106] A comparison of the *in vitro* aspects of these experiments is shown in Figure 1.2. The simplified nature of the setup using the tracheobronchial filter is attractive from the viewpoint of device development and method standardization, and these successful pilot studies suggest that such an approach may prove useful in expediting the development of innovative and generic inhalation products.

1.2.2 Inhalation Maneuver

In vivo inhalation maneuvers vary widely among the various types of devices: for some, the appropriate form is a sinusoidal-like tidal breath, for others, a fast and deep inhalation. With the advent of computer-controlled breathing machines (e.g., ASL 5000 Breathing Simulator, IngMar Medical, Pittsburg, PA, USA), it is often a straightforward matter to deliver physiologically realistic inhalation patterns when examining many inhalation devices *in vitro*. The following sections discuss appropriate inhalation profiles to use for the various classes of devices.

1.2.2.1 pMDIs and SMIs

The nominal inhalation maneuver for pMDIs consists of a slow and steady inhalation followed by an extended breath hold.[108] Ideally, the flowrate generated by a patient inhaling through a pMDI is as low as reasonably possible,[109] with a typical target of

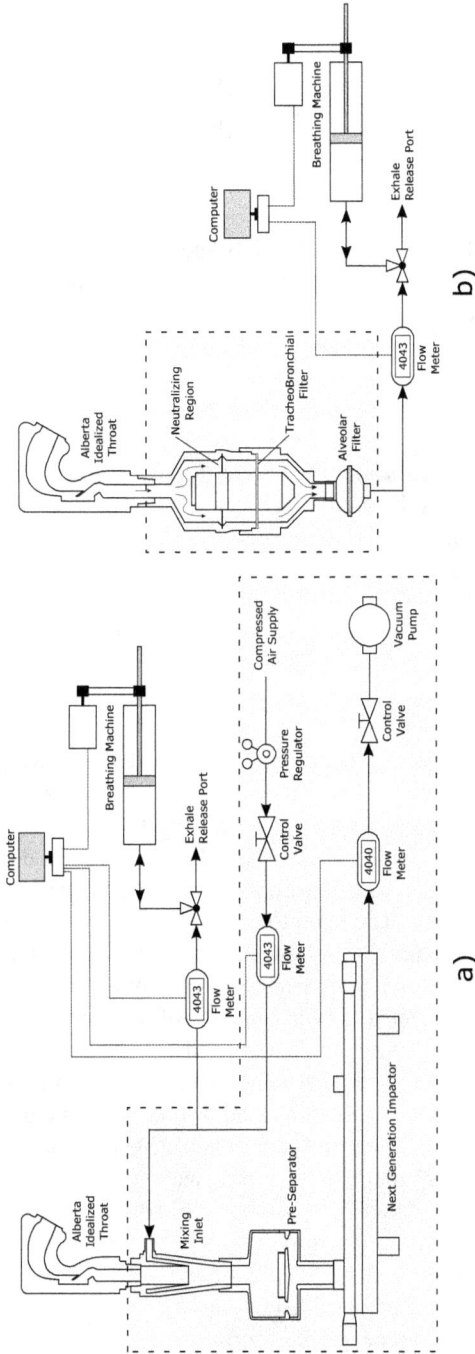

FIGURE 1.2 Schematic diagrams of the experimental apparatus for a) cascade impactor measurements or b) regional deposition filter measurements for characterizing inhaler performance *in vitro* using realistic inhalation profiles. Reproduced with permission from Tavernini et al.[106].

30 L/min.[22,110] pMDIs generally have a very low airflow resistance,[111] making it quite easy for most patient groups to generate 30 L/min through these devices. SMIs have a similarly low airflow resistance,[111] making 30 L/min a reasonable target flowrate here as well.[112] In some circumstances, a slow and deep inhalation (repeated three to five times) may be recommended when pMDIs and SMIs are used in conjunction with add-on devices such as spacers or valved holding chambers, although tidal inhalations are more common.[108,110]

In practice, *in vitro* examinations of pMDI and SMI performance are carried out using a constant inhalation flowrate generated by a vacuum source (i.e., a pump). This method is somewhat analogous to trained pMDI and SMI use, according to which the patient begins inhaling prior to actuating the device. One benefit of this approach is that it avoids issues coordinating the device actuation with a particular moment in the inhalation maneuver, as would otherwise be necessary when using more realistic inhalation profiles. Furthermore, droplet sizes initially generated by such devices are essentially independent of inhalation flowrate[108]; flowrate-dependent performance is instead caused by differing rates of impaction, turbulence levels, and hygroscopic effects that occur at different airflow velocities during transit through the airways.[87,113]

The aerosol spray emitted by a pMDI generally has a significant velocity exceeding that of the surrounding ambient air inhaled by the patient.[114] The development of this spray in a confined space (i.e., the oral cavity) and in the presence of a surrounding sheath of air (i.e., ambient air inhaled by the patient) is an extremely complex process[113] that can be influenced by the inhalation flowrate via shear-induced turbulence along the edges of the spray plume.[87] While the momentum of the spray alone can cause a significant amount of extrathoracic deposition owing to its inertia, these turbulent effects may play an additional role.[87]

The question then arises as to whether a constant inhalation flowrate is sufficient for capturing any of the aforementioned effects on pMDI performance *in vivo*, or if a fully realistic inhalation profile should be used instead. Limited work has explored the use of realistic inhalation profiles with pMDIs and SMIs. Drawing on data collected from several volunteers, Olsson et al.[68] developed a sophisticated *in vitro* setup incorporating a computer-controlled pneumatic hand to actuate pMDIs at specific moments in the inhalation maneuver. They found that volunteers actuated the pMDI an average of 0.25 seconds after the start of inhalation (noting a high degree of intra-subject variability) and selected three profiles they deemed as representative of the 5th, 50th, and 95th percentiles for (1) the flowrate at device actuation and (2) the average flowrate for a period of one second after actuation. Olsson et al.[68] then compared *in vitro* measurements of the ex-cast dose obtained with these inhalation profiles to *in vivo* lung doses estimated via plasma concentrations, finding a reasonable agreement. Unfortunately, no comparison was made to the use of steady inhalation flowrates, leaving this issue unresolved. There is evidence that extrathoracic deposition of a bolus of stable aerosol is governed more by the flowrate at which particles reach the site of deposition than by the flowrate at which they were inhaled, and that the process of bolus deposition for stable particles in the extrathoracic region can be considered quasi-steady.[115] With pMDIs and SMIs, however, large hygroscopic size changes can certainly occur.[113] If the effects of inhalation flowrate on these hygroscopic effects are negligible (i.e., if hygroscopic behavior is more or less the same at, for instance, 30 L/min as at 40 L/min, flowrates representing the average and maximum achieved by properly trained subjects [Olsson et al. 2013]), *in vitro* experiments using appropriately set steady inhalation flowrates with pMDIs and SMIs are likely indicative of deposition obtained with realistic inhalations *in vivo*.

The duration for which air is drawn through the pMDI/SMI *in vitro* is typically set to obtain an inhaled volume of 4.0 L.[45] This setting provides an ample volume of air to ensure that the bolus of aerosol emitted from these devices transits the entire volume of sizing instruments in use today.[116]

1.2.2.2 DPIs

Most DPIs are passive, relying on a patient's inhalation to generate the energy required for powder aerosolization, deagglomeration, and delivery into the respiratory tract. These devices tend to demonstrate high degrees of flowrate-dependent performance, and as such, are sensitive to the magnitude and shape of the inhalation profile used during their operation.[56] With DPIs, patients are typically instructed to inhale deeply, rapidly, and forcefully, and then follow up with a long breath hold.[108,110] The non-negligible airflow resistances of these devices necessitates a fair amount of effort on the part of the patient to achieve a strong inhalation, and typical use generates pressure drops of 1 to 6 kPa across the DPI.[56] Exactly how this pressure drop translates into an inhalation flowrate depends on the value of the airflow resistance of the specific device in question; a wide range of airflow resistances—anywhere from 0.015 to 0.06 $kPa^{1/2}min/L$[117]—are encountered with existing DPIs, resulting in a similarly wide range of inhalation flowrates.

Standard *in vitro* DPI tests use a solenoid valve to deliver a step inhalation through the device up to the peak inhalation flowrate.[45] This setup facilitates repeatability but provides no control over the acceleration of flowrate, a factor known to influence the performance of some DPIs.[118–120] The actual acceleration of flowrate developed across an inhaler using a step inhalation can vary with the magnitude of the peak flowrate and device resistance and is further influenced by the amount of "dead-space," or internal volume, of the sampling apparatus used during testing.[121–123] In effect, the acceleration of flowrate is more rapid when an inhaler is actuated with a solenoid valve directly into a filter than when it is actuated with a solenoid valve into an extrathoracic geometry attached to a Next Generation Impactor. In some circumstances, *in vitro* data obtained with these forms of inhalation can provide good predictions of *in vivo* deposition, provided inhalation flowrates are set appropriately.[124] For devices that demonstrate greater sensitivity to the acceleration of flowrate, however, more realistic inhalation patterns may be required to obtain predictive measures of *in vivo* performance.[125]

Realistic profiles can be delivered using programmable breathing machines, allowing for the direct replication of inhalation profiles generated by volunteers inhaling from various devices.[124] This method relies on *in vivo* data from subjects inhaling through devices and is somewhat cumbersome from a development perspective. A compromise may take the form of semi-realistic inhalation patterns that capture the general form of inhalations achieved *in vivo* through DPIs of varying resistance, as advocated by Delvadia et al.[126] For a device with a specific inhalation resistance *R*, this method provides tunable semi-realistic inhalation profiles of a sinusoidal form for the 10th, 50th, and 90th percentiles of peak inspiratory flowrate generated by adult volunteers that can be further modified for varying inhaled volume, duration of inhalation, and the time required to reach the peak inspiratory flowrate. The general form of these inhalation profiles follows Equation 1, where $Q_{DPI}(t)$ is the inhalation flowrate at time t, Q_{peak} is the peak inhalation flowrate, t_{peak} is the time required to reach Q_{peak}, and t_T is the duration of the inhalation (calculated as $t_T = 30\pi V/Q_{peak}$, where $_V$ is the inhaled volume).

$$Q_{DPI}(t) = \begin{cases} Q_{peak} \sin\left(\dfrac{\pi}{2} \dfrac{t}{t_{peak}}\right) & 0 \le t \le t_{peak} \\[2em] Q_{peak} \cos\left(\dfrac{\pi(t - t_{peak})}{2(t_T - t_{peak})}\right) & t_{peak} \le t < t_{total} \end{cases} \tag{1}$$

A caveat to using time-varying inhalation profiles *in vitro* is that cascade impactors must be operated at a constant flowrate to provide meaningful aerodynamic size classification data. The combination of a time-varying inhalation profile through a DPI and particle size measurements with a cascade impactor thus requires a more complicated *in vitro* setup incorporating a mixing inlet[68,75,106]—see Figure 1.2. The mixing inlet allows for a fully constant flowrate to be maintained through the cascade impactor that is balanced by an equal flow of bypass air before an inhalation through the DPI. Operating the breathing machine perturbs the mass balance of airflow across the mixing inlet, which is reestablished by airflow drawn through the DPI. Upon exiting the distal end of the throat, aerosol is diluted with the bypass airstream and enters the cascade impactor at a constant flowrate. Although the setup described in Figure 1.2 is more complicated than the pharmacopeial method for examining DPIs (i.e., using a step inhalation controlled via a solenoid valve), it is more likely to emulate DPI performance *in vivo* for devices that are sensitive to the effects of parameters such as the acceleration of flowrate. One limitation with the NGI is the maximum allowable flowrate of 100 L/min for which the NGI is properly characterized. Extension beyond this range without implementing a full compendial characterization of impactor performance (i.e., evaluating performance with well-characterized monodisperse particles) may result in off-spec impactor performance and mischaracterization of results.

1.2.2.3 Nebulizers, spacers, valved holding chambers, and facemasks

The administration of therapeutic aerosols using nebulizers occurs over several breaths and a timespan of minutes, with patients typically being instructed to breathe in a relaxed, normal manner.[22,108] Many nebulizers operate continuously during administration, with the drug delivered into the respiratory tract during inhalation and lost to the environment upon exhalation (through, for example, a one-way expiratory valve in the mouthpiece). Various designs are available, including traditional jet nebulizers (both vented and unvented), which are driven by a compressed air source, and vibrating mesh nebulizers, which generate droplets from a liquid solution via the action of a piezoelectric element on a fine mesh of nozzles. For such devices, primary droplet production is likely independent of inhalation flowrate, but the subsequent evolution of these droplets via impaction with interior baffles (when present), aerodynamic loading, and hygroscopic effects may be more sensitive.[113]

Spacers and valved holding chambers act to reduce the ballistic nature of the jet emitted from a pMDI upon actuation and provide additional time for the propellant to evaporate prior to inhalation. This delay results in a slower-moving aerosol comprised of smaller particles that are less likely to deposit in the extra thoracic region and more likely to penetrate into deeper airways.[127] Use of such devices also removes the need to coordinate device actuation and inhalation, making them an extremely useful tool for administering pharmaceutical aerosols to uncoordinated or uncooperative patients, and allows patients to inhale relatively normally during administration. Aerosol delivery to uncoordinated or non-compliant patients can be further facilitated using facemasks, as is standard practice with pediatrics,[128] again allowing the patient to inhale relatively normally during administration.

With respect to normal patient use, predictive *in vitro* tests for many types of nebulizers, spacers, valved holding chambers, and facemasks may best be performed using tidal inhalations over several breaths, including both the inhalation and exhalation portions of the breathing cycle. Depending on the parameter of interest, the full simulation of tidal breathing may be unnecessary; with unvented nebulizers, the inhaled dose can be estimated given knowledge both of the duration of inhalation relative to the full breath and of the total delivered dose measured using conventional methods.

While one can use realistic inhalations measured from patients directly, a more adaptable method involves the use of sinusoidal curves.[127] Roth, Lange, and Finlay[129] showed that sinusoidal inhalation profiles provide an excellent approximation of realistic inhalation profiles for subjects inhaling through vented nebulizers, as the *in vitro* particle size measurements they obtained with sinusoidal and realistic inhalations and subsequent simulations of regional lung deposition were essentially identical. Sinusoidal curves carry the added benefit of being easily modified to adjust the breathing pattern for the varying tidal volumes, duty cycles, and durations representative of various patient groups.[130] In practice, a full breath is typically modeled in two portions consisting of separate inhalations and exhalations, with pauses between cycles considered negligible. The mathematical form of the profile for the flowrate at a given time, $Q_{tidal}(t)$, is shown in Equation 2, where V_T is the tidal volume, f is the breathing frequency (expressed as the number of breathing cycles per minute), and δ_c is the duty cycle (the ratio of the durations of inhalation and exhalation) expressed in fractional form.

$$Q_{tidal}(t) = \begin{cases} \dfrac{\pi V_T}{\left(\dfrac{120\delta_c}{f}\right)}\sin\left(\dfrac{2\pi t}{\left(\dfrac{120\delta_c}{f}\right)}\right) & 0 \le t < \dfrac{120\delta_c}{f}\,; \text{inhale} \\[4ex] \dfrac{\pi V_T}{\left(\dfrac{120(1-\delta_c)}{f}\right)}\sin\left(\dfrac{2\pi\left(t+\dfrac{120\delta_c}{f}\right)}{\left(\dfrac{120(1-\delta_c)}{f}\right)}\right) & \dfrac{120\delta_c}{f} \le t < \dfrac{60}{f}\,; \text{exhale} \end{cases}$$

(2)

As with DPIs, the use of sinusoidal breath profiles to examine nebulizers in combination with particle sizing via cascade impactors requires the implementation of a mixing inlet. Additional consideration must be given to the hygroscopic nature of nebulized aerosols when measuring particle sizes with cascade impactors; considerable evaporative size changes often occur with these liquid aerosols during transit through cascade impactors, as noted in the following section.

For illustrative purposes, demonstrations of the various inhalation maneuvers discussed above are presented in Figure 1.3. These profiles have been chosen arbitrarily for qualitative comparison only, and care should be taken to ensure that appropriate inhalation parameter values (e.g., peak inhalation flowrates and device resistances for DPIs, breathing frequency and tidal volume for nebulizers, etc.) are used *in vitro*.

1.2.3 Hygroscopic Behavior

Hygroscopic size changes due to evaporation or condensation can significantly influence *in vitro* measurements of many inhaled pharmaceutical aerosols if not considered properly. A striking example is the substantial bias towards smaller particle sizes that occurs when nebulized aerosols are measured *in vitro* using cascade impactors without steps having been taken to mitigate evaporative size changes as the aerosol transits through the instrumentation.[131,132] The issue of evaporative size changes in cascade impactors with hygroscopic aerosols produced by nebulizers and SMIs, together with the time required to run routine cascade impactor measurements, has led to the preferential use of laser diffraction instrumentation to characterize these aerosols.[133,134]

The challenge lies first in determining the extent to which hygroscopic size changes are important for a given aerosol, and second in determining the extent to which hygroscopic behavior in a proposed *in vitro* test may differ from hygroscopic behavior *in vivo*. In many cases the relative importance of hygroscopic effects can be estimated via non-dimensional analysis,[135] which also provides some guidance on the steps required to mitigate or control such effects in a known manner. Yang et al.[136] used such methods in an *in vivo* scintigraphy study on respiratory tract deposition to mitigate hygroscopic size changes of nebulized aerosols via humidification of dilution air. This approach appreciably simplified their analysis.

In considering how hygroscopic size changes *in vitro* and *in vivo* may differ, it is important to recognize that one of the defining features of the human respiratory tract is the rapid heating and humidification of inhaled air as it transits through the upper airways.[137] Aerosols that are sensitive to hygroscopic size changes can see considerable growth via condensation in such conditions,[138,139] typically leading to greater respiratory tract deposition than would be assumed if the aerosol were treated as stable or constant in size. Early exploratory work described by Martonen[140] included *in vitro* surrogate airways designed to heat and humidify inhaled air in a manner similar to what occurs *in vivo*. Temperature and humidity gradients inside "growth chambers" representing generations of the tracheobronchial airways were controlled via heat and vapor transit from water circulating in concentric annular jackets. While this work did not extend much beyond the prototyping stage, *in vitro* measurements accounting for both hygroscopic effects and deposition in realistic airway geometries would be of great utility in better

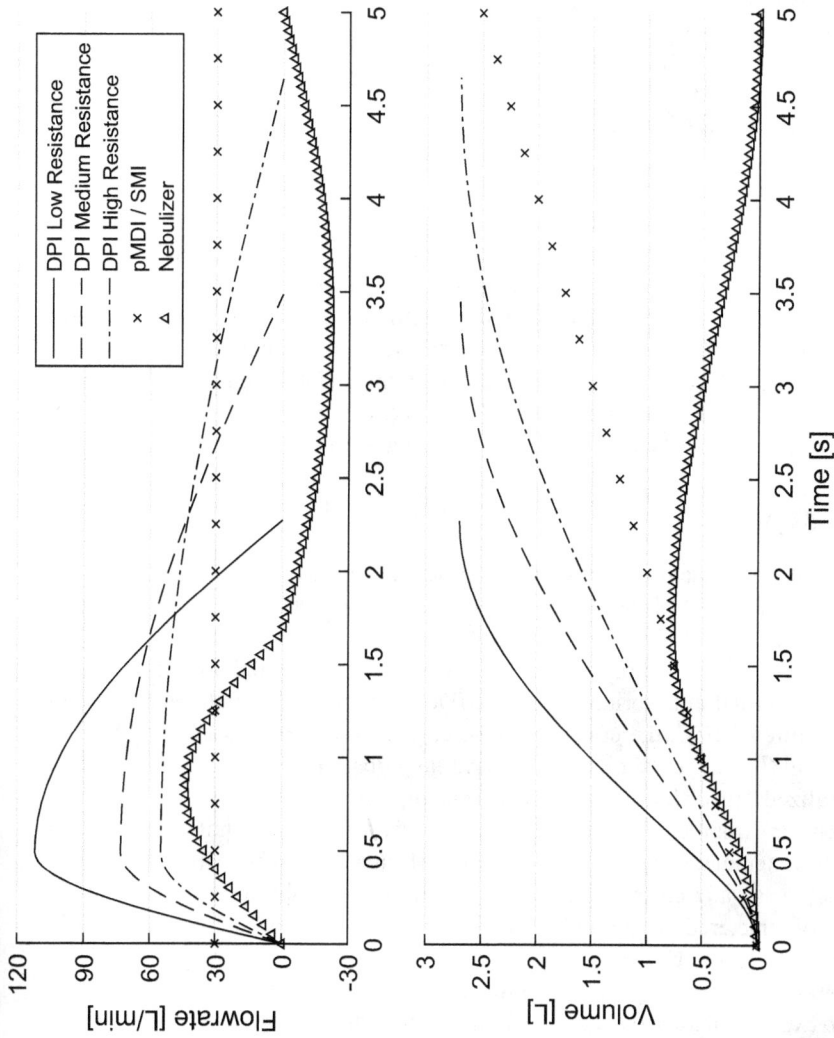

FIGURE 1.3 Examples of idealized inhalation maneuvers for *in vitro* performance evaluation of various devices. The top panel details the inhalation flowrate with respect to time, while the bottom details the inhaled volume with respect to time. For DPI profiles, device resistances of 0.02, 0.035, and 0.054 $kPa^{1/2}min/L$ were used as the low, medium, and high resistance DPIs, respectively, with the inhaled volume (2.7 L) and time to peak inhalation (0.49 s) chosen to match the average values in Delvadia et al.[126] for healthy adults. For the nebulizer, parameters were chosen to match the profile representative of an average adult in the Canadian Standard CAN/CSA/Z264 (Dolovich and Mitchell[130]).

characterizing aerosol behavior during inhalation. More recent work has seen the development of an *in vitro* setup designed to heat and humidify air during its transit through a simple induction-port-type geometry and into an Anderson Cascade Impactor,[141] but it is not clear how well such a setup can simulate the heat and mass transfer from airway walls that occurs *in vivo*, and the simple geometry of the induction port is a poor facsimile of the extrathoracic region. At present, hygroscopic behavior in the respiratory tract is perhaps best accounted for by numerical modeling using well-characterized *in vitro* data as input.[113]

1.2.4 Real-World Use

Environmental conditions, including temperature, humidity, and pressure, can influence the generation, transport, and evolution of inhaled pharmaceutical aerosols from the device to the site of deposition. Laboratory testing is often performed under controlled environmental conditions (relative humidity of ~50% at room temperature ~20 °C) and at altitudes near sea level (ambient air pressure of ~101.3 kPa), but these conditions can span a wide range of values in real-world use. With predictive *in vitro* testing, some focus may be placed on simulating the conditions under which an inhaler—particularly pMDIs and DPIs that are commonly carried with patients during day-to-day activities—will be used outside of a controlled clinical setting.

1.2.4.1 pMDIs

pMDI performance is sensitive to extreme variations in temperature. Morin et al.[84] found that relative to controls at 21°C the *in vitro* lung dose from four pMDIs measured downstream of an Alberta Idealized Throat decreased by an average of 70% at –12°C and increased by an average of 25% at 42°C when the inhaler and ambient environment were in thermal equilibrium. When pMDIs were instead maintained at a constant temperature of 21°C, the effects of ambient temperature decreased considerably. Shemirani et al.[87] observed similarly increased lung dose fractions downstream of an Alberta Idealized Throat for two beclomethasone dipropionate formulations (a solution and a suspension) when pMDIs were operated at 40°C in thermal equilibrium relative to 20°C. These temperature effects on pMDI performance can be explained by two mechanisms[84,87]: (i) altered propellant vapor pressures and subsequent effects on the atomization of a metered dose[142] and (ii) altered evaporative rates leading to variations in droplet/particle sizes. The first mechanism can be mitigated by keeping the pMDI at or near room temperature (e.g., stored within an inner coat pocket).

In vitro experiments also suggest that ambient humidity can influence the total lung dose achieved with some pMDIs.[87,89,93] Shemirani et al.[87] found that increasing relative humidity reduced the *in vitro* total lung dose obtained with pMDIs, with the effect being greater for suspension formulations than solution formulations. A possible explanation for the difference was the much greater number of residual drug particles generated by the solution formulation, which lent a larger total surface area for hygroscopic effects to occur over in the post-actuation stage. Ruzycki, Martin, and Finlay[89] confirmed the influence of relative humidity on suspension formulations, noting considerable reductions in *in vitro* lung doses at high relative humidity for two common suspensions (Ventolin™ Evohaler™ and Flixotide® HFA).

With respect to ambient pressure, Titosky et al.[143] found that the *in vitro* lung dose downstream of an Alberta Idealized Throat was not affected by altitudes up to 4300 m in five commercially available pMDIs, suggesting that pMDI performance is resistant to changes in altitude. This finding is well-explained by the fact that flow across a pMDI nozzle is choked, so altitude-dependent differences in the absolute pressure downstream of the pMDI nozzle have no effect on the initial atomization process.

1.2.4.2 DPIs

DPI performance can be negatively influenced by temperature and humidity during storage.[144] Microparticles formed by spray drying, for example, often have an energetically unfavorable state owing to their large surface areas, leaving them susceptible to conversion to more favorable states via crystallization, polymorph transition, crystal growth, or fusion of particles. Effects of temperature and humidity on device performance have been studied extensively,[145–148] with results showing that extended storage at atypical conditions leads to altered device performance. A variety of strategies have been employed to mitigate these effects during real-world use, for example, designing the glass transition temperature of an amorphous particle to be ~50°C greater than storage temperature, and using desiccants.[144]

Effects of temperature or humidity on a freshly primed dose from a multi-dose reservoir DPI are thought to be negligible in most scenarios given the less hygroscopic nature of inhaled powders than of liquid droplets produced by nebulizers and pMDIs, and the short timescales (seconds) between priming and delivery. Limited *in vitro* data from Ruzycki et al.[93] supports this hypothesis for one commercially available DPI, the Pulmicort® Turbuhaler®.

Ambient pressure may influence DPI performance through reductions in aerodynamic forces that occur due to decreased air density at increasing altitudes. Such effects have been examined in a number of *in vitro* studies on inhaler performance at varying altitudes.[58,143,149] Ruzycki et al.[58] demonstrated that while some DPIs are somewhat sensitive to altitude, effects are device-dependent and relatively minor, particularly at flowrates representative of patients capable of generating sufficient inspiratory efforts.

1.2.4.3 Inhaler orientation and other aspects of patient technique

Routine *in vitro* testing can be broadly described as the ideal use of inhalers in pharmacopeial experiments with well-defined and limited parameter spaces that focus on reductions in variability, providing a strong basis for quality control. More exploratory *in vitro* testing has begun to examine the effects of parameters that have typically gone unconsidered, like the effect of insertion angle of inhaler mouthpieces on extrathoracic deposition.[73,89] Insertion angle can significantly influence extra thoracic deposition and the *in vitro* lung dose for DPIs with high mouthpiece exit velocities and large particles, as well as for pMDIs with high momentum spray plumes.[89] Together with earlier *in vitro* observations of decreased extra thoracic deposition for pMDIs with lower momentum sprays,[60] these results suggest that refinement of devices and formulations may provide avenues for reducing variability in real-world use.

Aspects of real-world use related to improper operation or priming of inhalers are generally not explored experimentally, the expectation being that patients will use devices as intended by the manufacturers. As noted in the introduction, however, many patients demonstrate improper technique when using inhalers,[21] and this issue does not appear to have improved over time.[150] There remains room for improvement both in patient/clinician education and in device design to address improper real-world use and associated reduction in treatment efficacy.

1.3 DEPOSITION MODELS

Numerical models of deposition in the respiratory tract have numerous applications beyond inhalation drug delivery, including assessments of workplace and environmental exposure and characterization of disease transmission via airborne pathogens. The past few decades have seen extensive developments in numerical deposition models thanks to improvements in medical imaging, computational fluid dynamics simulations, and *in vitro* methods used to develop empirical correlations. These are summarized in a number of recent reviews.[17,53,151]

For inhaled therapies targeting the lungs, aerosol must first be generated by a device before being inhaled. The physical processes governing aerosol generation are so complex that quantitative modeling from first principles is not feasible. In practice, this necessitates the use of *in vitro* methods to provide the initial conditions for numerical models of respiratory tract deposition, but regardless of this limitation such models can provide a wealth of information for guiding the development of inhalation therapies. Inhaled pharmaceutical aerosols targeting the lungs must first transit the extrathoracic region, which acts as an efficient filter for large particles, and after reaching the thoracic airways must then deposit on airway walls to deliver the drug to target tissues without their being exhaled in any significant quantity. Addressing the unique challenge of avoiding wasted deposition in the extrathoracic airways while maximizing thoracic deposition (and even preferentially targeting specific regions of the lungs) can be aided through algebraic correlations of extra thoracic deposition and well-established one-dimensional lung deposition models, characteristics of which are discussed below.

1.3.1 Extrathoracic Deposition

The nose, mouth, and throat present a major obstacle for delivering inhaled therapeutics to the lungs without unwanted deposition in these extrathoracic airways. The high degree of inter-subject variability in lung deposition observed with some orally inhaled therapies is thought to be largely due to variation of mouth-throat deposition,[19] making this an extremely important parameter to characterize accurately when designing new devices and formulations. Historically, the impaction parameter d^2Q provided a means of incorporating the well-known dependence of inhalation flowrate and particle size on deposition in early algebraic correlations,[152,153] with scale factors and parameters like tidal volume incorporated to capture some elements of variability in deposition with age or sex.

In recent years, the understanding of how various factors influence extrathoracic deposition has grown considerably thanks largely to thorough *in vitro* characterizations of deposition in physical airway replicas. A number of reviews summarize many of the relevant studies.[17,154,155] Nondimensionalization of the equations governing fluid and particle behavior resulted in the identification of the Stokes and Reynolds numbers as important parameters for characterizing the deposition of many pharmaceutical aerosols of interest,[113] leading to their inclusion in modern extrathoracic deposition correlations. The Stokes number and Reynolds numbers, which characterize particle inertia and the relative importance of inertial and viscous effects on fluid behavior, respectively, are calculated as

$$\text{Stk} = \frac{\rho_{particle} d^2 C_c U}{18 \mu D} \tag{3}$$

$$\text{Re} = \frac{\rho_{fluid} U D}{\mu} \tag{4}$$

where $\rho_{particle}$ is the particle density, d is the particle diameter, C_c is the Cunningham correction factor, U, ρ_{fluid} and μ are the velocity, density, and dynamic viscosity of the gas phase, respectively, and D is some characteristic dimension of the geometry (note that the Stokes number is frequently written in terms of the aerodynamic diameter, with the reference density of 1000 kg/m^3 used in place of $\rho_{particle}$). Most correlations for extrathoracic deposition efficiency, η, are of the form

$$\eta = 1 - \frac{1}{1 + a \text{Re}^b \text{Stk}^c}. \tag{5}$$

The constants a, b, and c are typically determined by fitting Equation 5 to experimental data of deposition in realistic airway replicas corresponding to a particular age range (adults, children, infants, neonates), inhalation route (nasal, oral), and inhalation profile (constant flow rate or tidal); algebraic deposition correlations are thus empirical models. Various characteristic dimensions have been proposed for extrathoracic geometries spanning different age groups and routes of inhalation, such as the square root of the average cross sectional area of the oropharyngeal region[156] or the equivalent diameter obtained by dividing the mouth-throat volume by the centerline length.[157] In practice, these characteristic dimensions and the constants a, b, and c are chosen to collapse the scatter of *in vitro* data contained in Equation 5. Depending on the physics of the problem, Equation 5 can be further modified to include additional parameters.[17,154]

One of the major goals of the above work is the development of accurate *in vitro–in vivo* correlations. Yang et al.[136] recently demonstrated good agreement between *in vivo* scintigraphic measurements of extrathoracic deposition of tidally-inhaled nebulized aerosols in healthy adults and predicted extra thoracic deposition using the empirical correlation of Golshahi et al.[156]: average *in vivo* deposition of nebulized radiolabeled isotonic saline (0.193 ± 0.103, average $\pm$ standard deviation) agreed well with the average of predictions using a corrected version of the Golshahi et al.'s[156] correlation (0.182 ± 0.082), particularly when compared to correlations based on the impaction parameter. However, Yang et al.[136] also observed large errors in subject-specific predictions, with (at best) only weak correlations obtained between predictions and *in vivo* measurements of deposition in individual subjects for the five extrathoracic deposition models they used. This discrepancy was attributed to the breakdown of the assumption of geometric similarity that occurs with the transition from a limited number of well-characterized *in vitro* extrathoracic geometries used in the development of empirical correlations to the more complicated and variable situation *in vivo*.

The results of Yang et al.[136] indicate that a single characteristic-length scale will struggle to capture the full geometrical variation of the extrathoracic airways both within and between different subjects, with the consequence that *subject-specific* predictions of extrathoracic deposition using simple algebraic correlations of the type described in Equation 5 may be inherently limited in accuracy. However, *population-level* predictions of extrathoracic deposition, including inter-subject variability, may be achieved using algebraic correlations following the method proposed by Ruzycki et al.[18] In this method, inter-subject variability is presumed to arise from three factors:

1. Variations between subjects in the inhalation flowrate
2. Variations between subjects in the size of the extrathoracic region (captured by the characteristic dimension D)
3. Variations between subjects in the shape of the extrathoracic region, denoted as variation resulting from geometric dissimilarity.

Ruzycki et al.[18] describe how to obtain estimates of each source of variability based on the characteristics of the population under consideration (see also the subsequent pedagogical description by Finlay[113]), with the overall standard deviation of deposition in the extrathoracic region, $s\eta$, calculated as

$$s_\eta = \sqrt{s_Q^2 + s_D^2 + s_{gd}^2}. \tag{6}$$

Here, s_Q is the standard deviation in extrathoracic deposition due to variation in flowrate, s_D is the standard deviation due to variation in the characteristic dimension, and s_{gd} is the standard deviation arising from geometric dissimilarity. Variations in flowrate and characteristic dimensions can be measured or estimated for a given *in vivo* population, but determination of the variation due to geometric dissimilarity requires well-characterized *in vitro* data in realistic airway casts of varying shape (see Martin, Moore, and Finlay[17] for estimates of this factor for a number of deposition correlations). Note that if all geometries in a given population were simple isotropic scalings of a single mouth-throat shape, this factor would disappear, but the complexities and variation in airway shape observed between different subjects means this factor will always exist in real populations. As a case study, Ruzycki et al.[18] applied this method to the data of Yang et al.,[136] finding excellent agreement between predicted extrathoracic deposition (0.172 ± 0.101) and that measured *in vivo* (0.193 ± 0.103) considering the first-order nature of this analysis. Each of the three sources of variability mentioned above were found to contribute significantly to inter-subject variability, with the implication that knowledge of the characteristic dimension and flowrate alone is likely insufficient to fully characterize deposition with algebraic correlations of the form of Equation 5 that do not account for geometric dissimilarity.

Empirical correlations presented in the literature are generally developed using well-characterized stable particles, and most use large-diameter inlets into extrathoracic geometries that do not replicate the complicated jet effects from small mouthpiece diameter DPIs or spray plume effects from pMDIs. Numerous studies demonstrate the complications that arise when dealing with DPIs and pMDIs. As examples, DeHaan and Finlay[158] demonstrated substantially greater deposition of particles *in vitro* when delivered through small-mouthpiece-diameter DPIs than through large-diameter straight tubes, while Ruzycki, Martin, and Finlay[89] showed that insertion angle and ambient humidity can lead to large differences in *in vitro* deposition from pMDIs emitting high-momentum spray plumes. As a result, the extension of an algebraic correlation to a physical situation where parameters extend beyond the range used in its development can lead to erroneous or misleading predictions of device/formulation performance. Because of the complexity of modelling jet effects from small-mouthpiece-diameter DPIs and spray plume effects and subsequent hygroscopic behavior from pMDIs, current practice is to evaluate extrathoracic deposition from these devices *in vitro* using the mouth-throat geometries described in the previous section.

1.3.2 Thoracic Deposition

After a proper accounting of extrathoracic deposition comes the modeling of deposition within the lungs themselves. The thoracic airways can be broadly described as a fractal-branching structure consisting of some two dozen generations starting from the trachea and ending at the individual alveoli. Various deposition models have been proposed (see reviews by Hofmann[53] and Martin, Moore, and Finlay[17]), but the basic properties of the one-dimensional deposition models considered here are similar. The commonly used model described by the International Commission on Radiological Protection[152] separates the thoracic airways into distinct bronchial, bronchiolar, and alveolar regions, and treats each as a "filter" whose efficiency in removing particles from inhaled air is predicted using empirical formulae developed from analysis of *in vivo* deposition data and clearance rates.

Modern lung deposition models consider the influence on deposition in individual airways of such mechanisms as inertial impaction, gravitational sedimentation, and Brownian diffusion as air encounters an increasing number of smaller and smaller airways during inhalation. Analytical considerations of airflow properties and fluid dynamics in different regions of the lungs can direct the selection of appropriate expressions for different deposition mechanisms.[113] These can be mechanistic or empirical in nature. For example, Javaheri et al.[159] use the empirical correlation of Chan and Lippmann[104] for inertial impaction, the analytical correlations of Heyder[160] and Heyder and Gebhart[161] for sedimentation, and the empirical correlations of Ingham[162] for diffusion. One-dimensional models can be further modified to account for dynamic processes like hygroscopic growth and evaporation,[138,163,164] allowing for investigations of such processes that would be extremely difficult to study in a mechanistic fashion *in situ*.

Airflow in the more analytical one-dimensional models is often considered as well-mixed turbulent flow in the larger conducting airways, classical laminar Poiseuille flow in the smaller conducting airways, and laminar plug flow in the peripheral lung. The real nature of flow in the airways will vary somewhat from the ideal behavior assumed in one-dimensional models: transitions between turbulent, laminar, and plug flow must occur. Despite such variance, the favorable comparisons of predicted regional deposition in one-dimensional lung deposition models with available experimental data suggest that these models successfully capture the major factors influencing deposition in the lungs.[53] A more thorough validation of deposition at the level of individual airway generations, i.e., beyond the first few conducting airways, will require advances in medical imaging to address resolution and registration issues observed with modern technologies.[165]

One-dimensional lung deposition models can provide estimates of the mass of drug expected to deposit in various generations of the respiratory tract but not information on localized deposition "hotspots" that can occur on, e.g., airway bifurcations—elucidation here requires computational fluid and particle dynamics simulations. Bearing this in mind, a natural progression beyond one-dimensional deposition modeling is the incorporation of models of the airway surface liquid and mucociliary clearance in the tracheobronchial airways,[166,167] as the concentration of drug in the airway surface liquid is of more relevance for local drug action than the deposited mass alone. For example, Martin and Finlay[168] recently coupled a generational lung deposition model with an airway surface liquid and mucociliary clearance model to estimate whether (and for how long) the concentration of an inhaled antibiotic exceeded the minimum inhibitory concentration required for efficacious treatment of *Pseudomonas aeruginosa* infection in the airways. Such methods, particularly when coupled with pharmacokinetic models as discussed in the following section, may prove useful in predicting the performance of new formulations, as local effects in lung tissues will depend more on the concentration of free drug available than on the deposited mass alone.[169]

As a final note, for devices like DPIs and pMDIs where extrathoracic deposition is difficult to predict *a priori*, an emerging trend is to use one-dimensional lung deposition models "downstream" of *in vitro* extra thoracic deposition tests. In this approach, well-characterized experimental data provide the initial conditions for modeling what occurs after aerosol transits the extrathoracic region and enters the lungs themselves.[58,90,105,106]

1.4 PHARMACOKINETIC MODELS

Regional deposition models predict the initial distribution of drug throughout the respiratory tract. Thereafter, competing processes combine to determine the fate of deposited drug particles over time. The processes of drug dissolution or release, clearance, metabolism, and absorption from the lungs collectively influence both local and systemic exposure to inhaled drugs, with extensive reviews on these processes presented in the literature.[52,170–173] Models linking broad estimates of regional deposition to these pharmacokinetic (PK) processes date to the foundational work of Byron[174] and Gonda.[175] In recent years, models of regional or generational deposition have been combined with PK models to predict regional lung exposure and/or systemic exposure to inhaled drugs over time in a more detailed manner.[90,105,168,176–179] Such models have been described as physiologically based pharmacokinetic (PBPK) models, wherein mechanistic descriptions of deposition and disposition in the respiratory tract are integrated with systemic PK modeling.[17,178] In this manner, the influence of regional deposition pattern on clinically relevant parameters, such as local and systemic drug concentrations, can be predicted for a given drug product.

A number of recent studies have used PK modeling to extend and interpret predictions of regional deposition models. For example, Bäckman, Tehler, and Olsson[177] used the commercially-available Gastroplus™ model (SimulationsPlus Inc., Rochester, USA) to estimate systemic exposure to nebulizer and DPI formulations of a selective glucocorticoid receptor modulator. Regional deposition in the tracheobronchial airways, the smaller bronchiolar airways, and the alveolar spaces was predicted using a one-dimensional deposition model based on those described by the International Commission on Radiological Protection[152] and the National Council on Radiation Protection and Measurements.[180] Additional model calculations were included to predict particle dissolution in the ASL, as well as the competing processes of mucociliary clearance and absorption (use of a mechanistic dissolution model incorporating solubility-limited kinetics is critical when describing the dissolution of poorly soluble drugs in the ASL). The model of Bäckman, Tehler, and Olsson[177] was shown to accurately predict systemic exposure measured *in vivo* in healthy volunteers. Notably, predicted local exposure in the modeled lung regions was not well correlated with systemic exposure, suggesting that systemic PK data alone could not be used to infer local exposure for the poorly soluble drug that was studied.

Boger and Friden[179] have described a coupled deposition and PK model in which the lung was further divided into 24 airway generations, as described in the Weibel A lung model.[181] Individual lung generations were subdivided into three compartments, representing the ASL, the epithelium, and the sub-epithelium. Concentrations of inhaled salbutamol were compared in the sub-epithelium and the plasma, with higher free drug concentrations predicted in the lung tissue than in the plasma. Lung tissue concentration was also predicted to vary over lung generations, with the sub-epithelial concentration in the 6th generation (selected by the authors as a representative target generation based on its contribution to total airway resistance) found to correlate with pharmacodynamic response.

Martin and Finlay[168] described a three-part model in which previously developed regional deposition[159,182,183] and ASL[166,167,184] models provided input to a PK model incorporating drug dissolution/release, mucociliary clearance, and absorption from the lungs with traditional factors like oral absorption from the gastrointestinal tract and distribution within (and elimination from) the body. The combined model was used to compare the time course of local (ASL) and systemic (plasma) concentrations of the inhaled antibiotic ciprofloxacin following inhalation of nebulized liposomal formulations and a DPI formulation.[168] More recently, this model has been used to estimate local and systemic exposures to inhaled treprostinil and a prodrug form, treprostinil palmitil, through inclusion of the rate of conversion of prodrug to active drug within the lung.[185]

Ruzycki et al.[90] have recently presented a combined *in vitro-in silico* model used to predict both regional deposition and PK for budesonide DPIs. In this approach, *in vitro* experiments were conducted with the Alberta Idealized Throat and realistic inhalation maneuvers to measure the drug mass and aerodynamic particle size distribution of aerosol penetrating the throat, the latter being deemed the intrathoracic particle size distribution. Results of *in vitro* experiments were used in conjunction with regional deposition and mechanistic PK modeling to predict systemic drug concentrations for three distinct budesonide DPIs. By way of example, Figure 1.4 shows the predicted plasma concentration of budesonide for Pulmicort® Turbuhaler® compared with dose-normalized *in vivo* data reported in multiple studies. Notably, Ruzycki et al.[90] observed that significant differences between DPIs measured *in vitro* resulted in large differences in predicted drug masses depositing in the large (bronchial) airways and in the alveolar lung region. Conversely, less variation between DPIs was predicted in the drug mass depositing in the small (bronchiolar) airways. Furthermore, predicted PK parameters were influenced primarily by the alveolar dose or total lung dose but were poorly correlated with deposition in the large and small airways. These results suggest that PK data alone may fail to provide useful information describing drug delivery to the conducting airways, where inhaled corticosteroids such as budesonide are expected to have some therapeutic effect.[186] These results also reinforce the findings of Bäckman, Tehler, and Olsson[177] regarding local exposure as described above. A strength of the methodology proposed by Ruzycki et al.[90] is its ability to explore linkage between *in vitro* measured parameters, regional lung deposition, and PK parameters commonly evaluated in early-stage clinical studies. Such an approach may address limitations in similar studies that

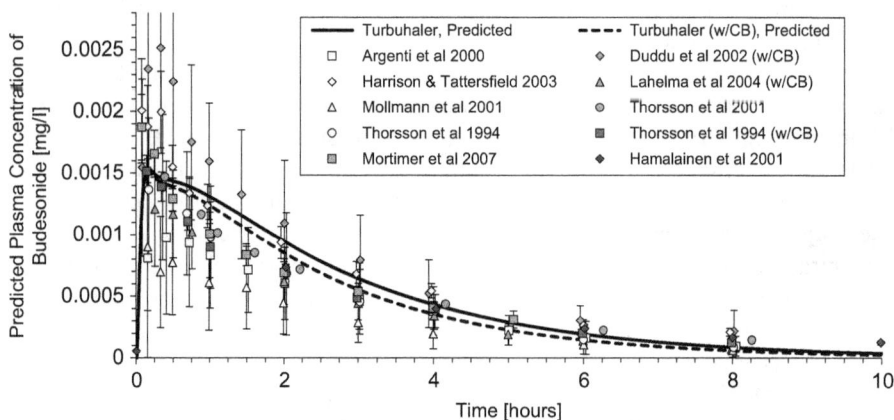

FIGURE 1.4 Budesonide plasma concentrations predicted using a combined *in vitro-in silico* model are shown for Pulmicort® Turbuhaler®. The dotted curve represents concentrations predicted for studies incorporating a charcoal block (w/ CB), where oral absorption was set to zero in the PK model. Data points represent concentrations reported from *in vivo* studies available in the archival literature. Where necessary, *in vivo* data are scaled to a nominal dose of 1000 μg budesonide. Adapted with permission from Ruzycki et al.[90]

rely on traditional *in vitro* measures (e.g., stage groupings of NGI data) to estimate regional deposition without mechanistic modeling.[187]

1.4.1 Characterizing Disposition

Accurate modeling of drug behavior after deposition in the lungs is a challenging topic owing to the various nuances that differentiate disposition in the respiratory tract and disposition in the more classical context of oral drug delivery via the gastrointestinal (GI) tract. Relative to delivery via the GI tract, drug delivery via the respiratory tract is typically associated with a given drug mass having a much larger specific surface area, the presence of smaller liquid volumes for dissolution, more moderate pH and milder hydrodynamic considerations, and additional interactions unique to the lung environment (e.g., macrophage uptake).[170] If an inhaled pharmaceutical aerosol is delivered in solid form (in powder form via a DPI or suspended particles in pMDIs), dissolution becomes a prerequisite for absorption and therapeutic effect, and the conditions to which a deposited particle are exposed depend on the location of deposition within the respiratory tract itself. Here, basic aspects of dissolution modeling are considered to identify important factors relevant for drug delivery via the respiratory tract.

1.4.1.1 Modeling dissolution

A proper accounting of dissolution in the ASL is important when considering the disposition of moderately or poorly soluble compounds after their deposition in the lungs.[170] While the current state of the art in dissolution testing *in vitro* is well summarized in recent reviews,[51,52] it is instructive to consider how current PK models consider dissolution in the respiratory tract, whether through mechanistic or empirical means. A classic mechanistic model of dissolution is the Nernst-Brunner type process.[188] This model assumes that the dissolution process is governed primarily by the diffusion of molecules across a stagnant film of liquid (called a diffusion layer) that surrounds submerged solid particles. The general equation defining Nernst-Brunner dissolution in ASL allows for the quantification of the change of mass, m, of a submerged particle with respect to time t:

$$\frac{dm}{dt} = -\frac{D_d S}{h}\left(c_s - c(t)\right). \tag{7}$$

Here, D_d is the diffusion coefficient of the drug in ASL, S is the surface area of the submerged particle, c_s is the solubility of the drug in ASL, $c(t)$ is the concentration of drug in the bulk of the ASL (outside of the diffusion layer), and h is the thickness of the diffusion layer itself.

An important characteristic of this model is the relation between the thickness of the diffusion layer and the size of the particle. For particles smaller than 60 μm in diameter, the thickness of the diffusion layer is thought to be well-approximated as the particle radius.[189,190] Therefore, for most inhaled pharmaceutical aerosols, where the pulmonary dose consists of particles roughly one to five micrometers in diameter, a diffusion layer thickness equal to the particle radius is likely a reasonable model. In the tracheobronchial airways, where the ASL has a depth on the order of 10 μm,[170] it is likewise reasonable to assume full immersion of particles in the ASL, especially given the observed tendency of particles to be displaced into the liquid phase due to the low surface tension of surfactant atop the mucus layer.[191] At the level of individual alveoli, however, the surface liquid layer is much thinner (~0.1 μm), meaning a critical assumption used in the derivation of the Nernst-Brunner model—the existence of a diffusion layer separating the particle from the bulk liquid—is not appropriate. Strictly speaking, dissolution kinetics in the periphery of the lung are likely not well described by as a classic Nernst-Brunner process because the alveolar lining fluid is too thin to accommodate the assumed thickness of the diffusion layer. Various modifications have recently been proposed to account for differences,[192,193] but, in the absence of an analytical model describing the dissolution of particles deposited in the very thin alveolar fluid, most PK models approximate particle dissolution and absorption in the alveolar region by a simple first order process, with a rate constant chosen to match available *in vivo* data (see e.g., Weber and Hochhaus).[176]

1.4.1.2 Solubility and permeability

The Nernst-Brunner model highlights the importance of drug solubility in the dissolution process. Drugs that are poorly soluble in airway surface liquid may easily saturate surrounding fluid after deposition, thereafter reducing the rate of dissolution (as per Equation 7) and effectively limiting the maximum rate at which drug is made available for subsequent absorption. Competing mechanisms such as mucociliary clearance in the conducting airways can then remove deposited particles before they completely dissolve, potentially reducing the bioavailability of such therapies.

In describing solubility and dissolution it can be useful to consider the dose number, Do, the dissolution number, Dn, and the absorption number, An, proposed by Amidon et al.[194] for use in biopharmaceutical classifications of dissolution. The dose number is calculated as

$$\text{Do} = \frac{M_0 / V_0}{c_S} \tag{8}$$

where M_0 is the dose (mass of drug), V_0 is the volume of dissolution fluid, and c_s is the solubility. Given the dependence of Do on the volume of dissolution fluid, its value is site-specific and will vary depending on the region of the respiratory tract where deposition occurs.[195] When Do<<1, the drug has sufficient solubility to be dissolved, and subsequent disposition depends primarily on permeability and absorption rates in relevant tissues. When Do>>1, the drug is considered to be dissolution-limited, and the more complicated interplay that occurs between dissolution, lung clearance mechanisms, and absorption determines local tissue concentrations and uptake into systemic circulation. In the conducting airways, V_0 is on the order of 10 to 30 mL, allowing for the definition of a band separating fully-soluble and dissolution-limited drugs based on the dose delivered to the conducting airways and the solubility in airway surface liquid.[170] Hastedt et al. note that while many drugs are not dissolution limited (including short-acting and long-acting bronchodilators), there are two classes of drugs that are: inhaled corticosteroids with a solubility less than 1 µg/mL (e.g., fluticasone propionate, beclomethasone dipropionate) and high dose anti-infectives with a nominal dose greater than 1 mg and a solubility less than 100 µg/mL (e.g., amphotericin B).[170] In such cases, the accurate modeling of disposition requires the consideration of dissolution in the airway surface liquid.

The dissolution number is calculated as

$$\text{Dn} = \frac{t_{res} 3 D_d c_s}{\rho_{particle} r_0^2} \tag{9}$$

where t_{res} is the mean residence time (in the lung) and r_0 is the particle diameter. The dissolution number informs what parameters can be varied to either increase or decrease dissolution rates. For example, halving the particle size increases the dissolution rate by a factor of four (though generally speaking such large differences in particle size will be associated with large differences in regional deposition that must be borne in mind). Alterations to e.g., particle density, morphology, and crystallinity (i.e., amorphous content) that can be achieved through particle engineering processes[144] may also provide some degree of control over dissolution *in vivo*.

Finally, the absorption number is calculated as

$$\text{An} = t_{res} k_a \tag{10}$$

where k_a is an absorption rate constant that is directly proportional to permeability and absorption surface area, but whose value is difficult to quantify *a priori* and can vary with time.[170,195] In practice, the difficulties in establishing k_a in the context of inhaled therapeutics (and effects of additional active-transport phenomena besides diffusion-based permeation) prevent much use of the absorption number, but the underlying relation between absorption and permeability remains useful to consider. Optimal permeability depends on the nature of the therapy. For locally acting medications in the respiratory tract, low permeability may aid in minimizing systemic exposure, particularly if coupled with low oral bioavailability. For systemic delivery, high permeability facilitates more rapid uptake. Dissolved low molecular weight drugs generally undergo fast absorption in the lungs (half-lives < 1 hr), with extremely fast absorption kinetics observed for lipophilic molecules (half-lives on the order of minutes or less).[12,196] Exceptions to this behavior can occur due to e.g., sustained binding and intracellular trapping.[170] Lipophilic drugs (with octanol-water partition coefficients, log P, being greater than 0) are absorbed primarily through the transcellular route, while hydrophilic drugs (log P < 0) are absorbed via the paracellular route. For larger macromolecules like peptides and proteins, the rates of absorption (generally on the order of hours) are tied primarily to size, with larger molecules undergoing slower absorption through various mechanisms including receptor-mediated transcytosis, paracellular diffusion, or non-specific pinocytosis.[197]

1.4.1.3 Lung-relevant dissolution testing

At present, no standardized method exists for *in vitro* dissolution testing of inhaled medications, be it for quality control, biorelevance, or clinical relevance.[51] As such, various approaches are proposed in the literature,[198] with some aiming to evaluate dissolution under essentially infinite sink conditions[189,199,200] and others utilizing smaller volumes of dissolution media that may be more representative of physiological conditions in airway surface liquid.[201–203] Even the most sophisticated *in vitro* apparatuses that aim to replicate air/blood barriers are typically of a much greater thickness than is representative of alveolar region,[203] and it is unclear how the balance between dissolution and absorption is best considered as one transitions from the very permeable alveolar region to the less permeable conductive airways.[170] As such, lung-relevant dissolution testing is an active area of research, and the interested reader is directed to a number of recent reviews on the topic.[51,52,195]

1.4.2 Considering Health or Disease

As with similar models, those proposed by Martin and Finlay[168] and Ruzycki et al.[90] predict regional deposition in lung geometries representative of healthy adults. These models are thus well suited for comparison with Phase 1 PK studies done in healthy subjects, and plasma drug concentration profiles predicted using these models have indeed been shown to agree well with data from Phase 1 trials.[90,168,185]

It is also of interest to develop models that can explore the influence of disease state on drug uptake due to, for example, heightened mucous production or reduced mucociliary clearance rates. The inclusion of a mechanistic ASL model for which daily mucous production rate and tracheal clearance velocity are input parameters allows the sensitivity of local and systemic drug concentrations to these parameters to be explored. For inhaled antibiotics such as ciprofloxacin, predicted drug concentrations in the ASL may be compared with minimum inhibitory concentrations against bacteria colonizing in the ASL, providing a means of estimating whether effective local drug concentrations are achieved. Figure 1.5 provides an example of such an analysis, where ASL concentrations of ciprofloxacin following inhalation of two different nominal doses delivered in a DPI formulation are modeled for three combinations of mucous production rate and tracheal clearance velocity.[168]

As seen in Figure 1.5, the longest residence times of drug in the airways are predicted for the combination of high mucous production and low clearance velocity, suggesting treatment efficacy for this class of drug may depend not only on formulation but also on physiological effects of disease. As impaired mucociliary clearance is observed in many respiratory diseases, poorly soluble drugs may be expected to persist longer in diseased lungs than in healthy lungs. Shapiro et al.[204] adapted the model presented by Martin and Finlay[168] to capture mucociliary clearance and ASL absorption dynamics in cystic fibrosis patients, including slow mucociliary clearance dynamics in small airways that had not been included in previous models. Such improvements may provide a method for examining the influence of cystic fibrosis treatments on mucous buildup and blockages, and on drug concentrations in ASL more generally. Evidently the influence of disease on natural clearance mechanisms in the lung such as mucociliary clearance can cause differences in drug concentrations in the lung over time, which may in turn influence drug action. Well-known challenges associated with modeling deposition in the context of respiratory disease[165,205] present additional barriers to predictive modeling

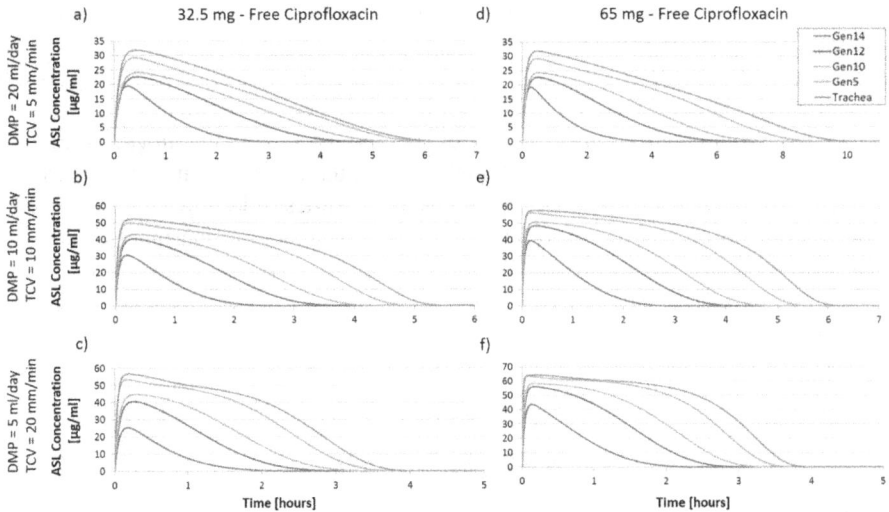

FIGURE 1.5 Predicted airway surface liquid (ASL) concentrations of free ciprofloxacin in the conducting airways of healthy adult subjects following inhalation of nominal dry powder doses of 32.5 mg (a–c) and 65 mg (d–f) ciprofloxacin. Results are shown for three combinations of daily mucous production (DMP) and tracheal clearance velocity (TCV). Gen *i* indicates tracheobronchial airway generation number *i*. Reprinted with permission from Martin, Moore, and Finlay[17.]

of local and systemic exposure to inhaled drugs in patients suffering from respiratory diseases that alter airway geometry or clearance mechanisms.

1.5 MOVING TOWARDS CLINICAL RELEVANCE

Of ongoing interest is the development of accurate *in vitro–in vivo* correlations for inhaled pharmaceutical aerosols. Recent research has moved towards treating *in vitro* data as the input or initial conditions for *in silico* models that can predict, through a mixture of mechanistic and empirical approaches, deposition, and disposition in the lungs. This chapter has identified some of the steps involved in such approaches, including the development of *in vitro* tests that provide a more realistic measure of device performance than compendial methods, deposition models for extra thoracic and thoracic deposition, and disposition models that consider the fate of drug after deposition and under competing mechanisms of liberation, absorption, distribution, metabolism, and excretion. At present, advanced *in vitro* measures can accurately replicate the dose of drug penetrating the extrathoracic airways and have provided critical insight into the factors that influence *in vivo* variability. Current regional lung deposition models elucidate general trends in deposition in geometries representative of broad population averages and, when coupled with disposition models, provide the necessary initial conditions for determining local concentrations of drug in target tissues within the respiratory tract and systemic exposure. Evolving methods for characterizing dissolution and absorption in physiologically-relevant manners may provide additional means for characterizing disposition *a priori* of *in vivo* pharmacokinetic studies.

The research reviewed here shows great potential for extending *in vitro* measurements beyond traditional compendial methods for quality control and into prediction of clinically relevant parameters. For novel therapeutics, additional study using *ex vivo* and *in vitro* cell models to inform, e.g., rate constants for pharmacokinetic and pharmacodynamics modeling will be of great use in early stage characterization of product performance, where the accurate prediction of treatment effects remains a perennial goal.

REFERENCES

1. Cazzola, M., Page, C. P., Calzetta, L. & Matera, M. G. Pharmacology and therapeutics of bronchodilators. *Pharmacol. Rev.* 64(3), 450–504 (2012).
2. Bateman, E. D. *et al.* Global strategy for asthma management and prevention: GINA executive summary. *Eur. Respir. J.* 31(1), 143–178 (2008).
3. Gross, N. J. & Barnes, P. J. New therapies for asthma and chronic obstructive pulmonary disease. *Am. J. Respir. Crit. Care Med.* 195(2), 159–166 (2017).
4. Quon, B. S., Goss, C. H. & Ramsey, B. W. Inhaled antibiotics for lower airway infections. *Ann. Am. Thorac. Soc.* 11(3), 425–434 (2014).
5. Döring, G., Flume, P., Heijerman, H. & Elborn, J. S. Treatment of lung infection in patients with cystic fibrosis: Current and future strategies. *J. Cyst. Fibros.* 11(6), 461–479 (2012).
6. Tarrant, B. J. *et al.* Mucoactive agents for chronic, non-cystic fibrosis lung disease: A systematic review and meta-analysis. *Respirology* 22(6), 1084–1092 (2017).
7. Santos Cavaiola, T. & Edelman, S. Inhaled insulin: A breath of fresh air? A review of inhaled insulin. *Clin. Ther.* 36(8), 1275–1289 (2014).
8. San, L. *et al.* PLACID study: A randomized trial comparing the efficacy and safety of inhaled loxapine versus intramuscular aripiprazole in acutely agitated patients with schizophrenia or bipolar disorder. *Eur. Neuropsychopharmacol.* 28(6), 710–718 (2018).
9. Tepper, S. J. Orally inhaled dihydroergotamine: A review. *Headache* 53(Supplement 2), 43–53 (2013).
10. Stapleton, K. W. Orally inhaled migraine therapy: Where are we now? *Adv. Drug Deliv. Rev.* 133, 131–134 (2018).
11. Olanow, C. W. & Stocchi, F. Levodopa: A new look at an old friend. *Mov. Disord.* 33(6), 859–866 (2018).
12. Patton, J. S. & Byron, P. R. Inhaling medicines: Delivering drugs to the body through the lungs. *Nat. Rev. Drug Discov.* 6(1), 67–74 (2007).
13. Wang, S. H., Thompson, A. L., Hickey, A. J. & Staats, H. F. Dry powder vaccines for mucosal administration: Critical factors in manufacture and delivery. In *Mucosal vaccines: Modern concepts, strategies, and challenges* (ed. Kozlowski, P. A.) 121–156. (Berlin, Heidelberg: Springer, 2012). https://doi.org/10.1007/82_2011_167.
14. Parumasivam, T. *et al.* Dry powder inhalable formulations for anti-tubercular therapy. *Adv. Drug Deliv. Rev.* 102, 83–101 (2016).
15. Agertoft, L. & Pedersen, S. Importance of the inhalation device on the effect of budesonide. *Arch. Dis. Child* 69(1), 130–133 (1993).

16. Buhl, R. Local oropharyngeal side effects of inhaled corticosteroids in patients with asthma. *Allergy Eur. J. Allergy Clin. Immunol* 61(5), 518–526 (2006).
17. Martin, A. R., Moore, C. P. & Finlay, W. H. Models of deposition, pharmacokinetics, and intersubject variability in respiratory drug delivery. *Expert Opin. Drug Deliv.* 15(12), 1175–1188 (2018).
18. Ruzycki, C. A., Yang, M., Chan, H.-K. & Finlay, W. H. Improved prediction of intersubject variability in extrathoracic aerosol deposition using algebraic correlations. *Aerosol Sci. Technol.* 51(6), 667–673 (2017).
19. Borgström, L., Olsson, B. & Thorsson, L. Degree of throat deposition can explain the variability in lung deposition of inhaled drugs. *J. Aerosol Med.* 19(4), 473–483 (2006).
20. Usmani, O. S. & Barnes, P. J. Assessing and treating small airways disease in asthma and chronic obstructive pulmonary disease. *Ann. Med.* 44(2), 146–156 (2012).
21. Fink, J. B., Faarc, R. R. T., Rubin, B. K. & Mba, M. Problems with inhaler use: A call for improved clinician and patient education. *Respir. Care* 50(10), 1360–1375 (2005).
22. Laube, B. L. *et al.* What the pulmonary specialist should know about the new inhalation therapies. *Eur. Respir. J.* 37(6), 1308–1331 (2011).
23. Hämmerlein, A., Müller, U. & Schulz, M. Pharmacist-led intervention study to improve inhalation technique in asthma and COPD patients. *J. Eval. Clin. Pract.* 17(1), 61–70 (2011).
24. Basheti, I. A., Reddel, H. K., Armour, C. L. & Bosnic-Anticevich, S. Z. Improved asthma outcomes with a simple inhaler technique intervention by community pharmacists. *J. Allergy Clin. Immunol* 119(6), 1537–1538 (2007).
25. Usmani, O. S., Biddiscombe, M. F. & Barnes, P. J. Regional lung deposition and bronchodilator response as a function of β2-agonist particle size. *Am. J. Respir. Crit. Care Med.* 172(12), 1497–1504 (2005).
26. Bjermer, L. Targeting small airways, a step further in asthma management. *Clin. Respir. J.* 5(3), 131–135 (2011).
27. Pellegrino, R. *et al.* Interpretative strategies for lung function tests. *Eur. Respir. J.* 26(5), 948–968 (2005).
28. Reddel, H. K. *et al.* An official American thoracic society/European respiratory society statement: Asthma control and exacerbations - Standardizing endpoints for clinical asthma trials and clinical practice. *Am. J. Respir. Crit. Care Med.* 180(1), 59–99 (2009).
29. Szczesniak, R., Heltshe, S. L., Stanojevic, S. & Mayer-Hamblett, N. Use of FEV(1) in cystic fibrosis epidemiologic studies and clinical trials: A statistical perspective for the clinical researcher. *J. Cyst. Fibros* 16(3), 318–326 (2017).
30. Kakavas, S. *et al.* Pulmonary function testing in COPD: Looking beyond the curtain of FEV1. *NPJ Prim. Care Respir. Med.* 31(1), (2021).
31. Daley-Yates, P. T. Inhaled corticosteroids: Potency, dose equivalence and therapeutic index. *Br. J. Clin. Pharmacol.* 80(3), 372–380 (2015).
32. Dahl, R. *et al.* A dose-ranging study of fluticasone propionate in adult patients with moderate asthma. *Chest* 104(5), 1352–1358 (1993).
33. Shapiro, G. *et al.* Dose-related efficacy of budesonide administered via a dry powder inhaler in the treatment of children with moderate to severe persistent asthma. *J. Pediatr.* 132(6), 976–982 (1998).
34. Montanaro, A., Weinstein, S., Beaudot, C., Scott, S. M. & Georges, G. Efficacy and safety of inhaled extrafine beclomethasone dipropionate in adults with asthma: A randomized, parallel-group, dose-ranging study (BEAM). *J. Asthma* 59(7), 1410–1419 (2022).
35. Daley-Yates, P. T. *et al.* Therapeutic index of inhaled corticosteroids in asthma: A dose–response comparison on airway hyperresponsiveness and adrenal axis suppression. *Br. J. Clin. Pharmacol.* 87(2), 483–493 (2021).
36. Caillaud, D., Le Merre, C., Martinat, Y., Aguilaniu, B. & Pavia, D. A dose-ranging study of tiotropium delivered via Respimat® Soft Mist™ inhaler or HandiHaler® in COPD patients. *Int. J. COPD* 2, 559–565 (2007).

37. Singh, D. *et al.* A dose-ranging study of the bronchodilator effects of abediterol (LAS100977), a long-acting β2-adrenergic agonist, in asthma; a Phase II, randomized study. *BMC Pulm. Med.* 14, 1–10 (2014).

38. Kerwin, E. M. *et al.* A dose-ranging study of epinephrine hydrofluroalkane metered-dose inhaler (Primatene® MIST) in subjects with intermittent or mild-to-moderate persistent asthma. *J. Aerosol Med. Pulm. Drug Deliv.* 33(4), 186–193 (2020).

39. Coates, A. L. *et al.* ERS technical standard on bronchial challenge testing: General considerations and performance of methacholine challenge tests. *Eur. Respir. J.* 49(5), 1–17 (2017).

40. Scichilone, N. *et al.* Alveolar nitric oxide and asthma control in mild untreated asthma. *J. Allergy Clin. Immunol* 131(6), 1513–1517 (2013).

41. Beasley, R. *et al.* Inhaled corticosteroid therapy in adult asthma time for a new therapeutic dose terminology. *Am. J. Respir. Crit. Care Med.* 199(12), 1471–1477 (2019).

42. Ramsey, B. W. *et al.* Intermittent administration of inhaled tobramycin in patients with cystic fibrosis. Cystic fibrosis inhaled tobramycin study group. *N. Engl. J. Med.* 340(1), 23–30 (1999).

43. Geller, D. E., Pitlick, W. H., Nardella, P. A., Tracewell, W. G. & Ramsey, B. W. Pharmacokinetics and bioavailability of aerosolized tobramycin in cystic fibrosis. *Chest* 122(1), 219–226 (2002).

44. Maselli, D. J., Keyt, H. & Restrepo, M. I. Inhaled antibiotic therapy in chronic respiratory diseases. *Int. J. Mol. Sci.* 18(5), 1062 (2017).

45. United States Pharmacopeia. USP 44(5) *General Chapter <601> Inhalation and Nasal Drug Products - Aerosols, Sprays, and Powders - Performance Quality Tests.* (2019).

46. United States Pharmacopeia. USP 45(2) *Informative Chapter <1604> Data Interpretation of Aerodynamic Particle Size Distribution Measurements for Orally Inhaled Products.* (2019).

47. European Pharmacopeia. *Ph Eur 9.8 general chapter 2.9.18 preparations for inhalation: Aerodynamic assessment of fine particles.* (2019).

48. US FDA Center for Drug Evaluation and Research (CDER). *Metered dose inhaler (MDI) and dry powder inhaler (DPI) products - Quality considerations guidance for industry* (draft). (2018).

49. European Medicines Agency Committee for Medical Products for Human Use. *Guidleline on the pharmaceutical quality of inhalation and nasal products* (2006). doi:EMEA/CHMP/QWP/49313/2005 Corr.

50. Shur, J. *et al.* Defining the dosage strength for labeling of DPIs: Use, limitations and relevance of in vitro data. *Inhal. Mag.* 13, 7–13 (2019).

51. Radivojev, S., Zellnitz, S., Paudel, A. & Fröhlich, E. Searching for physiologically relevant in vitro dissolution techniques for orally inhaled drugs. *Int. J. Pharm.* 556, 45–56 (2019).

52. Selo, M. A., Sake, J. A., Kim, K. J. & Ehrhardt, C. In vitro and ex vivo models in inhalation biopharmaceutical research — Advances, challenges and future perspectives. *Adv. Drug Deliv. Rev.* 177, 113862 (2021).

53. Hofmann, W. Regional deposition: Deposition models. *J. Aerosol Med. Pulm. Drug Deliv.* 33(5), 239–248 (2020).

54. Phalen, R. F., Oldham, M. J. & Wolff, R. K. The relevance of animal models for aerosol studies. *J. Aerosol Med. Pulm. Drug Deliv.* 21(1), 113–124 (2008).

55. Finlay, W. H. & Martin, A. R. Recent advances in predictive understanding of respiratory tract deposition. *J. Aerosol Med. Pulm. Drug Deliv.* 21(2), 189–206 (2008).

56. Weers, J. G. & Clark, A. The impact of inspiratory flow rate on drug delivery to the lungs with dry powder inhalers. *Pharm. Res.* 34(3), 507–528 (2017).

57. Wei, X. *et al.* In vitro tests for aerosol deposition. VI: Realistic testing with different mouth–throat models and in vitro—In vivo correlations for a dry powder inhaler, metered dose inhaler, and soft mist inhaler. *J. Aerosol Med. Pulm. Drug Deliv.* 31(6), 358–371 (2018).

58. Ruzycki, C. A., Martin, A. R., Vehring, R. & Finlay, W. H. An in vitro examination of the effects of altitude on dry powder inhaler performance. *J. Aerosol Med. Pulm. Drug Deliv.* 31(4), 221–236 (2018).

59. Byron, P. R. *et al.* In vivo – In vitro correlations: Predicting pulmonary drug deposition from pharmaceutical aerosols. *J. Aerosol Med. Pulm. Drug Deliv.* 23(Supplement 2), S59–S69 (2010).

60. Cheng, Y.-S., Fu, C. S., Yazzie, D. & Zhou, Y. Respiratory deposition patterns of salbutamol pMDI with CFC and HFA-134a formulations in a human airway replica. *J. Aerosol Med.* 14(2), 255–266 (2001).

61. Zhang, Y., Gilbertson, K. & Finlay, W. H. In vivo–in vitro comparison of deposition in three mouth–throat models with Qvar® and Turbuhaler® inhalers. *J. Aerosol Med.* 20(3), 227–235 (2007).

62. Zhou, Y., Sun, J. & Cheng, Y.-S. Comparison of deposition in the USP and physical mouth – Throat models with solid and liquid particles. *J. Aerosol Med. Pulm. Drug Deliv.* 24(6), 277–284 (2011).

63. Guilmette, R. A., Wicks, J. D. & Wolff, R. K. Morphometry of human nasal airways in vivo using magnetic resonance imaging. *J. Aerosol Med.* 2(4), 365–377 (1989).

64. McRobbie, D. W., Pritchard, S. & Quest, R. A. Studies of the human oropharyngeal airspaces using magnetic resonance imaging. I. Validation of a three-dimensional MRI method for producing ex vivo virtual and physical casts of the oropharyngeal airways During inspiration. *J. Aerosol Med.* 16(4), 401–415 (2003).

65. Pritchard, S. E. & McRobbie, D. W. Studies of the human oropharyngeal airspaces using the influence of mouthpiece diameter and resistance of inhalation devices on the oropharyngeal airspace geometry. *J. Aerosol Med.* 17(4), 310–324 (2004).

66. McRobbie, D. W. & Pritchard, S. E. Studies of the human oropharyngeal airspaces using magnetic resonance imaging. III. The effects of device resistance with forced maneuver and tidal breathing on upper airway geometry. *J. Aerosol Med.* 18(3), 325–336 (2005).

67. Burnell, P. K. P. *et al.* Studies of the human oropharyngeal airspaces using magnetic resonance imaging IV - The oropharyngeal retention effect for four inhalation delivery systems. *J. Aerosol Med.* 20(3), 269–281 (2007).

68. Olsson, B., Borgström, L., Lundbäck, H. & Svensson, M. Validation of a general in vitro approach for prediction of total lung deposition in healthy adults for pharmaceutical inhalation products. *J. Aerosol Med. Pulm. Drug Deliv.* 26(6), 355–369 (2013).

69. Delvadia, R. R., Longest, P. W. & Byron, P. R. In vitro tests for aerosol deposition. I : Scaling a physical model of the upper airways to predict drug deposition variation in normal humans. *J. Aerosol Med. Pulm. Drug Deliv.* 25(1), 32–40 (2012).

70. Xi, J. & Longest, P. W. Transport and deposition of micro-aerosols in realistic and simplified models of the oral airway. *Ann. Biomed. Eng.* 35(4), 560–581 (2007).

71. Yeh, H. C. & Schum, G. Models of human lung airways and their application to inhaled particle deposition. *Bull. Math. Viology* 42(3), 461–480 (1980).

72. Tian, G., Longest, P. W., Su, G., Walenga, R. L. & Hindle, M. Development of a stochastic individual path (SIP) model for predicting the tracheobronchial deposition of pharmaceutical aerosols: Effects of transient inhalation and sampling the airways. *J. Aerosol Sci.* 42(11), 781–799 (2011).

73. Delvadia, R. R., Longest, P. W., Hindle, M. & Byron, P. R. In vitro tests for aerosol deposition. III: Effect of inhaler insertion angle on aerosol deposition. *J. Aerosol Med. Pulm. Drug Deliv.* 26(3), 145–156 (2013).

74. Delvadia, R. R., Hindle, M., Longest, P. W. & Byron, P. R. In vitro tests for aerosol deposition II: IVIVCs for different dry powder inhalers in normal adults. *J. Aerosol Med. Pulm. Drug Deliv.* 26(3), 138–144 (2012).

75. Wei, X., Hindle, M., Delvadia, R. R. & Byron, P. R. In vitro tests for aerosol deposition. V: Using realistic testing to estimate variations in aerosol properties at the trachea. *J. Aerosol Med. Pulm. Drug Deliv.* 30(5), 339–348 (2017).

76. Kaviratna, A. *et al.* Evaluation of bio-relevant mouth-throat models for characterization of metered dose inhalers. *AAPS PharmSciTech* 20(3), 130 (2019).

77. Janssens, H. M. *et al.* The Sophia anatomical infant nose-throat (saint) model: A valuable tool to study aerosol deposition in infants. *J. Aerosol Med.* 14(4), 433–441 (2002).

78. Réminiac, F. *et al.* Nasal high flow nebulization in infants and toddlers: An in vitro and in vivo scintigraphic study. *Pediatr. Pulmonol.* 52(3), 337–344 (2016).

79. Laube, B. L., Sharpless, G., Shermer, C., Sullivan, V. & Powell, K. Deposition of dry powder generated by solovent in Sophia Anatomical Infant Nose-Throat (SAINT) model. *Aerosol Sci. Technol.* 46(5), 514–520 (2012).

80. Esposito-Festen, J. E. *et al.* Effect of a facemask leak on aerosol delivery from a pMDI-spacer system. *J. Aerosol Med.* 17(1), 1–6 (2004).

81. Minocchieri, S. *et al.* Development of the premature infant nose throat-model (PrINT-Model)-an upper airway replica of a premature neonate for the study of aerosol delivery. *Pediatr. Res.* 64(2), 141–146 (2008).

82. Stapleton, K. W., Guentsch, E., Hoskinson, M. K. & Finlay, W. H. On the suitability of k-epsilon turbulence modeling for aerosol deposition in the mouth and throat: A comparison with experiment. *J. Aerosol Sci.* 31(6), 739–749 (2000).

83. Weers, J. G. *et al.* In vitro–in vivo correlations observed With indacaterol-based formulations delivered with the Breezhaler®. *J. Aerosol Med. Pulm. Drug Deliv.* 28(4), 268–280 (2015).

84. Morin, C. M. D. *et al.* Performance of pressurized metered-dose inhalers at extreme temperature conditions. *J. Pharm. Sci.* 103(11), 3553–3559 (2014).

85. Fink, J. B. *et al.* Good things in small packages: An innovative delivery approach for inhaled insulin. *Pharm. Res.* 34(12), 2568–2578 (2017).

86. Ung, K. T., Rao, N., Weers, J. G., Huang, D. & Chan, H. K. Design of spray dried insulin microparticles to bypass deposition in the extrathoracic region and maximize total lung dose. *Int. J. Pharm.* 511(2), 1070–1079 (2016).

87. Shemirani, F. M. *et al.* In vitro investigation of the effect of ambient humidity on regional delivered dose with solution and suspension MDIs. *J. Aerosol Med. Pulm. Drug Deliv.* 26(4), 215–222 (2013).

88. Ciciliani, A. M., Langguth, P. & Wachtel, H. In vitro dose comparison of respimat® inhaler with dry powder inhalers for COPD maintenance therapy. *Int. J. COPD* 12, 1565–1577 (2017).

89. Ruzycki, C. A., Martin, A. R. & Finlay, W. H. An exploration of factors affecting in vitro deposition of pharmaceutical aerosols in the Alberta idealized throat. *J. Aerosol Med. Pulm. Drug Deliv.* 32(6), 405–417 (2019).

90. Ruzycki, C. A., Murphy, B., Nathoo, H., Finlay, W. H. & Martin, A. R. Combined in vitro-in silico approach to predict deposition and pharmacokinetics of budesonide dry powder inhalers. *Pharm. Res.* 37(10), 209 (2020).

91. Golshahi, L. & Finlay, W. H. An idealized child throat that mimics average pediatric oropharyngeal deposition. *Aerosol Sci. Technol.* 46(5), i–iv (2012).

92. Golshahi, L., Noga, M. L. & Finlay, W. H. Deposition of inhaled micrometer-sized particles in oropharyngeal airway replicas of children at constant flow rates. *J. Aerosol Sci.* 49, 21–31 (2012).

93. Ruzycki, C. A., Golshahi, L., Vehring, R. & Finlay, W. H. Comparison of in vitro deposition of pharmaceutical aerosols in an idealized child throat with in vivo deposition in the upper respiratory tract of children. *Pharm. Res.* 31(6), 1525–1535 (2014).

94. Javaheri, E., Golshahi, L. & Finlay, W. H. An idealized geometry that mimics average infant nasal airway deposition. *J. Aerosol Sci.* 55, 137–148 (2013).

95. Tavernini, S., Church, T. K., Lewis, D. A., Martin, A. R. & Finlay, W. H. Scaling an idealized infant nasal airway geometry to mimic inertial filtration of neonatal nasal airways. *J. Aerosol Sci.* 118, 14–21 (2018).
96. Keller, L. A., Merkel, O. & Popp, A. Intranasal drug delivery: Opportunities and toxicologic challenges during drug development. *Drug Deliv. Transl. Res.* 25, 1–25 (2021).
97. Kiaee, M., Wachtel, H., Noga, M. L., Martin, A. R. & Finlay, W. H. An idealized geometry that mimics average nasal spray deposition in adults: A computational study. *Comput. Biol. Med.* 107, 206–217 (2019).
98. Chen, J. Z., Kiaee, M., Martin, A. R. & Finlay, W. H. In vitro assessment of an idealized nose for nasal spray testing: Comparison with regional deposition in realistic nasal replicas. *Int. J. Pharm.* 582 (2020).
99. Kiaee, M., Wachtel, H., Noga, M. L., Martin, A. R. & Finlay, W. H. Regional deposition of nasal sprays in adults: A wide ranging computational study. *Int. J. Numer. Method. Biomed. Eng.* 34(5), 1–13 (2018).
100. Clark, A. R. Understanding penetration index measurements and regional lung targeting. *J. Aerosol Med. Pulm. Drug Deliv.* 25(4), 179–187 (2012).
101. Cheng, Y.-S., Zhou, Y. & Chen, B. T. Particle deposition in a cast of human oral airways. *Aerosol Sci. Technol.* 31(4), 286–300 (1999).
102. Borojeni, A. A. T., Noga, M. L., Martin, A. R. & Finlay, W. H. Validation of airway resistance models for predicting pressure loss through anatomically realistic conducting airway replicas of adults and children. *J. Biomech.* 48(10), 1988–1996 (2015).
103. Huynh, B. K. *et al.* The development and validation of an in vitro airway model to assess realistic airway deposition and drug permeation behavior of orally inhaled products Across synthetic membranes. *J. Aerosol Med. Pulm. Drug Deliv.* 31(2), 103–108 (2018).
104. Chan, T. L. & Lippmann, M. Experimental measurements and empirical modelling of the regional deposition of inhaled particles in humans. *Am. Ind. Hyg. Assoc. J.* 41(6), 399–409 (1980).
105. Bhagwat, S. *et al.* Predicting pulmonary pharmacokinetics from in vitro properties of dry powder inhalers. *Pharm. Res.* 34(12), 2541–2556 (2017).
106. Tavernini, S., Farina, D. J., Martin, A. R. & Finlay, W. H. Using filters to estimate regional lung deposition with dry powder inhalers. *Pharm. Res.* 38(9), 1601–1613 (2021).
107. Tavernini, S., Kiaee, M., Farina, D. J., Martin, A. R. & Finlay, W. H. Development of a filter that mimics tracheobronchial deposition of respirable aerosols in humans. *Aerosol Sci. Technol.* 53(7), 802–816 (2019).
108. Mitchell, J. P., Suggett, J. & Nagel, M. Clinically relevant in vitro testing of orally inhaled products—Bridging the gap between the lab and the patient. *AAPS PharmSciTech* 17(4), 787–804 (2016).
109. Pauwels, R., Newman, S. P. & Borgström, L. Airway deposition and airway effects of anti-asthma drugs delivered from metered-dose inhalers. *Eur. Respir. J.* 10(9), 2127–2138 (1997).
110. Broeders, M. E. A. C., Sanchis, J., Levy, M. L., Crompton, G. K. & Dekhuijzen, P. N. R. The ADMIT series - Issues in inhalation therapy. 2) Improving technique and clinical effectiveness. *Prim. Care Respir. J.* 18(2), 76–82 (2009).
111. Hira, D. *et al.* Assessment of inhalation flow patterns of soft mist inhaler co-prescribed with dry powder inhaler using inspiratory flow meter for multi inhalation devices. *PLOS ONE* 13(2), 1–12 (2018).
112. Newman, S. P., Brown, J., Steed, K. P., Reader, S. J. & Kladders, H. Lung deposition of fenoterol and flunisolide delivered using a novel device of inhaled medicines. *CHEST J.* 113(4), 957–963 (1998).
113. Finlay, W. H. *The mechanics of inhaled pharmaceutical aerosols: An Introduction.* (London: Academic Press, 2019).
114. Liu, X., Doub, W. H. & Guo, C. Evaluation of metered dose inhaler spray velocities using phase doppler anemometry (PDA). *Int. J. Pharm.* 423(2), 235–239 (2012).

115. Grgic, B., Martin, A. R. & Finlay, W. H. The effect of unsteady flow rate increase on in vitro mouth-throat deposition of inhaled boluses. *J. Aerosol Sci.* 37(10), 1222–1233 (2006).

116. Mohammed, H. *et al.* Effect of sampling volume on dry powder inhaler (DPI)-emitted aerosol aerodynamic particle size distributions (APSDs) measured by the next-generation pharmaceutical impactor (NGI) and the Andersen eight-stage cascade impactor (ACI). *AAPS PharmSciTech* 13(3), 875–882 (2012).

117. Frijlink, H. W. & De Boer, A. H. Dry powder inhalers for pulmonary drug delivery. *Expert Opin. Drug Deliv.* 1(1), 67–86 (2005).

118. Everard, M. L., Devadason, S. G. & Le Souef, P. N. Flow early in the inspiratory manoeuvre affects the aerosol particle size distribution from a Turbuhaler. *Respir. Med.* 91(10), 624–628 (1997).

119. Kamin, W. E. S. *et al.* Mass output and particle size distribution of glucocorticosteroids emitted from different inhalation devices depending on various inspiratory parameters. *J. Aerosol Med.* 15(1), 65–73 (2002).

120. Dorosz, A., Penconek, A. & Moskal, A. In vitro study on the aerosol emitted from the DPI inhaler under two unsteady inhalation profiles. *J. Aerosol Sci.* 101, 104–117 (2016).

121. Greguletz, R. *et al.* A collaborative study by the European pharmaceutical aerosol group (EPAG) to assess the flow-time profile of test equipment typically used for pMDI/DPI testing – Part 1: Volume test. *Ddl* 2010, 1–5 (2010).

122. Greguletz, R. *et al.* A cross-industry assessment of the flow rate-time profiles of test equipment typically used for dry-powder inhaler (DPI) testing: Part 1 – Compendial apparatuses. *Aerosol Sci. Technol.* 54(12), 1424–1447 (2020).

123. Versteeg, H. K. *et al.* A cross-industry assessment of the flow rate-elapsed time profiles of test equipment typically used for dry-powder inhaler (DPI) testing: Part 2 – analysis of transient air flow in the testing of DPIs with compendial cascade impactors. *Aerosol Sci. Technol.* 54(12), 1448–1470 (2020).

124. Finlay, W. H. & Gehmlich, M. G. Inertial sizing of aerosol inhaled from two dry powder inhalers with realistic breath patterns versus constant flow rates. *Int. J. Pharm.* 210(1–2), 83–95 (2000).

125. Ung, K. T. & Chan, H. K. Effects of ramp-up of inspired airflow on in vitro aerosol dose delivery performance for certain dry powder inhalers. *Eur. J. Pharm. Sci.* 84, 46–54 (2016).

126. Delvadia, R. R., Wei, X., Longest, P. W., Venitz, J. & Byron, P. R. In vitro tests for aerosol deposition. IV: Simulating variations in human breath profiles for realistic DPI testing. *J. Aerosol Med. Pulm. Drug Deliv.* 29(2), 196–206 (2016).

127. Mitchell, J. P. & Dolovich, M. B. Clinically relevant test methods to establish in vitro equivalence for spacers and valved holding chambers used with pressurized metered dose inhalers (pMDIs). *J. Aerosol Med. Pulm. Drug Deliv.* 25(4), 217–242 (2012).

128. Smaldone, G. C., Berg, E. & Nikander, K. Variation in pediatric aerosol delivery: Importance of facemask. *J. Aerosol Med.* 18(3), 354–363 (2005).

129. Roth, A. P., Lange, C. F. & Finlay, W. H. The effect of breathing pattern on nebulizer drug delivery. *J. Aerosol Med.* 16(3), 325–339 (2003).

130. Dolovich, M. B. & Mitchell, J. P. Canadian standards association standard CAN/CSA/Z264. *Can. Respir. J.* 11(7), 489–495 (2004).

131. Finlay, W. H. & Stapleton, K. W. Undersizing of droplets from a vented nebulizer caused by aerosol heating during transit through an Anderson impactor. *J. Aerosol Sci.* 30(1), 105–109 (1999).

132. Kwong, W. T. J., Ho, S. L. & Coates, A. L. Comparison of nebulized particle size distribution with Malvern laser diffraction analyzer versus Andersen cascade impactor and low-flow Marple personal cascade impactor. *J. Aerosol Med.* 13(4), 303–314 (2000).

133. Vecellio-None, L. *et al.* Validation of laser diffraction method as a substitute for cascade impaction in the European project for a nebulizer standard. *J. Aerosol Med. Depos. Clear. Eff. Lung* 14(1), 107–114 (2001).

134. Ziegler, J. & Wachtel, H. Comparison of cascade impaction and laser diffraction for particle size distribution measurements. *J. Aerosol Med.* 18(3), 311–324 (2005).

135. Finlay, W. H. Estimating the type of hygroscopic behavior exhibited by aqueous droplets. *J. Aerosol Med.* 11(4), 221–229 (1998).

136. Yang, M. Y. *et al.* Examining the ability of empirical correlations to predict subject specific in vivo extrathoracic aerosol deposition during tidal breathing. *Aerosol Sci. Technol.* 51(3), 363–376 (2017).

137. Ferron, G. A. The size of soluble aerosol particles as a function of the humidity of the air: Application to the human respiratory tract. *J. Aerosol Sci.* 8(4), 251–267 (1977).

138. Javaheri, E. & Finlay, W. H. Size manipulation of hygroscopic saline droplets: Application to respiratory drug delivery. *Int. J. Heat Mass Transf.* 67, 690–695 (2013).

139. Golshahi, L. *et al.* The use of condensational growth methods for efficient drug delivery to the lungs during noninvasive ventilation high flow therapy. *Pharm. Res.* 30(11), 2917–2930 (2013).

140. Martonen, T. B. Development of surrogate lung systems with controlled thermodynamic environments to study hygroscopic particles: Air pollutants and pharmacologic drugs. *Part. Sci. Technol.* 8(1–2), 1–20 (1990).

141. Majoral, C., Coates, A. L., Le Pape, A. & Vecellio, L. Humidified and heated cascade impactor for aerosol sizing. *Front. Bioeng. Biotechnol.* 8, 1313 (2020).

142. Ivey, J. W., Lewis, D., Church, T., Finlay, W. H. & Vehring, R. A correlation equation for the mass median aerodynamic diameter of the aerosol emitted by solution metered dose inhalers. *Int. J. Pharm.* 465(1–2), 18–24 (2014).

143. Titosky, J. T. F. *et al.* The effect of altitude on inhaler performance. *J. Pharm. Sci.* 103(7), 2116–2124 (2014).

144. Vehring, R. Pharmaceutical particle engineering via spray drying. *Pharm. Res.* 25(5), 999–1022 (2008).

145. Young, P. M. *et al.* Influence of humidity on the electrostatic charge and aerosol performance of dry powder inhaler carrier based systems. *Pharm. Res.* 24(5), 963–970 (2007).

146. Kwok, P. C. L. & Chan, H. K. Effect of relative humidity on the electrostatic charge properties of dry powder inhaler aerosols. *Pharm. Res.* 25(2), 277–288 (2008).

147. Janson, C., Lööf, T., Telg, G., Stratelis, G. & Nilsson, F. Difference in resistance to humidity between commonly used dry powder inhalers: An in vitro study. *npj Prim. Care Respir. Med.* 26(1), 1–5 (2016).

148. Yu, J., Wong, J., Ukkonen, A., Kannosto, J. & Chan, H. Effect of relative humidity on bipolar electrostatic charge profiles of dry powder aerosols. *Pharm. Res.* 1707–1715 (2017). https://doi.org/10.1007/s11095-017-2178-3.

149. Buttini, F. *et al.* Accessorized DPI: A shortcut towards flexibility and patient adaptability in dry powder inhalation. *Pharm. Res.* 33(12), 3012–3020 (2016).

150. Sanchis, J., Gich, I. & Pedersen, S. Systematic review of errors in inhaler use: Has patient technique improved over time? *Chest* 150(2), 394–406 (2016).

151. Nordlund, M. & Kuczaj, A. K. Aerosol dosimetry modeling using computational fluid dynamics. In *Computational systems toxicology* (eds. Hoeng, J. & Peitsch, M. C.) 393–427. (New York: Springer, 2015). https://doi.org/10.1007/978-1-4939-2778-4_16.

152. International Commission on Radiological Protection. Human respiratory tract model for radiological protection : A report of a task group of the international commission on radiological protection 24(1–3) 1–3, (published for the International Commission on Radiological Protection by Pergamon, 1994).

153. Cheng, Y.-S. Aerosol deposition in the extrathoracic region. *Aerosol Sci. Technol.* 37(8), 659–671 (2003).

154. Carrigy, N. B., Martin, A. R. & Finlay, W. H. Use of extrathoracic deposition models for patient-specific dose estimation during inhaler design. *Curr. Pharm. Des.* 21(27), 3984–3992 (2015).

155. Carrigy, N. B., Ruzycki, C. A., Golshahi, L. & Finlay, W. H. Pediatric in vitro and in silico models of deposition via oral and nasal inhalation. *J. Aerosol Med. Pulm. Drug Deliv.* 27(3), 149–169 (2014).

156. Golshahi, L., Noga, M. L., Vehring, R. & Finlay, W. H. An in vitro study on the deposition of micrometer-sized particles in the extrathoracic airways of adults during tidal oral breathing. *Ann. Biomed. Eng.* 41(5), 979–989 (2013).

157. Grgic, B., Finlay, W. H., Burnell, P. K. P. & Heenan, A. F. In vitro intersubject and intrasubject deposition measurements in realistic mouth – Throat geometries. *J. Aerosol Sci.* 35(8), 1025–1040 (2004).

158. Dehaan, W. H. & Finlay, W. H. Predicting extrathoracic deposition from dry powder inhalers. *J. Aerosol Sci.* 35(3), 309–331 (2004).

159. Javaheri, E. *et al.* Deposition modeling of hygroscopic saline aerosols in the human respiratory tract : Comparison between air and helium – Oxygen as carrier gases. *J. Aerosol Sci.* 64, 81–93 (2013).

160. Heyder, J. Gravitational deposition of aerosol particles within a system of randomly oriented tubes. *J. Aerosol Sci.* 6(2), 133–137 (1975).

161. Heyder, J. & Gebhart, J. Gravitational deposition of particles from laminar aerosol flow through inclined circular tubes. *J. Aerosol Sci.* 8(4), 289–295 (1977).

162. Ingham, D. B. Diffusion of aerosols from a stream flowing through a cylindrical tube. *J. Aerosol Sci.* 6(2), 125–132 (1975).

163. Ferron, G. A., Kreyling, W. G. & Haider, B. Inhalation of salt aerosol particles - II. *Growth Depos. Hum. Respir. Tract.* 19, 611–631 (1988).

164. Finlay, W. H. & Stapleton, K. W. The effect on regional lung deposition of coupled heat and mass transfer between hygroscopic droplets and their surrounding phase. *J. Aerosol Sci.* 26(4), 655–670 (1995).

165. Darquenne, C. *et al.* Bridging the gap between science and clinical efficacy: Physiology, imaging, and modeling of aerosols in the lung. *J. Aerosol Med. Pulm. Drug Deliv.* 29(2), 107–126 (2016).

166. Finlay, W. H., Lange, C. F., King, M. & Speert, D. P. Lung delivery of aerosolized dextran. *Am. J. Respir. Crit. Care Med.* 161(1), 91–97 (2000).

167. Lange, C. F., Hancock, R. E. W., Samuel, J. & Finlay, W. H. In vitro aerosol delivery and regional airway surface liquid concentration of a liposomal cationic peptide. *J. Pharm. Sci.* 90(10), 1647–1657 (2001).

168. Martin, A. R. & Finlay, W. H. Model calculations of regional deposition and disposition for single doses of inhaled liposomal and dry powder ciprofloxacin. *J. Aerosol Med. Pulm. Drug Deliv.* 31(1), 49–60 (2018).

169. Himstedt, A., Braun, C., Wicha, S. G. & Borghardt, J. M. Towards a quantitative mechanistic understanding of localized pulmonary tissue retention—A combined in vivo/in silico approach based on four model drugs. *Pharmaceutics* 12(5), (2020).

170. Hastedt, J. E. *et al.* Scope and relevance of a pulmonary biopharmaceutical classification system AAPS/FDA/USP Workshop March 16–17th, 2015 in Baltimore, MD. *Am. Assoc. Pharm. Sci. Open* 2(1), 1 (2016).

171. Olsson, B. *et al.* Pulmonary drug metabolism, clearance, and absorption. In *Controlled pulmonary drug delivery* (eds. Smyth, H. D. C. & Hickey, A. J.) 21–50. (New York: Controlled Release Society; Springer, 2011).

172. Sakagami, M. In vivo, in vitro and ex vivo models to assess pulmonary absorption and disposition of inhaled therapeutics for systemic delivery. *Adv. Drug Deliv. Rev.* 58(9–10), 1030–1060 (2006).

173. Hickey, A. J. Controlled delivery of inhaled therapeutic agents. *J. Control. Release* 190, 182–188 (2014).

174. Byron, P. R. Prediction of drug residence times in regions of the human respiratory tract following aerosol inhalation. *J. Pharm. Sci.* 75(5), 433–438 (1986).

175. Gonda, I. Drugs administered directly into the respiratory tract: Modeling of the duration. *J. Pharm. Sci.* 77(4), 340–346 (1988).
176. Weber, B. & Hochhaus, G. A pharmacokinetic simulation tool for inhaled corticosteroids. *Am. Assoc. Pharm. Sci. J.* 15(1), 159–171 (2013).
177. Bäckman, P., Tehler, U. & Olsson, B. Predicting exposure after oral inhalation of the selective glucocorticoid receptor modulator, AZD5423, based on dose, deposition pattern, and mechanistic modeling of pulmonary disposition. *J. Aerosol Med. Pulm. Drug Deliv.* 30(2), 108–117 (2017).
178. Bäckman, P. *et al.* Advances in experimental and mechanistic computational models to understand pulmonary exposure to inhaled drugs. *Eur. J. Pharm. Sci.* 113, 41–52 (2018).
179. Boger, E. & Fridén, M. Physiologically based pharmacokinetic/pharmacodynamic modeling accurately predicts the better bronchodilatory effect of inhaled Versus oral salbutamol dosage forms. *J. Aerosol Med. Pulm. Drug Deliv.* 32(1), 1–12 (2019).
180. National Council on Radiation Protection and Measurements. *Deposition, Retention, and Dosimetry of Inhaled Radioactive Substances: Recommendations of the National Council on Radiation Protection and Measurements* (Bethesda, MD: National Council on Radiation Protection and Measurements, 1997).
181. Weibel, E. R. *Morphometry of the Human Lung* (Springer, 1963).
182. Finlay, W. H., Stapleton, K. W., Chan, H.-K., Zuberbuhler, P. & Gonda, I. Regional deposition of inhaled hygroscopic aerosols: In vivo SPECT compared with mathematical modeling. *J. Appl. Physiol. (1985)* 81(1), 374–383 (1996).
183. Finlay, W. H. & Wong, J. P. Regional lung deposition of nebulized liposome-encapsulated ciprofloxacin. *Int. J. Pharm.* 167(1–2), 121–127 (1998).
184. Hoe, S. *et al.* Use of a fundamental approach to spray-drying formulation design to facilitate the development of multi-component dry powder aerosols for respiratory drug delivery. *Pharm. Res.* 31(2), 449–465 (2014).
185. Martin, A. R., Malinin, V. S., Cipolla, D. & Finlay, W. H. Modeling regional deposition and pharmacokinetics for inhaled prodrug treprostinil Palmitil. *J. Aerosol Med. Pulm. Drug Deliv.* 34, A-12 (2021).
186. Barnes, P. J. Inhaled corticosteroids. *Pharmaceuticals (Basel)* 3(3), 514–540 (2010).
187. Hochhaus, G. *et al.* Can pharmacokinetic studies assess the pulmonary fate of dry powder inhaler formulations of fluticasone propionate? *AAPS J.* 23(3), 1–14 (2021).
188. Dokoumetzidis, A. & Macheras, P. A century of dissolution research: From Noyes and Whitney to the biopharmaceutics classification system. *Int. J. Pharm.* 321(1–2), 1–11 (2006).
189. May, S. *et al.* Dissolution testing of powders for inhalation: Influence of particle deposition and modeling of dissolution profiles. *Pharm. Res.* 31(11), 3211–3224 (2014).
190. Hintz, R. J. & Johnson, K. C. The effect of particle size distribution on dissolution rate and oral absorption. *Int. J. Pharm.* 51(1), 9–17 (1989).
191. Schürch, S., Gehr, P., Im Hof, V., Geiser, M. & Green, F. Surfactant displaces particles toward the epithelium in airways and alveoli. *Respir. Physiol.* 80(1), 17–32 (1990).
192. Bäckman, P. & Olsson, B. Pulmonary drug dissolution, regional retention and systemic absorption: Understanding their interactions through mechanistic modeling. *Respir. Drug Deliv.* 2020(50), 113–122 (2020).
193. Eriksson, J. *et al.* Pulmonary dissolution of poorly soluble compounds studied in an ex vivo rat lung model. *Mol. Pharm.* 16(7), 3053–3064 (2019).
194. Amidon, G. L., Lennernäs, H., Shah, V. P. & Crison, J. R. A theoretical basis for a biopharmaceutic drug classification: The correlation of in vitro drug product dissolution and in vivo bioavailability. *Pharm. Res.* 12(3), 413–420 (1995).
195. Velaga, S. P. *et al.* Dry powder inhalers: An overview of the in vitro dissolution methodologies and their correlation with the biopharmaceutical aspects of the drug products. *Eur. J. Pharm. Sci.* 113, 18–28 (2018).

196. Patton, J. S., Fishburn, C. S. & Weers, J. G. The lungs as a portal of entry for systemic drug delivery. *Proc. Am. Thorac. Soc.* 1(4), 338–344 (2004).
197. Loira-Pastoriza, C., Todoroff, J. & Vanbever, R. Delivery strategies for sustained drug release in the lungs. *Adv. Drug Deliv. Rev.* 75, 81–91 (2014).
198. Floroiu, A., Klein, M., Krämer, J. & Lehr, C. M. Towards standardized dissolution techniques for in vitro performance testing of dry powder inhalers. *Technol.* 25(3), 6–18 (2018).
199. Rohrschneider, M. *et al.* Evaluation of the transwell system for characterization of dissolution behavior of inhalation drugs: Effects of membrane and surfactant. *Mol. Pharm.* 12(8), 2618–2624 (2015).
200. Price, R. *et al.* Development of an aerosol dose collection apparatus for in vitro dissolution measurements of orally inhaled drug products. *AAPS J.* 22(2), 1–9 (2020).
201. Arora, D., Shah, K. A., Halquist, M. S. & Sakagami, M. In vitro aqueous fluid-capacity-limited dissolution testing of respirable aerosol drug particles generated from inhaler products. *Pharm. Res.* 27(5), 786–795 (2010).
202. Tay, J. Y. S., Liew, C. V. & Heng, P. W. S. Dissolution of fine particle fraction from truncated Anderson cascade impactor with an enhancer cell. *Int. J. Pharm.* 545(1–2), 45–50 (2018).
203. Gerde, P., Malmlöf, M. & Selg, E. In vitro to ex vivo/in vivo correlation (IVIVC) of dissolution kinetics from inhaled particulate solutes using air/blood barrier models: Relation between in vitro design, lung physiology and kinetic output of models. *J. Aerosol Sci.* 151, 105698 (2021).
204. Shapiro, M. E., Corcoran, T. E., Bertrand, C. A., Serrano Castillo, F. & Parker, R. S. Physiologically-based model of fluid absorption and mucociliary clearance in cystic fibrosis. *IFAC PapersOnLine* 51(19), 102–103 (2018).
205. Darquenne, C. Aerosol deposition in health and disease. *J. Aerosol Med. Pulm. Drug Deliv.* 25(3), 140–147 (2012).

In Vitro Assessment of Drug Release, Dissolution, and Absorption in the Lung

2

Rajan S. Bhattarai, Virender Kumar,
Karthik Nagapudi, Ajit S. Narang,
and Ram I Mahato

Contents

DOI: 10.1201/9781003182566-3

2.1 INTRODUCTION

Administration of therapeutics to the lungs is being increasingly used to enable both local and systemic delivery of drugs.[1, 2] The large available surface area (50 m^2 to 100 m^2), mucosal surface, and rapid systemic absorption make the lungs a suitable "needleless" site for both local and systemic delivery of therapeutics.[2, 3] Currently, this route of administration is utilized for the treatment of cystic fibrosis,[4] asthma,[5] chronic obstructive pulmonary disease (COPD),[6] respiratory distress syndrome (RDS),[7] influenza,[8] and even diabetes.[9, 10] It should be noted that the pulmonary delivery of insulin was found to increase the risk of lung cancer, and the commercial product (Exubera) has been withdrawn from the market. Subsequently, companies working on inhalable insulin have terminated their product development efforts. Nevertheless, the insulin example shows the lungs' potential as a therapeutic delivery route.[10, 11]

Drug delivery to the lungs can either be in aqueous liquid or suspension form through nebulizers[12] and soft mist sprays[13] in non-aqueous forms through pressurized metered-dose inhalers (pMDI)[14] or in solid form through dry powder inhalers (DPI).[15] Though pMDIs form two-thirds of all the inhalers in the market, DPIs are gaining ground. While there has not been any systematic research to prove the superiority of one over the other, both pMDI and DPIs show dosing reliability, accuracy, and consistency compared to nebulizers.[16, 17] Inhalation devices have undergone technological advances, which have made them more effective in drug delivery. For example, the use of patient's breathing rate to trigger device activation sensitivity in Easibreathe®,[18] addition of dissolved carbon dioxide to decrease the droplet size,[19] addition of spacer in front of the mouth piece for ease of use in Azmacort®,[20] propellent free uniblock technology with decreased oropharyngeal deposition in Respimat®,[21] and low density hollow spheres of Pulmosphere™ increasing the amount of delivered drug, etc. have increased the acceptance of inhalation products by patients. In all these cases with technological advances, the best way to ensure the optimized drug delivery and adherence to therapy is to train the patient in the proper use of the device.[22]

The mist/particles/aerosols generated post-actuation by different inhalation devices are inhaled by the patient and get deposited on different sites in the lungs. Disposition of aerosolized particles in the lung and therefore the treatment efficacy is governed by multiple factors, including physicochemical properties of the drug (e.g., particle size, geometry, density, surface characteristics, and excipients) and the anatomical, physiological, and pathological factors of the patient (lung humidity, tidal volumes, and flow rates, structure of the epithelia, disease condition, and age).[23] After the inhalation of the DPI, the deposited particles are subjected to clearance mechanisms, absorption, and metabolism. Again, these physiological mechanisms are dependent on the physicochemical attributes of the inhaled drugs and the biological characteristics of the lungs. To understand the fate of the inhaled drug, various in vitro, ex vivo, in vivo, and computer modeling methodologies are used. In this review, we will focus on (a) the factors that affect performance of inhalation therapeutics and (b) the in vitro experiments that are utilized to understand drug release, dissolution, absorption, and permeation from the formulations designed for inhalation.

2.2 FACTORS AFFECTING DEPOSITION AND BIOAVAILABILITY

The deposition and bioavailability of the inhaled formulation on the different sites in the lungs is dependent on various factors described below.

2.2.1 Factors Affecting Bioavailability

2.2.1.1 Mucociliary clearance

Mucociliary clearance (MCC) is the primary innate defense mechanism in the upper respiratory tract of the body against the harmful particles getting into the airways. The lungs are functionally divided into two distinct zones: the conducting zone and the respiratory zone (Figure 2.1). Out of 23 generations of lung starting from trachea, 16 generations form the former while seven form the latter. The respiratory tract is lined with ciliated columnar epithelial cells which transition to ciliated cuboidal and finally to squamous cells in the alveoli. The cilia, mucus layer (produced by goblet cells), and surface liquid in the airway (ASL) act altogether to remove the inhaled particulate contaminants from the airways. The respiratory tract lining fluid (RTLF), especially in the proximal respiratory tract, is composed of periciliary sol layer surrounding the cilia, facilitating the ciliary movement and the mucus gel blanketing the cilia on top of periciliary liquid. Overall, the thickness of the RTLF (including sol) decreases as the generation numbers in the respiratory tract increases. The RTLF around the alveoli is the thinnest, devoid of any mucus but contains surfactants and phospholipids thus decreasing the surface tension. The sol layer is sufficient to cover the length of cilia and is around 7 μm in thickness while the mucus layer varies significantly in thickness.

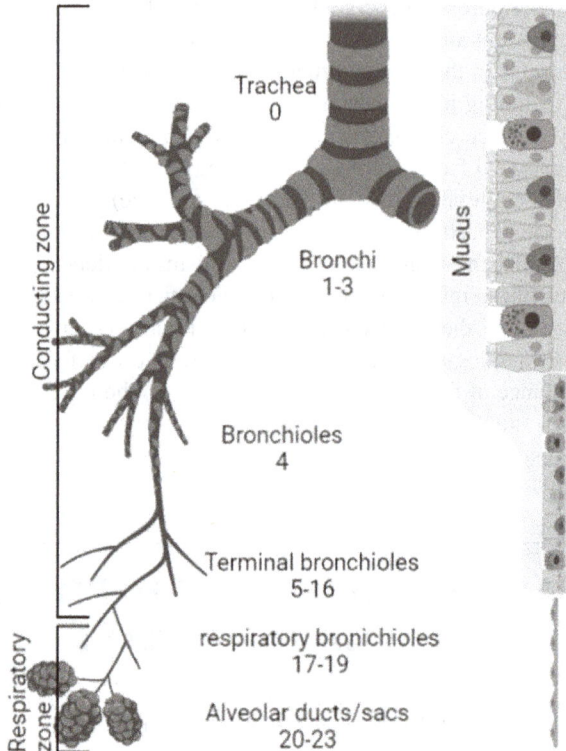

FIGURE 2.1   Structure of the lung. The airways generation is shown from the trachea (0) and goes down through the conducting airways (bronchi and bronchioles) to the respiratory zone (respiratory bronchioles and alveoli) which ends at 23rd generation. The ciliated epithelial cells form the lining of the respiratory tract covered by the mucus produced by goblet cells. The thickness of the mucus layer decreases along the respiratory tract and is missing in the alveoli and the type I and type II alveolar epithelial cells which line the alveolar sacs.

In general, the RTLF is 5–20 μm thick in upper respiratory tract, 1.8 μm in bronchioles, and 0.2–0.5 μm in the alveolar region of the lungs as determined by light microscopy, electron microscopy, and rapid freezing techniques.[24] The approximate volume of RTLF in conducting airways is 10–30 ml while that in the respiratory region is 7–20 ml.

Just like thickness, the composition of the RTLF is not the same throughout the respiratory tract. The RTLF in trachea, bronchi, and larger bronchioles consists mainly of water (95%), mucins/glycoproteins (2%), lipids (1%), proteins (1%), and salts (1%), while that in alveolar region is devoid of mucins and includes surfactants. The surfactant layer in alveolar region is composed of phospathidylcholine (PC) in the form of dipalmitoylphosphatidylcholine (DPPC) (41–70%), phosphotidylglycerol (~8–10%), phosphatidylethananolamine (~5%), phosphatidylinositol (~3%), sphingomyelin, phosphatidylserine, etc. Additionally, cholesterol, triglicerides, free fatty acids, and surfactant proteins A, B, C, and D (SP-A, -B, -C, -D) form the rest of surfactants. SP-A and -D support host defense, while SP-B and -C help reduce the surface tension of the alveolar fluid.

MCC forms a mechanical, chemical, and biological barrier. ASL traps the particles and removes them by ciliary action, and prevents adherence and circulation of particulates in the airway epithelium.[25] Antioxidative properties of the mucus create a chemical barrier against the oxides to protect the epithelial cells.[26, 27] The second layer of ASL, the periciliary layer underneath the mucus layer, provides liquid for clearance of particles from the trachea-bronchiolar region of the lungs towards the mouth.[28-30] In diseased lungs, the mucociliary activity is affected leading to an increase in the clearance of inhaled particles and reduction in their lung residence time thereby reducing the effectiveness of the drugs.[28, 29] The interaction between mucus and cilia decides the rate of MCC and fate of the particles. To put it in perspective, around 20–40 ml of mucus is secreted every day and transported to the pharynx region, which removes the particles with size range of 4.0–12.5 μm. The average MCC time for an adult is 7–15 min, and this can increase in case of rhinitis and allergies.[29]

Most of the marketed inhalable formulations are crystalline in nature, which have the advantages of purity and stability over the amorphous forms.[31] But due to their decreased solubility they get cleared by MCC while their amorphous counterpart exerts therapeutic effects due to rapid dissolution.[32]

2.2.1.2 Alveolar clearance

The alveoli (Figure 2.1) are the site of gaseous exchange in the lungs. They are composed of two types of epithelial cells, Type I and Type II, which are lined with the surfactants as discussed in the earlier section. The lung surfactants lower the surface tension of the fluid, making it possible for the gas exchange to take place in the air liquid interface. The alveolar clearance mechanism is observed in the deeper parts of the lungs, where alveolar macrophages (phagocytic cells derived from monocytes) clear the insoluble foreign particles in each alveolus.[33] The macrophages clear the deposited particle based on size (size range: 1.5–3.0 μm) either by translocating the particles for MCC towards the pharynx or by engulfing them.[34] Alveolar clearance can alter the half-life or residence time of drug which, in turn, can influence the pharmacokinetic properties and the efficacy of the inhaled particles. Size discrimination has been used as a basis for formulating inhalable drugs, which can escape the alveolar macrophages and provide a controlled drug release in the deep lung.[33] It is also important to note that the particle attachment to macrophages is size dependent while the rate of internalization is not.[35] This property of the macrophages is attributed to the ruffling of the membrane of the macrophages.

2.2.1.3 Enzymatic degradation

When designing inhalation drugs, one needs to consider the enzymatic degradation of the drugs in the lung by cytochrome P450 (CYP) family enzymes that represent Phase I metabolism. CYP enzymes are the defense mechanisms, and several isoforms – CYP1B1, CYP2B6, CYP2E1, CYP2J2, CYP3A5, and CYP1A1 (highly induced in smokers) – are commonly expressed in the lungs.[36-38] These CYPs not only degrade inhalable drugs but also are pollutants and toxic substances that are harmful to the body.[39] Several inhaled drugs such as salmeterol,[40] theophylline,[41] budesonide,[42] ciclesonide,[43] and fluticasone[44] are enzymatically degraded in the lung. In addition to the small molecule drugs, peptide/protein drugs such as insulin are highly vulnerable to peptidase and proteases present in the lung that represent the Phase II metabolism. Although the lung has low metabolic activity, compared to other organs such as the liver, enzymatic degradation significantly influences a drug's bioavailability in the lungs and hence should be carefully assessed during drug development.[45]

Treatment of local diseases:

- Direct delivery to disease site
- Rapid onset of action
- Minimum systemic side effects
- Bypasses GI track degradation and first pass metabolism in liver
- Decreased dose compared to systemic
- Enables delivery of poorly absorbed drugs

Treatment of systemic diseases:

- Non-invasive, needle free
- Fast onset of action
- Large surface area and highly permeable membrane
- Suitable for small molecules to large proteins
- Bypasses GI track degradation and first pass metabolism in liver
- Uniform and predictable absorption rate

2.2.1.4 Local vs systemic delivery

Local delivery to the lungs: Inhaled drugs can be used to treat disease that are either localized to the lung or in other parts of the body. For an ideal local effect, an inhaled drug must be absorbed in the lung, as systemic absorption might decrease the efficacy, enhance rapid elimination, and create adverse effects of the drugs. Owing to the large surface area, high epithelial permeability due to thinness of membrane, and high vascularity, systemic drug absorption becomes one of the challenges for formulations that are designed to treat local diseases such as COPD, cystic fibrosis, chronic bronchitis, asthma, etc. In the case of local treatment, the site of action in the lung will depend on the availability of the receptors for the drugs. This in turn will determine the design of the formulation for a particular disease. One of the earliest works on receptor mediated effect was reported for histamine where the drug was found to be more effective in increasing airway obstruction when deposited in the large conducting zone rather than in respiratory zone, as the receptors for the drugs are mainly in the large airway tracts.[46] Of note is the fact that it required an 11-fold higher dose of histamine to the respiratory zone to achieve the same impact as that seen for histamine deposited in the conducting zone. Similarly, the distribution of ß$_2$ adrenergic receptors and muscarinic-3 receptors (M3) in the respiratory tract influences the design of the formulation for bronchodilators. Autoradiographic visualization demonstrated that the β_2 adrenergic receptors are densely present in the epithelium of large bronchi and terminal bronchioles (Figure 2.1) while high density of M3 receptors is located in submucosal gland and airway ganglia.[47, 48] This in turn dictates that a β_2 adrenergic receptor agonist like salbutamol should target the periphery of the lungs while M3 receptor antagonists like ipratropium bromide should target the conducting airways. On the other hand, due to uniform distribution of inflammatory cells throughout the respiratory tract in case of asthma, it is suggested that the formulation should be able to evenly distribute in the respiratory tract (RT) for effective treatment.[49]

One of the diseases of the lungs which has benefited significantly from the local drug delivery is cystic fibrosis (CF). This is an autosomal recessive genetic disorder of various organs including lungs and is characterized by excessive production of mucus which blocks the RT and makes it hard to breathe. It is also characterized by exaggerated inflammatory response, progressive airway obstruction, endobronchial infection, bronchiectasis, and respiratory failure.[50] Various classes of drugs like bronchodilators, mucolytics, antibiotics, and anti-inflammatory medication are administered to manage the symptoms of CF. Antibiotics pose the biggest challenge for the formulators, as doses up to 1 g need to be delivered to the lungs to control the infection. Products like TOBI® (Tobramycin) and Cayston® (Aztreonam) delivered in nebulizers resulted in a high residual dose remaining in the nebulizer, while TOBI® in powder delivered by Podhaler™ deposited drug in the lungs much more efficiently, even if four capsules, each containing 28 mg of the drug, had to be used to deliver the same dose.[51] Pulmonary delivery of antibiotics delivers the high dose of drug directly to the microbes, which is not possible through systemic delivery without significant toxic effects.

Systemic delivery from the lungs: Small molecules (mw <1000 Da), peptides/proteins, and vaccines have been delivered by the pulmonary route for systemic delivery. Fentanyl citrate (Lazanda®) and Loxapine (Adasuve®) with MW of 336 Da and 328 Da respectively are currently approved for use in the United States. The former is pain management medication available as a metered nasal spray while the latter is for the treatment of psychiatric disorders in the form of dry powder inhaler. As with oral administration, bioavailability decreases with increasing molecular weight. Peptides/proteins with higher molecular weights have been given to patients through pulmonary route for many years. Exubera® was the first insulin inhalation product approved by the FDA for use in the United States. The DPI device used for the delivery system contained insulin and lactose, and was prepared by spray drying technology with 10–15% bioavailability. The product was a commercial failure and was withdrawn from the market, as it increased the chance of lung cancer. The second insulin product that is currently available in the market, Afrezza®, used fumaryl diketopiperazine as absorption enhancer which increased the bioavailability of insulin ($\leq$50% in first 3 h) and decreased the time to maximum plasma concentration (20–30 min).[52] Technosphere® technology was used for the design of the microspheres encapsulating insulin. This technology has the advantage of producing uniform small size particles (~2–3 µm) with good aerosolization properties and good dissolution in a neutral pH environment, with rapid absorption and deagglomeration in a basic plasma environment to immediately release insulin.[52]

There are very few studies that report the delivery of vaccines through the inhalation route, but they have shown promise. Inhalable vaccines are an attractive approach in the pharmaceutical field for two main reasons. First is the avoidance of the potential injury and disposal of needles in the developing countries. Second is the ability to avoid the cold storage chain during vaccine distribution in remote locations in the world. In a randomized clinical trial in Mexican school children, a four-fold increase in the neutralizing antibodies was observed in the aerosol treated group compared to the injection group when measles or measles-rubella vaccines were given by aerosol or injection.[53] In another study, DPI with the measles vaccine showed similar serological response as that of licensed subcutaneous measles vaccines in adult males aged 18 to 45 years.[54] Influenced by these promising studies, there are many ongoing vaccine studies on liquid as well as solid formulations for inhalation against tuberculosis,[55, 56] hepatitis B,[57] and COVID-19[58] among others.

For the systemic effect, the inhaled formulation must interact with the mucosa of tracheobronchial airways or alveolar region, which is influenced by the physicochemical properties of the drugs and determines whether the drug is absorbed or eliminated. For instance, the contact between peptide drugs and lung surfactant causes particle aggregations, which in turn compromise their dissolution and accelerate their clearance via alveolar macrophage. The contact between small molecular weight lipophilic drugs and lung surfactant improves their solubility and increases their rate and extent of absorption. Immediately below the lung surfactant layer, there is a 0.01–10 mm thick lining layer where the drug can diffuse to the epithelium, followed by interstitium, and eventually diffuse to the blood stream. The mechanisms of systemic drug absorption include passive and active transport mechanisms such as paracellular or transcellular transport pore formation, vesicular transport, and lymphatic drainage. The mechanisms of drug absorption across the epithelium are highly dependent on the physicochemical properties of drugs and the targeted site.

While hydrophobic drugs are efficiently absorbed within one to two minutes from the lung into the systemic circulation via passive diffusion, hydrophilic drugs are absorbed much slower through the tight junction. Hydrophilic and highly cationic small molecules exhibit a prolonged absorption. In contrast, the absorption of peptide drugs usually takes place either via transcytosis through caveolae or paracellularly through the tight junctions. Absorption through the tight junction is the predominant mechanism for most drugs. Consequently, the drug absorption site and mechanism should be considered when designing inhalation therapy for systemic delivery to achieve an optimum lung-tissue retention and permeability.

2.2.2 Factors Affecting Deposition

2.2.2.1 Formulation factors

Formulation design for inhalation must be done so as to achieve delivery to the intended site of action and to evade the clearance mechanisms and provide an effective therapy. The factors determining the suitability of formulations are discussed below:

2.2.2.1.1 Particle size
Particle size is one of the primary factors which determines where the particles will be deposited in the lungs after the application of the formulation. Particle size modulation can deliver the drug to the target site and evade the clearance mechanisms. The particle

size also determines the mechanism of deposition i.e., diffusion, sedimentation, impaction, and interception.[34, 45] Small particles with size < 0.5 mm are deposited in the alveoli by diffusion mechanism owing to their Brownian motion. But exhalation is the one major issue with these small particle sizes.[45, 59] With the particles of 1–5 μm in diameter, sedimentation is the primary mechanism of deposition especially in the bronchioles and alveoli. The rate of sedimentation is dependent on the gravitational forces, particle velocity, aerodynamic size, breathing pattern, etc. In addition, hygroscopic particles take up moisture in the airway and get deposited.

When the particle size is greater than 5 μM, they are usually deposited on the bronchial regions due to impaction, which is dependent on the mass and diameter of the particles and accounts for most of the particle deposition by mass. It is also the most common method of deposition for DPI and MDI at the bifurcation of bronchi. Yet, another method of deposition of particles is interception, where particle edge touches the airway wall surface, but the bulk of the particles does not deviate from air streamlines.[60] This mechanism associated with fibrous particles which have smaller aerodynamic diameter relative to their size.

2.2.2.1.2 Particle shape and orientation

Cellular uptake of particles by macrophages greatly depends on their shape and orientation. The rate of phagocytosis is much faster when macrophages are attached to the major axis of the elliptical disks while attachment on the minor axis or the flat surface significantly decreases the rate of phagocytosis. The local contact of particles is important as the shape of the contact position determined the actin structure complexity required to initiate phagocytosis and move the membrane over the particles.[61] So, macrophages uptake is more prominent for rectangular disks and ellipsoids than for spherical particles. This was also observed in another study where the spherical particles and worm-like particles of similar diameter were prepared, but the phagocytosis of the former was significantly higher than the latter. The worm-like particles were engulfed only when macrophages attached to the major axis of particles and not on the particle length.[62] Not only the macrophage uptake but also the deposition pattern changes with change in the shape of the particles. In a recent study, it was observed that elongated crystalline particles of Rifapentine avoided close packing and thus reduced cohesive Van der Waals forces and thereby penetrated deep into the lungs. The morphology prevented agglomeration, reduced deposition in the throat and residual content in capsules, and increased stability when compared to the amorphous particles of the same drug with dimpled spherical morphology.[63]

2.2.2.1.3 Electrostatic effect

Although the effect of the electrostatic nature of the particles on the deposition is not as well studied as other factors, it has proved to be significant in increasing the deposition of the particles in the lungs. Readers are directed to the review by Karner et al. for a more comprehensive understanding of electrostatic charge and its history in inhalation science.[64] Electrostatic effect can result in either repulsion (de-aggregate) or attraction between particles (re-aggregate) and the airway surfaces. Even though the airway surface is neutral, charge of the opposite polarity may be induced during the movement of charged particles in the small airways.[65] In addition, the attraction of charged particles to neutral surfaces is of significance in deeper regions of the lungs.[66] As reported in a recent study, the electrostatic charge increased the deposition fraction of small particles (0.1 µm) around the mouth and throat region while the increased flow rate had a relatively lesser impact on the charged particles, which were <2.5 µm compared to the larger particles. They also observed the increased deposition of sub-micron particles in the lungs suggesting electrostatic charge manipulation could increase the drug deposition in the conducting airways.[67] The electrostatic forces have stronger impact on low mass particles due to a high force-to-mass ratio.[66] It was also shown that controlling the amount of charge can cause deposition in predefined regions in the lungs. This could be achieved by combining the amount of charge with the pulsed volume in the inhaled airflow and a respiratory pause to increase the deposition.[68] To study the impact of the charge and the mass/size of the particles, the next generation impactors (NGI) are modified such that every stage is connected to an electrometer to measure the charge distribution. These types of impactors are referred to as electrical Next Generation Impactors (eNGI). For the commercial DPI products that only contain the drug, eNGI was able to characterize the particles based on electrostatics and size.[69]

2.2.2.1.4 Particle modifications

Stealth properties of particles extend the drug's half-life, prevent biofouling, and avoid immune recognition. Mucoadhesive polysaccharide hyaluronic acid is native to lungs and suppresses macrophage phagocytosis and prolongs the effect of drugs in the lungs. Similarly, dipalmitoylphosphatidyl choline (DPPC), polyethylene glycol (PEG) coating is shown to be effective in preventing macrophage uptake and biofouling leading to increased half-life of drugs in the lungs. These approaches have been used to deliver non-conventional proteins like insulin and peroxidase into the lungs. The most common physical modification for the DPI particles is to lower the density and increase the particle size to obtain large porous particles which tend to have less agglomeration compared to small non-porous particles. These particles escape the phagocytic clearance due to their size and release drug for a longer period to obtain sustained release behavior. The particles with densities <0.4 g/cm^3 and diameter >5 µm penetrated deep and escaped the clearance mechanism long enough to release the drug. Insulin in large porous form increased the systemic insulin level and controlled the glucose level for 96 h, while small-form insulin delivered through non-porous particles was able to control glucose levels for just 4 h. The increased bioavailability was also observed with 20 µm particles of testosterone and the formulations for both the molecules used 50:50 PLGA as the polymeric carrier.[70] The other common method of modifying the surface properties of the inhalable particles is to coat the particles with lubricant additives like magnesium stearate (Mgst) or glycerol monostearate (GMS).[71] The amount of Mgst needed for each DPI formulation will vary, but the optimized formulation is substantially improved in powder aerosolization efficiency.[72] Similar surface modifications have also been performed with different polymeric molecules like hydroxypropylmethylcellulose phthalate, colloidal silica, which led to changes in the hydrobhobic properties of the drug molecules and increased dispersibility thus leading to efficient inhalation.[73, 74] Looking at the chemical modification of the particles for the inhalation, the most common approach is thiolation. Thiol group in the particles behaves like mucolytics and decreases the viscosity of the bronchial secretions by disrupting disulfide bonds in the proteins. Several thiol-based drugs – N-acetyl L-cysteine (NAC), S-carboxymethyl-L-cysteine [3-(S-carboxymethylthio) alanine] (S-CMC), and N-(carboxymethylthioacetyl)-homocysteine thiolactone (erdosteine) – are common compounds for inhalation studies. Thiolated derivative of glycol chitosan was reported to have a two-fold increase in mucoadhesion and significantly increased pharmacological availability compared to unmodified glycol chitosan.[75]

2.2.2.2 Physiological factors

2.2.2.2.1 Airflow rates and volume

The deposition of particles across different generations of the lungs is dependent on the breathing flow rate. To understand the impact of the flow rate, Islam et al. did a 3D Computational Fluid Dynamics (CFD) study of an anatomically realistic 17-generation bronchial tree model and the impact of three different breathing rates (15, 30, and 60 L/min) on 1 µm, 5 µm, and 10 µm particle deposition.[76] They showed that 10 µm particles get deposited deeper with slow breathing rates in both the right and left lungs with higher deposition in the carinal region. 5 µm particles on the other hand, can penetrate deeper but not as much as 1 µm particles irrespective of flow rate. **Figure 2.2** shows the numerical model of deposition pattern of 5 µm particles at three different flow rates. The smaller particles have low inertia, and these particles can easily follow the air streamline irrespective of the obstacles on the way. Rate of airflow has significant impact on the deposition of larger particles but not on the deposition of small particles. This was also the conclusion drawn by another study where the deposition fraction of 2.5 and 5 µm particles increased with the increase in flow rate, while that of 0.1, 0.5, and 1µm particles remained similar at the given flowrate.[67] Similarly, higher inspiratory flow rates (60–90 L/min) deposited > 40% of albuterol through MDI. But the deposition was more significantly influenced by the coordination of actuation with inspiration rather than flow rate or the duration of inspiration.[77] Also, an increase in the inhalation volume results in increased penetration into the peripheral bronchial tree, and increasing the breath hold period increases the deposition due to gravity.[78, 79]

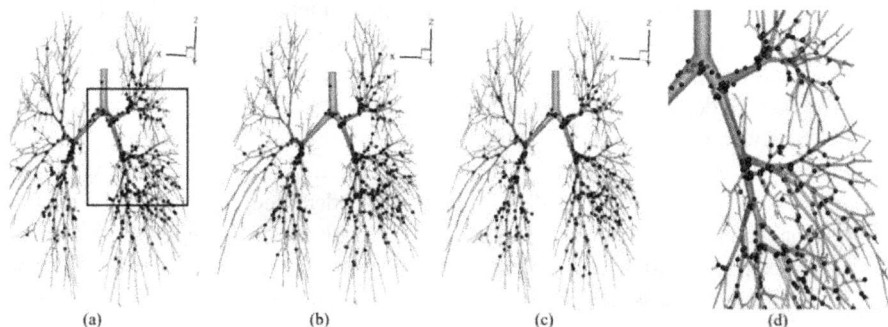

FIGURE 2.2 Numerical model of deposition pattern. Respiratory deposition patterns in up to 17th generation asymmetric pulmonary airways of 5-µm particles: (a) 15 lpm flow rate, (b) 30 lpm flow rate, (c) 60 lpm flow rate, and (d) the enlarged portion of Figure 8a. *Journal of Aerosol Science, 108, pp. 29–43.*

2.2.2.2.2 Airway geometry

One of the biological factors affecting the deposition of the particles in the RT is the geometry of the airway. The bifurcations, sharp bends, and decrease in the airway radius have significant impact on the deposition of the particles.[80] As the geometry of the airway varies between the individuals, it must be taken into consideration while designing the formulation for inhalation. Different simulated models of the airway geometry and the transport of particles have been utilized to better understand the mechanism, but until now there hasn't been a model which is universally acceptable.[81, 82]

2.2.2.2.3 Airway humidity and temperature

RT is highly humid with relative humidity of about 99.5%. The deposition of particles is dependent on the nature of particles. The moisture gets adsorbed onto the particles to increase the particle size, thereby leading to the deposition of particles. Low temperature and humidity are ideal for the delivery of very hygroscopic particles. The change in the size of the particles is the function of initial size of the particles. An earlier study[83] indicated that the smaller particles (<1 μm) have higher fold increase (five-fold) compared to slightly bigger (>2 μm) particles which have smaller fold increase (two- to three-fold) in diameter. Other studies estimated that the deposition of the hygroscopic aerosol particles of size 0.7–10 μm increases two-fold.[84, 85] Shedding further light into the matter was a study that showed no difference in deposition pattern of 0.1 μm (<0.2 μm) hygroscopic NaCl particles when compared with the non-hygroscopic particles; however, the total deposition was found to increase for the particles larger than 0.2 μm.[86] The increase in size of the finer particles was not sufficient to change the mechanism of deposition, while the larger particles change the mechanism of deposition from sedimentation to impaction with further increase in size. More recent studies by Xi et al. explored the impact of different thermo-humidity conditions on particle deposition. The conditions were cold-dry, cool-mild, warm-humid, and hot-humid, where a five- to eight-fold higher deposition was observed in warm and hot saturated conditions.[87] Similarly, Chang et al. reported that the cold-dry condition has the potential to increase the size forty-fold for a particle size of 0.2 μM. Though many modeling studies use a constant temperature of 37°C and 99.5% RH,[88, 89] this is typically not the case in RT. The temperature and RH of the upper RT depend on the inhaled air, and as such using constant temperature and %RH may not be ideal for predictions using. So, the better model should replicate the small variations in temperature, RH, and mass transfer during pulmonary delivery as their factors significantly impact the deposition of hygroscopic aerosols.[90]

In one study, micronized Salbutamol sulphate with lactose as carrier showed that the fine particle dose (FPD) and the fine particle fraction (FPF) increased with storage until 60% relative humidity (RH), after which it declined, as increasing moisture allowed for increased electron mobility (decreased tribo-electrification). To understand the impact of RH together with the electrostatic charge it is imperative that the whole picture of charge-to-mass ratio is understood and not one factor alone. The charge-to-mass ratio decreased with increasing storage humidity, and FPF increased due to reduction in charge-induced particle interaction. The decrease in aerosol charge was 25% while RH changed from 0 to 60%, and the decrease was 67% when RH was between 60 and 85% due to relative increase in moisture sorption by lactose and salbutamol sulphate at higher RH. The decrease in FPF (also efficacy) above 60% RH is likely due to increased capillary forces and adhesion to the carrier particles.[91]

2.3 IN VITRO PERFORMANCE TESTING FOR DPI PRODUCTS

2.3.1 Cascade Impactors

Cascade impactors (CI) are the devices used to determine the particle size ranges when they move through a mesh with decreasing pore size with the application of pressure. They are intended to simulate the path the inhaled formulation takes when actuated for lung delivery. These impactors are multi-stage and measure the aerosol aerodynamic particle size distribution based on inertial size fractionation and enable the quantitation of drugs at each stage using various analytical techniques. Different types of CIs are available and are used during formulation development from the bench-scale to commercial production.

2.3.2 Single-Stage Impactors

These are the most basic forms of the impactors where one or more nozzles of known diameter with an opening for the particles to impact a flat surface that may or may not be horizontal. Incoming particles are size classified based on their differing inertia, which reflects the resistance to a change in the direction of the flow. The laminar flow streamlines diverge on approach to the collection surface. Particles with greater inertia will tend to cross these streamlines more readily to impact the substrate, whereas finer particles with less inertia follow the streamlines and remain airborne as they pass the obstruction.

2.3.3 Multi-Stage Impactors

CIs are constructed by coupling several stages (≥ 7) together with progressively finer and reduced number of jets such that particle velocity and hence inertia is progressively increased (Figure 2.3). The scientific principles guide the aerodynamics of the CIs, which provide a consistent particle size fractionation behavior over the range of flow supported by the device. In this way, the device fractionates the incoming aerosol into particles covering discrete and well-defined size ranges. Andersen cascade impactor (ACI) is still the most widely used impactor for inhaler aerosol testing. However, the Next Generation Impactor (NGI) is becoming widely used as familiarity with its capabilities grows. NGI has been designed to meet the specific need of pharmaceutical inhalation product testing. Both CIs can operate in the flow rate range suitable for pMDI and DPI testing (30–100 L/min), but the ACI requires the removal of the lowermost stages (6 and/or 7) and insertion of new stages at the upper end (1 and 2) for use at flow rates of 60 and 100 L/min. On the other hand, the NGI can operate over the entire range with excellent size resolution. It can even be used without its pre-separator and with a back-up filter substituted

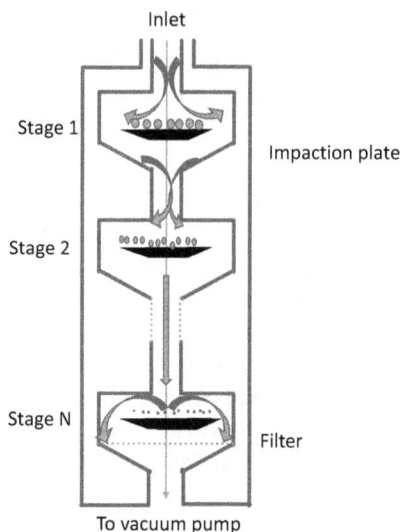

FIGURE 2.3   Schematics of multi-cascade impactors. The schematics show different layers of the multi-cascade impactors with filter for the final connection.

for the multi orifice collector for right-angle bend that represents a crude simulation of the human oropharynx. A pre-separator is usually inserted between the induction port and entry point to the CI for preventing entry of very coarse particulates, such as carrier particles from certain DPIs into the CI. NGI spans a cut size (D_{50}) range from 0.54 μm to 11.7 μm aerodynamic diameter at 30 L/min and 0.24 μm to 6.12 μm at 100 L/min. In an aerodynamic assessment study between three different marketed pMDI formulations and three different impactors, NGI and ACI analyzed particles uniformly for mass median aerodynamic diameter (MMAD), geometric standard deviation (GSD), and fine particles fraction of < 4.7 μm. Any slight variation was attributed to particle bounce, incomplete evaporation of volatile constituents, and the presence of surfactant particles.[92] The NGI has several features to enhance its utility for inhaler testing. One such feature is that particles are deposited on collection cups that are held in a tray. This tray is removed from the impactor as a single unit, facilitating quick sample turnaround times if multiple trays are used. For accomplishing drug recovery, the user can add up to approximately 40 ml of an appropriate solvent directly to the cups. Another unique feature is a micro-orifice collector (MOC) that captures microscopic particles normally collected on the final filter in other impactors.[92] The particles caught in the MOC cup can be analyzed in the same manner as the particles collected in the other cups at different impactor stages.

The fate of the drug post-deposition in RT is still not a well understood area for scientists. In this regard, in a recent study we utilized the NGI to understand the internalization of deposited particles by the Air-liquid-interface (ALI) monolayer of Calu-3 cells by modifying the collection cups to hold the transwell membranes with the cellular monolayer. Calu-3 cells inserted at different stages showed different rate of permeation indicting that the mechanistic, aerodynamic, and biophysical properties of the inhaled therapeutics determine the internalization process.[23] Figure 2.4a

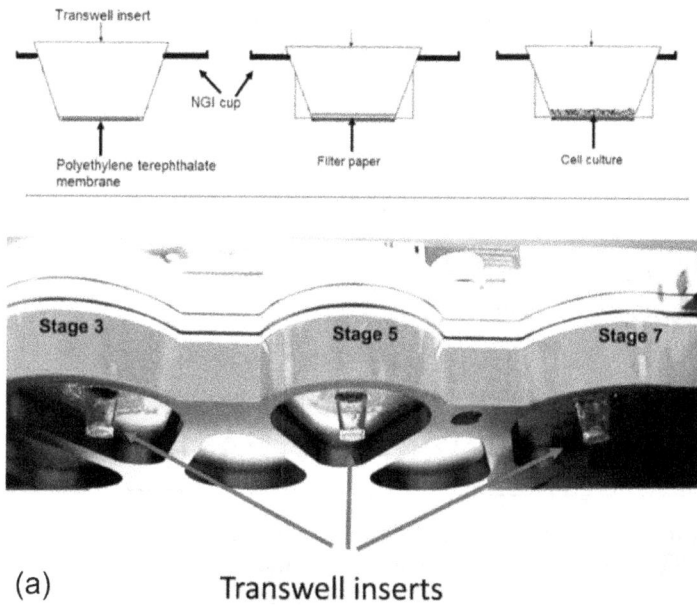

(a)   Transwell inserts

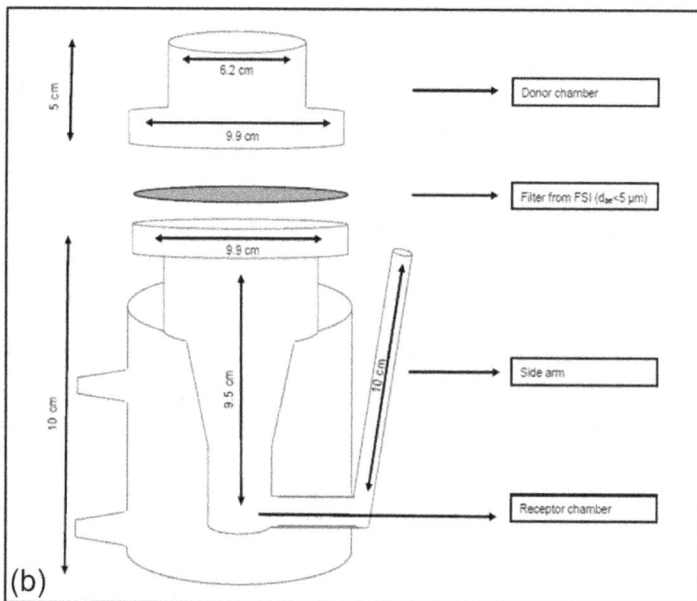

(b)

FIGURE 2.4 In vitro evaluation methods of dry powder inhalation products. a) Diagram of the NGI collection cups with Transwell membrane under the stage. Particles were aerosolized onto inserts using Flovent HFA and impinged for 30 s at 30 L/min. Upper panel: schematic diagram showing modified cups containing Transwell insert only (left), Transwell insert with filter paper (middle), and Transwell insert with cell monolayer (middle). Lower panel: NGI with modified cups containing Transwell inserts at stage 3, 5, and 7. b) Design of RespiCell® (EU registration No. 006649570-0001).

shows the NGI collection cups with transwell membrane fitted under the stage. Similarly, eNGI is the modified form of the instrument designed to measure the electrostatic charge in addition to the PSD measurement where NGI impaction cups are insulated and connected to the electrometer.[93, 94] Due to the complex interaction between the inhalation formulation and the devices used for the delivery, the aerosolized particles may be charged both negatively and positively; bp-NGI (bipolar-NGI) is incorporated with two electrostatic precipitators for collecting charged aerosols from stage 2 to stage 7.[94] The user-friendly, modifiable features and the aerodynamic design principles together make the NGI well suited to the needs of the inhaler testing community.

2.4 DRUG RELEASE

For a drug to be locally available it first needs to be released from its carrier formulation. For most of the coated/matrix formulations, the drug release primarily involves drug diffusion through the formulation into the fluid on the surface of the lungs. There could be different mechanisms depending upon the type of carrier involved in the delivery.[95] For drug delivery systems involving polymeric carriers, multiple different mechanisms may be operational depending upon the characteristics of the polymers. The drug might be released by diffusion through the polymeric matrix or the pores or by surface or bulk erosion of the carriers.[96, 97] Ideally the drug release from the formulation should neither be very fast or very slow. The "burst release" is usually due to high surface area-to-volume ratio of the polymeric formulation. On the other hand, the slow release of drug might increase the time required to exert the physiological effect of the drug. The common approaches to reduce the burst release are either to form a complex with the drug before incorporating into the formulation or to use lipid excipients to control the release from the formulation. In either case, overall drug loading in the formulation could also be improved.[98] The other types of formulation like the micelles or dendrimers utilize diffusion mechanisms, and the rate of release depends on the partition coefficient of the drug, the stability of the micelles or dendrimers, the rate of polymer degradation or stability of the formulation.[95, 99] Similarly, liposomes and solid lipid nanoparticles (SLN) utilize drug diffusion through the lipid bilayers or lipid matrix for the drug release, which in turn depends upon the lipid composition, the glass transition temperature of the phospholipids and the type of liposome used.[95] The fluidity of the membrane defines the drug release, as rigidity of phospholipids or cholesterol tends to decrease liposome membrane fluidity and thus decreases drug release.[100] The application of stimuli responsive systems for pulmonary drug delivery is limited except for temperature sensitive release. Thermo-sensitive and magnetic-sensitive delivery was obtained through superparamagnetic iron oxide nanoparticles (SPIONs) for targeted drug delivery.[101] Thermo-sensitive lipid system based on glyceryl behenate allowed slow drug release at body temperature, but fast release was observed at hyper-thermic temperatures.[102]

2.5 IN VITRO DISSOLUTION

Dissolution is the rate of mass transfer from a solid surface to the dissolution medium or solvent under defined conditions of the liquid or solid interface, temperature, and solvent composition. This kinetic parameter describes the solid erosion of the formulation either into ions, atoms, or molecules and its admixture with the dissolution medium. This testing reflects the drug release behavior of pharmaceutical dosage form and is used as a quality control test to differentiate between formulation batches and to estimate the dissolution behavior of the formulation in vivo. Though dissolution is critical for reflecting the in vivo efficacy of the formulation and facilitating the comparison between the inhalable formulations, there is no consensus on standard dissolution methods.[103] So, this quality attribute and its impact on the in vivo drug release and availability needs to be characterized, understood, and controlled during the early stages of the development process. There are different variations of the dissolution methods which can be utilized to distinguish the therapeutically relevant differences in the dissolution rate amongst the batches or the drug substances.

Several USP general chapters (711, 724, 1088, and 1092) discuss the dissolution tests to successfully estimate in vitro dissolution behaviors of solid or semi-solid dosage forms but not for the formulations designed for inhalation. The lack of dissolution testing guidelines for inhalation is not due to lack of research in this area. Developing a standardized method applicable to the lung is not an easy task, as the lung has several unique features which are difficult to replicate in vitro, such as the extremely small amount of aqueous fluid and the presence of endogenous lung surfactants. The Inhalation Ad Hoc advisory panel concluded that based on available information and data, the performance test for inhalation dosage form should only include 1) uniformity of dose and 2) aerodynamic particle size distribution, and does mention the need for dissolution tests.[104] The different types of dissolution tests employed for inhaled products in the literature are described below.

2.5.1 Traditional Dissolution Studies

Only a fraction of the active pharmaceutical ingredient (API) emitted from standard delivery devices is usually delivered to the target site of the deep lung, since most inhaler products are a mixture of fine API particles and coarse carrier particles or propellants. Thus, an ideal dissolution test procedure for inhalation formulations would involve particle classification followed by an evaluation of the dissolution behavior for the classified drug particles that may deposit at various sites in the respiratory tract. Additionally, a stagnant dissolution system would be required to estimate lung dissolution as the volume of lung fluid is approximately 10–20 ml/100 m^2.[105] Experimental difficulties exist in dose collection due to very fine powder being deposited and their electrostatic characteristics.[104] This has led to the use of traditional dissolution methods that have been developed for oral products to also be used for inhaled products.[106-108] Most dissolution procedures on powders have been performed in the absence of aerodynamic classification. Formulations have been directly dispersed into an apparatus II or modified basket dissolution testers to prevent drug particles from escaping directly into the dissolution medium. Huang et al. prepared itraconazole (ITZ) and mannose (MAN) DPI formulations and tested their dissolution in sink conditions using a USP 2 apparatus. The samples fractioned (~15 mg per vessel) at the NGI S3 plate were carefully transferred to 900 ml hydrochloric acid (pH 1.2) with 0.3% SDS at 37°C. The apparatus was operated at paddle speed of 100 rpm and the samples were withdrawn at different time points for HPLC analysis. For comparison, formulation dissolution was also done in non-sink conditions (300 ml), which simulated lung fluid (SLF). The dissolution of all samples reached a plateau after 360 min for all formulations. Notably, both the dissolution methods were able to differentiate the dissolution profile of formulations based on their wettability.[109]

These methods of dissolution using commercially available apparatus have the disadvantages of particles sticking to vessel wall/paddle/bucket during tests, inadvertent sampling of floating powder, and well-stirred environment. To overcome some of the shortfalls of testing using commercial apparatus, several diffusion-controlled cell systems, such as a custom-built diffusion cell, a twin-stage impinger (TSI)[110] and a dissolution cell[111] have been investigated. However, no single in vitro test system is the ideal choice for performing dissolution measurements for formulations designed to be inhaled. Some promising approaches are described below.

2.5.2 Flow-Through Cell

Several attempts to adapt a USP flow-through cell system (Apparatus 4) for evaluating in vitro dissolution behaviors of aerosol products have been made, since the flow-through apparatus offers specific sample cells associated with a filter system that may hold powder and granular dosage forms inside the cell.[112, 113] In the system, dissolution media is supplied by pump force, and dissolution profiles of a loaded drug inside the cell can be estimated from the amount of drug released from the flow-through cell. The flow-through cell system could possibly differentiate variables in dissolution patterns of several inhalation formulations.[114] However, there still remains issues with dose collection onto the flow-through cell and the hydrodynamic condition of the system in mimicking the dissolution behavior of delivered drug particles to the target lung site[115] In particular, the powder presentation inside the cell undoubtedly greatly influences the overall release/dissolution pattern, as the surface area and the wettability of the powder bed varies according to the loading method. To better utilize the system for the inhalation formulation, aerosol particles from DPI and pMDI devices were collected through aerodynamic classification using the Anderson Cascade Impactor onto a glass filter which was then placed inside the modified flow-through cell and subjected to dissolution testing.[115] The system consists of a reservoir and a HPLC pump for supplying a dissolution media and a flow-through cell. The impacts of dissolution media, flow rate, and surfactant on the dissolution of corticosteroids, budesonide, and fluticasone propionate among others were evaluated using this modified device. The data indicated that this method had a discriminatory capability. Moreover, the procedure employed a relatively lower flow rate (0.7 ml/min) than that commonly used in the USP apparatus (4–16 ml/min), which could potentially create more stagnant conditions for dissolution.

2.5.3 Membrane-Based Cell Systems

The concept of using a membrane holder to assess the dissolution profiles of aerodynami-cally separated drug particles is relatively recent.[116] This apparatus was designed to be easily incorporated into commercially available dissolution testers, where the membrane holder acts like a sinker device with a diffusion layer at its surface to enable dissolution testing. In these studies, dose collection was achieved after aerodynamic size-fraction-ation directly on to a polycarbonate membrane collection cup at each stage of the NGI. Following aerodynamic separation, the classified drug particles on their respective mem-branes were sandwiched underneath another identical membrane (presoaked with dis-solution medium). The drug, now contained within two membranes, is clamped into the holder and then placed into a dissolution vessel. The dissolution profiles were successively estimated by the amount of drug released from the membrane holder. It was found that there was a significant difference between the bulk formulation and an aerodynamically classified formulation in the dissolution profile.[116] However, in this dissolution setup, a modification of NGI was required to collect dispersed particles on the membrane, and the entire classified dose collected on the membrane cannot be used for dissolution testing due to a substantial limitation imparted by the prototype frame holder size. Subsequently, a modified membrane holder has been introduced by Son et al.[117] It was explicitly designed to be incorporated into the NGI for better dose collection performance than a previously reported prototype membrane holder. Two main components of the dissolution setup include USP dissolution apparatus 2 and a newly designed membrane holder. The mem-brane holder assembly consists of an NGI dissolution cup (a) which contains a removable impaction inset, (b) a securing ring, and (c) two sealing 0-rings, and a polycarbonate (PC) membrane to function as a highly porous diffusional powder retaining layer.

Dissolution depends on the diffusion-controlled drug release from the membrane holder. During the dissolution process, the drug disperses within the membrane holder as dissolution media migrates through the pores on the membrane surface. The dissolved drug is then released out to the bulk media by diffusion.[116] The membrane holder may impart optimally stagnant conditions for test compounds to be appropriate for compar-ing dissolution behaviors of formulations intended for lung administration. This mem-brane holder was designed to have a very thin liquid layer between the membrane, and the liquid layer was maintained to dissolve drug particles by continuous exchange of dissolution media through the pores by agitation. In other words, a dynamic equilibrium is rapidly established for solute exchange following the commencement of a given disso-lution test with the membrane holder. The dissolution profiles obtained in this study were shown to differ substantially between those from drugs having dissimilar hydrophobicity as well as the aerosols having different aerodynamic particle size distributions (APSD). Notably, this method can be used to examine the dissolution behaviors of inhalation dos-age forms with similar particle distribution by selecting drug particles accumulated in same collection plate. It would be anticipated that the dissolution of particles having a similar size distribution would provide more inter-formulation discrimination. However, a milestone study by Daley Yates at el. revealed that similar APSD does not always warrant bioequivalence.[118] They compared the in vitro and in vivo performance for two commercial DPIs (reservoir powder inhalation device (RPID) and the Diskus® multiple dose inhaler-delivering a combination of salmeterol 50 µg plus fluticasone propionate

(FP) 250 µg (SFC 50/250) to investigate assumptions of bioequivalence. They found that although the in vitro particle size distribution data were non-significant for both the products, they were not equivalent in terms of PK systemic exposure.

Later, a new approach has applied to the in vitro dissolution method, known as DissolvIt®, that simulates the dissolution and absorption of drugs from inhaled dry powders (Figure 2.4b). Dissolution in RespiCell occurs under air-liquid dissolution conditions with a limited volume of medium. The apparatus has two chambers: a customizable vertical diffusion cell able to accommodate a diffusive membrane, i.e., glass fiber filter, and an acceptor chamber which is filled with 170 ml of dissolution medium under constant stirring with a magnetic bead. The diffusion area between the two chambers is approximately 30.2 cm^2. In the initial study, RespiCell was able to differentiate in tobramycin release profiles induced by modifying the composition of the formulation by adding magnesium stearate and blending.[119] Further, generic products of Spiriva (Tiotropium bromide) as a water-soluble drug and Onbrez Breezhaler (Indacaterol maleate) were prepared with different parameters of the high shear mixing and evaluated with RespiCell. In the case of Spiriva, despite a similar APSD profile, only one generic formulation was found to have a significantly different dissolution profile. On the other hand, generic formulation of Onbrez Breezhaler, although with significant APSD, showed a similar dissolution profile.

Recently, an in vitro dissolution test method, DissolvIt®, was developed for inhaled particles, which simulates the physiological conditions in the lung and mimics the in vivo PK data. It is based on the air-blood barrier model, equipped with a precision-controlled pump for the blood simulant, and an inverted microscope with a high-resolution camera and a fraction collector. Particles are deposited on an exposure cover slip which encounters the mucus simulant applied to the underside of a hydrophilic polycarbonate membrane. The blood simulant is pumped above the polycarbonate membrane. The particle dissolution can be studied both from the "luminal" side through optical microscopy and from the "vascular" side by chemical analysis.[120] The DissolvIt® system was successfully used to evaluate dissolution of Budesonide and fluticasone propionate powders after aerosolized with Preciselnhale® aerosol generator. The collected particles on cover slips simulated mucus, and solute from the dissolving particles diffused through the barrier and was absorbed into the perfusate. This method simulates dissolution and absorption of drugs in the lung and also permits mimicing the pharmacokinetic data.

2.6 ASSESSMENT OF ABSORPTION AND DEPOSITION OF FORMULATION FOR INHALATION

Post dissolution, the rate and extent of drug absorption determines bioavailability. The respiratory epithelium is the principal barrier for the absorption of the molecules. The molecules can permeate through the epithelial cells in the lungs by one or more of the transport mechanisms: passive paracellular, transcellular, carrier-mediated, vesicular, or efflux transport. In the paracellular route, small hydrophilic compounds diffuse through the tight junction between the cells, through the intercellular pores according to their concentration gradient. The selectivity of the intercellular tight junction is controlled by many different proteins which could be actin-binding, cytoplasmic, or transmembrane adhesive function. Amongst those proteins, the claudin, family of transmembrane proteins, confers the barrier properties and selectivity for transport.[121] The transcellular route, on the other hand, supports partition of lipophilic compounds into the plasma membrane in unionized form through concentration dependent passive diffusion. The rate of drug transport is dependent on the concentration gradient, charge, size, and lipophilicity of the compound.[122] The limitation presented by the hydrophobic lipid bilayer can be overcome by utilizing the drug transporters present on the epithelial cell membranes. There are membrane transporters which impact the bioavailability of the drugs deposited in RT and are basically in divided in two classes, namely ATP-binding cassette (ABC) superfamily and solute linked carrier (SLC) superfamily.[123, 124] The active transporters facilitate the transfer of solutes against the concentration gradient using energy. However, a few transporters that facilitate diffusion do not utilize any energy like the transporters for amino acids, glucose (glucopyranose transporter), oxygen (myoglobin)[125] and carbon dioxide. The primary active transporters utilize energy from Adenosine Triphosphate (ATP) to drive the transport, like in the case of sodium-potassium (Na^+-K^+) channels, Ca^{2+} ion efflux in cardiac muscles, etc. But the secondary active transport utilizes the electrochemical gradient (membrane potential) established by the primary active transporter to drive the transport. For example, when Na^+-K^+ pump increases the concentration of Na^+ in the extracellular space, the concentration gradient is established which drives the movement of $Na+$ into the cell, and that drive is utilized by the glucose molecule to move into the cells using sodium glucose-linked transporter (SGLT).[126] The ABC superfamily of membrane transporters include P-glycoprotein (P-gp), multidrug resistance-associated proteins (MRP), and breast cancer resistant protein (BCRP) which are known to play significant roles in developing chemoresistance. P-gp is one of the important membrane transporters that decreases the concentration of its substrates intracellularly by eliminating them to the extracellular regions.[127] The last method of permeation includes the vesicle-mediated endocytosis, common in type I alveolar epithelial cells, where the membrane curves to entrap specific molecule, and the vesicles thus formed move across the cytoplasm and merge with the basolateral membrane to release the cargo.[128] The methods of permeation are captured in Figure 2.5.

The introduction of the Biopharmaceutics Classification System (BCS) into the FDA's regulatory guideline brought the in vitro cell culture models to the mainstream. This guidance helped to predict the intestinal absorption of test molecules from their solubility data and the apparent permeability coefficients obtained from the in vitro cell monolayer model.[129] The in vitro methods have the advantages of simplicity, robustness, better experimental and data acquisition control, and a reduction in operational costs and animal sacrifice. It is challenging to develop a model which can be universally validated and standardized, but attempts have been made for few decades to model the airway-to-blood barrier (ABB) with lung epithelial cell cultures. Although reproducibility and ease of use might vary between these primary and continuous culture models from lung epithelial cell monolayers, they enable the determination of transepithelial

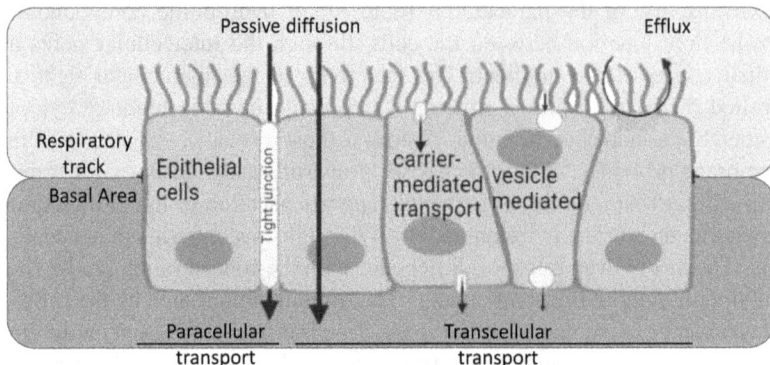

FIGURE 2.5 Schematics of mechanism of absorption. The schematics show different pathways of drug absorption through the epithelial monolayer.

transport kinetics of test molecules, possibly for the purpose of predicting in vivo lung absorption. Despite the popularity of these reconstructed single-cell barriers to represent complex lung tissue kinetics of absorption and disposition, their relevance is still open for debate.

The rate-limiting step for drug delivery for inhalation is the transportation of the API across the lung epithelium. The air-to-blood barrier (ABB) is constructed in the Transwell or Snapwell system with a monolayer of lung epithelial cells.[130, 131] The rate of drug transport across the lung cell monolayers is represented by the apparent permeation flux (J_a) or the apparent permeability coefficient (P_a). These parameters do not represent the extent of transport. The formulation with higher J_a or P_a values is deemed suitable for systemic delivery, while longer lung retention/residence time favors local delivery. Animal and human lung epithelial are utilized for the in vitro lung barrier models.[2, 131] The variety of human lung epithelial cells can either be differentiated based on their culture (immortalized or primary), origin (cancerous or non-cancerous), and lung region (trachea, bronchi, or alveoli). In vitro ALI culture systems of three dimensional (3D) human lung cell barriers like MucilAir,[132] SmallAir-29[133] EpiAirway[134] and EpiAlveolar[135] are of increasing interest in inhalation research. Figure 2.6a represents the schematic for the generation of ALI for various studies. The study of aerosol drug deposition into the in vitro lung cell monolayer, stem cell-derived lung epithelial cells, and "lung-on-a-chip" model technology is emerging.[136]

2.6.1 Calu-3 Cell Monolayer Model

Calu-3 cells are one of the most widely used cells to generate the in vitro lung cell barrier model to assess drug transport. These cells were grown to the confluent monolayers over one to three weeks in Transwell or Snapwell systems. Calu-3 cells were fed with the basolateral media, and the mucosa was left without the apical media to mimic the lung epithelia when compared to the conventional liquid submerged culture. The ALI cultured Calu-3 cells resulted in lower transepithelial electrical resistance (TEER) due

A)

B)

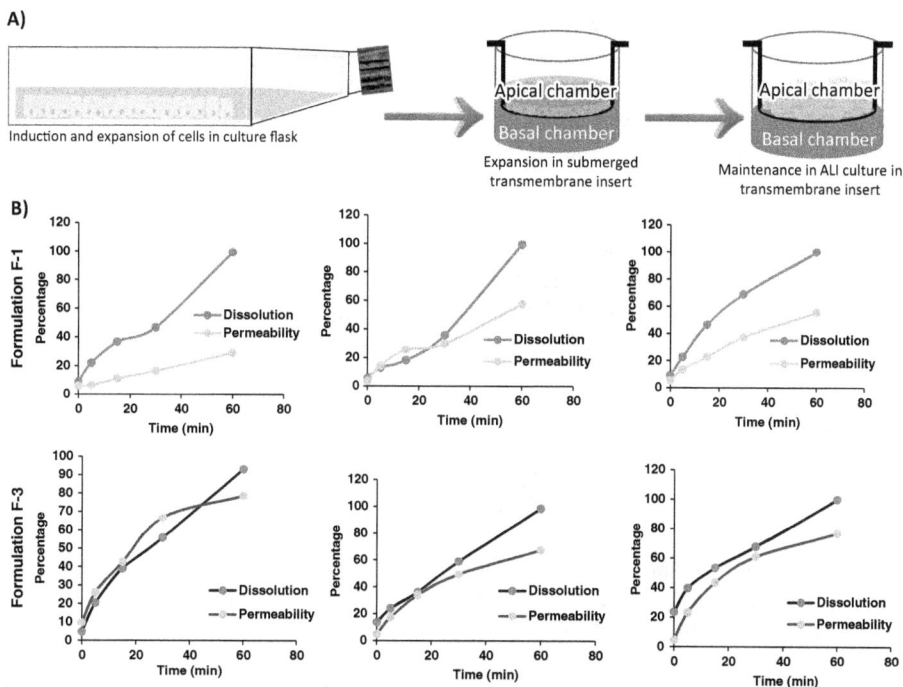

FIGURE 2.6 a) Schematics for the generation of air liquid interface (ALI). The ALI generation begins with expansion of the cells in culture flask followed by the growth of the cultured cells in liquid-liquid interface for a few days. The cells are then allowed to grow in ALI culture to form the mature monolayer for the respiratory studies. b) Correlation between percentage of drug dissolved and permeated through Calu-3 cell monolayer at different stages of NGI. Dissolution and permeation profiles for formulation F-1 and F-3.

to restricted barriers, but correlations between their outcome measures (J_a or P_a) and the rate parameters of in vivo lung absorption was strong and would enable prediction of the in vivo lung absorption rate for a drug entity. Reported tight junction properties greatly vary in the literature, ranging from 200 to 1200 $\Omega \cdot cm^2$ of TEER, mainly depending upon the growth duration.[137–140] Even so, within each cell monolayer, the P_a values were in line with Fick's law of diffusion, where the rate of diffusive absorption is inversely related to the size of the drug/molecule. Hence, ensuring consistent and sufficiently restricted barrier properties across Calu-3 cell monolayers of use is indispensable to obtain comparable J_a or P_a values. In fact, when the cell monolayers were formed with ≥800 $\Omega \cdot cm^2$ of TEER, the diffusive P_a values for hydrophilic drug moieties correlated well with molecular weights across the literature. Hence, there is a need to establish standards that consistently provide the restricted Calu-3 cell monolayers of desired TEER values for the studies. In addition, one also needs to consider that Calu-3 cells are cancerous bronchial epithelial cells and involve membrane transporters and/or local enzymatic degradation, which might reflect differences in lung absorption with useful in vivo applications.

Kumar et al. evaluated the APSD, dissolution, and permeation behavior of micronized fluticasone propionate (FP) and 2% magnesium stearate (MgSt) mixture prepared using different techniques. The physicochemical characterization and APSD data showed no significant difference between the MgSt mixed powder formulations. The dissolution behavior of the formulations was evaluated after collecting the fine particles on the Transwells insert incorporated into stages 3, 5, and 7 of the NGI. The acceptor chamber contained 300 ul of dissolution media to simulate lung conditions. Further, drug permeability after dissolution of formulations was assessed by directly depositing particles on Calu-3 cells at the air-liquid interface (ALI). Interestingly, despite no significant APSD, only one formulation (powder mixing with a RAM without heating) showed dissolution and permeation correlation (Figure 2.6b). It was concluded that the surface enrichment of hydrophobic MgSt improved aerosolization properties and the dissolution and permeability rate of micronized FP by reducing powder agglomerations.[141]

2.6.2 Human Alveolar Cell Monolayer Models

As 97% of the lung surface, which encounters the inhaled formulation, is covered by the alveolar epithelia, it was necessary to establish an in vitro model utilizing the alveolar epithelial cell monolayers. A549 cells are immortalized but cancerous and form unrestricted barriers with TEER value of ≤ 250 $\Omega \cdot cm^2$ so that the transport rates (J_a or P_a values) are hardly discriminative between drug moieties.[2] Human alveolar epithelial cells isolated from resected lungs form highly restricted cell monolayer barriers (TEER value $\geq 1,200$ $\Omega \cdot cm^2$), but they have limited division capacity. Furthermore, different lung cells have been studied as a prospective in vitro alveolar barrier models. One such cell is NCIH441 cells obtained from human lung adenocarcinoma with both alveolar epithelial type II and club cell characteristics.[142] In these cells, when treated with dexamethasone and insulin transferrin-sodium selenite in submerged culture, the cell monolayers became alveolar epithelial type I cell-like and formed restricted barriers (TEER ≥ 750 $\Omega \cdot cm^2$) in eight days and thus were able to discriminate drugs/molecules with the transport rates. On the other hand, their ALI culture resulted in a rather lower TEER (≤ 315 $\Omega \cdot cm^2$) and thus less discriminative transport barriers. NCIH441 cells, being primary cells, do not divide sufficiently to obtain consistent results. In contrast, the second cells, hAELVi, are lentivirus immortalized human alveolar epithelial cells, which expressed alveolar type I epithelial markers and formed highly restricted monolayers (TEER≥ 2000 $\Omega \cdot cm2$) in 14 days under ALI culture.[143] These cells show the stable expression of the markers up to 75 days. The TEER value for the cells when grown submerged was much lower (~1000 $\Omega \cdot cm^2$), unlike Calu-3 and NCI-H441 cells.

2.6.3 Human Primary ALI-Cultured 3D Lung Cell Barrier Models

Though the epithelial cell monolayer models represent the lung's most formidable transport barrier for drugs/molecules, the ABB in the human lungs is structurally 3D, composed of endothelial cells and extracellular matrix (ECM) of fibroblasts as well. The primary 3D human lung cell barriers ALI culture systems are now commercially available and are under investigation for their relevance. MucilAir, SmallAir, and EpiAirway systems are commercial tracheal/bronchial cell barrier models with or without lung fibroblast and can be developed under ALI culture in 14–45 days. Under the ALI culture without fibroblasts, the MucilAir and EpiAirway systems resulted in ~560 and ~391 $\Omega \cdot cm^2$ of moderate-to-low TEER, respectively,[144] showing less optimal discriminative barrier properties. Based on the donor's lungs, the EpiAirway system was reported to show a TEER value of <180 $\Omega \cdot cm^2$ similar to the MucilAir system.[145] On the other hand, the alveolar barrier model of the EpiAlveolar system, likely the first in vitro alveolar-like 3D barrier model, differentiates to form the three cell layers of alveolar epithelial cells, lung fibroblasts, and endothelial cells under ALI co-culture. The differentiated epithelial cells were shown to contain alveolar type I and type II cells similar to lung epithelia. This model maintained a TEER value[135] of >1000 $\Omega \cdot cm^2$, making it likely to sufficiently discriminate the rate of transport of drug moieties.

2.6.4 Stem Cell-Derived Lung Epithelial Cells

Human pluripotent stem cells (hPSCs), especially human embryonic stem cells (hESCs) and induced PSCs (iPSCs), can theoretically generate an unlimited somatic cells for in vitro predictive models and for large-scale screening of novel drugs and cell therapies.[146] But the large-scale production of alveolar epithelial cells is still a challenge. Recent development for hESC or iPSC to alveolar epithelial type II-like cells[147, 148] might make large-scale production feasible. Interestingly, the ALI culture induced the cell differentiation to form alveolar epithelial type I-like cells.[149] Similarly, iPSC-derived alveolar epithelial type II-like cells formed modestly restricted monolayers with 342–375 $\Omega \cdot cm2$ of the TEER.[149] Even though these cell monolayers are not as discriminative as the hAELVi cell monolayers in transport rates, further optimization may lead to generation of sufficiently restricted alveolar cell barriers from these stem cells for inhaled biopharmaceutics research.

2.6.5 "Lung-on-a-Chip" Model

The "lung-on-a-chip" model is a model of living human lungs in a microfluidic device with two flow channels separated by a thin, porous membrane which is coated with ECM. The human alveolar epithelial cells form the monolayer on the membrane in the apical channel while the vascular endothelial cells form the monolayer on the basolateral channels. Mucosal ALI is replicated by air flowing through the apical channel and the culture media flowing through the basolateral channel while controlled cell stretching can mimic in vivo breathing as represented in Figure 2.7. This device has primarily been used to predict absorption of airborne nanoparticles and to study the biological development and pathogenic responses to cause disease or toxicity.[150] However, within the scope of inhaled biopharmaceutics research, Artzy-Schnirman et al. reported a unique six-well "lung-on-a-chip" prototype, capable of integrating an in vitro aerosol deposition system. While the utility of this system is still being examined, this attempt

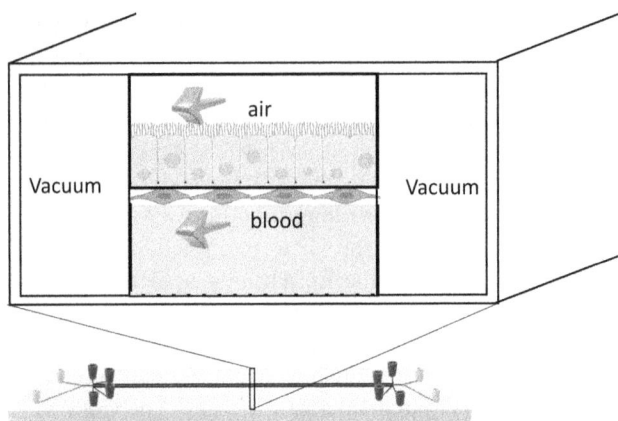

FIGURE 2.7 Schematics for "lung-on-a-chip" model. This small device is designed to grow the epithelial membrane on one side of the support and vascular epithelial cells on the other, mimicking the gaseous exchange in the alveoli.

sounds appealing if lung disposition behavior of drugs/molecules could be studied upon aerosol deposition in this physiologically relevant condition that includes the presence of air/media flow as well as breathing-like stretching. This microfluidics-based method assessing the permeability can utilize the traditional fluorescent tracer method as well as the relatively new electroactive tracer method similar to TEER. The electroactive tracer method has the advantage of online measurement of barrier function, eliminating the manual sampling and further processing of the samples, making the method much faster and reliable. In addition, dextran molecules of different molecular weights can be conjugated to the electroactive tracer to evaluate the size-selectiveness of the monolayers.[151]

2.7 CONCLUSION AND FUTURE PERSPECTIVES

Pulmonary drug delivery has gained much attention in recent years with new formulation techniques and drug delivery devices. The pulmonary route is now being used to deliver therapeutics for both local and systemic diseases. To reap the maximum benefit from this route of administration, the formulation, post-administration, should behave just the way it is intended. In this article, we have highlighted different factors to consider for the successful development of the inhalation formulation in terms of deposition and bioavailability. Next, we discussed the relevant instruments and the modifications which have made the in vitro testing of these products possible. Introduction of NGI has proven to be a milestone in inhalation therapy, and the number of studies exploring different aspects of NGI or increasing the functionality are exponentially increasing year after year. We have also explored release, dissolution, and subsequent absorption of the drug in the system and the diversity of techniques which can be utilized to reflect the same in vitro.

Previously, oral inhalation products were limited to low dose drugs and local treatments only. Therefore, powder APSD performance could be used as a surrogate for drug bioavailability. However, gradually, medicines that require high doses such as antibiotics and chemotherapies with hydrophobic molecules and for systemic delivery are being developed as for inhalation route. Further, the performance of inhalation pharmaceuticals are heavily affected by the device used for their administration. At the end of their innovative patent life, alternative versions are likely to be developed and possibly with different devices. The standards of alternative devices, although required to meet appropriate quality standards defined in regulatory guidelines, do not ensure equivalent delivery of medication to patients. There is a need to develop standard in vitro tests and bioequivalence methods to be more reflective of what happens in vivo in the lungs. None of the methods currently applied reflects the complexity and intricacy of what happens in the lungs post-administration, but they come close. As a result, the in vitro data alone do not support a claim of bioequivalence, and some regulatory agencies require pharmacokinetic study data.

As with all other routes of drug delivery, pulmonary drug delivery still needs to make many significant improvements to achieve the intended efficacy. Significant improvement is being made for venting device invention, formulation approaches, and delivery systems. The ultimate aim would be to have a good in vitro in vivo correlation (IVIVC) that will make inhalation therapy a highly effective and desired route of administration.

REFERENCES

1. Patton, J.S. & Byron, P.R. Inhaling medicines: Delivering drugs to the body through the lungs. *Nature Reviews Drug Discovery* 6(1), 67–74 (2007).
2. Nahar, K. *et al.* In vitro, in vivo and ex vivo models for studying particle deposition and drug absorption of inhaled pharmaceuticals. *European Journal of Pharmaceutical Sciences: Official Journal of the European Federation for Pharmaceutical Sciences* 49(5), 805–818 (2013).
3. Mathias, N.R. & Hussain, M.A. Non-invasive systemic drug delivery: Developability considerations for alternate routes of administration. *Journal of Pharmaceutical Sciences* 99(1), 1–20 (2010).
4. Nichols, D.P. *et al.* Developing inhaled antibiotics in cystic fibrosis: Current challenges and opportunities. *Annals of the American Thoracic Society* 16(5), 534–539 (2019).
5. Chan, H.K. & Chew, N.Y. Novel alternative methods for the delivery of drugs for the treatment of asthma. *Advanced Drug Delivery Reviews* 55(7), 793–805 (2003).
6. Mahler, D.A. *et al.* Effectiveness of fluticasone propionate and salmeterol combination delivered via the diskus device in the treatment of chronic obstructive pulmonary disease. *American Journal of Respiratory and Critical Care Medicine* 166(8), 1084–1091 (2002).
7. Polin, R.A., Carlo, W.A. & Committee on Fetus and Newborn; American Academy of Pediatrics. Surfactant replacement therapy for preterm and term neonates with respiratory distress. *Pediatrics* 133(1), 156–163 (2014).
8. Monto, A.S. *et al.* Zanamivir in the prevention of influenza among healthy adults: A randomized controlled trial. *JAMA* 282(1), 31–35 (1999).

9. Traynor, K. Inhaled insulin product approved. *American Journal of Health-System Pharmacy: AJHP: Official Journal of the American Society of Health-System Pharmacists* 71(15), 1238 (2014).

10. Greene, S.F., Nikula, K.J., Poulin, D., McInally, K. & Reynolds, J.A. Long-term nonclinical pulmonary safety assessment of afrezza, a novel insulin inhalation powder. *Toxicologic Pathology* 49(2), 334–348 (2021).

11. Heinemann, L. The failure of exubera: Are we beating a dead horse? *Journal of Diabetes Science and Technology* 2(3), 518–529 (2008).

12. Marqus, S. *et al.* High frequency acoustic nebulization for pulmonary delivery of antibiotic alternatives against Staphylococcus aureus. *European Journal of Pharmaceutics and Biopharmaceutics: Official Journal of Arbeitsgemeinschaft fur Pharmazeutische Verfahrenstechnik E.V* 151, 181–188 (2020).

13. Zhang, W. *et al.* Technical evaluation of soft mist inhaler use in patients with chronic obstructive pulmonary disease: A cross-sectional study. *International Journal of Chronic Obstructive Pulmonary Disease* 15, 1471–1479 (2020).

14. Sharma, K., Somavarapu, S., Colombani, A., Govind, N. & Taylor, K.M. Crosslinked chitosan nanoparticle formulations for delivery from pressurized metered dose inhalers. *European Journal of Pharmaceutics and Biopharmaceutics: Official Journal of Arbeitsgemeinschaft fur Pharmazeutische Verfahrenstechnik E.V* 81(1), 74–81 (2012).

15. Papaioannou, A.I. *et al.* Ability of using different dry powder inhalers during COPD exacerbations. *Pulmonary Pharmacology and Therapeutics* 48, 211–216 (2018).

16. Chandel, A., Goyal, A.K., Ghosh, G. & Rath, G. Recent advances in aerosolised drug delivery. *Biomedicine and Pharmacotherapy = Biomedecine and Pharmacotherapie* 112, 108601 (2019).

17. Yildiz-Pekoz, A. & Ehrhardt, C. Advances in pulmonary drug delivery. *Pharmaceutics* 12(10), (2020). https://doi.org/10.3390/pharmaceutics12100911.

18. Crompton, G.K. Breath-activated aerosol. *British Medical Journal* 2(5762), 652–653 (1971).

19. Kelkar, M.S. *Effervescent aerosols: A novel formulation technology for solution and suspension-type metered dose inhalers.* (2016).

20. Iula, A.K., Flynn, C.L. & Deluccia, F. Comparative study of the in vitro dose delivery and particle size distribution characteristics of an azmacort metered-dose inhaler in combination with four different spacer devices. *Current Therapeutic Research* 58(8), 544–554 (1997).

21. Dalby, R., Spallek, M. & Voshaar, T. A review of the development of respimat soft mist inhaler. *International Journal of Pharmaceutics* 283(1–2), 1–9 (2004).

22. Melani, A.S. Inhalatory therapy training: A priority challenge for the physician. *Acta Bio-Medica: Atenei Parmensis* 78(3), 233–245 (2007).

23. Kumar, V. *et al.* Functional similarity of modified cascade impactor to deposit drug particles on cells. *International Journal of Pharmaceutics* 583, 119404 (2020).

24. Bicer, E.M. *Compositional characterisation of human respiratory tract lining fluids for the design of disease specific simulants.* (2015).

25. Mall, M.A. Role of cilia, mucus, and airway surface liquid in mucociliary dysfunction: Lessons from mouse models. *Journal of Aerosol Medicine and Pulmonary Drug Delivery* 21(1), 13–24 (2008).

26. Cross, C.E., Halliwell, B. & Allen, A. Antioxidant protection: A function of tracheobronchial and gastrointestinal mucus. *Lancet* 1(8390), 1328–1330 (1984).

27. Wanner, A., Salathe, M. & O'Riordan, T.G. Mucociliary clearance in the airways. *American Journal of Respiratory and Critical Care Medicine* 154(6 Pt 1), 1868–1902 (1996).

28. Patton, J.S. *et al.* The particle has landed–Characterizing the fate of inhaled pharmaceuticals. *Journal of Aerosol Medicine and Pulmonary Drug Delivery* 23(Suppl 2), S71–S87 (2010).

29. Gizurarson, S. The effect of cilia and the mucociliary clearance on successful drug delivery. *Biological and Pharmaceutical Bulletin* 38(4), 497–506 (2015).
30. Hogg, J.C. Response of the lung to inhaled particles. *The Medical Journal of Australia* 142(13), 675–678 (1985).
31. Weers, J.G. & Miller, D.P. Formulation design of dry powders for inhalation. *Journal of Pharmaceutical Sciences* 104(10), 3259–3288 (2015).
32. Wang, Y.B. *et al.* In vitro and in vivo performance of dry powder inhalation formulations: Comparison of particles prepared by thin film freezing and micronization. *AAPS PharmSciTech* 15(4), 981–993 (2014).
33. El-Sherbiny, I.M., El-Baz, N.M. & Yacoub, M.H. Inhaled nano- and microparticles for drug delivery. *Global Cardiology Science and Practice* 2015, 2 (2015).
34. El-Sherbiny, I.M., Villanueva, D.G., Herrera, D. & Smyth, H.D.C. Overcoming lung clearance mechanisms for controlled release drug delivery. *Controlled Pulmonary Drug Delivery* 101–126 (Springer, 2011).
35. Champion, J.A., Walker, A. & Mitragotri, S. Role of particle size in phagocytosis of polymeric microspheres. *Pharmaceutical Research* 25(8), 1815–1821 (2008).
36. Ding, X. & Kaminsky, L.S. Human extrahepatic cytochromes P450: Function in xenobiotic metabolism and tissue-selective chemical toxicity in the respiratory and gastrointestinal tracts. *Annual Review of Pharmacology and Toxicology* 43, 149–173 (2003).
37. Hukkanen, J., Pelkonen, O., Hakkola, J. & Raunio, H. Expression and regulation of xenobiotic-metabolizing cytochrome P450 (CYP) enzymes in human lung. *Critical Reviews in Toxicology* 32(5), 391–411 (2002).
38. Raunio, H. *et al.* Expression of xenobiotic-metabolizing CYPs in human pulmonary tissue. *Experimental and Toxicologic Pathology: Official Journal of the Gesellschaft fur Toxikologische Pathologie* 51(4–5), 412–417 (1999).
39. Wiedmann, T.S., Bhatia, R. & Wattenberg, L.W. Drug solubilization in lung surfactant. *Journal of Controlled Release: Official Journal of the Controlled Release Society* 65(1–2), 43–47 (2000).
40. Cazzola, M., Testi, R. & Matera, M.G. Clinical pharmacokinetics of salmeterol. *Clinical Pharmacokinetics* 41(1), 19–30 (2002).
41. Ha, H.R., Chen, J., Freiburghaus, A.U. & Follath, F. Metabolism of theophylline by cDNA-expressed human cytochromes P-450. *British Journal of Clinical Pharmacology* 39(3), 321–326 (1995).
42. Tunek, A., Sjodin, K. & Hallstrom, G. Reversible formation of fatty acid esters of budesonide, an antiasthma glucocorticoid, in human lung and liver microsomes. *Drug Metabolism and Disposition: The Biological Fate of Chemicals* 25(11), 1311–1317 (1997).
43. Nave, R., Fisher, R. & Zech, K. In vitro metabolism of ciclesonide in human lung and liver precision-cut tissue slices. *Biopharmaceutics and Drug Disposition* 27(4), 197–207 (2006).
44. Pearce, R.E., Leeder, J.S. & Kearns, G.L. Biotransformation of fluticasone: In vitro characterization. *Drug Metabolism and Disposition: The Biological Fate of Chemicals* 34(6), 1035–1040 (2006).
45. Smola, M., Vandamme, T. & Sokolowski, A. Nanocarriers as pulmonary drug delivery systems to treat and to diagnose respiratory and non respiratory diseases. *International Journal of Nanomedicine* 3(1), 1–19 (2008).
46. Ruffin, R.E., Dolovich, M.B., Wolff, R.K. & Newhouse, M.T. The effects of preferential deposition of histamine in the human airway. *The American Review of Respiratory Disease* 117(3), 485–492 (1978).
47. Carstairs, J.R., Nimmo, A.J. & Barnes, P.J. Autoradiographic visualization of beta-adrenoceptor subtypes in human lung. *The American Review of Respiratory Disease* 132(3), 541–547 (1985).

48. Mak, J.C. & Barnes, P.J. Autoradiographic visualization of muscarinic receptor subtypes in human and guinea pig lung. *The American Review of Respiratory Disease* 141(6), 1559–1568 (1990).

49. Carroll, N., Cooke, C. & James, A. The distribution of eosinophils and lymphocytes in the large and small airways of asthmatics. *The European Respiratory Journal* 10(2), 292–300 (1997).

50. Bergeron, C. & Cantin, A.M. Cystic fibrosis: Pathophysiology of lung disease. *Seminars in Respiratory and Critical Care Medicine* 40(6), 715–726 (2019).

51. Geller, D.E., Weers, J. & Heuerding, S. Development of an inhaled dry-powder formulation of tobramycin using PulmoSphere technology. *Journal of Aerosol Medicine and Pulmonary Drug Delivery* 24(4), 175–182 (2011).

52. Pfutzner, A. & Forst, T. Pulmonary insulin delivery by means of the Technosphere drug carrier mechanism. *Expert Opinion on Drug Delivery* 2(6), 1097–1106 (2005).

53. Bennett, J.V. *et al.* Aerosolized measles and measles-rubella vaccines induce better measles antibody booster responses than injected vaccines: Randomized trials in Mexican schoolchildren. *Bulletin of the World Health Organization* 80(10), 806–812 (2002).

54. MVDP Author Group *et al.* Safety and immunogenicity of dry powder measles vaccine administered by inhalation: A randomized controlled phase I clinical trial. *Vaccine* 32, 6791–6797 (2014).

55. Gomez, M. *et al.* Development of a formulation platform for a spray-dried, inhalable tuberculosis vaccine candidate. *International Journal of Pharmaceutics* 593, 120121 (2021).

56. Jin, T.H., Tsao, E., Goudsmit, J., Dheenadhayalan, V. & Sadoff, J. Stabilizing formulations for inhalable powders of an adenovirus 35-vectored tuberculosis (TB) vaccine (AERAS-402). *Vaccine* 28(27), 4369–4375 (2010).

57. Thomas, C., Gupta, V. & Ahsan, F. Particle size influences the immune response produced by hepatitis B vaccine formulated in inhalable particles. *Pharmaceutical Research* 27(5), 905–919 (2010).

58. Zheng, B. *et al.* Inhalable nanovaccine with biomimetic coronavirus structure to trigger mucosal immunity of respiratory tract against COVID-19. *Chemical Engineering Journal (Lausanne, Switzerland: 1996)* 418, 129392 (2021).

59. Davies, C.N. & Muir, D.C. Deposition of inhaled particles in human lungs. *Nature* 211(5044), 90–91 (1966).

60. Boucher, R.C. Regulation of airway surface liquid volume by human airway epithelia. *Pflugers Archiv: European Journal of Physiology* 445(4), 495–498 (2003).

61. Champion, J.A. & Mitragotri, S. Role of target geometry in phagocytosis. *Proceedings of the National Academy of Sciences of the United States of America* 103(13), 4930–4934 (2006).

62. Champion, J.A. & Mitragotri, S. Shape induced inhibition of phagocytosis of polymer particles. *Pharmaceutical Research* 26(1), 244–249 (2009).

63. Chan, J.G. *et al.* A novel inhalable form of rifapentine. *Journal of Pharmaceutical Sciences* 103(5), 1411–1421 (2014).

64. Karner, S. & Anne Urbanetz, N. The impact of electrostatic charge in pharmaceutical powders with specific focus on inhalation-powders. *Journal of Aerosol Science* 42(6), 428–445 (2011).

65. Kwok, P.C. & Chan, H.K. Electrostatics of pharmaceutical inhalation aerosols. *The Journal of Pharmacy and Pharmacology* 61(12), 1587–1599 (2009).

66. Bailey, A.G. The inhalation and deposition of charged particles within the human lung. *Journal of Electrostatics* 42(1–2), 25–32 (1997).

67. Koullapis, P.G., Kassinos, S.C., Bivolarova, M.P. & Melikov, A.K. Particle deposition in a realistic geometry of the human conducting airways: Effects of inlet velocity profile, inhalation flowrate and electrostatic charge. *Journal of Biomechanics* 49(11), 2201–2212 (2016).

68. Bailey, A.G., Hashish, A.H. & Williams, T.J. Drug delivery by inhalation of charged particles. *Journal of Electrostatics* 44(1–2), 3–10 (1998).
69. Hoe, S., Young, P.M., Chan, H.K. & Traini, D. Introduction of the electrical next generation impactor (eNGI) and investigation of its capabilities for the study of pressurized metered dose inhalers. *Pharmaceutical Research* 26(2), 431–437 (2009).
70. Edwards, D.A. *et al.* Large porous particles for pulmonary drug delivery. *Science (New York, N.Y.)* 276(5320), 1868–1871 (1997).
71. Stank, K. & Steckel, H. Physico-chemical characterisation of surface modified particles for inhalation. *International Journal of Pharmaceutics* 448(1), 9–18 (2013).
72. Zhou, Q.T. *et al.* Effect of surface coating with magnesium stearate via mechanical dry powder coating approach on the aerosol performance of micronized drug powders from dry powder inhalers. *AAPS PharmSciTech* 14(1), 38–44 (2013).
73. Kawashima, Y., Serigano, T., Hino, T., Yamamoto, H. & Takeuchi, H. A new powder design method to improve inhalation efficiency of pranlukast hydrate dry powder aerosols by surface modification with hydroxypropylmethylcellulose phthalate nanospheres. *Pharmaceutical Research* 15(11), 1748–1752 (1998).
74. Serigano, T., Hino, T., Yamamoto, H., Takeuchi, H. & Kawashima, Y. The design of inhalation dry powders by the surface modification of drug particles. *Journal of the Society of Powder Technology, Japan* 33(7), 559–563 (1996).
75. Makhlof, A., Werle, M., Tozuka, Y. & Takeuchi, H. Nanoparticles of glycol chitosan and its thiolated derivative significantly improved the pulmonary delivery of calcitonin. *International Journal of Pharmaceutics* 397(1–2), 92–95 (2010).
76. Islam, M.S., Saha, S.C., Sauret, E., Gemci, T. & Gu, Y. Pulmonary aerosol transport and deposition analysis in upper 17 generations of the human respiratory tract. *Journal of Aerosol Science* 108, 29–43 (2017).
77. Biswas, R., Hanania, N.A. & Sabharwal, A. Factors determining in vitro lung deposition of albuterol aerosol delivered by ventolin metered-dose inhaler. *Journal of Aerosol Medicine and Pulmonary Drug Delivery* 30(4), 256–266 (2017).
78. Pavia, D., Thomson, M.L., Clarke, S.W. & Shannon, H.S. Effect of lung function and mode of inhalation on penetration of aerosol into the human lung. *Thorax* 32(2), 194–197 (1977).
79. Palmes, E.D. Measurement of pulmonary air spaces using aerosols. *Archives of Internal Medicine* 131(1), 76–79 (1973).
80. Newman, S.P. Aerosol deposition considerations in inhalation therapy. *Chest* 88(Suppl 2), 152S–160S (1985).
81. Kleinstreuer, C., Zhang, Z. & Li, Z. Modeling airflow and particle transport/deposition in pulmonary airways. *Respiratory Physiology and Neurobiology* 163(1–3), 128–138 (2008).
82. Byron, P.R. *et al.* In vivo-in vitro correlations: Predicting pulmonary drug deposition from pharmaceutical aerosols. *Journal of Aerosol Medicine and Pulmonary Drug Delivery* 23(Suppl 2), S59–69 (2010).
83. Swift, D.L. Aerosols and humidity therapy: Generation and respiratory deposition of therapeutic aerosols. *The American Review of Respiratorsease* 122(5 Pt 2), 71–77 (1980).
84. Ferron, G.A., Hornik, S., Kreyling, W.G. & Haider, B. Comparison of experimental and calculated data for the total and regional deposition in the human lung. *Journal of Aerosol Science* 16(2), 133–143 (1985).
85. Ferron, G.A., Oberdörster, G. & Henneberg, R. Estimation of the deposition of aerosolized drugs in the human respiratory tract due to hygroscopic growth. *Journal of Aerosol Medicine* 2(3), 271–284 (1989).
86. Xu, G.B. & Yu, C.P. Theoretical lung deposition of hygroscopic NaCl aerosols. *Aerosol Science and Technology* 4(4), 455–461 (1985).
87. Xi, J., Kim, J., Si, X.A. & Zhou, Y. Hygroscopic aerosol deposition in the human upper respiratory tract under various thermo-humidity conditions. *Journal of Environmental*

Science and Health. Part A – Toxic/Hazardous Substances and Environmental Engineering 48(14), 1790–1805 (2013).

88. Feng, Y., Kleinstreuer, C., Castro, N. & Rostami, A. Computational transport, phase change and deposition analysis of inhaled multicomponent droplet–vapor mixtures in an idealized human upper lung model. *Journal of Aerosol Science* 96, 96–123 (2016).

89. Chen, X., Feng, Y., Zhong, W. & Kleinstreuer, C. Numerical investigation of the interaction, transport and deposition of multicomponent droplets in a simple mouth-throat model. *Journal of Aerosol Science* 105, 108–127 (2017).

90. Chen, X., Ma, R., Zhong, W., Sun, B. & Zhou, X. Numerical study of the effects of temperature and humidity on the transport and deposition of hygroscopic aerosols in a G3-G6 airway. *International Journal of Heat and Mass Transfer* 138, 545–552 (2019).

91. Young, P.M. *et al.* Influence of humidity on the electrostatic charge and aerosol performance of dry powder inhaler carrier based systems. *Pharmaceutical Research* 24(5), 963–970 (2007).

92. Mitchell, J.P., Nagel, M.W., Wiersema, K.J. & Doyle, C.C. Aerodynamic particle size analysis of aerosols from pressurized metered-dose inhalers: Comparison of Andersen 8-stage cascade impactor, next generation pharmaceutical impactor, and model 3321 aerodynamic particle sizer aerosol spectrometer. *AAPS PharmSciTech* 4(4), E54 (2003).

93. Hoe, S., Traini, D., Chan, H.-K. & Young, P.M. Measuring charge and mass distributions in dry powder inhalers using the electrical next generation impactor (eNGI). *European Journal of Pharmaceutical Sciences* 38(2), 88–94 (2009).

94. Rowland, M. *et al.* Measuring the bipolar charge distributions of fine particle aerosol clouds of commercial PMDI suspensions using a bipolar next generation impactor (bp-NGI). *Pharmaceutical Research* 36(1), 15 (2018).

95. Bonacucina, G., Cespi, M., Misici-Falzi, M. & Palmieri, G.F. Colloidal soft matter as drug delivery system. *Journal of Pharmaceutical Sciences* 98(1), 1–42 (2009).

96. Beck-Broichsitter, M., Merkel, O.M. & Kissel, T. Controlled pulmonary drug and gene delivery using polymeric nano-carriers. *Journal of Controlled Release: Official Journal of the Controlled Release Society* 161(2), 214–224 (2012).

97. Fredenberg, S., Wahlgren, M., Reslow, M. & Axelsson, A. The mechanisms of drug release in poly(lactic-co-glycolic acid)-based drug delivery systems–A review. *International Journal of Pharmaceutics* 415(1–2), 34–52 (2011).

98. Bibby, D.C., Davies, N.M. & Tucker, I.G. Mechanisms by which cyclodextrins modify drug release from polymeric drug delivery systems. *International Journal of Pharmaceutics* 197(1–2), 1–11 (2000).

99. Klyashchitsky, B.A. & Owen, A.J. Nebulizer-compatible liquid formulations for aerosol pulmonary delivery of hydrophobic drugs: Glucocorticoids and cyclosporine. *Journal of Drug Targeting* 7(2), 79–99 (1999).

100. Beck-Broichsitter, M. *et al.* Correlation of drug release with pulmonary drug absorption profiles for nebulizable liposomal formulations. *European Journal of Pharmaceutics and Biopharmaceutics: Official Journal of Arbeitsgemeinschaft fur Pharmazeutische Verfahrenstechnik E.V* 84(1), 106–114 (2013).

101. Tewes, F., Ehrhardt, C. & Healy, A.M. Superparamagnetic iron oxide nanoparticles (SPIONs)-loaded Trojan microparticles for targeted aerosol delivery to the lung. *European Journal of Pharmaceutics and Biopharmaceutics: Official Journal of Arbeitsgemeinschaft fur Pharmazeutische Verfahrenstechnik E.V* 86(1), 98–104 (2014).

102. Upadhyay, D. *et al.* Magnetised thermo responsive lipid vehicles for targeted and controlled lung drug delivery. *Pharmaceutical Research* 29(9), 2456–2467 (2012).

103. Noriega-Fernandes, B. *et al.* Dry powder inhaler formulation comparison: Study of the role of particle deposition pattern and dissolution. *International Journal of Pharmacy* 607, 121025 (2021).

104. Shah, V.P., Smurthwaite, M.J., Veranth, J.M. & Zaidi, K. The inhalation Ad hoc advisory panel for the USP performance tests of inhalation dosage forms. *Pharmaceutical Forum* 34(4), 1068–1074 (2008).
105. Patton, J.S. Mechanisms of macromolecule absorption by the lungs. *Advanced Drug Delivery Reviews* 19(1), 3–36 (1996).
106. Asada, M., Takahashi, H., Okamoto, H., Tanino, H. & Danjo, K. Theophylline particle design using chitosan by the spray drying. *International Journal of Pharmaceutics* 270(1–2), 167–174 (2004).
107. Jaspart, S. *et al.* Solid lipid microparticles as a sustained release system for pulmonary drug delivery. *European Journal of Pharmaceutics and Biopharmaceutics: Official Journal of Arbeitsgemeinschaft fur Pharmazeutische Verfahrenstechnik E.V* 65(1), 47–56 (2007).
108. Learoyd, T.P., Burrows, J.L., French, E. & Seville, P.C. Chitosan-based spray-dried respirable powders for sustained delivery of terbutaline sulfate. *European Journal of Pharmaceutics and Biopharmaceutics: Official Journal of Arbeitsgemeinschaft fur Pharmazeutische Verfahrenstechnik E.V* 68(2), 224–234 (2008).
109. Huang, Z. *et al.* Dry powder inhaler formulations of poorly water-soluble itraconazole: A balance between in-vitro dissolution and in-vivo distribution is necessary. *International Journal of Pharmacy* 551(1–2), 103–110 (2018).
110. McConville, J.T. *et al.* Use of a novel modified TSI for the evaluation of controlled-release aerosol formulations. I. *Drug Development and Industrial Pharmacy* 26(11), 1191–1198 (2000).
111. Sdraulig, S. *et al.* In vitro dissolution studies of uranium bearing material in simulated lung fluid. *Journal of Environmental Radioactivity* 99(3), 527–538 (2008).
112. Azarmi, S., Roa, W. & Lobenberg, R. Current perspectives in dissolution testing of conventional and novel dosage forms. *International Journal of Pharmaceutics* 328(1), 12–21 (2007).
113. Siewert, M. *et al.* FIP/AAPS guidelines to dissolution/in vitro release testing of novel/special dosage forms. *AAPS PharmSciTech* 4(1), E7 (2003).
114. Taylor, M.K., Hickey, A.J. & VanOort, M. Manufacture, characterization, and pharmacodynamic evaluation of engineered ipratropium bromide particles. *Pharmaceutical Development and Technology* 11(3), 321–336 (2006).
115. Davies, N.M. & Feddah, M.R. A novel method for assessing dissolution of aerosol inhaler products. *International Journal of Pharmaceutics* 255(1–2), 175–187 (2003).
116. Son, Y.J. & McConville, J.T. Development of a standardized dissolution test method for inhaled pharmaceutical formulations. *International Journal of Pharmaceutics* 382(1–2), 15–22 (2009).
117. Son, Y.-J., Horng, M., Copley, M. & McConville, J.T. Optimization of an in vitro dissolution test method for inhalation formulations. *Dissolution Technologies* 17(2), 6–13 (2010).
118. Daley-Yates, P.T. & Parkins, D.A. Establishing bioequivalence for inhaled drugs; weighing the evidence. *Expert Opinion on Drug Delivery* 8(10), 1297–1308 (2011).
119. Sonvico, F. *et al.* RespiCellTM: An innovative dissolution apparatus for inhaled products. *Pharmaceutics* 13(10), 1541 (2021).
120. Gerde, P. *et al.* Dissolvit: An in vitro method for simulating the dissolution and absorption of inhaled dry powder drugs in the lungs. *Assay and Drug Development Technologies* 15(2), 77–88 (2017).
121. Diaz-Coranguez, M., Liu, X. & Antonetti, D.A. Tight junctions in cell proliferation. *International Journal of Molecular Sciences* 20(23), (2019). https://doi.org/10.3390/ijms20235972.
122. Burton, P.S., Conradi, R.A. & Hilgers, A.R. (B) Mechanisms of peptide and protein absorption: (2) Transcellular mechanism of peptide and protein absorption: Passive aspects. *Advanced Drug Delivery Reviews* 7(3), 365–385 (1991).

123. Bosquillon, C. Drug transporters in the lung–Do they play a role in the biopharmaceutics of inhaled drugs? *Journal of Pharmaceutical Sciences* 99(5), 2240–2255 (2010).

124. Nickel, S., Clerkin, C.G., Selo, M.A. & Ehrhardt, C. Transport mechanisms at the pulmonary mucosa: Implications for drug delivery. *Expert Opinion on Drug Delivery* 13(5), 667–690 (2016).

125. Wittenberg, J.B. On optima: The case of myoglobin-facilitated oxygen diffusion. *Gene* 398(1–2), 156–161 (2007).

126. Wood, I.S. & Trayhurn, P. Glucose transporters (GLUT and SGLT): Expanded families of sugar transport proteins. *The British Journal of Nutrition* 89(1), 3–9 (2003).

127. Bhattarai, R.S. *et al.* Nanoformulation design and therapeutic potential of a novel tubulin inhibitor in pancreatic cancer. *Journal of Controlled Release: Official Journal of the Controlled Release Society* 329, 585–597 (2021).

128. Takano, M., Kawami, M., Aoki, A. & Yumoto, R. Receptor-mediated endocytosis of macromolecules and strategy to enhance their transport in alveolar epithelial cells. *Expert Opinion on Drug Delivery* 12(5), 813–825 (2015).

129. Amidon, G.L., Lennernas, H., Shah, V.P. & Crison, J.R. A theoretical basis for a biopharmaceutic drug classification: The correlation of in vitro drug product dissolution and in vivo bioavailability. *Pharmaceutical Research* 12(3), 413–420 (1995).

130. Gordon, S. *et al.* Non-animal models of epithelial barriers (skin, intestine and lung) in research, industrial applications and regulatory toxicology. *Altex* 32(4), 327–378 (2015).

131. Fernandes, C.A. & Vanbever, R. Preclinical models for pulmonary drug delivery. *Expert Opinion on Drug Delivery* 6(11), 1231–1245 (2009).

132. George, I. *et al.* Toxicological assessment of ITER-like tungsten nanoparticles using an in vitro 3D human airway epithelium model. *Nanomaterials (Basel, Switzerland)* 9(10), (2019). https://doi.org/10.3390/nano9101374.

133. Huang, S. *et al.* Establishment and characterization of an in vitro human small airway model (SmallAir). *European Journal of Pharmaceutics and Biopharmaceutics: Official Journal of Arbeitsgemeinschaft fur Pharmazeutische Verfahrenstechnik E.V* 118, 68–72 (2017).

134. Rotoli, B.M. *et al.* Characterization of ABC transporters in EpiAirway, a cellular model of normal human bronchial epithelium. *International Journal of Molecular Sciences* 21(9), (2020). https://doi.org/10.3390/ijms21093190.

135. Barosova, H. *et al.* Use of EpiAlveolar lung model to predict fibrotic potential of multi-walled carbon nanotubes. *ACS Nano* 14(4), 3941–3956 (2020).

136. Stucki, A.O. *et al.* A lung-on-a-chip array with an integrated bio-inspired respiration mechanism. *Lab on a Chip* 15(5), 1302–1310 (2015).

137. Florea, B.I., Cassara, M.L., Junginger, H.E. & Borchard, G. Drug transport and metabolism characteristics of the human airway epithelial cell line Calu-3. *Journal of Controlled Release* 87(1–3), 131–138 (2003).

138. Matilainen, L. *et al.* In vitro toxicity and permeation of cyclodextrins in Calu-3 cells. *Journal of Controlled Release* 126(1), 10–16 (2008).

139. Kreft, M.E. *et al.* The characterization of the human cell line Calu-3 under different culture conditions and its use as an optimized in vitro model to investigate bronchial epithelial function. *European Journal of Pharmaceutical Sciences: Official Journal of the European Federation for Pharmaceutical Sciences* 69, 1–9 (2015).

140. Grainger, C.I., Greenwell, L.L., Lockley, D.J., Martin, G.P. & Forbes, B. Culture of Calu-3 cells at the air interface provides a representative model of the airway epithelial barrier. *Pharmaceutical Research* 23(7), 1482–1490 (2006).

141. Kumar, V. *et al.* Effect of magnesium stearate surface coating method on the aerosol performance and permeability of micronized fluticasone propionate. *International Journal of Pharmacy* 615, 121470 (2022).

142. Salomon, J.J. *et al.* The cell line NCl-H441 is a useful in vitro model for transport studies of human distal lung epithelial barrier. *Molecular Pharmaceutics* 11(3), 995–1006 (2014).

143. Kuehn, A. *et al.* Human alveolar epithelial cells expressing tight junctions to model the air-blood barrier. *Altex* 33(3), 251–260 (2016).

144. Furubayashi, T. *et al.* Comparison of various cell lines and three-dimensional mucociliary tissue model systems to estimate drug permeability using an in vitro transport study to predict nasal drug absorption in rats. *Pharmaceutics* 12(1), (2020). https://doi.org/10.3390/pharmaceutics12010079.

145. Hoffmann, W. *et al.* Establishment of a human 3D tissue-based assay for upper respiratory tract absorption. *Applied in Vitro Toxicology* 4(2), 139–148 (2018).

146. Scott, C.W., Peters, M.F. & Dragan, Y.P. Human induced pluripotent stem cells and their use in drug discovery for toxicity testing. *Toxicology Letters* 219(1), 49–58 (2013).

147. Van Haute, L., De Block, G., Liebaers, I., Sermon, K. & De Rycke, M. Generation of lung epithelial-like tissue from human embryonic stem cells. *Respiratory Research* 10, 105 (2009).

148. Ghaedi, M. *et al.* Alveolar epithelial differentiation of human induced pluripotent stem cells in a rotating bioreactor. *Biomaterials* 35(2), 699–710 (2014).

149. Tamo, L. *et al.* Generation of an alveolar epithelial type II cell line from induced pluripotent stem cells. *American Journal of Physiology Lung Cellular and Molecular Physiology* 315(6), L921–932 (2018).

150. Zhang, M., Xu, C., Jiang, L. & Qin, J. A 3D human lung-on-a-chip model for nanotoxicity testing. *Toxicology Research* 7(6), 1048–1060 (2018).

151. Wong, J.F. & Simmons, C.A. Microfluidic assay for the on-chip electrochemical measurement of cell monolayer permeability. *Lab on a Chip* 19(6), 1060–1070 (2019).

Lung-on-a-Chip and Lung Organoid Models

3

Muhammad H. Malik, Amer S. Alali,
Shalaleh Masoumi, Xue Zhou, and Xinli Liu

Contents

DOI: 10.1201/9781003182566-4

3.1 INTRODUCTION

Drug development is a lengthy and highly expensive process that generally takes at least ten years and \$2.6 billion to bring a new molecular entity to market.[1] A large amount of time and money are consumed on the human clinical trials. Reducing drug attrition rates in clinical development is a major challenge for the pharmaceutical industry. Many drug failures in clinical development are due to the poor predictive power of current preclinical models. Preclinical animal models have large inter-species variability. Organ systems in animals of different species generally differ from human organs in their morphology and physiology.[2] Even the closest of species like primates and humans differ, either slightly or significantly, depending upon the organ system. In addition, organ-systems' functionality is complemented by other tissues and organs, which makes the whole system biology more complicated. The conventional static two-dimensional (2D) cell culture models lack tissue-specific, differentiated functions and do not mimic in vivo biophysical, biochemical, and biomechanical cues.[3] As a result, these preclinical models do not always predict the correct clinical outcomes in humans.[4] More reliable and human relevant models are needed for better prediction of drug target engagement, drug efficacy and safety in the first-in-human testing in patients.

In the last decade, the development and maintenance of organs-on-chips and organoids, which can mimic the complex human tissue/organ in vitro, have been advanced to the center stage as physiologically relevant preclinical models. For lungs, a variety of microdevices and organoids culture protocols have been developed to integrate the mechano-physiological parameters of lungs to mimic lung tissue microarchitecture, lung functions, and disease phenotypes in vitro. These new models have shown an enormous potential for modeling various lung diseases, screening and testing various lung targeted therapeutics and drug carriers, and studying drug distribution in vitro. Organs-on-chips are in vitro hybrid engineered microdevices, usually about the size of an AA battery that contain continuously perfused microchannels in which fluids can run (microfluidics), and different cell types are seeded in these continuously perfused channels (Figure 3.1).[2] Due to the progress in engineering and biology, organs-on-chips have brought benefits by bringing complexities such as fluid shear stress,

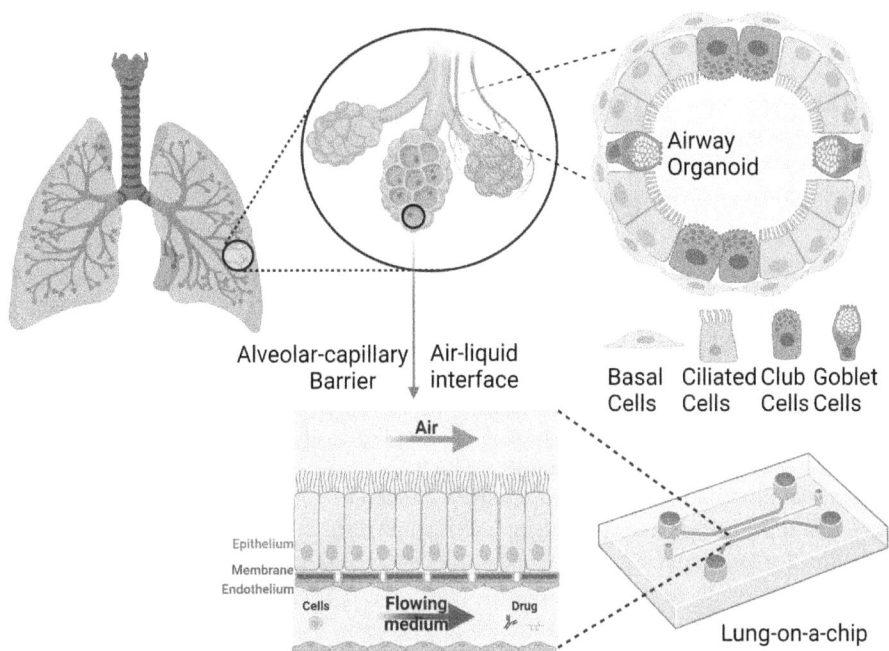

FIGURE 3.1 Schematic diagram of an airway organoid and lung-on-a-chip. The lung-on-a-chip microdevice recapitulates the microarchitecture of the alveolar-capillary barrier as a single layer of the alveolar epithelium grown at the upper air chamber and endothelial monolayers grown at the bottom fluid chamber, through which medium perfusion takes place.

mechanical compression, and diversity of cell types to the chip, which have assured that these miniatured devices can be employed to recreate natural physiological and/or pathological states of human tissue/organ, therefore can provide a plethora of information supporting preclinical drug development.[2,5] Organoids refer to three-dimensional (3D) organotypic structures composed of multiple cell types that originate from stem cells by means of self-organization and mimic the spatial and chemical complexity and the tissue architecture and functionality of native organs (Figure 3.1).[6,7] Development of novel biomimetic cell-based single organ-on-a-chip or integrated multi-organs-on-chips (body-on-a-chip) to reproduce physiologically relevant and complex organ-level system biology and disease models can potentially revolutionize medicine. The modular nature of organs-on-chips allows researchers to systemically study the response and behavior of a single organ (such as a lung) to different treatments by introducing drugs, chemicals, toxins, drug carriers, or immune cells to chips with a well-controlled microenvironment. Alternatively, multiple organs can be connected together via fluidics systems to form multiple organs-on-chips to study how different organs interact or respond to different treatments. These sophisticated organs-on-chips and organoids models are being deemed as increasingly useful and viable alternatives to the simple in vitro cell culture models or animal models, potentially improving the predictability of pre-clinical models.

3.2 LUNG-ON-A-CHIP AND ITS APPLICATION IN DRUG DISCOVERY AND DEVELOPMENT

3.2.1 Prevalence of Pulmonary Diseases

Lung diseases are some of the most common medical conditions that include airway diseases, lung tissue diseases, and lung circulation diseases and pose massive burden on health care in the world. Chronic lower respiratory diseases such as chronic obstructive pulmonary disease (COPD), chronic bronchitis, and emphysema are a leading cause of death in the United States. According to the American Lung Association, 16.4 million Americans were affected by any form of COPD, bronchitis, and emphysema in 2018.[8] Lung cancer is the second most common cancer worldwide and most common cause of cancer death in 2020.[9] Infectious lung diseases such as coronavirus (COVID-19), influenza, and tuberculosis are highly contagious illnesses that have widespread impacts on global health and economy.

3.2.2 Establishment of Air-Liquid Interface Model

The lung parenchyma comprises a large number of thin-walled alveoli that are involved with gas transfer via the rhythmic process of inspiration and expiration (Figure 3.1).[10] The alveolar wall comprises epithelium which lines the alveolus or air space, interstitium with connective and elastic tissues, and capillary endothelium.[11] Gas exchange occurs in the alveoli across the thin epithelial lining, fused basement membrane, and adjacent endothelium (air-blood barrier). The lung parenchyma has traditionally been considered relatively difficult to model in vitro. The development of lung-on-a-chip technology has evolved quickly to facilitate drug discovery and disease modeling of lungs. Air-liquid interface (ALI) is the basic unit of most in vitro biomimetic human respiratory system models. ALI replicates the human gaseous exchange paradigm in the lungs by exposing the basal layer of epithelial cells to the liquid, mimicking human alveolar epithelial-blood interface, whereas the apical end is exposed to air, mimicking exposure of alveolar cells to the air. This results in the formation of three layers that define the ALI, the respiratory airway niche, the respiratory epithelial/pseudo-epithelial cell layer beneath it and the liquid media (Figure 3.1). This simple unit has been employed since the late 1990s to develop relatively simple in vitro lung models to study epithelial cell-to-cell signaling, respiratory disease modelling, and respiratory regeneration, etc. For instance, a normal human tracheobronchial epithelial (NHTBE) cell-based ALI was developed by seeding NHTBE cells on a semi-permeable membrane to study the impact of different regulatory factors on airways secretion phenotypes, mucin, lysozyme, and secretory leukocyte protease inhibitor secretion, and gene expression.[12] A similar semi-permeable membrane seeded with human umbilical vein endothelial cells (HUVEC) on the basolateral side of the insert and epithelial cells on its apical surface was recently used to study the key signaling mechanisms between human airway epithelial and endothelial cells when exposed to double-stranded RNA to simulate viral lung infections.[13]

3.2.3 Evolution in Lung-on-a-Chip Fabrication and Complexity

3.2.3.1 Inception of microfluidics-based lung-on-a-chip model

Modern day lung-on-a-chip was developed based on the sophistication of microfluidics engineering technology, which allows the manipulation of fluids such as artificial blood at the sub-millimeter scale inside hollow microfluidic channels. Generally, a 3D network of hollow tubes inside of a silicone rubber with a size of microscope slide is produced by layering a photosensitive material onto silicon, and ultraviolet light is used to etch grooves in a pre-designed pattern into silicon rubber, and cells of the desired types are seeded and linked to pumps and external fluid source via inlets and outlets to mimic the blood flow. Blood is substituted by well controlled nutrients, and signaling molecules, immune cells, or drugs can be perfused to mimic the blood flow into tissues and the dynamic environment in organs (Figure 3.1). The chips are transparent to allow real-time imaging of cells.

One of the earliest examples of single-channel media flow models was developed by Anastacia M. Bilek et al. as they investigated the impact of mechanical ventilation (airway collapse and re-opening) in a lung model with low or no expression of surfactant in vitro. They developed a "parallel-plate chamber", whereby the cells derived from fetal rat pulmonary epithelial cell line were grown and sandwiched between two glass slides, along with the fluid channel created underneath the cell layer within the sandwich. This channel was connected with a syringe pump that made the fluids to flow through the channel. Airway opening was simulated by introducing an air bubble into the channel that flowed through the channel, exerting pressure on the epithelial cells. The resulting cellular injury(s) were quantified by exposing damaged/dead cells with ethidium homodimer-1 that binds to the DNA of damaged or dead cells and produces fluorescence.[14] Huh et al. reported a two microchannel media flow models, both interconnected by a thin polyester membrane with 400-nm pores. The top channel accommodated the epithelial cells layer, and once media was removed, it served as the ALI compartment, whereas lower channel was connected to the syringe pump, which made the media to flow continuously through it at 15 µl/hr. They introduced a liquid plug in the upper channel (ALI) and made it to flow through it, therefore exposing epithelial cells to the plug which led to injury of small airway epithelial cells by generating deleterious fluid mechanical stresses.[15]

The first organ-level human breathing lung-on-a-chip with a size of 1–2 cm in length was developed in Donald E. Ingber's lab (Figure 3.2)[16] This seminal work is considered as a landmark achievement not just in lung-on-a-chip development but also in organs-on-chips progress. This dynamic, mechanically relevant, and physiologically complex lung-on-a-chip was able to mimic human alveolar-capillary interface by separating a microfluidic channel by a 10-µm thick, porous poly(dimethylsiloxane) (PDMS) membrane, giving rise to two independent channels. The porous PDMS was

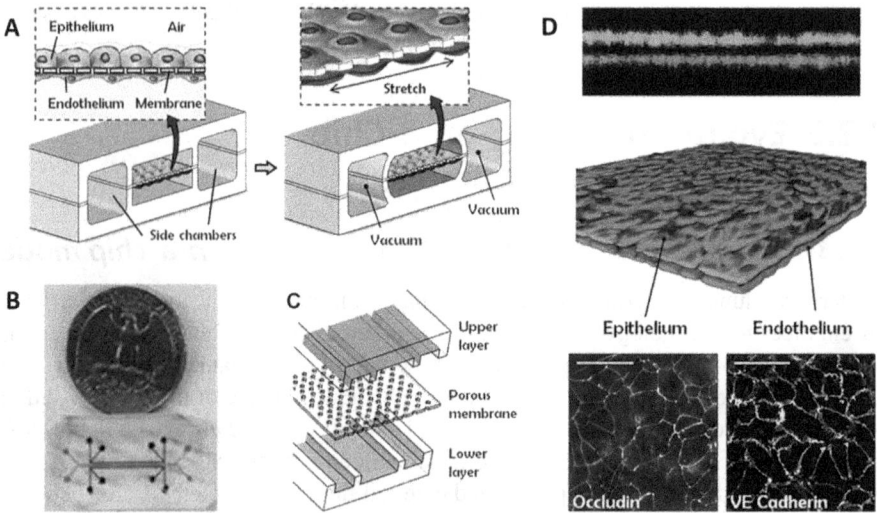

FIGURE 3.2 The schematic design and microfabrication of the first human breathing lung-on-a-chip. (A) The breathing lung-on-a-chip mimics the human alveolar-capillary interface by separating parallel microfluidic channels with a 10-µm thick, porous poly(dimethylsiloxane) (PDMS) membrane coated with an extracellular matrix. Vacuum was applied to the side chambers to cause mechanical stretching of the PDMS membrane to replicate the in vivo mechanical process of breathing. (B) Image of the size of lung-on-a-chip device of 1–2 cm in length and a few millimeters in width. (C) Three PDMS layers are aligned and bonded to form compartmentalized chambers. The PDMS membrane contains an array of microfabricated 10-µm diameter pores. (D) The breathing lung-on-a-chip forms an alveolar-capillary barrier on a PDMS membrane, and an intact single layer of the alveolar epithelium (stained with CellTracker Green) and microvascular endothelium (stained with CellTracker Red) were formed on the opposite side of the membrane. Intercellular junctional protein occludin or vascular endothelial cadherin (VE cadherin) were exhibited on epithelium or endothelium, respectively. Scale bar, 25 µm. (Reprinted with permission from Huh et al. (2010). Copyright 2021 AAAS).

employed because of its flexibility, inertness, and stress-bearing capacity. After coating PDMS membrane with extracellular matrix (ECM) proteins, the top side was seeded with human alveolar epithelial cells and the bottom side with human pulmonary microvascular endothelial cells. Since both channels were independent of each other, both cell types could have been exposed with their respective cell culture conditions. Two lateral microchambers were also included in the design to mimic alveolar events that occur during normal breathing. With the application and release of vacuum in the lateral chambers, the PDMS based system stretched and relaxed respectively, thereby replicating the in vivo mechanical process of breathing (Figure 3.2). Air flowed through the epithelial chamber, replicating ALI whereas endothelial chamber was continuously exposed to the flowing fluid, mimicking blood flow. They also demonstrated that on exposure to irritants, epithelial cells and endothelial cells expressed relevant biomarkers, as in vivo.[16] The tissue-tissue interface consisted of a monolayer of alveolar epithelium closely opposed to single layer microvascular endothelium, both of which contain the tight junction proteins such as occludin and vascular endothelial cadherin, thus preserving the permeability barrier function as in vivo (Figure 3.2).[16]

3.2.3.2 Challenges and further advancements in lung-on-a-chip fabrication, including 3D bioprinting

Lung-on-a-chip can be implemented in various stages of drug discovery and development such as disease modelling, drug screening, PK/PD modelling, drug delivery system evaluation, toxicology testing, and personalized therapy. Features and applications of most of the examples discussed below have been summarized in Table 3.1. A major shortcoming of the human breathing lung-on-a-chip was that there was no control over the exposure of oxygen and carbon dioxide in the airway channel. As alveoli are dynamic gas exchange units of the lungs, any system that would replicate alveoli should also be able to control oxygen and carbon dioxide exchange. To address this issue, Long et al. designed a PDMS microfluidic-based artificial alveolus. This "alveolus" was designed in such a way that the fluid entering the chamber mimicked venous blood (high carbon dioxide content) and the fluid exiting from the other side corresponded to arterial blood (high in oxygen content). They also connected the exiting channel with sensors to detect the dissolved gases.[17] Sellgren et al. reported the fabrication of a more complex lung-on-a-chip model comprising of three microfluidic channels, each with its own layer of primary cells. All three channels were stacked vertically, separated by nanoporous polymeric membranes. The apical channel had primary human airway epithelial cells layer running across its length; the central channel comprised of primary human lung fibroblasts and a layer of human lung microvascular endothelial cells were grown in the basolateral channel. This human lung airway (bronchiole) chip replicated the three layered (epithelia, fibroblasts, and endothelia) morphology in in vitro system, complemented with the microfluidic channels.[18]

Huang et al. fabricated a reversed-engineered human alveolar lung-on-a-chip using a 3D porous hydrogel.[19] They packed alginate microbeads into a cubic lattice pattern and filled the void spaces with 7% gelatin methacryloyl (scaffold due to its biocompatibility, ability to undergo photo cross-linking and gelatin's established profile as ECM polymer) to give rise to alveoli-like structures. After cross-linking gelatin methacryloyl, alginate microbeads were removed by treating the 3D system with ethylene diamine tetraacetic acid disodium (EDTA) solution, leaving behind the 3D alveolar structures of gelatin methacryloyl. The primary human alveolar epithelial cells were seeded to the 3D alveolar structure to form functional cells layer. Since these 3D alveolar sac structures were bonded in PDMS chip, they were also able to simulate the normal breathing patterns by forcing PDMS with rhythmic impulse by mechanical actuation. Hence the mechanical properties of the fabricated sacs were found to be closely related to that in vivo.[19]

Zamprogno et al. recently reported a second-generation lung-on-a-chip with an array of stretchable alveoli fabricated by replacing silicon based PDMS membrane with biodegradable and stretchable ECM based membrane made of collagen and elastin.[20] In contrast to the first-generation PDMS-based membrane made by the top-down approach (photolithography), this ECM membrane was fabricated based on a bottom-up approach

TABLE 3.1 Summary of the features of representative lung-on-a-chip models

EPITHELIAL LAYER CELL TYPE(S)	ENDOTHELIAL LAYER CELL TYPE(S)	INTERFACE MEMBRANE MATERIAL(S)	DEVICE DESIGN	APPLICATION(S)	REF
Human alveolar epithelial cells	Human pulmonary microvascular endothelial cells	PDMS	Two microchannels, one with epithelial and other with endothelial cells layers, separated by porous membrane	Emulate human lung functions in vitro	16
Primary human airway epithelial cells	Human lung microvascular endothelial cells	Polyetrafluoroethylene Polyester Polycarbonate	Three microchannels, apical with epithelial, middle with fibroblast and basolateral with endothelial cells layers, vertically stacked and separated by porous membranes	Relatively complex chip; to enhance physiological relevance	18
Primary human alveolar epithelial cells	Primary human lung endothelial cells	Collagen, elastin matrix	Drop-casting the solution of elastin and collagen on to a gold mesh, which formed a thin film within mesh, maintained by surface tension. The film is strong enough to seed and grow cells	Better lung biomimicking properties due to use of extracellular matrix mimetic membrane	20
Human airway epithelial cell line Calu-3	N/A	Polycarbonate	PDMS casted onto the 3D-printed mold and allowed to set, which possessed the desired patterns of microchannel and other parts	Emulate air-liquid interface Effects of cigarette smoke on epithelial layer inflammation	21

(Continued)

TABLE 3.1 (CONTINUED) Summary of the features of representative lung-on-a-chip models

EPITHELIAL LAYER CELL TYPE(S)	ENDOTHELIAL LAYER CELL TYPE(S)	INTERFACE MEMBRANE MATERIAL(S)	DEVICE DESIGN	APPLICATION(S)	REF
human bronchial epithelial cell line 16HBE, co-cultures with lung carcinoma epithelial cells A549	Human umbilical vein endothelial cells	PDMS	multi-organ microfluidic chip, "lung cancer organ" and three downstream "distant organ chambers"	Developed and demonstrated viability of lung cancer metastasis to bone, brain and liver	24
Co-cultured H1975 non-small cell lung cancer cell with human lung epithelial cells	human lung microvascular endothelial cells	Polyethylene terephthalate	Similar to[16]	The impact of changes in breathing movements on the tumor development within the chip microenvironment	25
Human alveolar epithelial cells	Human lung microvascular endothelial cells	PDMS	Similar to[16]	In vitro disease model of pulmonary edema Drug testing	27
Primary human airway epithelial cells	Primary human lung microvascular endothelial cells	Polyester	Similar to[16]	In-vitro disease model of pulmonary inflammation	28
Primary human alveolar epithelial cells	Human umbilical vascular endothelial cells	PDMS	Similar to,[16] however almost double the width of each chamber. Endothelial cells stimulated by inflammatory factors, then platelets containing blood introduced for thrombus formation	In vitro thrombus formation model Drug testing	29

(Continued)

TABLE 3.1 (CONTINUED)   Summary of the features of representative lung-on-a-chip models

EPITHELIAL LAYER CELL TYPE(S)	ENDOTHELIAL LAYER CELL TYPE(S)	INTERFACE MEMBRANE MATERIAL(S)	DEVICE DESIGN	APPLICATION(S)	REF
Primary human lung bronchial-airway epithelial basal stem cells	Primary human pulmonary microvascular endothelial cells	PDMS	Similar to[16]	In vitro Influenza A and SARS-CoV-2 model Drug testing	30
A549 pulmonary epithelial cells	Human umbilical vein endothelial cells	Polyester	Similar to[16]	Pharmacokinetic analysis of the aerosol formulation	31
Human Pulmonary Alveolar Epithelial Cells	Human umbilical vein endothelial cells	Matrigel	Matrigel channel serves as ECM-mimetic connection between epithelial (alveolar) and endothelial (vascular) channels	Evaluation of inhaled pollutants	34

by surface tension force. The ECM membrane was formed by drop-casting the solution of elastin and collagen on to a gold mesh. The proteins solution spread itself within the mesh as thin film, which was maintained by surface tension. These films were able to support the growth of primary human alveolar epithelial cells from patients co-cultured with primary human lung endothelial cells on both sides for weeks, and the epithelial cells on membrane expressed typical biomarkers of alveolar epithelia, including tight junction markers. As collagen is one of the most abundant type of ECM present in connective tissues, elastin can add elasticity which is important for maintaining continuous breathing motions of lung. By tuning the collagen and elastin ratios, the membrane was tailored to recreate the native viscoelastic microenvironment of the lung, with less nonspecific absorption and adsorption of small molecules encountered by the PDMS membranes. All these features rendered the device more biomimetic, thus employing it would yield more reliable and physiologically relatable models.[20]

A 3D bioprinting-based lung-on-a-chip was designed by fabricating the 3D-printed resin molds for PDMS casting using computer-aided-design (CAD) and a digital light processing (DLP) 3D-printer, which projects a UV wavelength through the resin on the resin bath. Once fabricated, the 3D-printed resin mold underwent surface treatment including oxygen plasma and silanization treatment to avoid PDMS sticking, then PDMS was cast onto the mold and allowed to set. The resulting PDMS chip possessed the desired patterns of microchannel and other parts.[21] This low-cost 3D printed fabrication technique allows the lung-on-a-chip to be fabricated in less a day and the molds can be used for repeated PDMS casting.

3.2.4 Application of Lung-on-a-Chip in Modeling of Lung Cancer Growth

Xu et al. developed an efficient lung-on-a-chip lung cancer model and showed the ability of the system to perform high-throughput screening of the drugs. They constructed a device with four microfluidic chip units integrated to each other via a common medium inlet pump. Each chip was further seeded with human non-small cell lung cancer cell (SPCA-1), co-culture of human lung fibroblast cells (HFL1) and SPCA-1 cells, and co-culture of freshly isolated primary lung cancer cells and stromal cells from patients with squamous carcinoma and adenocarcinoma. Each unit further had three cell culture chambers. The dynamic design allowed the perfusion of the drug(s) and media separately in each unit. They verified the viability of the cell-seeded chambers in each unit by assessing the cellular morphologies and squamous and adenocarcinomas biomarkers. In this way, they were able to establish the complex lung-on-a-chip lung cancer model system with four different cell groups in parallel.[22]

Jing Kong et al. developed an organ-on-a-chip model to replicate the metastasis of circulating tumor cells (CTC) to four organs, including lungs in vitro. The device consisted of four layers, with supporting base layer made from glass, over it the PDMS layer with four organ chambers, over which the porous membrane seeded with HUVECs and the top layer made of PDMS with four channels running over each organ chamber with CTCs. They used cells from MCF-7, MDA-MB-231, and ACC-M cell lines as CTCs.

To develop biomimetic organ chambers, primary cells derived from mouse organs were seeded in their respective organ chambers on the chip and the metastatic potential of the CTCs were assessed and compared among the organs.[23] Xu et al. also developed a simpler, but more effective, lung cancer metastasis lung-on-a-chip model. This micro-fluidic chip consisted of three PDMS layers, irreversibly bonded to each other in such a way that it gave rise to two organ-mimetic chambers; the upstream chamber replicated the lung tumor environment, and the downstream chamber established bone, brain and liver mimicking areas. They used A549 lung cancer cell line as model cells to assess the metastasis and verified the metastatic viability of the chip by immunofluorescence imaging of the epithelial-to-mesenchymal transition (EMT) and mesenchymal-to-epithelial transition (MET) markers.[24]

Hassell et al. developed an orthotopic lung cancer model. In the upper chamber, they seeded H1975 non-small cell lung cancer (NSCLC) with the alveolar epithelial cells at a ratio of approximately 1:100, whereas the lower chamber was seeded with endothelial cells to establish ALI. Because the chip had two side chambers, they used them to control breathing movements. The model was assessed for its viability by assessing the tumor density of GFP-labeled NSCLC cells via confocal microscopy. They also determined the impact of changes in breathing movements on the tumor development within the chip microenvironment.[25] Yang et al. used electro-spun poly(lactic-glycolic Acid) (PLGA) nanofibrous membrane as a substrate of cell attachment in a lung-on-a-chip to model lung cancer. To recapitulate the alveolar lung cancer microenvironment, they co-cultured A549 lung cancer cells, HFL1 cells, and HUVECs on the PLGA nanofibrous membrane. The cells viability was assessed by analyzing the morphology of cells and immunofluorescence staining of the respective markers of the cell lines used.[26] All these lung-on-a-chip have potential applications in modeling lung cancer in vitro.

3.2.5 Application of Lung-on-a-Chip in Modeling of Responses to Aerosolized Drugs and Nanoparticle Treatment

The first organ-level human breathing lung-on-a-chip developed in Donald E. Ingber's lab has been used to evaluate toxicity associated inhaled aerosol nanoparticles (Figure 3.2).[16] When alveolar epithelial cells with mechanical strain applied to mimic the breathing movement were exposed to ultrafine 12-nm silica nanoparticles, the reactive oxygen species (ROS) production was increased, the underlying endothelium in the microvascular channel became activated through up-regulation of leukocyte adhesion molecule ICAM-1 to induce endothelial capture of circulating neutrophils. This ROS response was not induced by treatment with gold nanoparticles, single-walled carbon nanotubes, polystyrene nanoparticles, or polyethylene glycol-coated quantum dots. This device demonstrates that physiological breathing movement enhances epithelial and endothelial uptake of nanoparticles that were introduced into the alveolar space; this observation was confirmed when a whole mouse lung ventilation-perfusion model showed the physiological breathing accentuates nanoparticle transport from the alveoli into the microvasculature.[16]

3.2.6 Application of Lung-on-a-Chip in Modeling of Pulmonary Edema and Lung Inflammation

The same lung-on-a-chip developed in Ingber's lab was adapted to model dose-limiting toxicity of interleukin-2 (IL-2)-induced edema.[27] The device contained human alveolar epithelial and pulmonary microvascular endothelial cells cultured in two parallel microchannels separated by a thin, porous membrane coated with ECM proteins. A clinically relevant dose of IL-2 was perfused through the microvascular channel, and an imaging study demonstrated that the IL-2 caused liquid in the microvascular channel to leak into the previously air-filled alveolar chamber and eventually fill the entire air space. IL-2, perfused together with human blood plasma proteins prothrombin and fluorescently labelled fibrinogen, induced formation of fibrin clots on the apical side of the alveolar epithelium. The chip also showed that direct toxic effects of IL-2 on endothelial and epithelial cells were amplified by mechanical breathing motions, which could not be discovered under static 2D culture condition. Based on this novel finding about the mechanical contribution to the IL-2-induced pulmonary edema, GSK2193874, an inhibitor of TRPV4 channel that were activated by mechanical strain, was found to prevent pulmonary edema induced by the IL-2 in the lung-on-a-chip model.[27] The study illustrated that in vitro lung-on-a-chip not only can model the lung disease but also produce mechanistic discovery of new pharmaceutical agents to treat lung disease.

Airway inflammatory diseases were modeled using a human lung small airway-on-a-chip in vitro model.[28] The microfluidic device contained fully differentiated pseudostratified mucociliary airway epithelium cultured on top of a porous collagen-coated membrane at an air-liquid interface in the upper channel and the pulmonary microvascular endothelium below the membrane with flowing medium that feeds both tissue layers (Figure 3.3A). The differentiated airway epithelium exhibited tight junctional connections, and the pulmonary endothelium also formed continuous adherens junctions between adjacent cells on chip. The epithelium formed from cells isolated from the primary airway epithelium of humans contained many ciliated epithelial cells and mucus-producing goblet cells, club cells, and basal cells, similarly to those found in humans (Figure 3.1), thus recapitulating human lung bronchioles. This airway-on-a-chip was used to model asthma by culturing the differentiated epithelium in the presence of IL-13, which led to significant increase in the number of goblet cells, secretion of the inflammatory cytokines G-CSF and GM-CSF into the vascular channel, and decrease in cilia beating frequency. This airway-on-a-chip was also used to model COPD by exposure of the airway epithelium to the viral mimic and lipopolysaccharide (LPS) endotoxin, which triggered proinflammatory responses such as increased secretion of IL-8 and M-CSF in the chip.[28] Jain et al. developed an alveolar lung-on-a-chip model system to replicate in vivo pulmonary thrombus formation, which results in high chances of mortality in humans. They established the ALI via alveolar epithelial cells and HUVECs seeded compartments separated by ECM coated porous membrane. All walls of the endothelial compartment were completely covered by the HUVECs, so that the platelets would not adhere to the ECM coating. The thrombus formation, instead, was initiated by stimulating endothelial cells by treating them with TNF-α before the blood flow. As a result of this stimulation, platelets started adhering to the endothelial

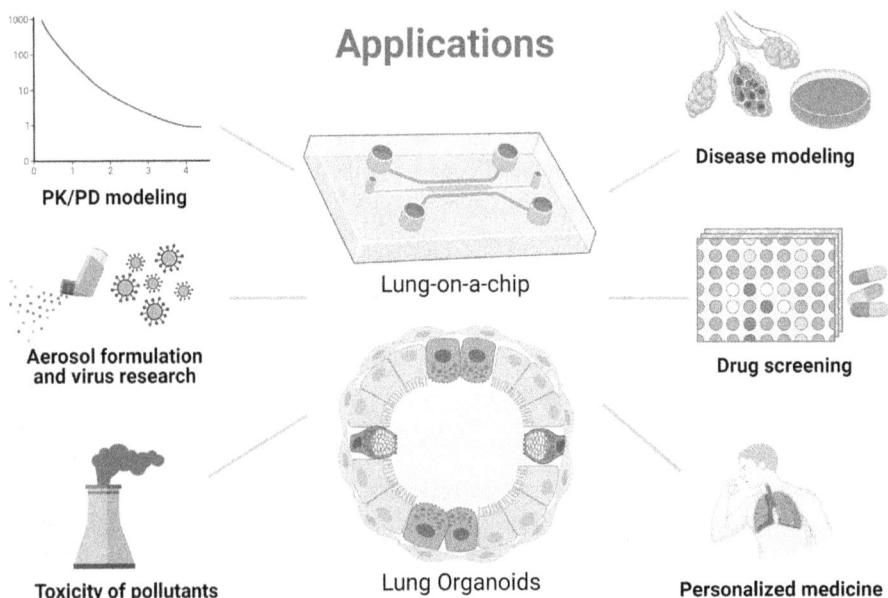

FIGURE 3.3 Utility of the lung-on-a-chip and lung organoids in basic drug discovery and development, and toxicology applications. The chip and organoid models share commons applications, except the PK/PD modeling which is thus far associated with lung-on-a-chip only.

linings and gradually grow, replicating the thrombus formation in this microfluidic device.[29] These studies demonstrate that lung-on-a-chip can be used as a discovery tool to study the mechanisms and identify therapeutic agents for various lung pathology, suggesting the potential of using the chip as a powerful tool for preclinical drug discovery.

3.2.7 Application of Lung-on-a-Chip in Modeling of Lung Infection and Identification of Antiviral Therapeutics

In 2021, Ingber et al. employed the strategy of lung-on-a-chip model developed previously in his lab[16] to develop influenza A and SARS-CoV-2 disease models and further test the antiviral drugs efficacy by biomimicking the in vivo disease environment.[30] The bronchial-airway-on-chip was developed by seeding epithelial compartment with differentiating human bronchial epithelial cells and pulmonary endothelial cells in the bottom compartment, which led to the establishment of ALI. To further replicate the in vivo bronchial microenvironment response to viruses, the chip was exposed to immune cells as well. Six strains of influenza A viruses were used to develop the influenza viral models, whereas SARS-CoV-2 pseudo-particles (SARS-CoV-2pp) were designed that contain the SARS-CoV-2 spike (S) protein assembled onto luciferase reporter gene-carrying retroviral core particles. By using SARS-CoV-2 pseudo-particles and not the full virus, they established the viability of the chip at BSL-2 culturing conditions, instead of much more expensive and stringent BSL-3 conditions required for virus study.[30] This chip was used for screening drugs that can prevent SARS-CoV-2 infection. While clinically relevant doses of the antimalarial drug amodiaquine inhibited infection in the chip, clinical doses of hydroxychloroquine that inhibit the entry of pseudotyped SARS-CoV-2 in cell lines under static condition did not inhibit SARS-CoV-2 infection in this human airway-on-a-chip model.[30] This application highlights the utility of lung-on-a-chip for rapid identification of antiviral therapeutics and prophylactics.

3.2.8 Application of Multi-Organ-Chip in Pharmacokinetics (PK) and Pharmacodynamics (PD) Modeling

The ability to quantitatively predict the drug PK (absorption, distribution, metabolism, and excretion) and PD in human based on in vitro analysis and animal PK studies is of paramount importance in drug development and drug regimen design for phase I clinical trials. Frost et al. generated aerosols of various compounds including dextran and insulin using a jet nebulizer. The aerosol flows were driven through a microfluidic bilayer device establishing an ALI to mimic the blood-air barrier. This microfluidic device consisted of two stacked microchannels and separated by a porous PDMS membrane. The aerosol system was connected to the top channel while the bottom channel was connected to a syringe pump to drive media across the microdevice. The permeability of several compounds across epithelial/endothelial barriers were measured. Concentration-time profiles were established in this microfluidic device with A549 cells; standard PK parameters such as the area under the curve (AUC), maximum concentration (C_{max}), and time to maximum concentration (T_{max}) were derived from the constructed curve.[31] Considering only A549 cells were used in this model, the PK analysis can be deemed as overly simplified.

In 2020, Ingber's research team showed that physiological PK modeling of the first-pass drug absorption, metabolism, and excretion of two drugs nicotine and cisplatin using in vitro data generated from multiple microfluidically linked two-channel organ chips.[32] They tested and simulated oral nicotine PK using human organ-chip of the gut, liver, and kidney as a first-pass model. This gut, liver, and kidney chip contained apical parenchymal and basal vascular compartments connected through their vascular endothelium-linked fluid channel. The arteriovenous reservoir was integrated into the fluid path to mimic the systemic circulation and enable mixing nicotine at clinically relevant concentration. The endothelium-lined vascular channels of multi-organ system was perfused with a common "blood substitute" comprising an optimized endothelial cell medium containing serum, while the parenchymal channel of each organ chip was perfused with different epithelium cell medium. This multi-organ-chip allowed the simulation of systemic drug transport between different organs and drug diffusion at the endothelium-parenchymal tissue interface. A major advantage of employing this chip is that drug concentrations within the vascular channels of the device can be frequently sampled and measured by mass spectrometry, which enables building an oral nicotine PK model by taking into consideration multiple factors including drug passive permeability, efflux, metabolism, plasma protein binding, pKa, pH, blood flow rates, and dimensions of major vessels to computationally predict nicotine PK and distribution in humans in a quantitative manner.[32] Similarly, a fluidically coupled, bone marrow, liver, and kidney multi-organ-chip was built to mimic the intravenous administered cisplatin by directly applying drug into the arteriovenous reservoir and carry out PK and PD analysis in vitro by detecting cisplatin-induced myeloid toxicity. Both chips and computer simulated PK models predicted the human PK reasonably well, yielding in vitro to in vivo extrapolation (IVIVE).[32] While this fluidically linked (vascularized) multi-organ chips did not contain lung chip, it is reasonable to assume that the integration of lung to the multi-organ chip is feasible to allow for quantitative prediction of human PK and PD of drugs, as Ingber's group has developed multiple vascularized organ chips (heart, lung, liver, kidney, intestine, skin, blood-brain barrier, and brain).[32]

3.2.9 Application of Lung-on-a-Chip in Toxicology Studies

Traditionally, the pulmonary toxicology assessment relies on histopathological and biochemical investigation of experimental animals following acute or long-term repeated inhalation exposures of inhalation hazards.[33] The lung-on-a-chip technology provides a low-cost, more efficient, and less complex model compared to animal models for pulmonary toxicity studies. The 3D chip can recapitulate the structural features of the air-blood barrier better than a cell monolayer (such as immortalized type II alveolar epithelial cells A549) that lack lung microenvironment when studying various air pollutants. Xu et al. used a lung-on-a-chip to study the toxicity of fine particle matters <2.5 μm (PM2.5) on the alveolar-capillary barrier.[34] The chip consisted of three parallel interconnected channels; the lung side was seeded with human pulmonary alveolar epithelial cells derived from primary type 2 pneumocytes, the vessel side was seeded with HUVECs, while the middle channel was used for Matrigel infusion to provide the extracellular matrix for the epithelial and endothelial cells. The chip allowed assessment of the barrier function after exposure to PM2.5 from the lung side. The dose-response relationship between PM2.5 exposure and permeability of the alveolar-capillary barrier was established. The observed cytotoxicity and ROS production of PM2.5 on endothelial and epithelial cells support PM2.5 induced lung injury. Also, immune and inflammatory responses triggered by PM2.5 toxicity were evidenced by TNF-α upregulation and cytokines secretion from alveolar epithelial cells, suggesting a direct communication between the lung epithelial cell and the endothelial cells in the chip.[34] Similarly, Guan et al. observed a significant increase in the secretion of the inflammatory cytokines, higher cells apoptosis, and increased levels of ROS when exposing the PM2.5 on an alveolar-capillary chip, constructed with A549 in the top chamber and HUVECs in the bottom chamber and separated by a layer of porous polycarbonate membrane.[35] The lung-on-a-chip model has also been used for studying the nanoparticle toxicity, as the small size of nanoparticles allows them to penetrate deeper in the alveolar cavity. Zhang et al. used a human pulmonary alveolar epithelial cell and HUVECs based alveolar-capillary chip to investigate the inorganic nanoparticles' pulmonary toxicity.[36] They exposed the alveolar side to ZnO nanoparticles and found that ZnO nanoparticles caused disruption of the alveolar-capillary barrier function, decreased expression of adherent junction proteins, and increased the permeability of the barrier on the chip in a dose-dependent manner. In contrast, TiO_2 nanoparticles showed a limited effect on the barrier integrity in the same chip model. These results are consistent with the notion that that ZnO nanoparticles are more toxic than TiO_2 nanoparticles against mammalian cells; TiO_2 nanoparticles are recognized as a relative safer nanomaterial.[36] Together, these studies demonstrate that the lung-on-a-chip can be a valuable tool for investigating the toxicity of environmental pollutants and nanoparticles.

The conventional rodent-based animal models are not suitable for studying the human immunotoxicity due to the species differences in the immunological responses. Organ-on-chip model can potentially overcome this limitation and offers a tool for toxicological studies of immunotherapy. In 2021, Kerns et al. developed an alveolus lung-on-a-chip for safety assessment of a T-cell engaging bispecific antibody, an immune-oncology agent, as the chip-controlled environment could better capture the interaction between the antibody, immune cells, and antigen-expressing cells. The chip consisted of a top channel seeded with epithelial cells, a bottom channel seeded with endothelial cells, and a porous membrane coated with an ECM between the two parallel channels. They added peripheral mononuclear blood cells to the epithelial channel to have direct contact with the mature alveolar cells, rendering chip immunocompetent and allowing antibody to exert its action. The safety profile of antibody was evaluated through quantifying apoptosis in epithelial cells, T-cell activation, measurements of multiplex cytokines in the epithelial channel supernatant, and quantification of immune cells present in chip and their attachment to target epithelium cells post-treatment.[37] This immunocompetent chip model could reproduce and predict antigen target-dependent safety liabilities of the antibody. The ability of lung-on-a-chip to recreate complex multifactorial immune microenvironment of lung will allow modeling immune-related toxicities, facilitating the safety evaluation of immuno-oncology drugs, and providing mechanistic insights of immunotoxicity.

3.2.10 Further Challenges and Future Directions in Lung-on-a-Chip Development

While lung-on-a-chip developed thus far can emulate in-vivo bioenvironment in in-vitro settings. it is still in its nascent to adolescent stage. To fully recapitulate the in vivo microenvironment, the chip would have to be constructed with the increased level of complexity. Tissues and organs are usually a mix of multiple cell types, orderly arranged together in a very specific way by the ECM. Intercellular signaling or crosstalk via biochemical and/or biophysical cues also impact hugely in the way each cell behaves. Better control over distribution of cells of different types within the chip can be implemented. Multiple other factors such as the mechanical strength of the tissue that can impact the anatomy and physiological functioning of organs should be taken into consideration when constructing chips. More physiologically relevant, chemically defined ECM biomaterials other than PDMS should be explored. An ideal, biomimetic organ-on-a-chip would have an epithelial layer in 3D, with the histologically similar arrangement of epithelial cells of all cell types found in the tissue/organ. Although organoids are yet to fully recapitulate the human organs, they are usually complex enough to be used as models for the organs. Therefore, a biomimetic organoids-on-a-chip device that combines the strengths of both microfluidic properties of the chip and biologic complexity of the organoids will bring new levels of innovation and broad application as potential pre-clinical models for organ and disease models.

3.3 APPLICATION OF LUNG ORGANOIDS IN DISEASE MODELING AND DRUG TARGETING

In addition to organs-on-chips, organoids are another alternative 3D model to mimic organs in the laboratory. Organoids represent self-organizing 3D functional units that consist of multiple cell types originated from stem cells to mimic the physiological state of the original tissue including 3D architecture, cell-type composition, and genetic and molecular characteristics.[6,7,38] Organoids are usually a few millimeters across, much smaller than the actual organ. Organoids often promote and maintain the physiological relevant cell differentiation, morphological and biochemical features, and tissue organization, not possible in conventional 2D cell culture model. Thus, organoids can complement 2D cell culture and animal models in studying diseases, human development, drug therapies, and facilitating personalized therapy design.

3.3.1 Human Lung Organoids Derived from Primary Human Lung Epithelium Cells and Human Bronchioalveolar Stem Cells

Organoids build on a foundation of stem cell technology and can be established from induced pluripotent stem cells (iPSCs) or isolated organ progenitors that differentiate to an organ-like tissue.[38] A variety of organoids have been developed including lung organoids.[39–42] Human airways are covered with a continuous epithelial sheet. From the developmental perspective, the lung epithelium is derived from the endodermal germ layer, which undergoes a complex series of signaling events to generate the network of airways (bronchi, bronchioles) and gas-exchanging units (alveoli).[42] The respiratory epithelium in trachea and bronchi consists of cell types including a layer of basal cells, secretory cells including goblet cells and club cells, and cilia cells (Figure 3.1). The basal cells are stem/progenitor cells that differentiate into other cell types of normal epithelium to maintain and restore a healthy epithelial cell layer. Goblet cells and club cells secrete mucins and glycoproteins to trap airway pathogens and debris. The ciliated cells are located across the apical surface of respiratory epithelium and facilitate the movement of mucus across the respiratory track. The mucociliary clearance system helps to remove lung pathogens and large particulates inhaled from the environment.[7,42]

In the lung, a variety of culture protocols have been developed in the last decade to generate and culture lung organoids to mimic structure and function of lung. Lung organoids are generated mainly by cultivating human primary airway cells or precisely directing the differentiation of iPSCs.[7] In 1993, Benali et al. developed the first self-organizing 3D cultures of adult human airway epithelium. Human surface respiratory epithelial cells from nasal polyps were cultured within 3D collagen gel and soluble factors such as epidermal growth factor (EGF) in a serum-free defined medium for 12 days. Tubular lumens formed with ciliated cells, secretory cells, and undifferentiated cells.[43] In 2012, Wong et al. described an in vitro directed differentiation protocol for generation of lung organoids from human iPSCs. Carefully timed treatment by exogenous growth factors followed by air-liquid interface culture resulted in maturation of patches of a tight junction-coupled differentiated airway epithelium.[44] In 2014, Dye et al. described a stepwise differentiation of human iPSCs into lung organoids by careful manipulation of developmental signaling pathways of human iPSCs.[45] This lung organoid possessed an upper airway-like epithelium with basal cells and immature ciliated cells surrounded by smooth muscle and myofibroblasts and resembled human fetal lung based on global transcriptional analysis.[45] In 2017, Chen et al. reported the generation from human iPSCs of lung bud organoids that contained mesoderm and pulmonary endoderm and develop into branching airway and early alveolar structure when cultured with Matrigel in transwell culture. RNA-seq analysis showed that lung organoids express lung specific genes and markers.[46]

One of the most most-utilized procedures of lung organoids construction from human iPSCs was published in *Nature Protocols* by Miller et al.[42] The human lung organoids were generated in 50–85 days, and bud tip progenitor organoids were built up in 22 days. The resultant human lung organoids included structures and types of cells similar to the bronchial of the growing human respiratory system surrounded by lung mesenchyme and alveolar cells. The bud tip progenitor organoids also included a population of highly proliferative multipotent cells, possessing potential to differentiate into several lineages in vitro and engraft in vivo. As a result, the human lung organoids may be utilized to simulate epithelial–mesenchymal crosstalk during human lung development, whereas the bud tip progenitor organoids are suitable for studying epithelial fate choices. Prior to 2019, most of the culture methods only allow a short time (a few days to a few months) expansion of airway epithelium from adult human individuals in vitro. Sachs et al. developed a culture condition for long-term expansion of healthy, hereditary disease and malignant human airway epithelial organoids.[47] They collected lung tissue from patients undergoing surgery and isolated epithelial cells through mechanical and enzymatic tissue disruption, then embedded isolated cells in basement membrane extract and submerged in a well optimized medium containing specific cocktail of small molecules to activate or inhibit the major signaling pathways involved in lung differentiation. The formed pseudostratified airway organoids consisted of basal cells, mucus-producing secretory cells, and functional multi-ciliated cells. These lung organoids were shown to recapitulate morphology and function, maintaining their features for at least one year.[47]

3.3.2 Application of Patient-Derived Lung Cancer Organoids in Testing and Screening Anticancer Drugs

3D lung organoids derived from healthy and tumor tissue from lung cancer patients were established and used for a high throughput drug screening. In 2019, Kim et al. derived lung cancer organoids from patient primary lung cancer tissues and normal bronchial organoids from paired non-neoplastic airway tissues. They created a biobank containing of 80 lung cancer organoids lines from five histological subtypes of lung cancer and five normal bronchial organoids as in vitro model representing individual patients.[48] The 3D lung cancer organoids were cultured in Matrigel using minimum basal medium containing epidermal growth factor, basic fibroblast growth factor and supplement for insulin and transferrin. These lung cancer organoids were shown to maintain the histology of original cancer tissues by H&E staining and immunohistochemistry analysis and retain genetic characteristics of cancer tissues by genotyping. The lung cancer organoids recapitulated the tissue architecture of primary lung tumors and genomic alternations during long-term expansion, thus enabling in vitro patient-specific drug sensitivity testing. These lung cancer organoids responded to molecularly targeted anticancer drugs based on their genomic alternations, for instances, a BRCA2-mutant organoid respond to PARP inhibitor olaparib, and an EGFR-mutant organoid responded to EGFR inhibitor erlotinib.[48] Another report described protocols for the development of NSCLC organoids[49] from surgically resected NSCLC primary patient tissues and previously established patient-derived xenografts (PDX). These NSCLC organoids preserve mutation, copy number, and gene expression profiles of the parental tumors as evidenced by whole exome and RNA sequencing analysis and retained tumorigenicity. Combination therapy of FGFR and MEK inhibitors were selected in the FGFR1-amplifed NSCLC organoids as positive combination; organoid drug response is similar to that of the matched PDX, which is an expensive and time-consuming in vivo model. In 2021, Hu et al. developed an integrated superhydrophobic microwell array chip for high-throughput 3D culture and analysis of lung cancer organoids derived from 103 surgically resected lung tumor samples, including adenocarcinomas, squamous cell carcinomas, and small cell lung cancers.[50] This microwell array chip containing 108 microwells replaced the conventional 96-well microplate for culturing organoids and measuring the responses of lung cancer organoids to various anticancer drugs in the nanoliter scale, thus improving the throughput. One-week drug sensitivity tests recapitulate patient responses to the chemotherapies and targeted therapy drugs.[50] Together, these results support the research that lung cancer organoids can be used as reliable in vitro tools for preclinical drug testing of effective drugs in a personalized setting.

3.3.3 Application of Lung Organoids in Modeling Lung Infections and Antiviral Drugs

In the era of COVID-19 pandemic and the increased importance of respiratory viruses nowadays, Salahudeen et al. established a long-term chemically defined culture system for distal lung progenitors as organoids derived from single adult human alveolar epithelial type II cells or basal cells. These lung organoids were used to model SARS-CoV-2 infection.[51] The basal cell organoids developed lumens lined with differentiated club and ciliated cells. The expression of SARS-CoV-2 receptor angiotensin converting enzyme receptor 2 (ACE-2) and processing protease TMPRSS2, which is important for virus entry were observed in club cells and alveolar epithelial type II cells. SARS-CoV-2 infected the cells that cover the air-exposed surface, which are rich in ACE2 receptor. SARS-CoV-2 infected about 10% of basal organoids and virus nucleocapsid protein appeared by 96 h after infection, suggesting that this organoid model can facilitate investigation of mechanisms of SARS-CoV-2 lung infection.[51] Han et al. developed a lung organoid model using human iPSCs with specific signaling agents (activin A, Y-27632, BMP4, and bFGF) to screen drugs targeting SARS-CoV-2.[52] Gene expression profiles revealed that lung organoids, specifically alveolar type II cells, were susceptible to infection with SARS-CoV-2 through the ACE-2 receptor. Using these lung organoids, they performed a high-throughput screening of FDA-approved drugs and identified imatinib and mycophenolic acid as potentially useful agents for inhibiting viral entry.[52] Other than SARS-CoV-2, various lung organoids have been used as models to study other lung pathology including respiratory viruses such as influenza virus and respiratory syncytial virus (RSV).[47,52]

3.3.4 Application of Lung Organoid in Toxicological Studies

The lung organoid model is emerging as an attractive species-specific in vitro tool for human pulmonary toxicological studies. The 3D highly ordered multicellular structures consist of a fully differentiated and functional human respiratory epithelium, including cilia and mucus layer, similar to the lining of the human airway, which enables toxicity assessment of inhaled toxicants and drug-induced lung injury.[53,54] In 2020, Narsue et al. developed mouse lung and liver organoid-based carcinogen models induced by genotoxic chemicals treatment.[55] Lung tissue was dissected from mice at five weeks of age, and lung organoids were cultured in vitro in the presence of various signaling proteins such as Noggin, Jagged-1, R-Spondin, and Matrigel ECM. The mouse lung organoids were treated with known genotoxic chemicals such as acrylamide and ethyl methanesulfonate, and the tumorigenic potential of each compound was confirmed based on histopathological evaluation of the detected enlargement of the subcutaneous nodules of lung organoids.[55] This study suggests the advantages of the application of normal tissue-derived organoids to investigate the chemical carcinogenesis comparing to the costly and laborious animal carcinogenesis model. In another study, Yamamoto et al. reported efficient generation and long-term expansion of alveolar organoids harboring alveolar stem cells derived from human iPSCs. This alveolar iPSC organoids can recapitulate alveolar epithelial type II cell-specific phenotype for drug toxicology studies. They investigated the toxicity of amiodarone (an anti-arrhythmia agent) and GNE7915 (a kinase inhibitor) that induced alveolar injury and observed lamellar bodies enlargement and morphological changes in cells in response to drug-induced toxicity.[56] Kim et al. also used human pluripotent stem cell-derived alveolar organoids to investigate the toxicity of diesel PM2.5 exposure during alveolar epithelial cells differentiation and 3D alveolar organoid development. The exposure of diesel PM2.5 caused alveolar cell differentiation disruption and led to potential alveolar toxicity. Notably, they also observed upregulation of ACE-2 (receptor for SARS-CoV-2) and its cofactor transmembrane protease serine 2 in alveolar organoids treated with diesel PM2.5,[57] suggesting the organoids are a useful model for virus research. Thus, lung organoids are considered valuable tools to perform toxicological studies and provide insights into key mechanisms of toxicity at a cellular and molecular level.

3.4 CONCLUDING REMARKS

Organs-on-chips and organoids can mimic the complex human tissue/organ in vitro and have emerged as physiologically relevant preclinical models for disease modeling, drug screening, toxicology evaluation, PK/PD modeling, drug formulation testing, and individualized therapy design (Figure 3.3). Organs-on-chips and organoids represent different yet complementary state-of-the-art approaches for mimicking the complex organs in vitro. There is a trend to combine the strength of the two technologies to build organoids-on-a-chip. Together, these emerging technologies will complement cell lines and mouse models as versatile tools to facilitate drug discovery and personalized therapy design.

COMPETING INTERESTS

The authors declare that they have no competing interests.

REFERENCES

1. Mullard, A. How much do phase III trials cost? *Nature Reviews Drug Discovery* 17(11), 777 (2018).
2. Low, L. A., Mummery, C., Berridge, B. R., Austin, C. P. & Tagle, D. A. Organs-on-chips: Into the next decade. *Nature Reviews Drug Discovery* 20(5), 345–361 (2021).
3. Jensen, C. & Teng, Y. Is it time to start transitioning from 2D to 3D cell culture? *Frontiers in Molecular Biosciences* 7, 33 (2020).
4. Hay, M., Thomas, D. W., Craighead, J. L., Economides, C. & Rosenthal, J. Clinical development success rates for investigational drugs. *Nature Biotechnology* 32(1), 40–51 (2014).
5. Ingber, D. E. Reverse engineering human pathophysiology with organs-on-chips. *Cell* 164(6), 1105–1109 (2016).

6. Ballard, D. H., Boyer, C. J. & Alexander, J. S. Organoids - Preclinical models of human disease. *The New England Journal of Medicine* 380(20), 1981–1982 (2019).
7. Paschini, M. & Kim, C. F. An airway organoid is forever. *The EMBO Journal* 38(4), e101526 (2019).
8. http://phrma-docs.phrma.org/sites/default/files/pdf/rd_brochure_022307.pdf.
9. https://www.who.int/news-room/fact-sheets/detail/cancer.
10. Suki, B., Stamenović, D. & Hubmayr, R. Lung parenchymal mechanics. *Comprehensive Physiology* 1(3), 1317–1351 (2011).
11. Knudsen, L. & Ochs, M. The micromechanics of lung alveoli: Structure and function of surfactant and tissue components. *Histochemistry and Cell Biology* 150(6), 661–676 (2018).
12. Yoon, J. H., Gray, T., Guzman, K., Koo, J. S. & Nettesheim, P. Regulation of the secretory phenotype of human airway epithelium by retinoic acid, triiodothyronine, and extracellular matrix. *American Journal of Respiratory Cell and Molecular Biology* 16(6), 724–731 (1997).
13. Blume, C. *et al.* Cellular crosstalk between airway epithelial and endothelial cells regulates barrier functions during exposure to double-stranded RNA. *Immunity, Inflammation and Disease* 5(1), 45–56 (2017).
14. Bilek, A. M., Dee, K. C. & Gaver, D. P. Mechanisms of surface-tension-induced epithelial cell damage in a model of pulmonary airway reopening. *Journal of Applied Physiology* 94(2), 770–783 (2003).
15. Huh, D. *et al.* Acoustically detectable cellular-level lung injury induced by fluid mechanical stresses in microfluidic airway systems. *Proceedings of the National Academy of Sciences of the United States of America* 104(48), 18886–18891 (2007).
16. Huh, D. *et al.* Reconstituting organ-level lung functions on a chip. *Science* 328(5986), 1662–1668 (2010).
17. Long, C. *et al.* Design optimization of liquid-phase flow patterns for microfabricated lung on a chip. *Annals of Biomedical Engineering* 40(6), 1255–1267 (2012).
18. Sellgren, K. L., Butala, E. J., Gilmour, B. P., Randell, S. H. & Grego, S. A biomimetic multicellular model of the airways using primary human cells. *Lab on a Chip* 14(17), 3349–3358 (2014).
19. Huang, D. *et al.* Reversed-engineered human alveolar lung-on-a-chip model. *Proceedings of the National Academy of Sciences* 118(19), e2016146118 (2021).
20. Zamprogno, P. *et al.* Second-generation lung-on-a-chip with an array of stretchable alveoli made with a biological membrane. *Communications Biology* 4(1), 168 (2021).
21. Shrestha, J. *et al.* A rapidly prototyped lung-on-a-chip model using 3D-printed molds. *Organs-on-a-Chip* 1, 100001 (2019).
22. Xu, Z. *et al.* Application of a microfluidic chip-based 3D co-culture to test drug sensitivity for individualized treatment of lung cancer. *Biomaterials* 34(16), 4109–4117 (2013).
23. Kong, J. *et al.* A novel microfluidic model can mimic organ-specific metastasis of circulating tumor cells. *Oncotarget* 7(48), 78421–78432 (2016).
24. Xu, Z. *et al.* Design and construction of a multi-organ microfluidic chip mimicking the in vivo microenvironment of lung cancer metastasis. *ACS Applied Materials and Interfaces* 8(39), 25840–25847 (2016).
25. Hassell, B. A. *et al.* Human organ chip models recapitulate orthotopic lung cancer growth, therapeutic responses, and tumor dormancy in vitro. *Cell Reports* 2, 508–516 (2017).
26. Yang, X. *et al.* Nanofiber membrane supported lung-on-a-chip microdevice for anti-cancer drug testing. *Lab on a Chip* 18(3), 486–495 (2018).
27. Huh, D. *et al.* A human disease model of drug toxicity-induced pulmonary edema in a lung-on-a-chip microdevice. *Science Translational Medicine* 4(159), 159ra147 (2012).
28. Benam, K. H. *et al.* Small airway-on-a-chip enables analysis of human lung inflammation and drug responses in vitro. *Nature Methods* 13(2), 151–157 (2016).

29. Jain, A. *et al.* Primary human lung alveolus-on-a-chip model of intravascular thrombosis for assessment of therapeutics. *Clinical Pharmacology and Therapeutics* 103(2), 332–340 (2018).
30. Si, L. *et al.* A human-airway-on-a-chip for the rapid identification of candidate antiviral therapeutics and prophylactics. *Nature Biomedical Engineering* 5(8), 815–829 (2021).
31. Frost, T. S., Jiang, L. & Zohar, Y. Pharmacokinetic analysis of epithelial/endothelial cell barriers in microfluidic bilayer devices with an air-liquid interface. *Micromachines* 11(5), 536 (2020).
32. Herland, A. *et al.* Quantitative prediction of human pharmacokinetic responses to drugs via fluidically coupled vascularized organ chips. *Nature Biomedical Engineering* 4(4), 421–436 (2020).
33. https://www.oecd.org/officialdocuments/publicdisplaydocumentpdf/?cote=env/jm/mono(2009)28/rev1&doclanguage=en.
34. Xu, C. *et al.* Assessment of air pollutant PM2.5 pulmonary exposure using a 3D lung-on-chip model. *ACS Biomaterials Science and Engineering* 6(5), 3081–3090 (2020).
35. Guan, M. *et al.* Development of alveolar-capillary-exchange (ACE) chip and its application for assessment of PM(2.5)-induced toxicity. *Ecotoxicology and Environmental Safety* 223, 112601 (2021).
36. Zhang, M., Xu, C., Jiang, L. & Qin, J. A 3D human lung-on-a-chip model for nanotoxicity testing. *Toxicology Research* 7(6), 1048–1060 (2018).
37. Kerns, S. J. *et al.* Human immunocompetent organ-on-chip platforms allow safety profiling of tumor-targeted T-cell bispecific antibodies. *eLife* 10, e67106 (2021).
38. Lancaster, M. A. & Knoblich, J. A. Organogenesis in a dish: Modeling development and disease using organoid technologies. *Science* 345(6194), 1247125 (2014).
39. Hofer, M. & Lutolf, M. P. Engineering organoids. *Nature Reviews Materials* 6(5), 402–420 (2021).
40. Rookmaaker, M. B., Schutgens, F., Verhaar, M. C. & Clevers, H. Development and application of human adult stem or progenitor cell organoids. *Nature Reviews Nephrology* 11(9), 546–554 (2015).
41. Drost, J. & Clevers, H. Organoids in cancer research. *Nature Reviews Cancer* 18(7), 407–418 (2018).
42. Miller, A. J. *et al.* Generation of lung organoids from human pluripotent stem cells in vitro. *Nature Protocols* 14(2), 518–540 (2019).
43. Benali, R. *et al.* Tubule formation by human surface respiratory epithelial cells cultured in a three-dimensional collagen lattice. *The American Journal of Physiology* 264(2 Pt 1), L183–L192 (1993).
44. Wong, A. P. *et al.* Directed differentiation of human pluripotent stem cells into mature airway epithelia expressing functional CFTR protein. *Nature Biotechnology* 30(9), 876–882 (2012).
45. Dye, B. R. *et al.* In vitro generation of human pluripotent stem cell derived lung organoids. *eLife* 4, e05098 (2015).
46. Chen, Y.-W. *et al.* A three-dimensional model of human lung development and disease from pluripotent stem cells. *Nature Cell Biology* 19(5), 542–549 (2017).
47. Sachs, N. *et al.* Long-term expanding human airway organoids for disease modeling. *The EMBO Journal* 38(4), e100300 (2019).
48. Kim, M. *et al.* Patient-derived lung cancer organoids as in vitro cancer models for therapeutic screening. *Nature Communications* 10(1), 3991 (2019).
49. Shi, R. *et al.* Organoid cultures as preclinical models of non-small cell lung cancer. *Clinical Cancer Research: An Official Journal of the American Association for Cancer Research* 26(5), 1162–1174 (2020).
50. Hu, Y. *et al.* Lung cancer organoids analyzed on microwell arrays predict drug responses of patients within a week. *Nature Communications* 12(1), 2581 (2021).

51. Salahudeen, A. A. *et al.* Progenitor identification and SARS-CoV-2 infection in human distal lung organoids. *Nature* 588(7839), 670–675 (2020).
52. Han, Y. *et al.* Identification of SARS-CoV-2 inhibitors using lung and colonic organoids. *Nature* 589(7841), 270–275 (2021).
53. Pfuhler, S. *et al.* Use of in vitro 3D tissue models in genotoxicity testing: Strategic fit, validation status and way forward. Report of the working group from the 7(th) international workshop on genotoxicity testing (IWGT). *Mutation Research/Genetic Toxicology and Environmental Mutagenesis* 850–851, 503135 (2020).
54. Matsui, T. & Shinozawa, T. Human organoids for predictive toxicology research and drug development. *Frontiers in Genetics* 12, 767621 (2021).
55. Naruse, M. *et al.* An organoid-based carcinogenesis model induced by in vitro chemical treatment. *Carcinogenesis* 41(10), 1444–1453 (2020).
56. Yamamoto, Y. *et al.* Long-term expansion of alveolar stem cells derived from human iPS cells in organoids. *Nature Methods* 14(11), 1097–1106 (2017).
57. Kim, J.-H. *et al.* Diesel particulate matter 2.5 induces epithelial-to-mesenchymal transition and upregulation of SARS-CoV-2 receptor during human pluripotent stem cell-derived alveolar organoid development. *International Journal of Environmental Research and Public Health* 17(22), 8410 (2020).

Interaction between Inhalable Nanomedicines and Pulmonary Surfactant

4

Xin Pan, Zhengwei Huang, Chuanbin Wu

Contents

DOI: 10.1201/9781003182566-5

4.1 INTRODUCTION

The collaboration of nanotechnology and medicine gives birth to the concept of nano-medicines. In the recent decades, the research and development of nanomedicines have been boosted, and it is widely believed that the 21st century is a century of nanomedicines. In the literature, nanomedicines have been employed in various administration routes, including but not limited to oral,[1] intravenous,[2] transdermal,[3] and pulmonary routes,[4] which all demonstrate promising outcomes.

In the area of pulmonary drug delivery, inhalable nanomedicines are under intensive exploitation. They exhibit ample potential for the clinical treatment of respiratory diseases like asthma,[5] chronic obstructive pulmonary disease (COPD),[6] cystic fibrosis (CF),[7] bacterial/fungal/viral infections,[8] and lung cancers.[9] Compared to systemic drug delivery of nanomedicines, inhalable nanomedicines can directly transport the active pharmaceutical ingredients into the lesion site, overcoming the first-pass effects and reducing the systemic adverse reactions[10]; when compared with pulmonary delivery of non-nanoparticulate systems, the drug release rate can be controlled and the targeting ability can be enhanced[11] by inhalable nanomedicines.

Although less reported, it is worth noticing that inhalable nanomedicines can also be utilized in systemic disease treatment. For example, nanomedicines have been used in treating diabetes,[12] osteoporosis,[13] and vascular diseases[14] in previous studies, which showed promising preclinical outcomes. The superiorities for systemic disease treatment mainly lay in that the thin alveolar epithelium facilitates the translocation of inhaled nanomedicines into the circulation.[15]

According to the literature, there are many kinds of nanomedicines involved in the fundamental research of respiratory and systemic diseases therapy, for instance, liposomes,[16] micelles,[17] dendrimers,[18] and metallic nanoparticles,[19] where the active pharmaceutical ingredients are physically incorporated or chemically linked.[20] Besides this, drug-polymer conjugates[21] are also reported. Amongst these nanomedicines, liposomes and micelles with satisfactory biocompatibility and high loading capacity[22] are the most promising candidates for clinical translation.

Although possessing great superiority, the clinical translation of inhalable nanomedicines lags far behind. Up till now, there are no relevant commercialized products on the market. The bottleneck issues impeding the clinical translation of inhalable nanomedicines mainly lay in (1) the difficulties in scale-up manufacture and (2) the vague biological fate.[23] The continuous development of materials science and pharmaceutical science is creating opportunities to upgrade the scale-up techniques for inhalable nanomedicines by introducing new production theories[24] and processing machines.[25] Therefore, the difficulties in scale-up manufacture are being mitigated.

Nevertheless, the ambiguous biological fate is still an unneglectable hurdle hindering the clinical translation of inhalable nanomedicines. In brief, how will the nanomedicines be disposed of after administration? To address this question, the anatomic structure of the respiratory tract should be considered.[26, 27]

The anatomic structure of the respiratory tract is mainly composed of three parts: The extrathoracic airway, tracheobronchial airway, and alveolar interstitium (Figure 4.1a). The extrathoracic airway and part of the tracheobronchial airway are regarded as the conducting airways, which begin with the nasal epithelium, then the pharynx and larynx, and followed by the trachea and bronchial tree. Part of the tracheobronchial airway and alveolar interstitium are perceived as the respiratory zone, mainly consisting of

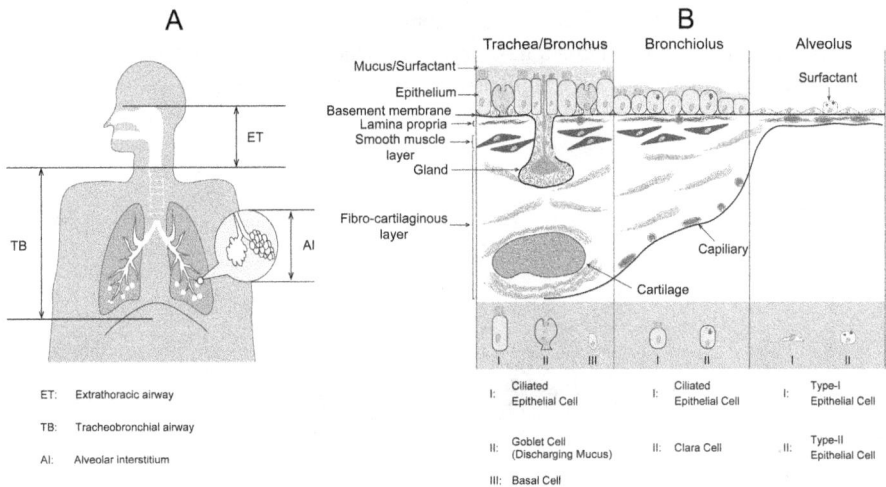

FIGURE 4.1   Anatomic structure of respiratory tract, macroscopic (A) and microscopic (B). Modified from the literature.[26, 27]

respiratory bronchioles and alveoli, mediating the gas exchange process. The trachea and bronchial tree mainly consist of mucus, bronchial epithelium, and endothelium. The cilia are embedded in the periciliary layer (PCL) and active to clear the xenobiotics. The tips of cilia drive the self-renewal of mucus every 20 minutes, a synergistic barrier composed by the secretory cells, especially goblet cells (Figure 4.1b).[28] In the alveolar region, the alveolar epithelial type I and type II cells constitute the alveolar epithelium. The osmiophilic multilamellar body, a special secretory organelle, is located in alveolar epithelial type II cells and secrete the pulmonary surfactant.

Inhaled nanomedicines can successively pass through several organs and tissues: Firstly, the nanomedicines enter the nasal or oral cavity during administration. Then, they are pushed forward by the airflow into the pharynx region. The nanomedicines are heated and humidified when entering the pharynx. They continue to pass through the trachea and bronchus, reaching the lung. Microscopically, there are bronchiolus and alveolus in the lung, where the inhaled nanomedicines may deposit.

Noticeably, the lung is a critical organ associated with the fate of nanomedicines *in vivo*. As mentioned before, for those intended for respiratory diseases therapy, the lesion site is in the lung region, and the nanomedicines should enter the targeted cells.[29] As for systemic diseases therapy, inhaled nanomedicines need to be absorbed by alveolar epithelial cells and transported into the circulation. The lung is somehow a "terminate" or "interchange" of inhaled nanomedicines, and the biological disposal occurs there is a dominant scenario of the *in vivo* fate.

To be specific, the pulmonary surfactant is a dominant factor for the biological disposal of the lung, because pulmonary surfactant plays a critical part in both "terminate" and "interchange" situations. Pulmonary surfactant is homogeneously distributed in the lining fluid of alveolar cavities: in other words, the air-liquid interface of the lining fluid.[30] The distribution profile is illustrated in Figure 4.2. Because inhaled nanomedicines, whether for respiratory diseases or systemic disease treatment, must interact with lung cells and pulmonary surfactant exists in the superficial layer of alveolar lining fluid, the contact of inhalable nanomedicines and pulmonary surfactant can be foreseen. Since nanomedicines have a large surface area and surface energy,[31] and pulmonary surfactant possesses high surface activity,[31] such contact undoubtedly is a consequence of the interaction between them, i.e., nanomedicine-pulmonary surfactant interaction.

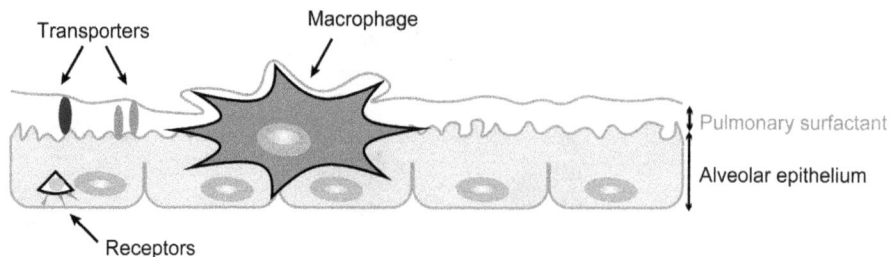

FIGURE 4.2 Distribution of pulmonary surfactant in the alveolar region. Modified from the literature.[32]

Owing to nanomedicine-pulmonary surfactant interaction, the biological fate of inhalable nanomedicines is less predictable. During real-world clinical administration, the predicted pharmacodynamics effects of nanomedicines may be manipulated, and the normal physiological functions of pulmonary surfactant may be influenced, and finally, safety issues may be provoked. These results are not acceptable in pharmaceutical development. We must figure out the effect of this interaction on the *in vivo* fate and drug delivery outcomes of inhalable nanomedicines, and demonstrate the underlying mechanisms. Only then the clinical translation of inhalable nanomedicines can be facilitated, and novel pulmonary delivery nano-strategies will be established.

This chapter will introduce the basic information of pulmonary surfactants, highlight the impact of nanomedicine-pulmonary surfactant interaction upon both counterparts, and review the characterization methods for nanomedicine-pulmonary surfactant interaction. The implication of such an interaction in pulmonary drug delivery will be discussed as well. It is anticipated that this work can serve as guidance for the future design, development, and evaluation of inhalable nanomedicines, and accelerate the clinical translation of related products.

4.2 BASIC INFORMATION OF PULMONARY SURFACTANT

4.2.1 Physiological Functions

Pulmonary surfactant is a kind of surf-active substance found in the pulmonary region. It acts as a biological barrier for the body to defend against the inhaled xenobiotic,[33] like pathogens, organic particles, and inorganic particles. The physiological activities and functions of pulmonary surfactant are as follows[34] and are mostly associated with its surface tension reducing capacities.

(1) Pulmonary surfactant supplies alveolar surface tension which prevents alveolar collapse at the end of the expiratory process. By spreading in the alveolar lining in a thin liquid pattern, pulmonary surfactant reduces the surface tension of the air-liquid interface. The collapsed alveoli will expand under low inhalation pressure, and maintain the plump shape during the entire respiration stage. As a result, the collapse of alveoli is prevented at the end of the expiratory process.

(2) Pulmonary surfactant maintains lung compliance. It is also endowed by the lung surface tension reducing properties. In addition to avoiding the collapse of the alveoli during exhalation, the pulmonary surfactant can effectively prevent excessive expansion of the alveoli during inhalation. Thus, the relative stability of the alveolar volume is maintained, the alveolar tissues can be physically protected from overexpansion, and lung compliance is improved.

(3) Pulmonary surfactant prevents pulmonary edema and achieves a fluid balance between alveoli and capillaries. The pulmonary surfactant can transfer the excess fluid in the alveoli to the interstitial sites through the blood-gas barrier and maintain the hemostasis of the alveolar fluid. Also, the pulmonary surfactant can weaken the contraction force of the alveolar by reducing the alveolar surface tension, decreasing the "suction" effects[35] of pulmonary capillaries upon the plasma and the lung tissue fluid, to prevent the occurrence of pulmonary edema.

(4) Pulmonary surfactant participates in respiratory immune regulation and increases respiratory defense function. The biomolecules consisting of the pulmonary surfactant form a powerful defense against inhaled xenobiotics, especially pathogens. Pulmonary surfactant also regulates inflammatory responses to microbial components[26] and can reduce tissue damage in multiple organs by inhibiting a variety of pro-inflammatory mediators.

4.2.2 Components

Pulmonary surfactant, chemically, is a biomolecular complex consisting of lipids (90%, mass proportion) and proteins (10%).[30] Among them, dipalmitoyl phosphatidylcholine (DPPC) is the major lipid species,[36] and the proteins are mainly referred to as surfactant-associated proteins (SP). The components of pulmonary surfactant are depicted in Figure 4.3.

DPPC accounts for about 41% weight of pulmonary surfactants. The tight intermolecular packing state of DPPC endows it with the attributes of ultra-low surface tension upon compression,[36] which is regarded to be largely responsible for the surface tension reducing activity that guards against alveolar collapse, especially at end of expiration.

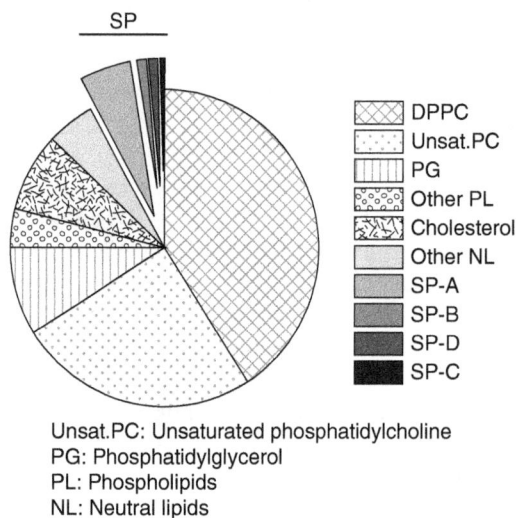

Unsat.PC: Unsaturated phosphatidylcholine
PG: Phosphatidylglycerol
PL: Phospholipids
NL: Neutral lipids

FIGURE 4.3 Components of pulmonary surfactant. Modified from the literature.[37]

Besides this, in some cases, DPPC can facilitate particle entry into alveolar epithelial cells by binding to the particles and acting as a non-receptor carrier for cell penetration.[38] It should be noticed that other lipids like unsaturated phosphatidylcholine and phosphatidylglycerol also participate in surface tension reduction.

SP mainly includes SP-A, SP-B, SP-C, SP-D, SP-G, and SP-H, all of which play critical roles in the physiological functions of the lung. SP-A and SP-D are large molecules of hydrophilic nature, participating in the immunoregulation of the respiratory system.[30] For instance, SP-A and SP-D can bind a variety of viruses, including influenza A virus (IAV), respiratory syncytial virus (RSV), and human immunodeficiency virus (HIV), and subsequently promote their clearance of mucosal entry points and regulate the antiviral immune response of the host. In addition, through induction of aggregation, opsonization, modulation of inflammatory pathways, and macrophage activation, SP-A and SP-D can assist in pathogen recognition and elimination, and then up-regulate or down-regulate the inflammatory factors, playing a role in maintaining pulmonary immune homeostasis.[39] As for low-molecular hydrophobic SP, SP-B and SP-C can regulate the surface activity and prevent the alveoli from collapse,[40] with a similar function to the lipids. During inhalation, SP-B and SP-C together assist in the redistribution of pulmonary surfactant in the alveolar surface;[41] during exhalation, SP-B stabilizes the three-dimensional structure of pulmonary surfactant, while SP-C induces some lipid-protein complexes to detach from the pulmonary surfactant and adjusts the surface tension. Besides reducing surface tension, SP-B exhibits a certain level of antibacterial activity and can protect the lung from hypoxic lung injury.[42] Newly identified, SP-G and SP-H show similar activities with their SP analogs.[43] The chemical structure is quite different from SP-A, B, C, and D, but they not only show similar physical and chemical properties to SP-B and SP-C[44] but also possess the immune modulation function of SP-A and SP-D.[43] Hence, SP-G and SP-H have the function of regulating alveolar surface tension and immune regulation and may strengthen the activities of SP-A, B, C, and D.

4.2.3 Biosynthesis and Biodegradation

It has been proven that pulmonary surfactant is mainly synthesized and secreted by the alveoli.[36] Type-II alveolar epithelial cells contain key enzymes for pulmonary surfactant synthesis and are the major bio-factory for the lipids and SP. DPPC and other family members of phosphatidylcholine are synthesized in the endoplasmic reticulum of type-II alveolar epithelial cells, while phosphatidylglycerol is mostly synthesized in mitochondria of those cells.[45] After the preliminary synthesis, these lipids are transported to the Golgi apparatus and transformed into the lamellar body. The lamellar body is secreted by exocytosis into the alveolar cavity and then rapidly transformed into double-layered tubular myelin which finally adsorbs onto the alveoli as a lipid monolayer.[46] Also, SP is synthesized by the endoplasmic reticulum of type-II alveolar epithelial cells. The mature SP are translocated from the endoplasmic reticulum in the manner of budding vesicles and then biologically activated.[47]

Genetically, recent studies demonstrated that multiple gene expression and synthesis pathways were involved in the pulmonary surfactant secretion process. Lung lysoPC acyltransferase (LPCAT1) expression is restricted in type-II alveolar epithelial cells, regulating the remodeling process of existing monosaturated phosphatidylcholine species, which was estimated to dominate ~55%–75% of those species.[48] In addition, the calcineurin b1 (Cnb1) gene was also found to control the structural maturation of the peripheral pulmonary region by regulating surfactant biosynthesis.[49] Other genes like signal transducer and activator of transcription 3 (STAT3) expression in type-II alveolar epithelial cells were also proved to regulate the synthesis of pulmonary surfactant.[50]

The biosynthesized pulmonary surfactant will be metabolized or eliminated by the human body to maintain a relatively stable concentration of it. Interestingly, most of the produced pulmonary surfactant is re-absorbed by type-II alveolar epithelial cells through cellular engulfment and re-transported to the lamellar bodies for storage.[51] It has also been reported that pulmonary surfactants become vesicles after ingestion.[52] Some vesicles fuse with primary lysosomes and are degraded into choline and fatty acids which enter the endoplasmic reticulum for the re-synthesis of pulmonary surfactant, while other vesicles combine with the lamellar bodies for direct recycling. Pulmonary surfactants secreted into the alveolar cavities can be quickly cleared. The clearance is dominantly achieved through the trachea, whereas a certain proportion will be cleared through the lymphatic system and blood circulation system. Alveolar macrophage phagocytosis after degradation is sometimes involved.[53]

In some rare cases (e.g., pulmonary surfactant administration for the therapy of atelectasis[54]), exogenous pulmonary surfactant is brought into the lung region. For the exogenous species, tracheal infusion takes place. After that, they are filtrated into the alveoli and cleared from the lung. An interesting fact is that the same exogenous pulmonary surfactant has a constant clearance rate, independent of the dose given.[55]

4.3 INTERACTION BETWEEN INHALABLE NANOMEDICINES AND PULMONARY SURFACTANT: A BIOMOLECULAR CORONA-ASSOCIATED PROCESS

4.3.1 Inevitableness of Nanomedicine-Pulmonary Surfactant Interaction

After inhaled nanomedicines enter the lung, they will firstly suspend in the alveolar lining fluid. Since pulmonary surfactant is distributed in the air-liquid interface, the interaction between nanomedicines and pulmonary surfactant takes place. The alveolar lining fluid serves as the interaction medium for both counterparts. It is anticipated that nanomedicines are wrapped by pulmonary surfactant, and the complex resembles an "endosome" (Figure 4.4). With the formation of this "endosome", some ingredients of pulmonary surfactant will spontaneously and inevitably be absorbed onto the surface of nanomedicines.[56] Based on the physicochemical attributes of nanomedicines, different

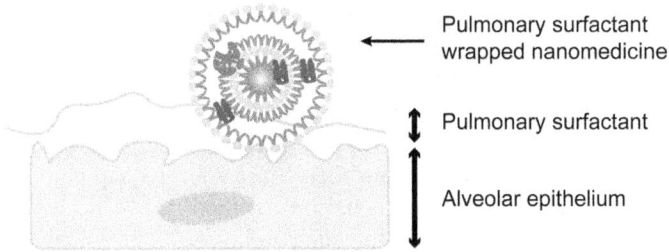

FIGURE 4.4   Inhaled nanomedicines wrapped by pulmonary surfactant.

pulmonary surfactant ingredients are involved in the nanomedicine-pulmonary surfactant interaction. It was reported that the nanomedicines with the same components yet different surface chemistry may cause the adsorption of different kinds of biomolecules on them; when nanoparticles with different components are exposed to the pulmonary surfactant environment, different kinds of biomolecules will be adsorbed.[57]

4.3.2 Connection between the Interaction with Biomolecular Corona

Interestingly, the spontaneous adsorption of pulmonary surfactant onto the surface of nanomedicines is similar to a recently defined phenomenon in nanoscience, viz. the formation of the biomolecular corona. Biomolecular corona refers to the corona-like layer of biomolecules accumulated around nanomedicines, which is formed upon the interaction between nanomedicines and biological fluids.[58] The formation of the biomolecular corona is related to two sets of bindings: (1) Nanomedicines-biomolecules binding and (2) biomolecules-biomolecules binding (herein, the biomolecules were those already adsorbed on the nanoparticles).[59] A schematic illustration of the biomolecular corona is shown in Figure 4.5.

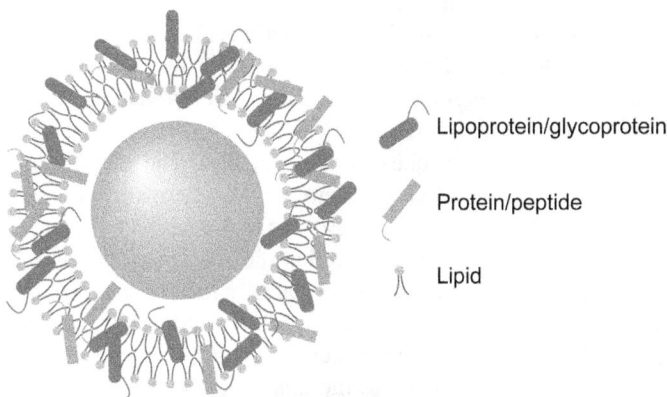

FIGURE 4.5   Biomolecular coronated nanomedicines.

The formation of biomolecular corona may change the characteristics of both nano-medicines or biomolecules, which further affects their functions of them.[57] Specifically, the formation of biomolecular corona will alter the surface chemistry of nanomedicines since the pristine nanomedicines possess a surface consisting of nanomaterials, whilst it is the adsorbed biomolecules present on the surface for the coronated ones. As a result, the biochemical characteristics of nanomedicines are affected, and ultimately the phar-macokinetics and pharmacodynamics behaviors are modified. It has been documented that the biodistribution, drug leakage, targeting ability, immunogenicity, and biotrans-formation of nanomedicines would be influenced when the biomolecules were bound.[60]

(1) Biomolecular corona influences biodistribution. The generated corona will impact the organs accumulating tendencies of nanomedicines. The associa-tion of gold nanoparticles with plasma proteins such as albumin and apolipo-protein E significantly reduces the translocation to the spleen, compared to protein-uncoated systems.[61] It was reported that an increase in the number of apolipoprotein A-1 and A-2 in the biomolecular corona resulted in the spe-cific accumulation of hollow mesoporous silica nanoparticles in the liver, and there was no accumulation in other reticuloendothelial system organs, such as the spleen or lungs.[62]

(2) Biomolecular corona induces drug leakage. On one hand, the abundant plasma proteins can replace proteins cargoes loaded on the outer layer of the nanomedicines during biomolecular corona formation, making them easy to dissociate from the corona and thus cause leakage issues.[63] On the other hand, the formation of biomolecular corona may interfere with the integrity of nanomedicines and lead to drug leakage. For example, the integrity of Doxove, a lipid-based nano-drug for doxorubicin delivery, was destructed upon biomolecular corona formation, finally provoking a fraction of doxoru-bicin leakage.[64]

(3) Biomolecular corona undermines the targeting ability. K.A. Dawson et al.[65] demonstrated that when a biomolecular corona was adsorbed, the transferrin-functionalized silica nanoparticles lose their targeting capabili-ties. Transferrin-functionalized small polymer-coated iron-platinum (FePt) nanoparticles also showed the loss of targeting functions.[66] Meanwhile, in the case of monoclonal antibodies conjugated with ultra-small superparamag-netic iron oxide nanoparticles, the targeting ability in vivo was lost although remained under in-vitro conditions.[67]

(4) Biomolecular corona provokes immunogenicity. The biomolecular corona enriched in opsonins and clotting proteins can activate immune cells and promote phagocytosis, which causes nanomedicines to be cleared from cir-culation.[68] It has been demonstrated that the adsorption of opsonins on cat-ionic gold nanoparticle surfaces could augment macrophages recognition and subsequent uptake of the nanoparticles.[69,70,71] In addition, opsonins and other components in the complement system can induce an immune response by recognizing proteins adsorbed to the nanomedicine surface.[72] Interestingly, protein interaction with the nanomedicine surface promotes the deformation of its tertiary structure and even aggregation, and the immunogenicity of

endogenous proteins will increase then, thereby inducing an autoimmune response.[73, 74] Also, this will make the antigens of nanomedicines more immunogenic.[75]

(5) Biomolecular corona affects the biotransformation of nanomedicines. It is reported that the strongly attached proteins on silver nanoparticles can act as a sulphidation site that promotes biotransformation,[76] resulting in decreased toxicity. In addition, with human serum albumin adsorption, signal-wall carbon nanotubes exhibit a higher biodegradation rate in neutrophils.[77] Thus, more attention should be paid to the optimization of nanomedicines' biodegradation rate by regulating biomolecular corona formation.

In the scenario of inhalable nanomedicines, the pulmonary surfactant-containing lining fluid is a typical biological fluid, and the biomolecules of pulmonary surfactant (lipids and SP) are prone to interact with nanomedicines and finally generate a biomolecular corona. From this perspective, nanomedicine-pulmonary surfactant interaction can be regarded as a biomolecular corona-associated process. Consequently, the theories of biomolecular corona can be imported herein to obtain a better interpretation of the interaction. For example, the fact that biomolecular corona influences biodistribution can explain the following example. It was expected that the graphene oxide (~100–500 nm) could readily enter the pulmonary capillary and evade the lung because the particle size is significantly smaller than the capillary diameter (~7 μm). Nevertheless, the interaction between graphene oxide and proteins yielded a nanocomposite, which cannot enter the pulmonary capillary and then was trapped in the lung.[78]

The absorption and desorption kinetics of the biomolecular formation process is qualitatively defined by the Vroman effect,[56] which can be extrapolated to nanomedicine-pulmonary surfactant interaction. According to the Vroman effect, the biomolecular corona formation process is time-associated.[79] The biomolecules with higher abundance yet lower affinity are adsorbed initially, which are later substituted by those with lower abundance yet higher affinity.[79] After a certain period, the time evolution of the adsorption-desorption balance reaches a plateau. For an equilibrated nanoparticle, the yielded biomolecular corona is named "full corona", the high-affinity biomolecule species located at a short distance from nanomedicines surface and the low-affinity ones distributed at a long distance from nanomedicines surface are called "hard corona" and "soft corona", respectively. Compared to the hard corona, the soft corona represents a more dynamically exchangeable layer of proteins that will easily detach under changeful microenvironments.[57, 80] A scheme is displayed in Figure 4.6.

When it comes to nanomedicine-pulmonary surfactant interaction, lipids and proteins (especially DPPC and SP) will be adsorbed onto the surface of nanomedicines obeying the Vroman effect. There is an adsorption-desorption equilibrium, and subsequently, a full corona (consisting of the hard corona and soft corona) of pulmonary surfactant will be generated. What's different from the commonly reported biomolecular corona formation is that the lipid content of the pulmonary surfactant is approximately 90%,[82] and hence lipids may account for a considerable proportion of the full corona in this case. In light of this, one must consider lipid species when studying the nanomedicine-pulmonary surfactant interaction.

Time evolution

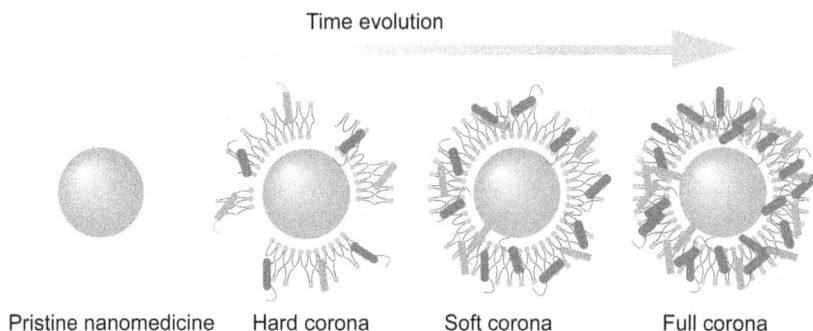

Pristine nanomedicine   Hard corona   Soft corona   Full corona

FIGURE 4.6   The formation of the hard, soft, and full corona. Modified from the literature.[81]

In addition to corona generation, biomolecular adsorption sometimes leads to the aggregation of the nanomedicine-biomolecule complex. The aggregation can be viewed as an "overreacted" corona formation. Some factors can disrupt the colloidal interface stability of nanomedicines, and lead to the formation of aggregates, namely the electrostatic interaction and the non-covalent crosslinks.

(1) The aggregation could be caused by the electrostatic interaction between biomolecules and nanomedicines with opposite charges. The route of this is the weakening of electrostatic repulsion between nanomedicines. When the positively-charged proteins are adsorbed on the negatively-charged surface of ferroferric oxide (Fe_3O_4) and zinc-doped magnetite ($Zn_{0.4}Fe_{2.6}O_4$) nanoparticles, the repulsive forces provided by negative charges reduced, leading to the aggregation of them.[83] Positively-charged proteins are easily absorbed onto the negatively-charged carboxymethyl-coated magnetic nanoparticles by electrostatic interaction, and the negative charges were partially neutralized which caused the aggregation of the nanoparticles.[84]

(2) Proteins adsorbed on the surfaces of nanomedicines may drive the aggregation *via* non-covalent crosslinks.[85] The adsorbed proteins, which are composed of multiple active functional groups and complicated tertiary spatial structures, could be cross-linked by hydrogen bonding and Van der Waals force to drive nanoparticles aggregation. S. Dominguez-Medina et al.[86] observed that the adsorption of bovine serum albumin on gold nanorods induced protein unfolding and then induced the nanomedicine aggregation *via* the unfolded protein-protein interactions. R. Cukalevski et al.[87] demonstrated that immunoglobulin G (IgG) and fibrinogen could act as a protein bridge between nanoparticles and drive the aggregation of sulfonated polystyrene nanoparticles in the circulation.

It should be noticed that many ions (cations and anions) coexist with pulmonary surfactant in the alveolar lining fluid,[88, 89] e.g., sodium (Na^+), potassium (K^+), calcium (Ca^{2+}), magnesium (Mg^{2+}), and chloride (Cl^-), and they can to some degree form electrostatic interaction with the inhaled nanomedicines. Under some circumstances, SP may be susceptible to forming non-covalent crosslinks. Therefore, these components may render the inhaled nanomedicines possible to aggregation.

Nevertheless, it is worth mentioning that the outcome of nanomedicine-pulmonary surfactant interaction is the formation of biomolecular corona in most scenarios, and commonly the aggregation tendency is not remarkable. Only nanomedicines with poor intrinsic colloidal stability, for example, those having too high hydrophobicity,[90] may undergo an aggregation process. Generally, the stronger the hydrophobicity of nanomedicines, the more proteins will be adsorbed, and the trend for aggregation is lifted.[91]

4.3.3 Categories of the Interaction

In parallel to the biomolecular formation, nanomedicine-pulmonary surfactant interaction is associated with multiple driving forces (Figure 4.7). The dominant driving forces are Van der Waals forces, electrostatic interaction, hydrogen bonding, and hydrophobic forces. Rarely would the driving force be covalent bonding. The following section launches a visit not limited to the inhalation scenario, which can serve as guidance for the nanomedicine-pulmonary surfactant interaction.

According to the literature,[92] if the interface morphology matched well, the Van der Waals interaction is usually the main contributor of biomolecules-nanomedicines interaction. This is because the molecular weight of nanomedicines (viewed as integrity) and biomolecules is typically large. The Van der Waals interaction represents an attraction force when the distance of two atoms is close to the sum of their Van der Waals radii. In general, the closer the atomic pair is, the stronger the Van der Waals interaction is. A too-close distance will reverse the Van der Waals interaction into a repulsion force, but this is unlikely to occur in an actual case.

For the electrostatic interaction, the opposite charges of the biomolecules and nanomedicine surface serve as a bridge to the interaction.[93, 94] It is easy to find the electrostatic

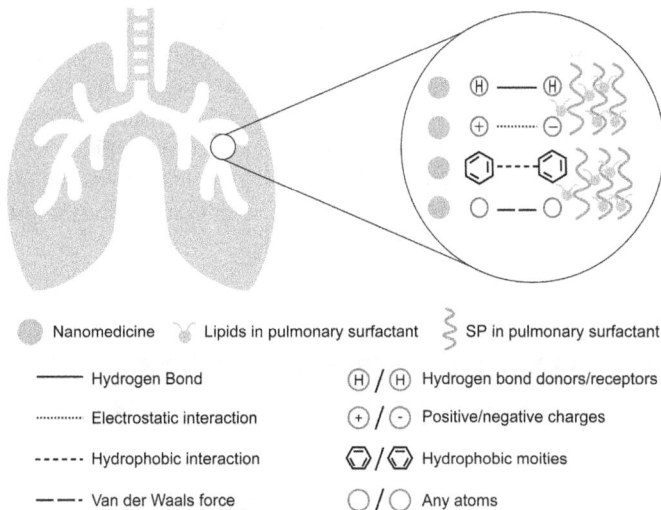

| ● Nanomedicine | ⋎ Lipids in pulmonary surfactant | ⧘ SP in pulmonary surfactant |

────── Hydrogen Bond	Ⓗ / Ⓗ Hydrogen bond donors/receptors
·········· Electrostatic interaction	⊕ / ⊖ Positive/negative charges
- - - - - Hydrophobic interaction	⬡ / ⬡ Hydrophobic moities
— —· Van der Waals force	○ / ○ Any atoms

FIGURE 4.7   Driving forces of nanomedicine-pulmonary surfactant interaction.

interactions between biomolecules and nanomedicines. The interaction intensity mostly depends on the surface charge of nanomedicines, and thus the pH value of the solution can sometimes determine the electrostatic interaction because it controls the surface charge state.[95] Nevertheless, it should be noticed that biomolecules adsorbed on the surface of nanomedicine may remain folded to form monolayers that do not generate electrostatic interaction but instead induce Van der Waals interaction, particularly in the case of proteins.[96]

Hydrogen bonding plays an important role in biomolecules-nanomedicines interactions. While biomolecules (especially proteins) have many hydrogen donors and receptors on the surface, the number of hydrogen donors and receptors on the surface of nanomedicines varies widely. Although the hydrogen bonding is intrinsically stronger than the Van der Waals interaction, the number of hydrogen bonds between nanomedicines and biomolecules is limited. Therefore, the importance of hydrogen bonding is subsidiary.[97] However, because the hydrogen bonding is directional, it enables direction-specific interactions.[98]

Hydrophobic interaction is also very important in biomolecule-nanomedicine interaction. Nanomedicines with a large hydrophobic surface are easy to bind to the partially exposed nonpolar moieties of biomolecules.[99] As the nonpolar moieties of biomolecules are generally less than the polar ones, the contribution of such an interaction is relatively low.

As the high surface energy and complicated nanomedicines compositions, multiple interaction forces collectively drive the biomolecular corona formation process upon nanomedicines. Van der Waals forces universally exist in different systems. For nanomedicines with positive/negative surface potential, the negatively/positively charged biomolecules are susceptible to being adsorbed. The hydrogen bonding dominates the biomolecular formation process of nanomedicines with rich hydrogen bond donors (like protein or some polymeric nanoparticles). Hydrophobic interaction may take place between hydrophobic nanomedicines and lipids.

Noticeably, the intensity of various interactions is quite different. In the interaction between nanomedicines and biomolecules, the intensity of Van der Waals forces is the strongest, followed by hydrogen bonding and electrostatic interaction, and that of hydrophobic interaction is the weakest. This can be interpolated into the case of nanomedicine-pulmonary surfactant interaction, but the importance of hydrophobic interaction needs to be elevated, since hydrophobic substances like DPPC, SP-B, and SP-C may induce strong hydrophobic interactions. The mechanisms of different interactions between nanomedicines and biomolecules should be considered during the design and development of related pharmaceutical products.

4.4 THE IMPACT OF INTERACTION UPON NANOMEDICINES

Compared to plasma or other biological fluids, the content of lipids is significantly higher in pulmonary surfactants, which causes that the adsorbed biomolecules in the pulmonary region are remarkably different from those in other anatomic environments.

The kinds of adsorbed biomolecules are dependent on the key physicochemical properties, like hydrophobicity and charge. After interacting with a pulmonary surfactant, these physicochemical attributes are greatly changed, which may turn to be similar to those of adsorbed biomolecules and can also induce instability issues. Subsequently, the biological fate like targeting region and cellular uptake can be altered as well.

In brief, various properties of nanomedicines including hydrophobicity, surface charge, colloidal stability, pulmonary surfactant layer permeability, targeting region, and cellular uptake may change after the interaction. The detailed discussion is as follows.

4.4.1 Hydrophobicity

The adsorbed biomolecules alter the hydrophobicity of nanomedicines. The changed hydrophobicity may provoke the interaction with other substances. A previous study showed that silicon dioxide (SiO_2) and zinc dioxide (ZrO_2) nanoparticles did not directly interact with pure lipids, but could interact with lipid-protein complex. It was speculated that the nanomedicines-lipids interaction was mediated by proteins:[100] The adsorption of proteins on the nanomedicine surface alters the surface hydrophobicity, and probably the hydrophobic residues stretched out and favored the interaction with lipids. Also, the adsorption of SP-D or antimicrobial peptides on the surface of nanomedicines was believed to trigger the interaction with lipids.[100–102]

The change in hydrophobicity is determined by the original hydrophobicity of nanomedicines. According to the like-dissolves-like principle,[103] hydrophobic and hydrophilic nanomedicines tend to adsorb hydrophobic and hydrophilic moieties of biomolecules, respectively. Then, the system represents the apparent hydrophobicity of the adsorbed biomolecules. The effect of nanomedicine hydrophobicity on the capture probability of pulmonary surfactant was demonstrated by G. Hu et al.[25] Using hydroxyapatite nanoparticles (HA-NPs) and polystyrene nanoparticles (PST-NPs) as model nanomedicines, the results showed that the hydrophobicity of nanomedicines determined the degree of displacement on the natural pulmonary surfactant membrane. HA-NPs did not interact remarkably with the pulmonary surfactant membrane, and thus they were not sufficiently lipid-modified. However, PST-NPs exhibited strong interaction with the membrane and a high degree of lipid modification, and even a part of them was captured by the membrane. Besides this, SP-A is more likely to interact with lipophilic NPs, while SP-D is more likely to interact with hydrophilic surfaces;[104] the former and the latter result in a hydrophobic and hydrophilic corona, respectively.

4.4.2 Surface Charge

The surface charge of nanomedicines is likely to be altered upon the interaction. To be specific, the surface charge of nanomedicines may be replaced by that of the adsorbed biomolecules. It was reported that citric acid-stabilized silver nanoparticles intrinsically had a certain tendency towards aggregation, especially due to the influence of pH shift.[105] However, when incubated with lipids such as DPPC, the aggregation tendency is drastically reduced. As lipids were less ionizable in the aqueous system, the adsorption of lipids constructed a layer whose surface charge was less influenced by environmental pH. Therefore, the alteration of surface charge may further impact the colloidal stability of nanomedicines.

Similar to the case of hydrophobicity, the change in surface charge is determined by the original surface charge of nanomedicines. Theoretically, nanomedicines are apt to interact with the biomolecule moieties of opposite charges. Nonetheless, a previous study showed that the actual electrostatic interaction might be tuned by the hydrophobicity of both counterparts, and equilibrium was reached.[25] This is probably due to that the nanomedicines and biomolecules with different hydrophobicities are hardly miscible to establish electrostatic interactions.

4.4.3 Colloidal Stability

Inspired by the case of citric acid-stabilized silver nanoparticles in Section 4.4.2, the colloidal stability of nanomedicines can change upon the interaction. The main manifestation of colloidal instability is the aggregation phenomenon, and the aggregate is the nanomedicines-biomolecules complex.

As mentioned in Section 4.3.2, the circumstances where the aggregation is triggered by pulmonary surfactant are typically rare. The occurrence of aggregation is dependent on the hydrophobicity of nanomedicines. One can refer to the reports that SP-A interacted with mannose-decorated nanoparticles to form a strong aggregate state by C.A. Ruge et al.,[106] and the existence of pulmonary surfactant accelerated the aggregation of nanocarbon particles by Q. Zhao et al.[107] Moreover, the hydrophilic SP, but neither the hydrophobic SP nor the lipids, induced agglomeration of the silver nanowires.[108]

4.4.4 Pulmonary Surfactant Layer Permeability

Distributing on the surface of pulmonary lining fluid, the pulmonary surfactant can be regarded as a "vulnerable" barrier for the delivered nanomedicines to reach the alveolar epithelium.[109] Inhaled nanomedicines can be retarded and even retained by the pulmonary surfactant layer, and a successful delivery demands an acceptable permeability of the nanomedicines. Of note, the interaction with biomolecules may alter the permeability. Y. Xu et al. developed a model nanodrop for aerosolization and used molecular dynamics simulation to study the interplay between the nanodrops and the pulmonary surfactant layer.[110] Herein, the nanodrops were hydrophilic, and a lipid-coating modification was performed on them to obtain a hydrophobic group. The results of this study revealed that the naïve nanodrops rapidly permeated the pulmonary surfactant layer, while the coating of lipids on the nanodrops slowed down the permeation. It was inferred that pre-incubation with lipids would decrease the permeability of nanomedicines in pulmonary surfactants.

Further, the pulmonary surfactant layer permeability enhancement of hydrophobic nanomedicines may also be driven by adsorbing SP-B and SP-C.[111] As hydrophobic proteins, the SP-B and SP-C are susceptible to being adsorbed on hydrophobic nanomedicines. The SP-B and SP-C could disturb the barrier structure of the pulmo-nary surfactant layer, especially at a high concentration. From this perspective, the nanomedicines with potent interaction with SP-B and SP-C may exhibit high perme-ability and further have more access to the alveolar epithelium.

4.4.5 Targeting Region

The interaction with biomolecules in pulmonary surfactants can change the targeting region of inhalable nanomedicines. On one hand, the prerequisite for local or systemic absorption of nanomedicines is nanomedicines entering the deep lung. For some nano-medicines, only if they adsorb pulmonary surfactant can they be transported into the epithelial cells. On the other hand, microscopically, there are many classes of cells in the respiratory tract that can be the targets of nanomedicines, viz. macrophages, type-I, and type-II alveolar epithelial cells, etc., considering different disease situations. The interaction with pulmonary surfactant sometimes improves the targetability to a certain cell.

Based on the above rationale, as endogenous biomaterial, the pulmonary surfac-tant components could also be employed as biomimetic nanoparticulate systems. For example, T. Kato et al. injected lecithin-coated and uncoated polystyrene microspheres into the trachea of rats.[112] The results showed that both kinds of microspheres could be absorbed by alveolar macrophages, but only lecithin-coated microspheres could enter type-I and type-II alveolar epithelial cells. The study by C.A. Ruge et al. revealed that the interaction of SP-A, one of the relevant proteins recognized by macrophages, with mannosylated nanoparticles enhanced the targeting ability of macrophages.[106] The rea-son behind the above results is that the adsorbed biomolecules have different affinities to the cells in the respiratory tract. Alveolar epithelial cells, in particular the type-II cells, tend to re-absorb the lipids in pulmonary surfactant, as mentioned in Section 4.2.3. As a result, the lecithin-coated microspheres accumulated more in alveolar epi-thelial cells. SP-A participates in pulmonary immunity (Section 4.2.2), and thus the adsorption of it may contribute to the promoted phagocytosis. These phenomena may have implications in the design of targeted delivery nanomedicines.

4.4.6 Cellular Uptake

The outcome of the biological fate of inhaled nanomedicines is the level of cellular uptake, and hereto the impact of the interaction on the cellular uptake is discussed. Generally, the interaction with lipids and SP-B may markedly improve the cellular uptake. For instance, the pulmonary surfactant layer could easily wrap the lipid-deco-rated nano drops to form a bubble-like structure, which might promote the fusion with the cell membrane, thereby elevating the uptake.[110] Recently, pulmonary surfactant-modified liposomes were proposed to enhance cellular uptake. D. Backer et al. observed that pulmonary surfactant-coated dextran nanogels delivered small interfering ribonu-cleic acid (siRNA) to different types of cells more efficiently than the uncoated nanogels *in vitro* and *in vivo*.[113, 114] The team also reported that the SP-B may be a key factor enhancing the delivery efficiency of siRNA. Besides this, P. Merckx et al. established an acute lung injury model induced by mouse lipopolysaccharide (LPS), where the role of SP-B in promoting transport *in vivo* was also proven.[115]

As discussed above, the interaction with biomolecules may sometimes lead to aggregation. It should be noticed that the formation of nanomedicine aggregates substantially affects cell uptake. It was elucidated that compared with dispersed gold nanoparticles, the uptake of aggregated gold nanoparticles in A549 cells was decreased up to 25%.[116] This reminds the investigators to consider the influence of interaction-induced aggregation.

4.5 THE IMPACT OF INTERACTION UPON PULMONARY SURFACTANT

The nanomedicine-pulmonary surfactant interaction includes two counterparts, and thus it not only impacts the nanomedicines but also influences the pulmonary surfactant. If nanomedicines-biomolecules complex provokes oxidative and/or inflammatory damages to the alveolar epithelial cells, the biosynthesis of pulmonary surfactants will be hampered. The interaction also can directly change the components and surface activity of pulmonary surfactant.

In summary, the interaction affects the biosynthesis, components, and compactness of pulmonary surfactant, and is scrutinized below.

4.5.1 Biosynthesis

The impact of the nanomedicine-pulmonary surfactant interaction on the biosynthesis of pulmonary surfactant is seldom discussed in the published documents, which remains a mystery to some degree, and the authors suggest that this is an unneglectable issue deserving more attention. To figure out this issue, the harmfulness and producing mechanisms of nanomedicine-biomolecule complexes related to reactive oxygen species (ROS) should be analyzed.

The direct outcome of nanomedicine-pulmonary surfactant interaction is the generation of nanomedicine-biomolecule complexes. Inhaled nanomedicines *per se* are associated with ROS, and the nanomedicine-biomolecule complexes may also cause the generation of ROS in some scenarios. ROS is a collective term that describes the chemical species formed upon incomplete reduction of oxygen (O_2), including superoxide anion (O^{2-}), peroxides (H_2O_2 and $ROOH$), singlet oxygen ($^1O_2$), radicals ($HO\cdot$ and $RO\cdot$), and so forth.[117]

In general, excessive ROS will cause damage to biological macromolecules such as proteins, nucleic acids, and lipids, thus affecting their normal physiological and biochemical functions.[118] A continuously high level of ROS can lead to pathological and even fatal results, including inflammation, hypertrophy, fibrosis, metaplasia, genotoxicity, carcinogenesis, apoptosis, and necrosis.[119] In the case of pulmonary delivery, the production of ROS will impair type-II alveolar epithelial cells and provoke inflammations. The main function of type-II alveolar epithelial cells in the biosynthesis, secretion, and re-absorption of pulmonary surfactants, as stated in Section 4.2.3. The damages and inflammations will directly influence the biosynthesis and metabolism of pulmonary surfactants. Another important function of these cells is their participation in epithelial regeneration processes. Following epithelial injury, type-II alveolar epithelial cells migrate to the wounded area, proliferate into alveolar type-II cells, and differentiate into type-I alveolar epithelial cells.[120] In this context, type-II alveolar epithelial cells are recognized as the progenitors of alveolar epithelial cells.[121] Therefore, the biosynthesis of pulmonary surfactants will be affected further.

The next task is to claim the generation mechanisms of ROS and the impact of nanomedicine-pulmonary surfactant interaction. In physiological conditions, ROS is a natural response to normal oxygen metabolism,[122] which is produced in the endoplasmic reticulum (ER), peroxisomes, and most especially in the mitochondria.[123] However, when cells are exposed to nanomedicines, the generation of ROS is a stress response. The large specific surface area and high reactivity of surface molecules make the nanomedicines possess high oxidation capacity. In general, ROS can be produced by nanomedicines through several different mechanisms:

(1) When exposed to acidic environments (e.g., lysosomes), chemical degradation of nanomedicines often takes place. The released ions from the nanomedicines join in catalyzing the production of ROS, and the reactive nanomaterials or the degraded products and byproducts thereof will cause the generation of ROS as well.[124]

(2) Nanomedicines interact with mitochondria and destroy their outer membrane, resulting in the collapse of mitochondrial membrane potential. The electron transfer chain (ETC) for oxidative phosphorylation was therefore interfered, finally leading to the yield of ROS.[125]

(3) The interaction between nanomedicines and the cellular reduction/oxidation (REDOX) system upregulates the expression of nicotinamide adenine dinucleotide phosphate (NADPH) oxidase (NOX), which causes an increase in ROS levels.[126]

(4) Nanomedicines bind with receptors on the cell membrane to activate the intracellular signaling channels, ultimately leading to the massive expression of stress-responsive genes that can up-regulate ROS levels.[127]

The nanomedicine-pulmonary surfactant interaction resulting in nanomedicine-biomolecule complexes can have double-edged effects on the above four mechanisms, compared with pure nanomedicines. For one thing, the degradation of adsorbed biomolecules in the lysosomes may facilitate the generation of ROS, and the adsorption of some biomolecules may enhance the interaction with mitochondria, REDOX system, and receptors, and therefore the ROS level is raised.[128] For another thing, the formation of biomolecular corona may cover the ROS-inducing nanomaterials and reduce the reactivity, which inhibits such four mechanisms.[129]

Hence, it is indicated that for nanomedicines *per se* with high potential to produce ROS, the possibility of the biosynthesis of pulmonary surfactant being impacted is relatively high, unless the adsorbed biomolecules surmount ROS generation; nano-medicines *per se* with low potential in ROS generation have negligible effects on the biosynthesis of pulmonary surfactant, but under some circumstances, the adsorbed bio-molecules promote the ROS production and strengthen the effects. The influence on biosynthesis should consider both counterparts.

4.5.2 Components

The cooperation of lipids and SP ensure the normal physiological functions of pulmo-nary surfactant. If some components of pulmonary surfactant (e.g., DPPC or SP) were removed, the physiological functions would be severely impaired. In the absence of DPPC, alveolar surface tension at the end of exhalation cannot approach zero,[130] which can lead to lung dysfunction. The deficiency of other lipids may cause similar results. The complete or partial lack of hydrophilic SP (mainly SP-A and SP-D) may exert the weakening of the pulmonary innate immune system.[40] When the content of hydropho-bic SP (mainly SP-B or SP-C) drops below a certain threshold, the distribution of pul-monary surfactant at the air-liquid interface decreases, limiting its surface activity.[115] If SP-G is removed, the insertion of newly-synthesized lipids into the air-fluid interface of the existing system will be affected, and the stability of the pulmonary surfactant monolayer will be reduced.[131] The absence of SP-H affects the release of pro-inflamma-tory cytokines to modulate immune defense, and phagocytic and opsonic processes.[132,][133] During nanomedicine-pulmonary surfactant interaction, some biomolecules attach upon the surface of nanomedicines and are thus removed from the pulmonary surfac-tant, which should be tackled carefully in nanomedicine development.

Due to the physicochemical characteristics of nanomedicines, several components of pulmonary surfactant will be selectively adsorbed. For instance, single-walled car-bon nanotubes could selectively adsorb SP-A and SP-D in animal models.[134] Metal oxide nanoparticles tended to adsorb SP-A, while gold nanoparticles tended to adsorb SP-D.[105] The selectivity roughly adheres to the like-dissolves-like principles.

4.5.3 Surface Activity

As noncovalent bonding is associated with the nanomedicine-pulmonary surfactant interaction, the conformation of biomolecules is highly likely to alter, to adapt to the corresponding binding sites of nanomedicines.[135] As a result, the microscopic mechani-cal properties (compressibility, ductility, etc.) of pulmonary surfactant may change, manifesting in the alteration of surface activity.

It is perceived that the influence on surface activity varies in nanomedicines with different hydrophilicity and sizes. The underlying mechanisms are as follows.

For one thing, a previous study showed that hydrophobic nanomedicines were able to interact with pulmonary surfactant and aggregate around the lipid-condensed domain, rendering a fluidization effect on the pulmonary surfactant membrane.[101] As for hydrophilic nanomedicines, it was confirmed that they could also form aggregates but interfere with the phase transformation and re-adsorption of subphase, and increase the compressibility of the pulmonary surfactant film.[25, 101] It should be noted that although hydrophilic nanomedicines increased compressibility, the actual effect was not significant. Seemingly, hydrophobic nanomedicines possess a stronger influence on surface activity.

For another thing, the size-dependent effects had been shown on pulmonary surfactants. Dwivedi et al. investigated the effects of poly(organosiloxane) nanoparticles with different particle sizes on pulmonary surfactant films and observed that nanoparticles with 12 nm and 20 nm in size had little effect on the films.[136] However, it was shown that 136-nm nanoparticles increased the compressibility of the model film, which was due to the formation of a multilayer convex structure that prevented the acquisition of minimum surface activity. Under the experimental conditions, it can be concluded that nanoparticles with a larger size have a more significant effect on the surface activity of pulmonary surfactants than those with a smaller size.

4.6 CHARACTERIZATION METHODS FOR THE INTERACTION

As discussed above, the nanomedicine-pulmonary surfactant interaction has a significant impact on both nanomedicines and pulmonary surfactants. Hence, it is necessary to investigate such an interaction, to evaluate the biocompatibility and therapeutic efficacy of inhalable nanomedicines, and to scrutinize the effects of nanomedicines on the physiological functions of the lung. The mainstream characterization methods for nanomedicine-pulmonary surfactant interaction are summarized hereby. The following examples all pertain to or are associated with the nanomedicine-pulmonary surfactant characterization, which can offer valuable guides to this field.

4.6.1 Morphology

Transmission electron microscopy (TEM), atomic force microscopy (AFM), and Brewster angle microscopy (BAM) are generally adopted to study the morphology of pulmonary surfactant-adsorbed nanomedicines.

TEM is an electron-optical microscope-based technology with high resolution that uses an electron beam with an extremely short wavelength as the illumination source and an electromagnetic lens to focus the image.[137] At present, the resolution of the TEM can reach 0.1 nm. It has been widely used in medicinal, biological, and material sciences.[138] For example, H. Elham et al. used TEM to observe the morphological state of the complex formed by the tannic acid and lung fluid. They found that the tannic acid-lung fluid complex could self-assemble into spherical particles with a particle size of < 30 nm.[139] R.E. Cristian et al. used TEM to observe the morphology of silica nanoparticles after the interaction with serum albumin. The system has a spherical appearance with a diameter of less than 10 nm.[140]

AFM, also known as scanning force microscope, employs an atomic probe tip to physically scan the sample at the submicron level, and provides nanometer resolution in particle size measurement.[141] It can image non-conductive samples without any special treatment. Therefore, AFM is widely used for the imaging of nanostructures and microstructures. For example, H. Zhang et al. used AFM to observe and compare the nanostructures and microstructures of four animal-derived exogenous pulmonary surfactant preparations, thereby revealing significant differences in the microscopic structure and molecular organization of these preparations.[142] A.K. Sachan et al. used AFM to observe the changes in the accumulation status of pulmonary surfactants caused by nanoparticles at the molecular level. On the level of individual nanoparticles, the coating or combination of surfactants around the nanoparticles was demonstrated.[143] L. Xu and others used AFM to study the effect of heavy metal ions on the pulmonary surfactant monolayer and observed that copper (Cu^{2+}), ferric ion (Fe^{3+}), and mercury (Hg^{2+}) would form a complex with the polar microdomain of the pulmonary surfactant monolayer, changing the membrane structure.[144]

BAM is a microscope commonly used to study thin films on air-liquid interfaces. It can observe single molecules on the interface and obtain strong contrast images with high sensitivity.[145] In the research on nanomedicine-pulmonary surfactant interaction, it is often used to study Langmuir-Blodgett film. For example, E. Guzmán et al. used BAM to characterize the mixed phosphatidylcholine film. Under BAM, it was revealed that hydrophilic silica nanoparticles modified the film structure and dispersed in the subphase.[146]

4.6.2 Biomolecules Separation and Identification

To separate and identify the adsorbed biomolecules after nanomedicine-pulmonary surfactant interaction, a couple of methods can be selected.[147, 148] Amongst them, size exclusion chromatography (SEC) and hydrodynamic interaction chromatography (HIC) can be utilized for separation, and liquid chromatography-mass spectroscopy (LC-MS) and sodium dodecyl sulfate-polyacrylamide gel electrophoresis (SDS-PAGE) can be adopted for separation and identification.

SEC is a liquid chromatography technique that employs a column filled with porous particles for separation. The components with large size are discharged whilst those with small size are blocked, to achieve the purpose of separation.[149] This technique is often used for the separation of biological matrices. For example, R.Q.U. Ain et al. used the SEC method to effectively separate a group of diversified lipid bilayer surrounded nanoparticles from the bovine follicle fluid samples.[150] P. Setzer et al. used the SEC method to separate the proteins bound to nanoparticles and the free proteins for analyses.[151]

HIC is also a liquid chromatography that separates biomolecules based on their size. Different from SEC, HIC columns are filled with non-porous solid particles. For example, J.P.F.G. Helsper et al. used the HIC method to separate liposomal nanoparticles and other biomolecules from the food matrix.[152]

LC-MS is a combined method of liquid chromatography (LC) and mass spectrometry (MS). The eluent is separated by LC and assayed by MS, to realize the separation and identification of complex systems. For example, S. Tenzer et al. used this method to identify more than 300 different protein components adsorbed on the surface of the silicon nano-drug delivery system.[153] A. Hamidu et al. used the LC-MS method to isolate and identify the protein products of breast cancer cell lines treated with doxorubicin and doxorubicin-calcium carbonate nanoparticles.[154] A.L. Dar et al. used this method to determine the composition of protein corona and identified about 100 proteins from the LC-MS data.[155]

SDS-PAGE is a well-known analytical technique to separate and identify proteins with different molecular weights. The main principle is to denature proteins into negatively charged linear chains via sodium dodecyl sulfate (SDS), and then separate them in polyacrylamide gels through electrophoresis.[156] For example, S. Lian et al. used SDS-PAGE technology to separate the SP-B and SP-C from calf pulmonary surfactant.[157] When studying the interaction between nanoparticles and human/bovine serum albumins, R.E. Cristian et al. used SDS-PAGE to separate the albumin adsorbed on the nanoparticles and found that human serum albumin is more easily absorbed than bovine serum albumin.[140] P. Katrin et al. used SDS-PAGE to separate the protein corona formed by the nanoparticles in different volumes of serum, and determined the composition of the corona, and elucidated that the composition varied as the serum volumes increased.[158]

4.6.3 Conformational Change

The conformation changes of pulmonary surfactant components (usually SP) can be examined by circular dichroism (CD), fluorescence correlation spectroscopy (FCS), Fourier Transform infrared spectroscopy (FTIR), and surface-enhanced Raman spectroscopy (SERS).

CD is a spectroscopic method for the determination of proteins. Chiral molecules like proteins show different absorption degrees for left-handed circularly polarized light and right-handed circularly polarized light. Using this characteristic, the CD is widely used in the study of the conformation of proteins.[159] For example, A.L. Dar et al. used this method to determine the conformational changes of proteins adsorbed on the surface of magnetic fluorescent nanoparticles.[155] M. Voicescu et al. used this method to determine a large degree of change in the secondary structure of human serum albumin-bound to silver nanoparticles.[160] X. Xu et al used this method to study the conformational changes after graphene oxide-silver nanocomposites (GO-AgNCP) interacted with bovine serum albumin. The results showed that the interaction changed the secondary structure of bovine serum albumin, and at the same time the model protein lost helical stability.[161]

FCS is a fluorescence-based technology, where the diffusion information can be transformed to size information. Based on this, the thickness of adsorbed proteins on nanomedicines can be obtained, and the binding confirmation can be speculated.[162] For example, A. Silvestri et al. used this method to study the effect of surface coatings on the protein adsorption of nanomedicines *in vivo*.[163] S. Li et al. used FCS as an *in-situ* technique to detect the interaction between nanoparticles and proteins in biological matrices.[164] H. Elham et al. used this method to describe the complexing process between tannic acid and lung fluid.[139]

FTIR can generate structure-specific spectra by detecting the vibration mode of molecules and measuring the frequency of sample absorption, providing information about the conformation.[165] For example, R.E. Cristian et al. used FTIR to study the effect of nanoparticles on the secondary structure of proteins.[140] R. Wojnarowska-Nowak et al. used FTIR to determine protein conformation when studying the interaction between gold nanoparticles and cholesterol enzymes.[166] When studying the effect of silver nanoparticles on *Escherichia coli* (*E. coli*), FTIR was employed by H. Li et al.[167]

SERS uses light to generate enhanced Raman scattering on the surface of nanomedicines to analyze the conformation of adsorbed biological macromolecules.[168] For example, Y. Lin et al. used SERS to analyze the scattering signal of target proteins adsorbed by hydroxyapatite particles for breast cancer diagnosis.[169] X. Cao et al. developed a potential label-free SERS platform to analyze the adsorbed proteins in the plasma to diagnose non-small cell lung cancer.[170]

4.6.4 Surface Tension

In order to detect the surface tension changes of pulmonary surfactant caused by the combination with nanomedicines, Langmuir-Blodgett trough study and oscillating bubble technique (OBT) are usually used.

Langmuir-Blodgett trough is usually used to prepare a monolayer of biomolecules deposited on subphase, called Langmuir-Blodgett films. The interaction between the monolayer and nanomedicines is further investigated.[171] U. Azam et al. used Langmuir-Blodgett trough to process pulmonary surfactants when studying the interaction-induced surface tension alteration in soft nanoparticle vesicles-pulmonary surfactant monolayers system.[172]

OBT is a method for measuring the mass transfer kinetics of pulmonary surfactants at the air-liquid interface.[173] The change in surface tension upon interaction between pulmonary surfactant and poly(styrene), poly(D,L-lactide-co-glycolide), or poly(butyl methacrylate-co-(2-dimethylaminoethyl)   methacrylate-co-methyl   methacrylate) nanoparticles was evaluated by M. Beck-Broichsitter et al.[174]

4.6.5 Kinetics and Thermodynamics

Quantitative investigation of kinetics and thermodynamics is quite important to characterize nanomedicine-pulmonary surfactant interaction. Quartz crystal microbalance (QCM) is an emerging method for kinetics study based on the determination of the vibration frequency of materials.[175] For example, F. Wan et al analyzed the data of QCM through the Langmuir adsorption equation, determined the kinetic and equilibrium parameters, and clarified the nature of the interaction between liposomes and pulmonary surfactant.[176] U. Azam et al. clarified the interaction kinetics between soft nanoparticle vesicles and pulmonary surfactants by observing the frequency changes of lipid bilayer injected into QCM.[172]

Isothermal titration calorimetry (ITC) can accurately characterize nanomedicine-biomolecule interaction by calculating thermodynamic parameters.[177] The major advantage of ITC technology is that it provides a large number of thermodynamic information in a single experiment. For example, V. Parikh et al. used this method to analyze the thermodynamics of the interaction between recombinant human growth hormone (r-hGH) and polymer nanoparticles.[178] N. Gal et al. used ITC to study the interaction between serum proteins and nanoparticles grafted with dense polymeric brushes and found that albumin could be adsorbed on the nanoparticle surface.[179]

4.6.6 *In-silico* Interaction Model

In-silico coarse-grained molecular dynamics can be considered to visualize the interaction. The coarse-grained process preserves the essential details of molecular structure, omits the unessential information, and establishes a meaningful interaction model.[180] For example, F. Jiao et al. applied this method to preliminarily study the mechanical mechanism of the interaction between nanomedicines and pulmonary surfactants.[181] It is advisable to prove the simulation results with experimental evidence to improve the credibility.

4.7 IMPLICATIONS FOR PULMONARY DRUG DELIVERY OF NANOMEDICINES

4.7.1 Impact of the Interaction on Drug Delivery

After the inhalation of nanomedicines, they are firstly suspended in the alveolar lining fluid where pulmonary surfactant was distributed, and hence nanomaterials will interact with pulmonary surfactant. Pulmonary surfactant spontaneously adsorbs to the surface of the nanomedicines, forming a biomolecular corona.

For nanomedicines, this interaction will change the physical and chemical properties of them, or at least the physicochemical attributes of the surface will be altered. This is reflexed by the change in hydrophobicity, surface charge, and colloidal stability of nanomedicines. These changes, in turn, impact the pulmonary surfactant layer permeability, targeting region, and cellular uptake of nanomedicines. In this context, the pharmacokinetic and pharmacodynamic behaviors will be ultimately influenced. For pulmonary surfactants, this interaction can induce changes in the biosynthesis of pulmonary surfactant, which is an ROS-related process: Nanomedicine-biomolecule complexes can boost or attenuate the production of ROS in type-II alveolar epithelial cells. The components and surface activity of pulmonary surfactant may also be affected by the interaction.

From this perspective, the nanomedicine-pulmonary surfactant interaction exerts an impact on both counterparts, and the impact is typically unwanted. On one hand, the basic properties of nanomedicines may be severely changed by interactions with the pulmonary surfactant, which remarkably compromises the desired multi-functions of well-designed nanomedicines. On the other hand, by interaction with nanomedicines, the critical physiological functions and even basic components of pulmonary surfactants may fall into an abnormal state. Without being controlled, the interaction may make the biological fate of inhalable nanomedicines complicated, and even lead to treatment failure by reduced lesion site accumulation and raised adverse effects.

Regretfully, as most developed nanomedicines do not seriously consider this aspect, the controlling capacity of such an interaction is far from satisfaction. Although great therapeutic effects are revealed in the reported nanomedicines in the *in vitro* model and even animal models, the translation from lab to clinical trials are still lag far behind. According to the abovementioned reports, the pulmonary surfactant-nanomedicines interactions should partially account for this fact. Before considering the well-known issues like large-scale productions and *in vivo* safety, the basic but key factors including nanomedicine-pulmonary surfactant interaction should be incorporated into the *ab initio* design.

Therefore, acquiring in-depth knowledge of nanomedicine-pulmonary surfactant interaction, taking advantage of the alteration of nanomedicines properties, and manipulating such interaction to minimize the interference on safety and efficacy of nanomedicines and physiological functions of pulmonary surfactant is of great significance for the promotion of clinical translation of inhalable nanomedicines, and they are gradually becoming utmost priorities in the design and development of relevant products.

4.7.2 Manipulation of the Interaction

So how to regulate the interaction between nanomedicines and pulmonary surfactants? The prerequisite to understanding is what factors are involved in this interaction. As indicated in the former sections, the key parameters affecting the interaction are the surface properties, mainly referred to as hydrophobicity and charge.

In theory, hydrophobic nanomedicines have stronger interaction with the pulmonary surfactant, which is mainly composed of hydrophobic substances like DPPC.[182] On the other hand, hydrophilic nanomedicines exhibit a lower tendency to interact with pulmonary surfactants. Y. Xu et al. employed the molecular dynamics simulations method to study the translocate behavior of nanoparticles on pulmonary surfactant film with different surface hydrophilicity.[183] It was observed that the hydrophilic nanoparticles translocated directly across the film, while the hydrophobic NPs were wrapped by a pulmonary surfactant layer, demonstrating that the hydrophobic surface is more favorable to interact with pulmonary surfactant rather than the hydrophilic one. Herein, to mitigate the interaction, one can consider modifying the nanomedicines with a hydrophilic surface.

There are cationic and anionic biomolecules in pulmonary surfactants, and therefore nanomedicines with either cationic or anionic surface will adsorb biomolecules with opposite charges. To this end, non-ionizable or zwitterionic nanomaterials without distinct trends to attract charged biomolecules can be chosen to reduce biomolecule adsorption.[184] It is suggested that nanomedicines with hydrophilic and non-ionizable or zwitterionic surfaces are promising to attenuate the interaction with pulmonary surfactants. Hydrophilic and non-ionizable or zwitterionic nanomaterials can be directly fabricated into nanomedicines, or used as the coating zone for nanomedicines.

Currently, surface modification by poloxamer[185] and polyethylene glycol (PEG)[186] (hydrophilic plus non-ionizable materials) are the main reported strategies. Poloxamer 407 had been utilized to shield the surface with the hydrophilic property. It was reported that the pulmonary surfactant function was hindered upon contact with bare polymeric nanoparticles due to the depletion of the SP content.[186] In contrast, the poloxamer 407 modification exerted the opposite effect, protecting the normal functions of pulmonary surfactants. M. Beck-Broichsitter et al. modified the plain poly(lactide) nanoparticles surface with PEG chains to avoid pulmonary surfactant interactions.[187] By determining the surface tension behavior of Alveofact®, the naturally derived pulmonary surfactant, the PEGylation nanoparticles showed better pulmonary surfactant function compatibility than control. Additionally, for pharmaceutical development, it is necessary to control the content of these modifiers during the preparation of nanomedicines, to prevent their unpredicted dose-dependent toxicities of them.

4.7.3 Application of Pulmonary Surfactant in Nanomedicine Design

The nanomedicine-pulmonary surfactant interaction has been intensively discussed in this chapter. Thinking outside the box is suggested herein. Due to its excellent surface activity, pulmonary surfactant is a prospective alternative for surfactants, emulsifiers, or amphiphilic carriers in drug delivery systems. In recent years, some studies have examined the possibility of incorporating a pulmonary surfactant into nanomedicines. It was shown that pulmonary surfactant-containing complexes could facilitate the effective distribution of drug delivery systems along with the air-liquid interface and promote the diffusion process.[188]

By surface coating of entire pulmonary surfactant, the prepared pulmonary delivered bio-inspired nanomedicines can obtain better biocompatibility, improved therapeutic efficiency, and elevated stability. L. De Backer et al. reported a hybrid pulmonary surfactant (Curosurf®)-coated nanogels for siRNA pulmonary delivery to murine alveolar macrophages.[189] It was proved that both the surfactant-coated and uncoated nanogels achieved high levels of siRNA uptake but only the surfactant-coated formulation could significantly reduce gene expression on the protein level. Further, the authors also found that the decoration of siRNA-loaded dextran nanogel with a surfactant shell enhanced the colloidal stability and prevented siRNA release in the presence of competing polyanions, which are abundantly present in biofluids.[190]

As one of the most important components of pulmonary surfactants, DPPC has been used in the modification of liposomes to acquire better pulmonary delivery outcomes.[191] The designed DPPC-coated lipid nanoparticles (DPPC-LNS) were composed of solid natural lipid core, stabilized by a shell of pulmonary surfactant. The physical and chemical stability of DPPC-LNS were significantly improved.[192] Another study showed that DPPC-LNS had the advantages of effective deposition, high local concentration, rapid therapeutic onset, and long retention time in the lung.[193] It is anticipated that more pulmonary surfactant decorated nanomedicines will be developed shortly.

4.8 CONCLUDING REMARKS AND OUTLOOK

Nanomedicines possess many advantages in drug delivery and are attracting more attention in pulmonary disease treatment. There is plenty of fundamental research, however, no commercial products have reached the market. The main reason behind it is that the *in vivo* fate of nanomedicines after inhalation is still unclear. Particularly, the interaction between inhaled nanomedicines and pulmonary surfactant is scarcely visited.

In sight of this, recent studies intensively investigate the nanomedicine-pulmonary surfactant interaction, whose influence on the *in vivo* fate of nanomedicines is revealed. The concept of biomolecular corona adds to the understanding of the interaction. These provide a firm basis for the design, fabrication, and application of functional nanomedicines. At the same time, lots of interaction characterization methods are put forward, offering new strategies for the clarification of nanomedicine-pulmonary surfactant interaction from a microscopic perspective.

Even though it is a challengeable commission to master the detailed mechanisms of nanomedicine-pulmonary surfactant interaction. Exploring these mechanisms will become the next task for scientists in biochemistry, pharmacology, and toxicology. Soon, demonstration of the influencing factors for the interaction and establishment of precise interaction models should be conducted, and the active modification of nanomedicines towards manipulation of pulmonary surfactant adsorption will be the potential hotspot.

4.9 ACKNOWLEDGMENT

The authors would like to appreciate the financial supports from the National Natural Science Foundation of China (grants No. 82073774 and 81973263) and the Key Areas Research and Development Program of Guangdong Province (Grant No. 2019B020204002), during the preparation of this book chapter.

4.10 APPENDICES

4.10.1 Representative Cases Summary of the Interaction

The aforementioned cases are about the interaction between nanomedicines and pulmonary surfactants. For simplicity and clarity, a tabular summary (Table 4.1) is provided, listing the interaction counterparts and main conclusion.

TABLE 4.1   Representative case summary of the interaction between inhalable nanomedicine and pulmonary surfactant

NO.	INHALABLE NANOMEDICINE	PULMONARY SURFACTANT	MAIN CONCLUSION	REFERENCE
1	Mannosylated nanoparticles	SP-A	Uptake of nanoparticles is enhanced	106
2	SiO_2 and ZrO_2 inhaled nanomedicine	Pure lipid samples	Nanomedicine don't interact with pure lipid samples	102
3	Silver nanomedicine	Lipids such as DPPC	Reduce the tendency of nanomedicine's aggregation	101
4	Silver nanowires	Entire pulmonary surfactant	Restrain the nanomedicine's aggregation	108
5	Polystyrene microspheres	Lecithin	Lecithin-coated microspheres can enter alveolar epithelial cells	194
6	Nanodroplets	Entire pulmonary surfactant	Changes nanomedicine's ability to penetrate the pulmonary surfactant film and elevating cellular uptake	195
7	Mannosylated nanoparticles	SP-A	Enhance the targeting ability to macrophages	106
8	Dextran nanogels	Entire pulmonary surfactant	Promote absorption and transport of nanogels	189, 190
9	Single-walled carbon nanotubes	SP-A and SP-D	Resulting in a loss of lung function	50
10	Metal oxide nanoparticles	Entire pulmonary surfactant	Metal oxide nanoparticles tended to adsorb SP-A	196
11	Gold nanoparticles	Entire pulmonary surfactant	Gold nanoparticles tended to adsorb SP-D	196
12	Hydrophobic SP	Entire pulmonary surfactant	Fluidization of the interface membrane	100
13	Nanomedicines of different sizes	Entire pulmonary surfactant	136 nm NMs has more significant effect on PS than 12 nm NMs	40
14	Gold nanomedicine	Entire pulmonary surfactant	Cell uptake decrease	116
15	HA-NPs and PST-NPs	Entire pulmonary surfactant	Hydrophobicity of nanomedicines determines the degree of displacement on the natural pulmonary surfactant membrane	25

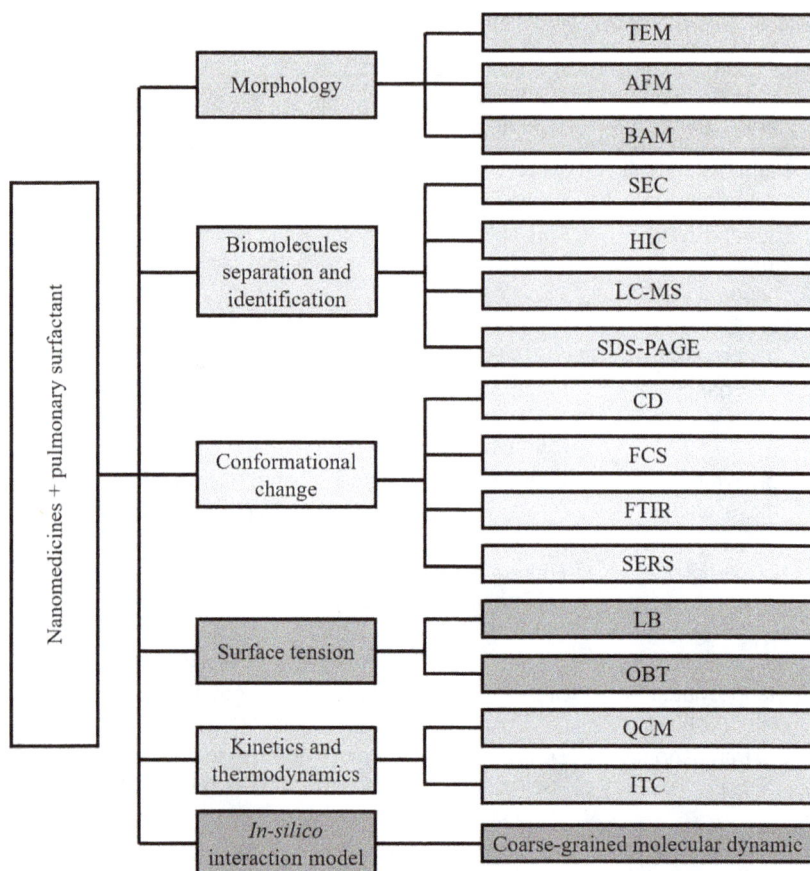

FIGURE 4.8 Summary of characterization methods for inhalable nanomedicine-pulmonary surfactant interaction.

4.10.2 Summary of Characterization Methods for the Interaction

The characterization methods for the interaction between inhalable nanomedicines and pulmonary surfactants are summarized in Figure 4.8. The methods are categorized into six classes, i.e., morphological, biomolecules identification, conformational change, surface tension, kinetics and thermodynamics, and *in-silico* interaction model.

REFERENCES

1. Nie, X. et al. Oral nano drug delivery systems for the treatment of type 2 diabetes mellitus: An available administration strategy for antidiabetic phytocompounds. *Int J Nanomed* 15, 10215–10240 (2020).

2. Nikravesh, N. et al. Factors influencing safety and efficacy of intravenous iron-carbohy-drate nanomedicines: From production to clinical practice. *Nanomed* 26, 102178 (2020).

3. Ramadon, D., McCrudden, M.T.C., Courtenay, A.J. & Donnelly, R.F. Enhancement strategies for transdermal drug delivery systems: Current trends and applications. *Drug Deliv Transl Res* 12–4), 758–791 (2021).

4. Al-Halifa, S., Gauthier, L., Arpin, D., Bourgault, S. & Archambault, D. Nanoparticle-based vaccines Against respiratory viruses. *Front Immunol* 10, 22 (2019).

5. Huang, C.H., Chen, X.Y., Xue, Z.J. & Wang, T. Effect of structure: A new insight into nanoparticle assemblies from inanimate to animate. *Sci Adv* 6(20), (2020).

6. Passi, M., Shahid, S., Chockalingam, S., Sundar, I.K. & Packirisamy, G. Conventional and nanotechnology based approaches to combat chronic obstructive pulmonary disease: Implications for chronic airway diseases. *Int J Nanomed* 15, 3803–3826 (2020).

7. Ong, V., Mei, V., Cao, L., Lee, K. & Chung, E.J. Nanomedicine for cystic fibrosis. *SLAS Technol* 24(2), 169–180 (2019).

8. Heinrich, M.A., Martina, B. & Prakash, J. Nanomedicine strategies to target coronavirus. *Nano Today* 35, 100961 (2020).

9. Hussain, S. Nanomedicine for treatment of lung cancer. *Adv Exp Med Biol* 890, 137–147 (2016).

10. Patra, J.K. et al. Nano based drug delivery systems: Recent developments and future prospects. *J Nanobiotechnology* 16(1), 71 (2018).

11. Kamaly, N., Yameen, B., Wu, J. & Farokhzad, O.C. Degradable controlled-release polymers and polymeric nanoparticles: Mechanisms of controlling drug release. *Chem Rev* 116(4), 2602–2663 (2016).

12. Zhao, Y.Z. et al. Experiment on the feasibility of using modified gelatin nanoparticles as insulin pulmonary administration system for diabetes therapy. *Acta Diabetol* 49(4), 315–325 (2012).

13. Sultana, S. et al. Inhalation of alendronate nanoparticles as dry powder inhaler for the treatment of osteoporosis. *J Microencapsul* 29(5), 445–454 (2012).

14. Miller, M.R. et al. Inhaled nanoparticles accumulate at sites of vascular disease. *ACS Nano* 11(5), 4542–4552 (2017).

15. Yang, W., Peters, J.I. & Williams, R.O. Inhaled nanoparticles - A current review. *Int J Pharm* 356(1–2), 239–247 (2008).

16. Elhissi, A. Liposomes for pulmonary drug delivery: The role of formulation and inhalation device design. *Curr Pharm Des* 23(3), 362–372 (2017).

17. Long, M. et al. Enhanced delivery of artesunate by stimuli-responsive polymeric micelles for lung tumor therapy. *J Drug Deliv Sci Technol* 66, 102812 (2021).

18. Chauhan, A.S. Dendrimers for drug delivery. *Molecules* 23(4), 938 (2018).

19. Wang, L. et al. Manipulation of macrophage polarization by peptide-coated gold nanoparticles and its protective effects on acute lung injury. *J Nanobiotechnology* 18(1), 38 (2020).

20. Wang, C. et al. Carrier-free platinum nanomedicine for targeted cancer therapy. *Small* 16(49), e2004829 (2020).

21. Wadhwa, S. & Mumper, R.J. Polymer-drug conjugates for anticancer drug delivery. *Crit Rev Ther Drug Carrier Syst* 32(3), 215–245 (2015).

22. Bassetti, M., Vena, A., Russo, A. & Peghin, M. Inhaled liposomal antimicrobial delivery in lung infections. *Drugs* 80(13), 1309–1318 (2020).

23. Qi, J.P. et al. Towards more accurate bioimaging of drug nanocarriers: Turning aggregation-caused quenching into a useful tool. *Adv Drug Deliv Rev* 143, 206–225 (2019).

24. Shi, J., Kantoff, P.W., Wooster, R. & Farokhzad, O.C. Cancer nanomedicine: Progress, challenges and opportunities. *Nat Rev Cancer* 17(1), 20–37 (2017).

25. Hu, G. et al. Physicochemical properties of nanoparticles regulate translocation across pulmonary surfactant monolayer and formation of lipoprotein corona. *ACS Nano* 7(12), 10525–10533 (2013).

26. Ching, J. & Kajino, M. Aerosol mixing state matters for particles deposition in human respiratory system. *Sci Rep-Uk* 8(1), 1–11 (2018).

27. Hittinger, M. et al. Preclinical safety and efficacy models for pulmonary drug delivery of antimicrobials with focus on in vitro models. *Adv Drug Deliv Rev* 85, 44–56 (2015).

28. das Neves, J., Arzi, R.S. & Sosnik, A. Molecular and cellular cues governing nanomaterial-mucosae interactions: From nanomedicine to nanotoxicology. *Chem Soc Rev* 49(14), 5058–5100 (2020).

29. Eskandari, Z., Bahadori, F., Celik, B. & Onyuksel, H. Targeted nanomedicines for cancer therapy, from basics to clinical trials. *J Pharm Pharm Sci* 23(1), 132–157 (2020).

30. Han, S. & Mallampalli, R.K. The role of surfactant in lung disease and host defense against pulmonary infections. *Ann Am Thorac Soc* 12(5), 765–774 (2015).

31. Li, J. et al. Nanomaterials for the theranostics of obesity. *Biomaterials* 223, 119474 (2019).

32. Haghi, M., Ong, H.X., Traini, D. & Young, P. Across the pulmonary epithelial barrier: Integration of physicochemical properties and human cell models to study pulmonary drug formulations. *Pharmacol Ther* 144(3), 235–252 (2014).

33. Parra, E. & Perez-Gil, J. Composition, structure and mechanical properties define performance of pulmonary surfactant membranes and films. *Chem Phys Lipids* 185, 153–175 (2015).

34. Ji, J. et al. Potential therapeutic applications of pulmonary surfactant lipids in the host defence Against respiratory viral infections. *Front Immunol* 12, 730022 (2021).

35. Welde, M.A., Sanford, C.B., Mangum, M., Paschal, C. & Jnah, A.J. Pulmonary hemorrhage in the neonate. *Neonatal Netw* 40(5), 295–304 (2021).

36. Autilio, C. & Perez-Gil, J. Understanding the principle biophysics concepts of pulmonary surfactant in health and disease. *Arch Dis Child Fetal Neonatal Ed* 104(4), F443–F451 (2019).

37. Guagliardo, R., Perez-Gil, J., De Smedt, S. & Raemdonck, K. Pulmonary surfactant and drug delivery: Focusing on the role of surfactant proteins. *J Control Release* 291, 116–126 (2018).

38. Sanaki, T. et al. Inhibition of dengue virus infection by 1-stearoyl-2-arachidonoyl-phosphatidylinositol in vitro. *FASEB J* 33(12), 13866–13881 (2019).

39. Ji, J. et al. Potential therapeutic applications of pulmonary surfactant lipids in the host defence Against respiratory viral infections. *Front Immunol* 12, 730022 (2021).

40. Lopez-Rodriguez, E. & Perez-Gil, J. Structure-function relationships in pulmonary surfactant membranes: From biophysics to therapy. *Biochim Biophys Acta* 1838(6), 1568–1585 (2014).

41. Albert, R.K. The role of ventilation-induced surfactant dysfunction and atelectasis in causing acute respiratory distress syndrome. *Am J Respir Crit Care Med* 185(7), 702–708 (2012).

42. Vieira, F., Kung, J.W. & Bhatti, F. Structure, genetics and function of the pulmonary associated surfactant proteins A and D: The extra-pulmonary role of these C type lectins. *Ann Anat* 211, 184–201 (2017).

43. Schicht, M. et al. SFTA3, a novel protein of the lung: Three-dimensional structure, characterisation and immune activation. *Eur Respir J* 44(2), 447–456 (2014).

44. Rausch, F. et al. "SP-G", a putative new surfactant protein–Tissue localization and 3D structure. *PLOS ONE* 7(10), e47789 (2012).

45. Ji, Y., Ma, M. & Pei, Y. Research progress and application of pulmonary surfactant. *Chin Pharamceutical J* 40, 1449–1453 (2005).

46. Sever, N., Milicic, G., Bodnar, N.O., Wu, X.D. & Rapoport, T.A. Mechanism of lamellar body formation by lung surfactant protein B. *Mol Cell* 81(1), 49–66 (2021).

47. Voorhout, W.F., Weaver, T.E., Haagsman, H.P., Geuze, H.J. & Van Golde, L.M. Biosynthetic routing of pulmonary surfactant proteins in alveolar type II cells. *Microsc Res Tech* 26(5), 366–373 (1993).

48. Bridges, J.P. et al. LPCAT1 regulates surfactant phospholipid synthesis and is required for transitioning to air breathing in mice. *J Clin Invest* 120(5), 1736–1748 (2010).

49. Dave, V. et al. Calcineurin/Nfat signaling is required for perinatal lung maturation and function. *J Clin Invest* 116(10), 2597–2609 (2006).

50. Echaide, M., Autilio, C., Arroyo, R. & Perez-Gil, J. Restoring pulmonary surfactant membranes and films at the respiratory surface. *Biochim Biophys Acta Rev Biomembr* 1859(9 Pt B), 1725–1739 (2017).

51. Young, S.L. & Tierney, D.F. Dipalmitoyl lecithin secretion and metabolism by the rat lung. *Am J Physiol* 222(6), 1539–1544 (1972).

52. Chroneos, Z.C., Sever-Chroneos, Z. & Shepherd, V.L. Pulmonary surfactant: An immunological perspective. *Cell Physiol Biochem* 25(1), 13–26 (2010).

53. Wright, J.R. & Dobbs, L.G. Regulation of pulmonary surfactant secretion and clearance. *Annu Rev Physiol* 53, 395–414 (1991).

54. Silva, L.C.G. et al. Exogenous surfactant replacement immediately at birth as preventive therapy for lung prematurity in neonatal lambs. *Theriogenology* 171, 14–20 (2021).

55. Torresin, M. et al. Exogenous surfactant kinetics in infant respiratory distress syndrome: A novel method with stable isotopes. *Am J Respir Crit Care Med* 161(5), 1584–1589 (2000).

56. Wang, H., Lin, Y., Nienhaus, K. & Nienhaus, G.U. The protein corona on nanoparticles as viewed from a nanoparticle-sizing perspective. *Wiley Interdiscip Rev Nanomed Nanobiotechnol* 10(4), e1500 (2018).

57. Chen, D.Y., Ganesh, S., Wang, W.M. & Amiji, M. Plasma protein adsorption and biological identity of systemically administered nanoparticles. *Nanomed-UK* 12(17), 2113–2135 (2017).

58. Monopoli, M.P., Aberg, C., Salvati, A. & Dawson, K.A. Biomolecular coronas provide the biological identity of nanosized materials. *Nat Nanotechnol* 7(12), 779–786 (2012).

59. Zanganeh, S., Spitler, R., Erfanzadeh, M., Alkilany, A.M. & Mahmoudi, M. Protein corona: Opportunities and challenges. *Int J Biochem Cell Biol* B 75, 143–147 (2016).

60. Cai, R. & Chen, C.Y. The crown and the scepter: Roles of the protein corona in nanomedicine. *Adv Mater* 31(45), 1805740 (2019).

61. Konduru, N.V. et al. Protein corona: Implications for nanoparticle interactions with pulmonary cells. *Part Fibre Toxicol* 14(1), 1–12 (2017).

62. Pochert, A., Vernikouskaya, I., Pascher, F., Rasche, V. & Linden, M. Cargo-influences on the biodistribution of hollow mesoporous silica nanoparticles as studied by quantitative F-19-magnetic resonance imaging. *J Colloid Interf Sci* 488, 1–9 (2017).

63. Wu, J.J. et al. Binding-mediated formation of ribonucleoprotein corona for efficient delivery and control of CRISPR/Cas9. *Angew Chem Int Edit* 60(20), 11104–11109 (2021).

64. Caracciolo, G. et al. Human biomolecular corona of liposomal doxorubicin: The overlooked factor in anticancer drug delivery. *ACS Appl Mater Inter* 10(27), 22951–22962 (2018).

65. Salvati, A. et al. Transferrin-functionalized nanoparticles lose their targeting capabilities when a biomolecule corona adsorbs on the surface. *Nat Nanotechnol* 8(2), 137–143 (2013).

66. Jiang, X. et al. Quantitative analysis of the protein corona on FePt nanoparticles formed by transferrin binding. *J R Soc Interface* 7, S5–S13 (2010).

67. Shanehsazzadeh, S. et al. Monoclonal antibody conjugated magnetic nanoparticles could target MUC-1-positive cells in vitro but not in vivo. *Contrast Media Mol Imaging* 10(3), 225–236 (2015).

68. Ahsan, S.M., Rao, C.M. & Ahmad, M.F. Nanoparticle-protein interaction: The significance and role of protein corona. *Adv Exp Med Biol* 1048, 175–198 (2018).

69. Sakulkhu, U. et al. Ex situ evaluation of the composition of protein corona of intravenously injected Superparamagnetic nanoparticles in rats. *Nanoscale* 6(19), 11439–11450 (2014).

70. Mahmoudi, M., Sant, S., Wang, B., Laurent, S. & Sen, T. Superparamagnetic iron oxide nanoparticles (SPIONs): Development, surface modification and applications in chemotherapy. *Adv Drug Deliv Rev* 63(1–2), 24–46 (2011).

71. Walkey, C.D., Olsen, J.B., Guo, H.B., Emili, A. & Chan, W.C.W. Nanoparticle size and surface chemistry determine serum protein adsorption and macrophage uptake. *J Am Chem Soc* 134(4), 2139–2147 (2012).

72. Dobrovolskaia, M.A. & Mcneil, S.E. Immunological properties of engineered nanomaterials. *Nat Nanotechnol* 2(8), 469–478 (2007).

73. Goy-Lopez, S. et al. Physicochemical characteristics of protein-NP bioconjugates: The role of particle curvature and solution conditions on human serum albumin conformation and fibrillogenesis inhibition. *Langmuir* 28(24), 9113–9126 (2012).

74. Zhang, D.M. et al. Gold nanoparticles can induce the formation of protein-based aggregates at physiological pH. *Nano Lett* 9(2), 666–671 (2009).

75. Han, H. et al. Versatile controllability of non-axisymmetric magnetic perturbations in KSTAR experiments. *Fusion Eng Des* 108, 60–66 (2016).

76. Miclaus, T. et al. Dynamic protein coronas revealed as a modulator of silver nanoparticle sulphidation in vitro. *Nat Commun* 7, 1–10 (2016).

77. Lu, N.H., Li, J.Y., Tian, R. & Peng, Y.Y. Binding of human serum albumin to single-walled carbon nanotubes activated neutrophils to increase production of hypochlorous acid, the oxidant capable of degrading nanotubes. *Chem Res Toxicol* 27(6), 1070–1077 (2014).

78. Liu, J.H. et al. Effect of size and dose on the biodistribution of graphene oxide in mice. *Nanomed-UK* 7(12), 1801–1812 (2012).

79. Vroman, L., Adams, A.L., Fischer, G.C. & Munoz, P.C. Interaction of high molecular weight kininogen, factor XII, and fibrinogen in plasma at interfaces. *Blood* 55(1), 156–159 (1980).

80. Pearson, R.M., Juettner, V.V. & Hong, S. Biomolecular corona on nanoparticles: A survey of recent literature and its implications in targeted drug delivery. *Front Chem* 2, 108 (2014).

81. Huang, Z.W. et al. Relationship between particle size and lung retention time of intact solid lipid nanoparticle suspensions after pulmonary delivery. *J Control Release* 325, 206–222 (2020).

82. Hu, Q.L., Bai, X., Hu, G.Q. & Zuo, Y.Y. Unveiling the molecular structure of pulmonary surfactant corona on nanoparticles. *ACS Nano* 11(7), 6832–6842 (2017).

83. Wang, X.Q. et al. Adsorption of proteins on oral Zn2+ doped iron oxide nanoparticles in mouse stomach and in vitro: Triggering nanoparticle aggregation. *Nanoscale* 12(44), 22754–22767 (2020).

84. Bohorquez, A.C. & Rinaldi, C. In situ evaluation of nanoparticle-protein interactions by dynamic magnetic susceptibility measurements. *Part Part Syst Charact* 31(5), 561–570 (2014).

85. Curnutt, A., Smith, K., Darrow, E. & Walters, K.B. Chemical and microstructural characterization of pH and [Ca2+] dependent sol-gel transitions in mucin biopolymer. *Sci Rep-Uk* 10(1), 1–12 (2020).

86. Dominguez-Medina, S. et al. Adsorption and unfolding of a single protein triggers nanoparticle aggregation. *ACS Nano* 10(2), 2103–2112 (2016).

87. Cukalevski, R., Ferreira, S.A., Dunning, C.J., Berggard, T. & Cedervall, T. IgG and fibrinogen driven nanoparticle aggregation. *Nano Res* 8(8), 2733–2743 (2015).

88. Matalon, S. Mechanisms and regulation of ion transport in adult mammalian alveolar type II pneumocytes. *Am J Physiol* 261(5 Pt 1), C727–C738 (1991).

89. Saumon, G. & Basset, G. Electrolyte and fluid transport across the mature alveolar epithelium. *J Appl Physiol (1985)* 74(1), 1–15 (1993).

90. Kankala, R.K. et al. Nanoarchitectured structure and surface biofunctionality of mesoporous silica nanoparticles. *Adv Mater* 32(23), 1907035 (2020).

91. Tenzer, S. et al. Nanoparticle size is a critical physicochemical determinant of the human blood plasma corona: A comprehensive quantitative proteomic analysis. *ACS Nano* 5(9), 7155–7167 (2011).

92. Yang, S.T., Liu, Y., Wang, Y.W. & Cao, A.N. Biosafety and bioapplication of nanomaterials by designing protein-nanoparticle interactions. *Small* 9(9–10), 1635–1653 (2013).
93. Bharti, B., Meissner, J. & Findenegg, G.H. Aggregation of silica nanoparticles directed by adsorption of lysozyme. *Langmuir* 27(16), 9823–9833 (2011).
94. Bharti, B., Meissner, J., Klapp, S.H.L. & Findenegg, G.H. Bridging interactions of proteins with silica nanoparticles: The influence of pH, ionic strength and protein concentration. *Soft Matter* 10(5), 718–728 (2014).
95. Zhang, M.Z., Chen, X.X., Li, C. & Shen, X. Charge-reversal nanocarriers: An emerging paradigm for smart cancer nanomedicine. *J Control Release* 319, 46–62 (2020).
96. Okyem, S., Awotunde, O., Ogunlusi, T., Riley, M.B. & Driskell, J.D. Probing the mechanism of antibody-triggered aggregation of gold nanoparticles. *Langmuir* 37(9), 2993–3000 (2021).
97. O'Brien, J. & Shea, K.J. Tuning the protein corona of hydrogel nanoparticles: The synthesis of abiotic protein and peptide affinity reagents. *Acc Chem Res* 49(6), 1200–1210 (2016).
98. Chen, P.Y. et al. Amyloidosis inhibition, a new frontier of the protein corona. *Nano Today* 35 (2020).
99. Pishkar, L. et al. Studies on the interaction between nanodiamond and human hemoglobin by surface tension measurement and spectroscopy methods. *J Biomol Struct Dyn* 35(3), 603–615 (2017).
100. Wohlleben, W. et al. Influence of agglomeration and specific lung lining lipid/protein interaction on short-term inhalation toxicity. *Nanotoxicology* 10(7), 970–980 (2016).
101. Arick, D.Q., Choi, Y.H., Kim, H.C. & Won, Y.Y. Effects of nanoparticles on the mechanical functioning of the lung. *Adv Colloid Interface Sci* 225, 218–228 (2015).
102. Raesch, S.S. et al. Proteomic and lipidomic analysis of nanoparticle corona upon contact with lung surfactant reveals differences in protein, but not lipid composition. *ACS Nano* 9(12), 11872–11885 (2015).
103. Zhuang, B.L., Ramanauskaite, G., Koa, Z.Y. & Wang, Z.G. Like dissolves like: A first-principles theory for predicting liquid miscibility and mixture dielectric constant. *Sci Adv* 7(7), (2021).
104. Guagliardo, R., Perez-Gil, J., De Smedt, S. & Raemdonck, K. Pulmonary surfactant and drug delivery: Focusing on the role of surfactant proteins. *J Control Release* 291, 116–126 (2018).
105. Theodorou, I.G., Ryan, M.P., Tetley, T.D. & Porter, A.E. Inhalation of silver nanomaterials–Seeing the risks. *Int J Mol Sci* 15(12), 23936–23974 (2014).
106. Ruge, C.A. et al. Pulmonary surfactant protein A-mediated enrichment of surface-decorated polymeric nanoparticles in alveolar macrophages. *Mol Pharm* 13(12), 4168–4178 (2016).
107. Zhao, Q. et al. Interaction of nano carbon particles and anthracene with pulmonary surfactant: The potential hazards of inhaled nanoparticles. *Chemosphere* 215, 746–752 (2019).
108. Theodorou, I.G. et al. Static and dynamic microscopy of the chemical stability and aggregation state of silver nanowires in components of murine pulmonary surfactant. *Environ Sci Technol* 49(13), 8048–8056 (2015).
109. Hidalgo, A., Cruz, A. & Perez-Gil, J. Barrier or carrier? Pulmonary surfactant and drug delivery. *Eur J Pharm Biopharm* 95(A), 117–127 (2015).
110. Xu, Y. et al. Role of lipid coating in the transport of nanodroplets across the pulmonary surfactant layer revealed by molecular dynamics simulations. *Langmuir* 34(30), 9054–9063 (2018).
111. Parra, E. et al. A combined action of pulmonary surfactant proteins SP-B and SP-C modulates permeability and dynamics of phospholipid membranes. *Biochem J* 438(3), 555–564 (2011).
112. Kato, T. et al. Evidence that exogenous substances can be phagocytized by alveolar epithelial cells and transported into blood capillaries. *Cell Tissue Res* 311(1), 47–51 (2003).

113. De Backer, L. et al. Bio-inspired pulmonary surfactant-modified nanogels: A promising siRNA delivery system. *J Control Release* 206, 177–186 (2015).

114. De Backer, L. et al. Hybrid pulmonary surfactant-coated nanogels mediate efficient in vivo delivery of siRNA to murine alveolar macrophages. *J Control Release* 217, 53–63 (2015).

115. Merckx, P. et al. Surfactant protein B (SP-B) enhances the cellular siRNA delivery of proteolipid coated nanogels for inhalation therapy. *Acta Biomater* 78, 236–246 (2018).

116. Albanese, A. & Chan, W.C. Effect of gold nanoparticle aggregation on cell uptake and toxicity. *ACS Nano* 5(7), 5478–5489 (2011).

117. Yang, B., Chen, Y. & Shi, J. Reactive oxygen species (ROS)-based nanomedicine. *Chem Rev* 119(8), 4881–4985 (2019).

118. Mary, V.S., Theumer, M.G., Arias, S.L. & Rubinstein, H.R. Reactive oxygen species sources and biomolecular oxidative damage induced by aflatoxin b1 and fumonisin B1 in rat spleen mononuclear cells. *Toxicology* 302(2–3), 299–307 (2012).

119. Yu, Z. et al. Reactive oxygen species-related nanoparticle toxicity in the biomedical field. *Nanoscale Res Lett* 15(1), 115 (2020).

120. Ruaro, B. et al. The history and mystery of alveolar epithelial type II cells: Focus on their physiologic and pathologic role in lung. *Int J Mol Sci* 22(5), 2566 (2021).

121. Sugahara, K., Tokumine, J., Teruya, K. & Oshiro, T. Alveolar epithelial cells: Differentiation and lung injury. *Respirology* 11, S28–S31 (2006).

122. Liu, Y.Y. & Imlay, J.A. Cell death from antibiotics without the involvement of reactive oxygen species. *Science* 339(6124), 1210–1213 (2013).

123. Murphy, M.P. How mitochondria produce reactive oxygen species. *Biochem J* 417(1), 1–13 (2009).

124. Grabowska-Jadach, I. et al. Cytotoxicity studies of selected cadmium-based quantum dots on 2D vs. 3D cell cultures. *New J Chem* 42(15), 12787–12795 (2018).

125. Chipuk, J.E., Bouchier-Hayes, L. & Green, D.R. Mitochondrial outer membrane permeabilization during apoptosis: The innocent bystander scenario. *Cell Death Differ* 13(8), 1396–1402 (2006).

126. Dayem, A.A. et al. The role of reactive oxygen species (ROS) in the biological activities of metallic nanoparticles. *Int J Mol Sci* 18, 120 (2017).

127. Fisher, A.B. Redox signaling across cell membranes. *Antioxid Redox Signal* 11(6), 1349–1356 (2009).

128. Ma, Z., Bai, J. & Jiang, X. Monitoring of the enzymatic degradation of protein corona and evaluating the accompanying cytotoxicity of nanoparticles. *ACS Appl Mater Interfaces* 7(32), 17614–17622 (2015).

129. Cai, R. & Chen, C. The crown and the scepter: Roles of the protein corona in nanomedicine. *Adv Mater* 31(45), e1805740 (2019).

130. Meyer, K. Lung surfactants: Basic science and clinical applications. *Crit Care Med* 30(1), 266 (2002).

131. Rausch, F., Schicht, M., Brauer, L., Paulsen, F. & Brandt, W. Protein modeling and molecular dynamics simulation of the two novel surfactant proteins SP-G and SP-H. *J Mol Model* 20(11), 1–12 (2014).

132. Sano, H. & Kuroki, Y. The lung collectins, SP-A and SP-D, modulate pulmonary innate immunity. *Mol Immunol* 42(3), 279–287 (2005).

133. Tschernig, T. et al. The importance of surfactant proteins-new aspects on macrophage phagocytosis. *Ann Anat Anat Anz* 208, 142–145 (2016).

134. Kapralov, A.A. et al. Adsorption of surfactant lipids by single-walled carbon nanotubes in mouse lung upon pharyngeal aspiration. *ACS Nano* 6(5), 4147–4156 (2012).

135. Bai, X., Xu, M., Liu, S.J. & Hu, G.Q. Computational investigations of the interaction between the cell membrane and nanoparticles coated with a pulmonary surfactant. *ACS Appl Mater Interfaces* 10(24), 20368–20376 (2018).

136. Dwivedi, M.V., Harishchandra, R.K., Koshkina, O., Maskos, M. & Galla, H.J. Size influences the effect of hydrophobic nanoparticles on lung surfactant model systems. *Biophys J* 106(1), 289–298 (2014).

137. Rauwel, P., Kuunal, S., Ferdov, S. & Rauwel, E. A review on the green synthesis of silver nanoparticles and their morphologies studied via TEM. *Adv Mater Sci Eng* 2015, 682749 (2015).

138. Li, Y., Huang, H., Zhang, X., Deng, R. & Lin, P. Current application of transmission electron microscope in biology. *Chin J Trop Agric* 39, 58–67 (2019).

139. Elham, H. et al. Tannic acid-lung fluid assemblies promote interaction and delivery of drugs to lung cancer cells. *Pharmaceutics* 10, (2018).

140. Cristian, R.E. et al. Analyzing the interaction between two different types of nanoparticles and serum albumin. *Materials (Basel)* 12(19), (2019).

141. Sitterberg, J., Ozcetin, A., Ehrhardt, C. & Bakowsky, U. Utilising atomic force microscopy for the characterisation of nanoscale drug delivery systems. *Eur J Pharm Biopharm* 74(1), 2–13 (2010).

142. Hong, Z. et al. Comparative study of clinical pulmonary surfactants using atomic force microscopy. *Biochim Biophys Acta* 1808, (2011).

143. Sachan, A.K. & Galla, H.J. Understanding the mutual impact of interaction between hydrophobic nanoparticles and pulmonary surfactant monolayer. *Small* 10(6), (2014).

144. Xu, L. et al. Effect of heavy metal ions on the surface activity of pulmonary surfactant monolayer membrane. *China Environ Sci* 40, 857–864 (2020).

145. Dopierala, K., Bojakowska, K., Karasiewicz, J., Maciejewski, H. & Prochaska, K. Interfacial behaviour of cubic silsesquioxane and silica nanoparticles in Langmuir and Langmuir-Blodgett films. *RSC Adv* 6(97), 94934–94941 (2016).

146. Guzman, E., Liggieri, L., Santini, E., Ferrari, M. & Ravera, F. DPPC-DOPC Langmuir monolayers modified by hydrophilic silica nanoparticles: Phase behaviour, structure and rheology. *Colloids Surf A* 413, 174–183 (2012).

147. Raha, A.K. et al. Surface chemistry of photoluminescent F8BT conjugated polymer nanoparticles determines protein corona formation and internalization by phagocytic cells. *Biomacromolecules* 16, (2015).

148. Ahmad, K.R. et al. Interactions of stealth conjugated polymer nanoparticles with human whole blood. *J Mater Chem*, B 3, (2015).

149. Garcia-Alvarez, R., Hadjidemetriou, M., Sanchez-Iglesias, A., Liz-Marzan, L.M. & Kostarelos, K. In vivo formation of protein corona on gold nanoparticles: The effect of their size and shape. *Nanoscale* 10(3), 1256–1264 (2018).

150. Ain, R.Q.U., Mehedi, H.M., Keerthie, D. & Alireza, F. Isolation of extracellular vesicles (EVs) using benchtop size exclusion chromatography (SEC) columns. *Methods Mol Biol (Clifton NJ)* 2273, (2021).

151. Satzer, P., Wellhoefer, M. & Jungbauer, A. Continuous separation of protein loaded nanoparticles by simulated moving bed chromatography. *J Chromatogr A* 1349, (2014).

152. Helsper, J.P.F.G., Peters, R.J.B., Brouwer, L. & Weigel, S. Characterisation and quantification of liposome-type nanoparticles in a beverage matrix using hydrodynamic chromatography and MALDI–TOF mass spectrometry. *Anal Bioanal Chem* 405(4), (2013).

153. Tenzer, S. et al. Rapid formation of plasma protein corona critically affects nanoparticle pathophysiology. *Nat Nanotechnol* 8(10), (2013).

154. Hamidu, A. et al. LC-MS/MS proteomic study of MCF-7 cell treated with dox and dox-loaded calcium carbonate nanoparticles revealed changes in proteins related to glycolysis, actin signalling, and energy metabolism. *Biology* 10, (2021).

155. Dar, A.I., Walia, S. & Acharya, A. Molecular recognition based rapid diagnosis of immunoglobulins via proteomic profiling of protein-nanoparticle complexes. *Int J Biol Macromol* 138, (2019).

156. Rath, A., Glibowicka, M., Nadeau, V.G., Chen, G. & Deber, C.M. Detergent binding explains anomalous SDS-PAGE migration of membrane proteins. *Proc Natl Acad Sci U S A* 106(6), 1760–1765 (2009).

157. Lian, S. et al. Comprehensive characterization and proteoform analysis of the hydrophobic surfactant proteins B and C in calf pulmonary surfactant. *J Pharm Biomed Anal* 174, (2019).

158. Katrin, P., Robin, K., Dennis, M., Hans-Ulrich, H. & Klaus, L. Serum type and concentration both affect the protein-corona composition of PLGA nanoparticles. *Beilstein J Nanotechnol* 10, (2019).

159. Cheng, H., Yan, D., Wu, L. & Wang, M. Application of circular dichroism spectroscopy in pharmaceutical analysis. *J Pharm Anal* 41, 559–571 (2021).

160. Voicescu, M., Ionescu, S., Manoiu, V.S., Anastasescu, M., Craciunescu, O. & Moldovan, L. et al. Synthesis and biophysical characteristics of riboflavin/HSA protein system on silver nanoparticles. *Mater Sci Eng C Mater Biol Appl* 96, (2019).

161. Xu, X.Y. et al. Study on the interaction of graphene oxide silver nanocomposites with bovine serum albumin and the formation of nanoparticle-protein corona. *Int J Biol Macromol* 116, 492–501 (2018).

162. Moustaoui, H. et al. A protein corona study by scattering correlation spectroscopy: A comparative study between spherical and urchin-shaped gold nanoparticles. *Nanoscale* 11(8), 3665–3673 (2019).

163. Silvestri, A et al. Influence of surface coating on the intracellular behaviour of gold nanoparticles: A fluorescence correlation spectroscopy study. *Nanoscale* 9(38), (2017).

164. Li, S. & Ulrich, N.G. In situ characterization of protein adsorption onto nanoparticles by fluorescence correlation spectroscopy. *Acc Chem Res* 50, (2017).

165. Sinha, S., Li, Y.S., Williams, T.D. & Topp, E.M. Protein conformation in amorphous solids by FTIR and by hydrogen/deuterium exchange with mass spectrometry. *Biophys J* 95(12), 5951–5961 (2008).

166. Wojnarowska-Nowak, R., Polit, J. & Sheregii, E.M. Interaction of gold nanoparticles with cholesterol oxidase enzyme in bionanocomplex—Determination of the protein structure by Fourier transform infrared spectroscopy. *J Nanopart Res* 22(5), (2020).

167. Li, H. et al. A comparative study of the antibacterial mechanisms of silver ion and silver nanoparticles by fourier transform infrared spectroscopy. *Vib Spectrosc* 85, (2016).

168. Sharma, B., Frontiera, R.R., Henry, A.I., Ringe, E. & Van Duyne, R.P. SERS: Materials, applications, and the future. *Mater Today* 15(1–2), 16–25 (2012).

169. Yamin, L. et al. A microsphere nanoparticle based-serum albumin targeted adsorption coupled with surface-enhanced Raman scattering for breast cancer detection. *Spectrochim Acta A Mol Biomol Spectrosc* 261, (2021).

170. Cao, X., Wang, Z., Bi, L., Zheng, J. & Cheng, Z. Label-free detection of human serum using surface-enhanced Raman spectroscopy based on highly branched gold nanoparticle substrates for discrimination of non-small cell lung cancer. *J Chem* 2018, (2018).

171. Li, X.L. et al. Highly conducting graphene sheets and Langmuir-Blodgett films. *Nat Nanotechnol* 3(9), 538–542 (2008).

172. Azam, U. Investigation of interaction of soft nanoparticles based vesicles with lung surfactant via Langmuir-Blodgett trough and quartz crystal microbalance study. *J Nanomed Nanotechnol* 9(3), (2018).

173. Johnson, D.O. & Stebe, K.J. Experimental confirmation of the oscillating bubble technique with comparison to the pendant bubble method: The adsorption dynamics of 1-decanol. *J Colloid Interface Sci* 182(2), (1996).

174. Beck-Broichsitter, M. et al. Biophysical investigation of pulmonary surfactant surface properties upon contact with polymeric nanoparticles in vitro. *Nanomed Nanotechnol* 7(3), 341–350 (2011).

175. Chen, Q., Xu, S.M., Liu, Q.X., Masliyah, J. & Xu, Z.H. QCM-D study of nanoparticle interactions. *Adv Colloid Interface Sci* 233, 94–114 (2016).

176. Wan, F. et al. Qualitative and quantitative analysis of the biophysical interaction of inhaled nanoparticles with pulmonary surfactant by using quartz crystal microbalance with dissipation monitoring. *J Colloid Interface Sci* 545 (2019).

177. Cedervall, T. et al. Understanding the nanoparticle-protein corona using methods to quantify exchange rates and affinities of proteins for nanoparticles. *Proc Natl Acad Sci U S A* 104(7), 2050–2055 (2007).

178. Parikh, V. & Gupta, P. Thermodynamic analysis of r-hGH-polymer surface Interaction using isothermal titration calorimetry. *Growth Horm IGF Res* 42–43, (2018).

179. Noga, G., Martina, S. & Erik, R. Stealth nanoparticles grafted with dense polymer brushes display adsorption of serum protein investigated by isothermal titration calorimetry. *J Phys Chem B* 122, (2018).

180. Wang, J. et al. Machine learning of coarse-grained molecular dynamics force fields. *ACS Cent Sci* 5(5), 755–767 (2019).

181. Jiao, F., Sang, J., Liu, C. & Li, Y. The mechanism of the interaction between nanoparticle and lipids monolayer of pulmonary surfactant. *Mech Eng* 42, 424–429 (2020).

182. Beck-Broichsitter, M., Ruppert, C., Schmehl, T., Gunther, A. & Seeger, W. Biophysical inhibition of synthetic vs. naturally-derived pulmonary surfactant preparations by polymeric nanoparticles. *Biochim Biophys Acta* 1838(1 Pt B), 474–481 (2014).

183. Xu, Y. et al. Transport of nanoparticles across pulmonary surfactant monolayer: A molecular dynamics study. *Phys Chem Chem Phys* 19(27), 17568–17576 (2017).

184. Debayle, M. et al. Zwitterionic polymer ligands: An ideal surface coating to totally suppress protein-nanoparticle corona formation? *Biomaterials* 219, (2019).

185. Beck-Broichsitter, M., Ruge, C.A. & Bohr, A. Impact of triblock copolymers on the biophysical function of naturally-derived lung surfactant. *Colloids Surf B Biointerfaces* 156, 262–269 (2017).

186. Beck-Broichsitter, M., Ruppert, C., Schmehl, T., Gunther, A. & Seeger, W. Biophysical inhibition of pulmonary surfactant function by polymeric nanoparticles: Role of surfactant protein B and C. *Acta Biomater* 10(11), 4678–4684 (2014).

187. Beck-Broichsitter, M. Compatibility of pegylated polymer nanoparticles with the biophysical function of lung surfactant. *Langmuir* 34(1), 540–545 (2018).

188. Canadas, O., Garcia-Garcia, A., Prieto, M.A. & Perez-Gil, J. Polyhydroxyalkanoate nanoparticles for pulmonary drug delivery: Interaction with lung surfactant. *Nanomater-Basel* 11(6), (2021).

189. De Backer, L. et al. Hybrid pulmonary surfactant-coated nanogels mediate efficient in vivo delivery of siRNA to murine alveolar macrophages. *J Control Release* 217, 53–63 (2015).

190. De Backer, L. et al. Bio-inspired pulmonary surfactant-modified nanogels: A promising siRNA delivery system. *J Control Release* 206, 177–186 (2015).

191. Murphy, A., Sheehy, K., Casey, A. & Chambers, G. The surfactant dipalmitoylphophatidylcholine modifies acute responses in alveolar carcinoma cells in response to low-dose silver nanoparticle exposure. *J Appl Toxicol* 35(10), 1141–1149 (2015).

192. Scalia, S., Young, P.M. & Traini, D. Solid lipid microparticles as an approach to drug delivery. *Expert Opin Drug Deliv* 12(4), 583–599 (2015).

193. Li, Z. et al. DPPC-coated lipid nanoparticles as an inhalable carrier for accumulation of resveratrol in the pulmonary vasculature, a new strategy for pulmonary arterial hypertension treatment. *Drug Deliv* 27(1), 736–744 (2020).

194. Kato, T. et al. Evidence that exogenous substances can be phagocytized by alveolar epithelial cells and transported into blood capillaries. *Cell Tissue Res* 311(1), 47–51 (2003).

195. Xu, Y. et al. Role of lipid coating in the transport of nanodroplets across the pulmonary surfactant layer revealed by molecular dynamics simulations. *Langmuir* 34(30), 9054–9063 (2018).

196. Theodorou, I.G., Ryan, M.P., Tetley, T.D. & Porter, A.E. Inhalation of silver nanomaterials-seeing the risks. *Int J Mol Sci* 15(12), 23936–23974 (2014).

SECTION II

Particle Design Understanding

Particle Engineering for Pulmonary Drug Delivery

5

Vikram Karde and Jerry Y.Y. Heng

Contents

DOI: 10.1201/9781003182566-7

5.1 INTRODUCTION

More often than not, whenever one thinks of pulmonary drug delivery, the first thing that comes to one's mind is the aerosolized drug delivery systems. Aerosolized delivery of drugs to the lungs is highly favored for the treatment of respiratory and other ailments. It is used for the delivery of a wide range of therapeutic agents to the lungs. Aerosolized pulmonary delivery offers advantages like faster drug absorption, improved local and systemic bioavailability, and non-invasiveness and ease of administration, allowing faster treatment and quick relief to patients. This is why the global respiratory inhalers market cap is estimated to be around $33.9 billion in 2020 and is projected to reach around $51 billion by 2027. This is primarily driven by the likely rise in respiratory-related illnesses during this period owing to increasing air pollution levels and lifestyle changes.

There are three main types of aerosolized systems commonly available for pulmonary drug delivery: dry powder inhalers (DPI), nebulizers and pressurized metered-dose inhalers (pMDI). In these aerosolized systems, the formulation and the delivery device are the two main components affecting the therapeutic efficacy of these drug delivery systems.[1-3] Hence, a combination of innovative formulation strategies and advanced device design approaches is required for optimized targeting of therapeutics to the lungs.[4,5] In this chapter, we focus on the formulation aspects and particle engineering strategies for targeted pulmonary drug delivery.

Among the inhalation delivery systems, DPIs are the most preferred system, dominate the drug delivery through pulmonary route and are employed for a diverse range of drugs and diseases.[6] Also, from the sustainability point of view and ease of drug administration, there is a gradual inclination to shift from other aerosolized systems to DPI-based delivery systems. The DPI dosage forms are powder-based formulations, often consisting of an active pharmaceutical ingredient (API) and a carrier excipient. These frequently comprise formulations of highly potent low-dose therapeutic agents for pulmonary targeting. There are also efforts being directed towards the development of targeted administration of high-dose drugs for rapid and improved therapeutic effects. Moreover, despite several challenges involved in the drug delivery of large molecules through the pulmonary route, a few successful products have been developed and commercialized as listed in Table 5.1. In view of such a significant impact on drug delivery routes and the advancements in pulmonary drug delivery, a comprehensive understanding of the powders and particulate properties is indispensable for pulmonary drug delivery development. This is due to the complex nature of the interplay of several of these particle and powder properties and its effect on the final product's quality and performance. These include particle level properties like size, shape, density, mechanical properties, surface properties like surface energy and surface roughness, as well as bulk properties like powder flow, dispersibility, etc. By investigating various physicochemical properties of particles and studying their relevance to drug delivery efficiency and therapeutic efficacy, the groundwork for smooth pharmaceutical manufacturing could be laid down for competent pulmonary drug delivery and products thereof. This also helps us in understanding the underlying mechanisms

TABLE 5.1   Marketed biologics using inhalation-based delivery system.

NO.	BIOTHERAPEUTIC FOR LUNG DELIVERY	CLASS OF DRUG	BRAND NAME	INDICATION
1	Insulin	Hormone (protein)	Exubera® (Pfizer and Sanofi-Aventis)	Diabetes
2	Insulin	Hormone (protein)	Afrezza® (MannKind)	Diabetes
3	Tobramycin	Antibiotic (aminoglycoside)	TOBI Podinhaler® (Novartis)	Cystic fibrosis
4	rhDNase (recombinant human deoxyribonuclease I)	Enzyme (protein)	Dornase alfa Pulmozyme® (Genentech)	Cystic fibrosis

guiding particulate behavior, rather than looking for desperate solutions at the later stages of product development.

More importantly, particle engineering to generate, design and control particles with desired properties is key in formulating micronized drugs for delivery to the lungs. Therefore, this chapter of the book is devoted to the existing and upcoming particle engineering approaches, some of which are being developed into a platform technology. Such particle engineering and design aspects of the product development help in providing a quick and cost-effective solution for tailoring particles and allowing desired interparticle interactions to deliver the favored drug to the lungs for local or systemic effects.

The cohesion and adhesion interactions of the particles remain central to the fundamental understanding of particulate behavior. To highlight the underlying mechanisms for these interactions of the particles in the pulmonary drug delivery, the next section describes briefly some of the fundamental interparticle forces with an emphasis on the particle interactions at the interfaces or surfaces for aerosol-based targeted delivery to the lungs.

5.2 INTERPARTICLE INTERACTIONS IN AEROSOL-BASED DELIVERY SYSTEMS

The need for studying the interparticle interactions becomes even more important considering that the delivery systems to the lungs regularly involve carrier-based powder formulations, with API and a carrier excipient. Interparticle interactions are broadly classified into cohesive and adhesive interactions. An optimal balance, called cohesive-adhesive balance (CAB), between these interactions is desired for efficient drug delivery to the lungs using inhaler-based systems.

The adhesion or attractive interparticle interaction occurs between the particles at different operations during the manufacturing processes. This is particularly desired during carrier-based formulations which involve the coating or adhesion of low dose APIs over a carrier like lactose monohydrate. However, it could also prove to be undesirable during the initial stages of product development and create handling or processing issues as well as inefficient API detachment and pulmonary deposition. For example, high cohesivity in API particles could create dispersibility and deposition problems which in turn will reduce its loading over the carrier particle surfaces leading to poor product quality and performance. Also, the attractive interactions during the size reduction processes of APIs and carrier particles could be exacerbated. This becomes problematic as it can diminish the grinding effect, lengthen the grinding time and increase the energy requirement due to the undesired agglomeration tendencies of the particles.[7]

From the powder bulk behavior perspective, these lopsided interparticle interactions are especially undesirable during transport, storage and feeder systems. As stated, the dominance of interparticle forces in fine particles often results in a number of processing and manufacturing problems with respect to their flowability and dispersibility, etc. Poor or variable powder flow and packing can result in various processing and formulation problems like content uniformity and dispersibility problems in potent low dose dosage forms from DPIs[8] and blend uniformity issues during mixing.[9]

It is clear that interparticle interaction forces like van der Waals (vdW) forces, electrostatic force, capillary force and solid bridge force affect properties like cohesion-adhesion, powder flow, dispersibility, etc. Mostly in a dry system, the total adhesion force can be attributed to the vdW forces and electrostatic forces. Compared to vdW and capillary forces, the strength of the electrostatic force is less at smaller distances but does not decrease much with the increasing distance.[10] Thus, in a dry uncharged powder system of a small size fraction, the powder flow is dominated by vdW forces.[11] The magnitude of these interparticle forces can be directly determined from the detachment force (also called pull-off force) measurements using techniques like atomic force microscopy (AFM) and surface force apparatus (SFA). Other indirect methods employ surface energy or surface tension measurements, and static charge measurement can also be used to back-calculate the interparticle adhesion forces. The different types of interparticle forces and their significance for drug delivery to the lungs are briefly discussed in Table 5.2.

5.3   PARTICLE PROPERTIES AND INTERFACES

This section appreciates the fact that the role of particle morphological properties like size and shape; mechanical properties like hardness; solid-state properties like crystallinity and amorphous nature; as well as the surface properties like surface energy, surface roughness, surface moisture, etc., are important for effective and efficient pulmonary drug delivery formulation strategies.[22,23] All these factors could modulate the interparticle interaction forces which eventually affect the particle and bulk behavior of powders with subsequent effects on pulmonary dose delivery and bioavailability. These physicochemical properties also drastically influence the targeting capabilities of the drug delivery system. Table 5.3 presents the important particle properties from the

TABLE 5.2 Interparticle forces and their influence in pulmonary drug delivery

NO.	INTERPARTICLE FORCE	DETERMINISTIC MODELS	SIGNIFICANCE FOR PULMONARY DRUG DELIVERY
1	*van der Waals (Vdw) force* Quantum mechanical origin. Constitutes the attractive and repulsive components. Types: Keesom, Debye and London components of vdW.	The vdW force (F_{vw}) between two spherical bodies of radius (R) and separated by a distance (a) can be expressed as follows, $$F_{vw} = \frac{AR}{12a^2} \qquad (1)$$ where, A is the Hamaker's constant. JKR [12]: $F_{vw} = 3\pi\gamma R$ (2) DMT [13]: $F_{vw} = 4\pi\gamma R$ (3)	noindent Dispersibility and dose reproducibility problems in low dose dosage forms from DPIs.[8]
2	*Capillary force* Attractive capillary forces develop due to the formation of liquid bridges between contacting particles. These forces are also sensitive to particle properties like shape, size or surface roughness.[14]	For two spherical particles in the pendular state, the maximum static liquid bridge or capillary force (F_{cf}) is given by $$F_{cf} = 2\pi R\gamma \qquad (4)$$ where, γ is the surface tension of liquid, and R is the radius of the spherical particles.	Decreased aerosolization or dispersibility of fine powders exposed to high humidity conditions owing to increased capillary forces.[8,15]
3	*Electrostatic force* Electrostatic charging can occur by contact or friction. In contact charging, the two bodies come in contact and subsequently separated without rubbing. Frictional (tribocharging) is due to the relative movement between two contacting bodies. Static charge can be generated during the operations like sizing, fluidization, hopper flow, mixing.	The electrostatic force (F_e) between two charged dielectric spheres of diameter (D) having charges (Q_1) and (Q_2) in a medium with permittivity (ϵ) is given by: $$F_e = \frac{Q_2^2}{4\pi\epsilon D^2}\left[\alpha\left(\frac{Q_2^2}{Q_2^2+1}+1\right) - \beta\frac{Q_1}{Q_2}\right] \qquad (5)$$ where, α and β are the constants.[16]	Triboelectrification is affected by the particle size, relative humidity (RH),[17,18] temperature, surface impurities,[19] surface roughness, nature of contact[20] and various other factors.
4	*Mechanical interlocking (solid bridge force)* Force due to morphological characteristics. Sometimes an extension of liquid bridge formation between the particles part-solubilization followed by recrystallization also lead to caking phenomenon.		Strong adhesion interaction between the carrier and API particles (Salmeterol xinafoate) particles exposed to high humidity conditions is reported due to formation of irreversible solid bridges.[21]

TABLE 5.3 Different particle properties of significance in pulmonary drug delivery

NO.	PARTICLE PROPERTIES	INFLUENCE IN PULMONARY DRUG DELIVERY
1	Particle size and size distribution	Aerosolization behavior, cohesion-adhesion interactions, drug deposition, bioavailability
2	Particle shape	Aerosolization behavior, cohesion-adhesion interactions, drug deposition, blend uniformity
3	Solid state characteristics	Stability, bioavailability, biosafety
4	Surface energy	Powder handling, inhaler filling, drug loading
5	Surface roughness	Carrier-API interactions, drug delivery performance
6	Surface charge	Powder handling, inhaler filling, dose metering
7	Surface moisture	Stability, drug deposition and delivery

perspective of drug delivery to the lungs. Furthermore, these particle properties become critical during downstream pharmaceutical processing, transport and manufacturing, with a continuous tendency towards the introduction of finer nonhomogeneous entities in pharmaceutical formulations.

5.3.1 Size

Particle size is the most important property in designing the formulations for the pulmonary drug delivery as it affects almost every aspect of the function including the CAB, drug loading, deposition, dispersibility, flow properties as well as pharmacokinetic aspects like drug dissolution, cell transport, uptake and clearance. This becomes particularly significant considering that the size of the particles involved in pulmonary drug delivery formulation is usually in the micron, submicron to sometimes even nanoscale range. The particle size is generally expressed as aerodynamic diameter (d_a), which is dependent on the shape and particle density. The aerodynamic diameter (d_a) of a particle is the diameter of a sphere of unit density that settles in the airstream at the same velocity as that of the test particle. This size descriptor is specifically used to represent the pulmonary particle deposition mechanism and can be calculated as below,

$$da = \sqrt{\frac{18\mu u_s}{g\rho o}} \tag{6}$$

where, μ is the coefficient of air viscosity, u_s is the settling velocity, ρ_0 is the unit density and g is the acceleration due to gravity.

Typically, for DPI formulations, the API particles are desired to have the aerodynamic diameter (d_a) of 1–5 μm for the pulmonary delivery and deposition. For carrier-based inhalation drug delivery systems, the size of the carrier influences the aerosolization performance of the drug from a drug–carrier formulation. It is reported that the aerosolization performance of the carrier-API blend is inversely proportional to the carrier particle size.[24,25]

Milling is the most preferred and popular route for particle size reduction of API and the excipients. This can be achieved using different milling techniques like fluid energy mill, ball mill, cone mill, etc. Other approaches like spray drying were also found to be effective in attaining the desired particle size for effective drug delivery to the lungs.[26] The micron to the submicron size range of the APIs offers primary benefits in terms of improved dissolution, increased absorption and high bioavailability. However, going down in the particle size has its fair share of complications involved. The associated increase in the surface area of the particles normally tilts the balance in the favor of interparticle interaction forces, as mentioned in the previous sections. The subsequent effects related to the adverse powder flow and increased cohesion-adhesion tendencies of these fine particles could lead to handling and processing problems during the formulation stages. These could also have adverse effects on the product performance, for example, suboptimal dosing or inability to deliver drugs to the lungs in a reproducible manner.

5.3.2 Shape

To incorporate a predictable performance or powder behavior during formulation and manufacturing, particle shape or crystalline habit control is very important as far as micronized APIs or the carrier excipients are concerned. However, unlike the particle size, controlling particle shape is a very difficult task that could involve complex and cumbersome primary or secondary particle processing approaches. Some of these involve chemical synthesis, crystallization, spray drying, granulation, etc. Different particle generation methods will produce particles of different shapes or habits. Various parameters such as solvent environment, precursor or solute concentration, stabilizing agents, temperature, pH, etc. demand extra care while synthesizing and crystallizing APIs or excipients with controlled shapes.

From the perspective of particle attachment-detachment propensities too, particle shape plays an important role. More regular the particle shape more predictable would be the bulk powder behavior. Particles closer to a more spherical geometry provide an added advantage of avoiding anisotropy in the surface properties of solids. However, a majority of the powders employed in formulations contain primary particles having irregular shapes and sizes. Also, most of these particles involved are obtained from secondary processing like milling, sizing, etc. The irregularities in particle geometry should be given adequate attention as they strongly influence the particle cohesion-adhesion properties.[27] These irregularities in particle shape can be effectively expressed with the help of different shape descriptors. Any deviation from the regular spherical shape can be described by the shape factor of the particle in terms of its sphericity index or circularity index. The aspect ratio defined as the ratio of length to width and circularity index, which provides a degree of closeness of particle shape to a circle, is the most common dimensionless descriptor used to describe particle shape irregularities.

As stated earlier, the differences in particle shape could significantly affect the interparticle cohesion forces between carrier excipient particles, micronized drug particles as well as the adhesion forces between the drug and carrier. These forces decrease with the separation distance, hence particles with irregular sharp edges and high local surface curvature would lead to a decrease in the interparticle forces due to decreased interfacial contact area. On the other hand, with elongated or flat particles there is an overall increase in the interparticle forces due to the subsequent increase in the contact area. This is the case especially when the particles are oriented flat to maximize the interparticle contact. Also other possible orientations, particle rearrangement and mechanical interlocking may lead to different magnitude forces acting on these particles. From the formulation standpoint, particle shape could influence the surface area available for API loading, drug deposition, mechanism of attachment to the cell lining, drug dissolution and absorption. Also, from the drug targeting perspective, it can evidently dictate some of the biological particle-cell interactions like absorption, phagocytosis and clearance.

5.3.3 Solid-State Properties

Solid-state property (crystalline and amorphous nature) and surface chemistry are the important factors that affect the molecular and particle level adhesive and cohesive interactions. It is well known that the crystalline forms of APIs and excipients are often preferred in pharmaceutical industries due to the reasons of purity and stability. Researchers have found that often the solid-state stability appears to correspond to the crystallinity or contrarily, to the extent of disorder in that material.[28] The particle engineering approaches employed for pulmonary drug delivery development like milling, spray drying, etc. can often lead to crystalline transformations and disorders. These associated effects depend on the material properties and process operation parameters.

Size reduction operations like milling can cause numerous changes in a crystalline solid, and the majority of these begin at the surface, which may later propagate to the bulk of the particle. The most commonly observed adjunct change in milled crystalline materials is the occurrence of a small degree of amorphization, especially in the vicinity of the surface stress event.[29,30] The length scales and domains over which such order and disorder persist are also important. As can be conceived, even in amorphous materials, a short-range order exists due to chemical constraints. This particle processing can thus induce disorder in the crystalline form but induce order in its amorphous form. Also, mechanical treatment associated thermodynamic vulnerability of the activated solids can result in spontaneous recrystallization with time.[31] Ward and Schultz reported a phase transformation from amorphous to crystalline state in the case of micronized salbutamol sulfate aided by temperature and humidity exposure. Such an instability created in turn could dramatically affect the effectiveness of powder inhalation products. The performance indicators of DPI products like the fine particle fraction (FPF) drastically decreased for salbutamol sulfate formulations with its high amorphous content as against the formulations containing higher crystalline drug.[32]

Another phenomenon that has intrigued researchers over the years is that processing prompted polymorphic transformation in crystalline solids. In crystalline solids, polymorphism and the presence of different crystal habits influence surface energetics and wetting behavior that could affect dissolution. Descamps et al. have reported such polymorphic conversions in a wide variety of crystalline materials.[33,34] Studies have also proposed that anhydrous forms of crystalline solids are more prone to amorphization as compared to their hydrate forms.[35] Besides this, it has been found that the high mechanical stresses could also lead to the release of bound water in some cases. As stated, such mechanical treatments expose the solids to a large variety of perturbations in the physicochemical properties. The altered interfacial interactions (adhesion/cohesion) in particles could result in problems like processing delays, increased costs and lower yields.

5.3.4 Surface Properties of Solids

A tendency and a need of moving towards finer particulate domain often shift the balance in favor of interfacial or surface phenomena. In such cases, the crucial surface information obtained, like material surface energy characteristics, critical roughness, interparticle cohesion, surface adsorbed moisture, etc. can be effectively utilized for analyzing and predicting the powder bulk behavior of fine powders during pharmaceutical manufacturing. The following three surface or interfacial properties of solid particulates appear to have a significant impact on drug delivery and targeting.

5.3.4.1 Surface energy

In Section 5.2 of this chapter, we briefly touched upon the significance of different interparticle forces in pulmonary drug delivery. Surface energy is a property whose origin lies in some of these molecular forces, predominantly vdW forces, influencing particle or powder behavior. Thus, it is considered to be one of the most critical particle properties to be taken into consideration for the functionality of the product. The criticality of particle surface energy applies to both the components of the pulmonary drug development process, i.e., formulation and development and manufacturing.

Surface energy characterization of powders plays an important role in discerning their physicochemical properties such as wettability, flowability, dispersibility, surface chemistry, etc.[36–39] Solid surface energy, expressed in J/m^2, includes a contribution from the dispersive non-polar interactions, also known as Lifshitz–van der Waals or dispersive (γ^d) components, and the specific polar interactions also known as acid-base (γ^{ab}) components of the total surface energy(γ^t). The dispersive (γ^d) component of total solid surface energy is from the London-van der Waals interaction forces and is ubiquitous. On the other hand, the γ^{ab} component of solid surface energy arises due to all other interaction forces such as dipole-dipole interactions, hydrogen bonding, etc. However, the author must admit that there exists plenty of confusion on terminologies to be used to categorize different surface energy components in the literature. A detailed study of the contribution from the polar and non-polar surface energy components becomes especially important when dealing with the hydrophobic and hydrophilic surface chemistry changes. The surface energy of powders can be determined from analytical techniques based on thermodynamic principles such as contact angle determination, inverse gas chromatography (IGC) and microcalorimetry. However, the two former methods are the most popular. There are also other available measurement techniques using mechanical approaches like AFM, SFA, Drop Test methods, etc., for the surface energy measurements of solids. In recent times, a new IGC approach called Finite Dilution Inverse Gas Chromatography (FD-IGC) is widely employed for the energetic heterogeneity characterization of the particle surfaces. In this approach, an increasing amount of probes are injected to interact with a wider range of energy sites on the surface.[40]

A detailed discussion on each of these mentioned surface energy determination techniques can be found elsewhere.

The surface energy of particles can be affected by factors like particle size, shape, solid-state properties, surface roughness, processing or handling, surface functionalization, environmental conditions, etc. Fundamentally, the differences in surface energy of the solids due to variations in these particle attributes can be observed owing to the surface molecules existing in different energy states. The ability to decouple contributions of surface vs bulk is key in developing an understanding of the respective transformations in processed solids. Particle size reduction using approaches like milling cause an increase in surface area and surface energy of particles, which consequently promotes the adhesion of particles. An extensive amount of work has been done to understand the effect of the size reduction or milling operation on the surface energy changes of different materials. The presence of surface energy hotspots or active sites offers adsorption sites for itself (cohesion) as well as to foreign surfaces (adhesion). Through this adsorption (cohesion or adhesion) mechanism, lower energy and thermodynamically stable particle surface are achieved. Moreover, the influence of other transformational effects in particle shape, crystalline facets and surface chemistry could be elucidated using the surface energy investigation of the powders. For pulmonary drug delivery applications, surface energy characteristics of excipients or APIs have been widely studied and correlated to aerosolization behavior and product performance.[41-46] An expression (Equation 7) relating surface area (S_a), surface energy (γ) and a closely associated parameter known as cohesive energy density (CED) (δ) of carrier particles was proposed to predict and optimize the dispersion behavior of API-carrier formulations by Sethuraman and Hickey.[47] Overall, an intimate correlation between the surface energy and the functionality of the product for pulmonary administration can be observed.

$$Dispersion = k \frac{\left(\delta^2\right)j}{S_a l \gamma^m} \tag{7}$$

Here, k is the parameter representing molar volume of the carrier and the number of molecules present at the surfaces of the carrier particles, l and m are the surface energy exponents and j is dependent on the arrangement of atoms or molecules in space.

5.3.4.2 Surface roughness

Surface roughness is another particle surface property that has a considerable effect on interparticle interaction. The surface roughness decreases the interparticle contact area between the interacting particles. The roughness associated asperities can also act as a spacer and increase the distance between contacting particles. Both these factors can lead to a reduction of the attractive interparticle interactions. Surface roughness parameters include rugosity, root mean square deviation and maximum peak to valley height. The rugosity (R_a), also known as the center line average (CLA) height, is the arithmetic mean average distance of all points of the profile from the center line, given by,

$$R_a = \frac{1}{n} \sum_{i=1}^{n} |Y_i| \tag{8}$$

where n is the number of points and Y_i is the distance of point i from the center line.

The root mean square (RMS or R_q) deviation describes the variability of the profile from the center line.

$$R_q = \sqrt{\frac{1}{n}\sum_{i=1}^{n}Y_i^2}$$

(9)

The maximum peak-to-valley height is the difference between the maximum and minimum points of the profile.

Several reported studies assert the influence of particle surface roughness on the carrier-API interactions for DPI formulation performance.[48–50] Although a majority of these studies are focused on engineering and/or investigating the carrier particle roughness on the DPI performance, particle engineering approaches can be utilized to modify the surface roughness of the therapeutic agents or API. Adi et al. were able to produce rough corrugated protein particles with reduced adhesion and increased deagglomeration behavior with subsequent enhancement in its dispersibility compared to its smoother counterpart.[51]

However, the scale of surface roughness is also an important consideration while contemplating the benefits of surface roughness and the consequential decrease in the interparticle cohesion or adhesion. In some cases, smoothing of roughened particle surfaces has led to an improvement in powder flow attributed to the decreased mechanical interlocking and reduced friction between interacting particles.[52] A decrease in the emitted dose (ED) and FPF of L-Leucine coated salbutamol powders was reported due to mechanical interlocking as the surface asperity size was changed from a few nanometers to hundreds of nanometers.[53]

5.3.4.3 Surface charge

Micronized fine powders are prone to surface charge accumulation. The surface static charge decreases as the particle size increases. The organic nature of the APIs and excipients involved in the pulmonary drug development means there is increased resistance to charge flow and slow charge dissipation. Surface charge accumulation or transfer in fine powders occurs by contact between the powder particles and the equipment surface, therefore the nature of the contacting surface influences the electrostatic charge generated. A study on the effect of surface material on electrostatic charge generation in powders reported that lactose, when passed through a cyclone apparatus with PVC as the internal material, accumulated a positive surface charge compared to a negatively charged surface when PVC was replaced with stainless steel. Also, the roughness of the contacting surface has an effect on the magnitude of the charge developed on the surface. Smooth surfaces tend to produce slightly higher charges than rough stainless steel, but the difference is smaller than that between different material types.[20] Mostly, there is a direct proportionality between the energy involved in a process and the surface static charge generation.

Impurities present on the surface also affect the magnitude of the surface static charges generated. It was found that the charging of lactose powders decreased with the use of an uncleaned surface of stainless steel.[54] Also, the particle surface charge decays rapidly with increasing ambient relative humidity (RH). This can be explained by the fact that at higher humidity levels the dissipation or leakage of electric charge occurs due to a decrease in electrical resistance on the particle surface.

Frequently, an interplay of different particle properties is observed on particle behavior. For example, particle surface roughness can influence the charging behavior of particles during the blending process. An increase in charge saturation and lower mixing homogeneity was reported with rough mannitol carrier particles as compared to the smoother particles.[55]

5.3.4.4 Surface moisture

As much as we highlight the importance of the physicochemical properties of the solid particulates for the safety, performance and efficacy in the inhalation drug delivery system, there is no denying the fact that surface moisture is also one of the important considerations for the same. Powder flow is the most important and frequently studied bulk powder property which is affected by the capillary forces at high RH conditions. The altered cohesion or adhesion behavior of the particles due to capillary bridge formation could subsequently affect the properties like dispersibility of dose from DPIs.[56] These changes also affect the blend uniformity and the overall drug content delivered to the lungs. Apart from the external RH conditions, the humidity within the respiratory tract presents added complexities in terms of particulate interactions and pulmonary drug delivery. The high levels of humidity in the alveolar lumen can alter the particle size of the dispersed material. Also, the moisture-sensitive particles can show higher particle adhesion due to the development of capillary forces, further affecting the drug detachment and alveolar deposition. In addition, the overall production and manufacturing capacity is affected by the undesirable powder bulk behavioral changes of the formulated blend containing moisture-sensitive components.

On the other hand, as stated earlier, surface moisture can improve the surface conductivity of the particles promoting the accumulated charge dissipation. The effect of relative humidity on the electrostatic charging of powders can vary depending on the hygroscopic tendency of the powder. It was observed that the relative humidity had a negligible effect on powder charging for low hygroscopic powders whereas for high hygroscopic powders the relative humidity and powder charging were inversely related.[17]

5.4 PARTICLE ENGINEERING APPROACHES

Particle engineering has become a mainstay during the drug delivery development process for efficient processing and product performance enhancement. It is clear that understanding and engineering the physicochemical properties of the materials and processes in aerosol-based delivery technology will allow us to influence and control the aerodynamic efficiency and therapeutic efficacy. Intrinsically, the particle engineering part applied to the pulmonary development process is predominantly aimed at powder flow improvement, enhanced dispersibility, reproducible delivery, content uniformity, stability and safety aspects.

The particle engineering approaches for the development of pulmonary drug delivery applications can be applied to the drug as well as to the excipient (carrier) particles. Distinct drug and excipient particle modification techniques could render different effects on the physicochemical properties of these solids. Recently, carrier-free DPI formulations for high dose drug delivery to the lungs have been in trend for their noticeable benefits. The primary focus of particle engineering for carrier-free DPI formulations is to control the interparticle interactions and reduce the cohesivity of the fine API particles. This is to improve the dispersibility, deposition and delivery of API to the lungs upon inhalation and avoid or mitigate any unintended adverse bulk behavior problems of the powders in these high-dose DPIs.

This section will review the current state-of-the-art approaches for particle engineering for inhalation delivery to the lungs including some of the novel and exploratory methods. Figure 5.1 depicts the major particle engineering approaches being employed for pulmonary drug delivery development. Also, some of the advantages and limitations of these engineering approaches are reported in Table 5.4.

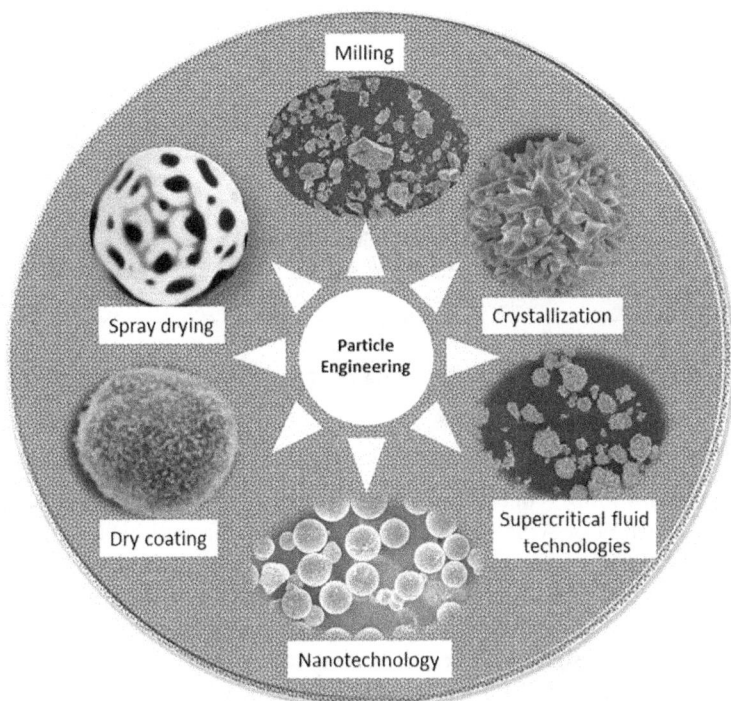

FIGURE 5.1 Particle engineering approaches being employed for pulmonary drug delivery development.

TABLE 5.4 Particle engineering and design approaches for beneficial inhalation therapeutics

NO.	PARTICLE ENGINEERING TECHNOLOGIES	ADVANTAGES	DISADVANTAGES
1	Milling or particle sizing	Particles in the chosen size range to achieve better drug loading, drug dissolution and bioavailability.	Stability issues, phase change (crystalline to amorphous), poor aerosolization due to high surface energy and/or surface charge.
2	Crystallization	Control over the crystal habit (shape), purity and stability.	Solubility limitations.
3	Spray drying	Precise control over a range of critical particle attributes like size, shape, density, roughness, solid-state. Increased bioavailability and stability of the processed particles.	Often not suitable for thermosensitive materials, amorphization of materials.
4	Supercritical fluid technology	Suitable for heat sensitive materials, good control over size distribution and solid state.	Limited by material properties, expensive, scale-up issues.
5	Surface modification through dry coating	Modulation of interfacial interactions to optimize the cohesive-adhesive balance. Improved drug loading, dispersibility and deposition.	Limitations with the size of the guest and host particles.
6	Nanotechnology	Targeted drug delivery, better bioavailability, extended release.	Expensive, toxicity issues, process complexity.

5.4.1 Conventional Approaches

5.4.1.1 Particle sizing

Particle sizing or milling is one of the most common and popular top-down approaches for the micronization of APIs or excipients in the pharmaceutical industry. As mentioned earlier, controlling particle size is one of the parameters of utmost importance for aerosolized drug delivery to the lungs. Thus, sizing operations like milling and sieving form an important component of the particle engineering approach aimed at processing and formulation design for these pulmonary drug dosage forms. Air jet milling is regularly used for the micronization of APIs of desirable size for inhaled drug delivery formulations, although other milling techniques can also be used.

Apart from the benefits to the drug delivery aspect of the size reduction operation in pulmonary drug delivery, it has a significant impact in improving the dissolution of crystalline APIs and consequently improving other biopharmaceutical properties like absorption, bioavailability, etc. Usually, pulmonary formulation compositions consist of a combination of micronized API with other delivery aiding components like carrier excipients in DPIs, propellants and surfactants in pMDIs and solvents for nebulizers. Recently, even micronized API-only marketed DPI formulations such as Pulmicort Turbuhaler containing micronized budesonide were found to show enhanced deposition and pharmacokinetics. The reduction in particle size and the consequential increase in surface area due to micronization is the primary factor responsible for dissolution improvement. The association between the surface area increase and the dissolution rate can be found in the proposed Nernst–Brunner relationship as below.

$$\frac{dQ}{dt} = DA\frac{(Cs - Cb)}{h} \tag{10}$$

Thus, according to the Nernst-Brunner model, the dissolution rate (dQ/dt) is given by the concentration gradient (Cs-Cb) from the surface of the exposed solid with surface area (A), and the diffusivity across a hydrodynamic boundary layer of thickness (h).

While a size reduction approach, it is frequently accompanied by associated, uncontrollable changes in the particle and bulk powder properties. These include alterations in the particle shape, surface energy, surface roughness as well as changes in the bulk behavior like powder flow, dispersibility, particle agglomeration, etc. as depicted in Figure 5.2.

In the case of crystalline to amorphous transformation in these micronized drugs, the lack of the long-range order leads to higher surface reactivity and faster dissolution. Furthermore, it is observed that milling results in the generation of new surfaces exposing different crystal facets varying in facet specific surface energy, defects and creation of high energy amorphous regions, or a combination of any of these. These mechanically induced perturbations in crystalline solids also play a crucial role in dissolution improvement. On the flip side, the increased surface energies and the subsequent off-shift in the CAB of the formulation composition could cause unintended

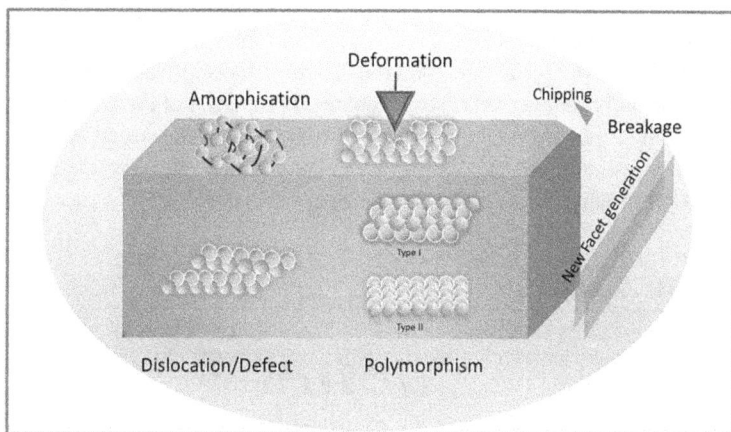

FIGURE 5.2   Milling-induced transformations in solid particulates.

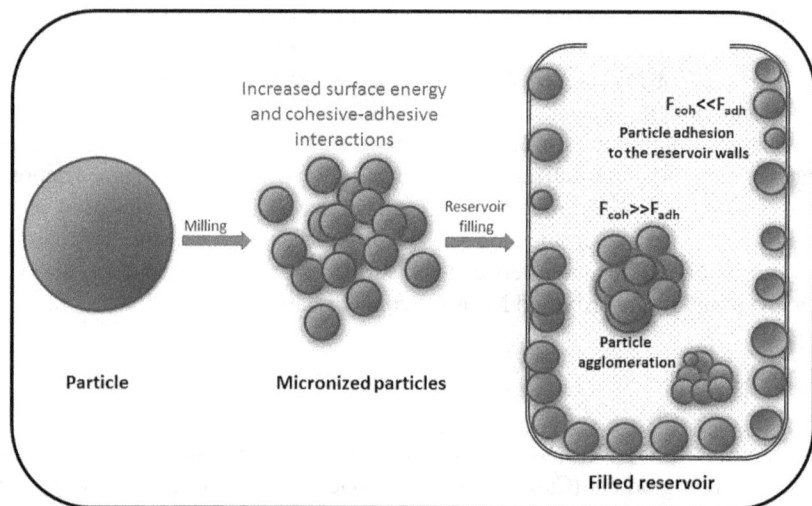

FIGURE 5.3 Size reduction effects on the cohesion-adhesion tendencies of the micronized particles.

handling, processing and performance issues for the drug delivery development. This is depicted in Figure 5.3 for the micronized particles filled in the inhaler reservoir. Also, the importance of crystal habit and crystal anisotropy changes induced from milling and breakage cannot be understated and is discussed later.

The breakage behavior of these solids is dependent on the material properties such as particle mechanical properties (hardness, elastic moduli) as well as the process parameters like energy input (milling time, speed). When it comes to the predictive approaches, the majority of reported literature is focused on the utilization of the energy input-size reduction relationship. As a result, early attempts have led to the development of several empirical size-reduction laws (Rittinger's, Kick's and Bond's law) as listed in Table 5.5, correlating energy input with the particle size parameters. However, from a critical viewpoint, seldom do these laws apply well in practical situations. From a molecular perspective, researchers have also tried to explore the use of crystal inter-planar d-spacings and slip-plane interaction energies for the prediction and characterization of mechanical properties of crystalline solids.[57] Sun and Kiang (2008) proposed that precautions must be taken in the selection of appropriate force fields while using attachment energy calculations for identifying the slip planes or cleavage planes in organic crystals on milling.[58] Specific to the crystalline cleavage planes, it

TABLE 5.5 Size reduction laws based on energy input of the comminution process

SIZE REDUCTION THEORY	EMPIRICAL EQUATION	
Kick's	$E = K_k f cln(L1/L2)$	(11)
Rittinger's	$E = K\_R f cln(1/L2 - 1/L1)$	(12)
Bond's	$E = E_i(100/L2)^{1/2}[1-(1/q)^{1/2}]$	(13)

is often argued that the crystals fracture along the weakest attachment energy planes, which are known to be the most hydrophobic. However, morphological factors like size and shape should also be given due consideration in the prediction or estimation of breakage behavior. Also, the process operation conditions like temperature and humidity could affect the particle properties. Particles milled at cryogenic temperatures showed significantly higher surface area compared to room temperature milled particles. This is attributed to the changes in the mechanical properties (elasticity/brittleness) of the drug particles.[59]

Certainly, comprehensive strategies to carefully control milling-induced transformations in particulate solids and employing suitable technique/s to probe milled solids are needed for effective and efficient formulation design for the pulmonary drug delivery. Thus, designing the methods and selecting the conditions that create different degrees of disorder and/or in distinct domains as well as analyzing them at this level is important.

5.4.1.2 Spray drying

Among the different available technologies, spray drying is the most well-established technology for particle engineering in the field of drug delivery for inhalation applications. Spray drying is a single-step process of obtaining solid particulates by atomization and rapid drying or evaporation of liquid feedstock in a hot airstream. Further, the process can be divided into subprocesses that comprise feedstock formulation, atomization, drying and particle collection. The fine particles are produced during this process by rapid heat and mass transfer.

Spray drying is regarded as one of the robust and scalable technologies accessible and can be applied to a wider range of small and large molecule APIs for pharmaceutical development and manufacturing. The advantages offered for particle engineering include control over particle size, size distribution, shape, density, solid-state, surface energy and moisture content, etc. The feedstock used can be in the form of solutions, suspensions or emulsions. The technique also offers flexibility to atomize the API and excipient particles together (co-spraying). Furthermore, the encapsulation capabilities of spray drying technology provide an additional dimension to the particle design and engineering characteristics. This becomes particularly important for the physical and chemical stability of molecules during the development of biologics or other heat or RH sensitive APIs.[60,61] In fact, all of the commercially marketed DPI products for administering biotherapeutics, as mentioned in Table 5.1, use spray drying techniques for particle engineering designed for product development. All these benefits of providing control over a range of significant particle attributes to boosting product stability render the spray drying technology as having an unprecedented edge over the rest of the approaches.

In the spray drying process, the particle size is controlled by the atomized droplet size, solid content of the slurry, solid particle and liquid densities. Thus, the final particle size ($d_{particle}$) can be assessed from the droplet size ($d_{droplet}$), particle density (ρ_p) and solute concentration (C) using the below equation.[62]

$$d_{particle} = \left(\frac{C}{\rho_p} \right)^{\frac{1}{3}} d_{droplet} \qquad (14)$$

It is clear that controlling the initial atomized droplet size is key to producing spray-dried particles with desired size range, which is critical for inhalation-based drug delivery systems. Further, the spray drying process generally produces particles with high circularity index. This is due to the dynamics of droplet creation (atomization) and droplet drying under the hot airstream in the drying chamber inherent to the spray drying process. The sphericity and shape regularity afforded can remove the disadvantages and uncertainty associated with the anisotropic crystalline solids. The shape regularity and the associated homogeneity in the surface properties offer uniform cohesion-adhesion interaction opportunities.

Moreover, the particle size and shape can be affected by the incorporation of additives in the feedstock. In one study, co-spraying the API with lactose produced smaller and denser particles. In comparison, the particles produced from a co-sprayed drug-albumin combination generated larger, lighter particles with sponge-like shapes.[63] Particles with desired solid-state characteristics, particularly for the generation of amorphous particles with enhanced bulk behavior can be obtained using the spray drying technique.[64]

Referring back to Equation 6, it is clear that one way to reduce the particle aerodynamic diameter (d_a) is to reduce the particle density. Particles with low density and aerodynamic size are desired for enhanced aerosolization efficiencies (FPF~60–70%).[65] On the other hand, large porous particles (LPP), typically >5µm, afford the benefits of low particle aggregation tendencies, fewer phagocytotic losses in the lungs and increasing bioavailability.[66] Spray drying has been successfully utilized to generate porous or hollow particles with low density. Due to the instantaneous nature of the heat and mass transfer during the drying stage of the aerosolized droplets, porous particles with low particle density can be generated. TOBI® Podhaler, one of the commercial DPI formulations containing tobramycin, is a spray-dried engineered particle formulation for the treatment of cystic fibrosis. It consists of light porous particles with a phospholipid-based shell and the amorphous antibiotic (tobramycin) in the core.[67] Contrary to such a core-shell assembly, a structured particle assembly consisting of large porous particles (LPP) loaded with the small dense API particles can also be engineered using an optimized feedstock formulation consisting of excipients. The LPP particles are produced usually by additives, such as a porogen in the feedstock.[68] Incorporating water-miscible propellant or a polymer in the feedstock solution, particles can be designed with a porous matrix for faster or sustained release dissolution profiles respectively.

From the particle formation perspective, a lot of emphasis has been placed on the droplet evaporation rate and the diffusion kinetics of the solutes during the drying process.[69,70] The ratio of the evaporation rate to diffusion rate, termed as Peclet number, was utilized to explain and even predict the morphological changes in the spray-dried particles. In the processes with low Peclet number (>1), the solute diffusion rate is faster compared to the receding evaporating surfaces, and the solutes remain well distributed within the droplet. In this case, the spray-dried particles have similar densities as that of the dry components. On the other hand, for high Peclet numbers (<1), the rate of evaporation is faster than the solute diffusion. As a result, the surface moves faster compared to the solutes and becomes enriched with the high Peclet number constituent. This proposed particle formation mechanism is depicted in Figure 5.4. A range of particle morphologies is possible in such cases depending on the properties of the enriched

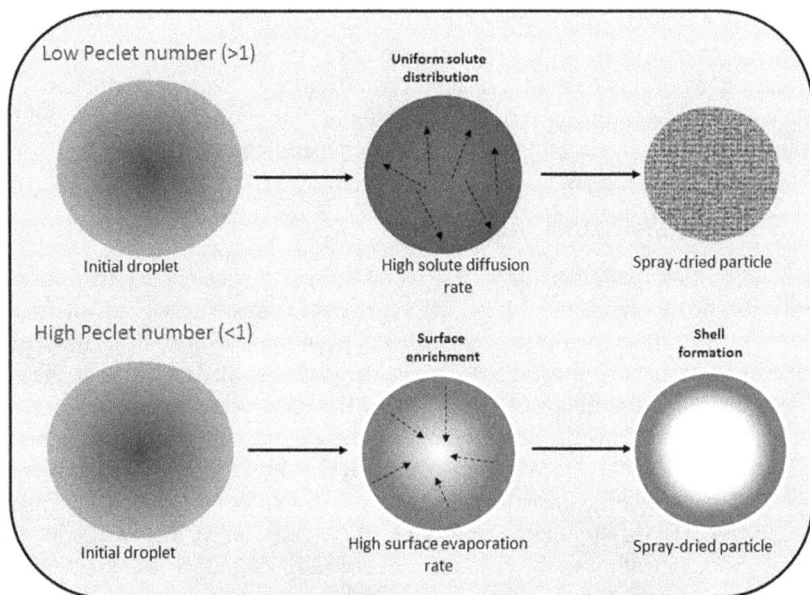

FIGURE 5.4   Particle formation during spray drying process.[69]

component. Hollow solid shell particles, or dimpled or wrinkled particles are some of the morphologies that are commonly observed. Therefore, it is clear that spray drying also alters the surface topographical features of a particle. This can be achieved via optimizing the formulation of feedstock solutions or by varying the process operating parameters.

The spray drying process parameters such as air-flow rate, feed-flow rate, inlet and outlet temperatures have a direct impact on the particle properties. The effect of these spray drying process parameters on the particle size and shape is well reported.[71] Particularly the inlet temperature is shown to have a significant impact on the particle size and shape. On the other hand, it has been shown that particle morphology can be altered by employing varying outlet air temperatures during spray drying. Spray-dried crystalline particles with varying degrees of surface roughness can be produced by using different outlet air temperature conditions.[71] As stated earlier, the kinetics of the particle formation within the drying chamber induces surface level stresses giving rise to the creation of textured surfaces of the spray-dried product. The detailed aspects of the particle formation process in spray drying and its dependence on the parameters like droplet size, evaporation rate, solid content of the feedstock, etc., is a complex topic of study covered elsewhere.[69] Such process parameters dependent on the surface texturing of the particles provide the opportunity to modify and modulate the interparticle contacts and could play an important role in optimizing the CAB.

Overall, the engineered particles obtained with precise control over the above-mentioned particle attributes result in powders with better flow properties and bulk behavior. Several studies focused on particle engineering for DPI drug delivery report an improved flowability coupled with better aerosolization performance for spray-dried formulations. A similar improvement in the functionality of the DPI formulation was highlighted by Pilcer et al. while working with lipid-coated tobramycin particles generated using a spray drying method. The lipid-coated antibiotic particles exhibited desired particle size range with the narrower size distribution, improved flowability and better aerosolization performance with improved deagglomeration behavior and higher FPF.[72]

5.4.1.3 Crystallization

Crystallization is an essential particle generation and downstream purification unit operation for the development of drug delivery dosage forms. Particle growth and control from the crystallization process have always been the backbone of pharmaceutical drug development and engineering. Mechanistically, the detailed concepts of nucleation and crystal growth are well covered elsewhere.[73] During crystallization, the faceting of crystals is observed during the growth process where the crystal tries to create surfaces or facets with minimum surface energy. This provides an opportunity to intervene and modulate the facet-specific growth to obtain crystals with desired habits, size and surface properties. The different techniques for particle engineering and design in pulmonary drug development using the fundamental crystallization approach are depicted in the schematic in Figure 5.5.

Crystal habit modification and regulating crystal size are some of the most aspired-to targets for particle design, especially as these crystalline properties are of particular significance in the surface area-driven kinetic processes like adhesion, dissolution and absorption.[74,75] It has been shown that crystalline solids have anisotropic properties owing to the multifaceted nature of the morphology.[76,77] These anisotropic properties of crystalline solids have a significant impact on a number of unit operations like milling, mixing, granulation and tableting. In addition, anisotropic crystalline properties can affect certain critical quality attributes like wettability, dissolution rate, drug loading, etc.[74] Moreover, as stated earlier, crystalline solids with defects and disorders like ledge, kinks and vacancy, i.e., high surface energy, are also chemically reactive.[78] This can have a direct impact on the chemical and physical stability of the generated particles.

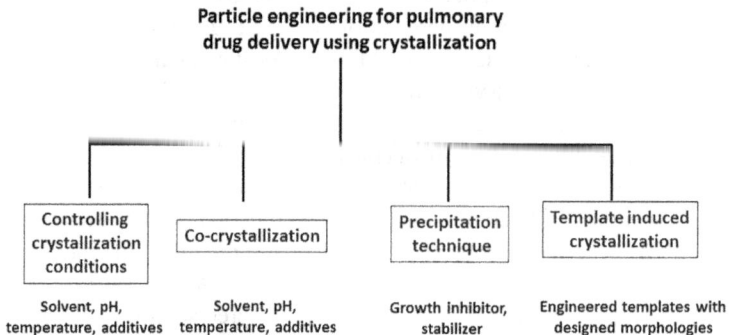

FIGURE 5.5 Particle engineering for pulmonary delivery through crystallization approaches.

The primary route of attaining crystalline particles with desired properties for inhalation drug delivery using a bottom-up approach like crystallization is by careful control of the process parameters and conditions. The crystallization process is influenced by various parameters, the most important of which appears to be the solvent environment for crystal growth. The interfacial interaction at the liquid-solid interface during crystal growth is very important as such a multiphase system becomes stabilized due to the molecular attachment and the associated energy transfer occurring at these interfaces. Other parameters like supersaturation, additives, growth inhibitors as well as crystallization conditions like pH and temperature have a substantial importance in the nucleation and crystal growth process. The solvent environment is found to be one of the prime factors in altering the crystal habit.[79] Apart from this, varying the supersaturation or controlling the temperature profile during the crystallization process has also found success in gaining a handle over the crystal size.

Additionally, direct-controlled crystallization for particle size control can be employed through precipitation techniques to generate micronized crystals or with different crystalline habits. An antisolvent precipitation technique using a crystal growth inhibitor like hydroxypropyl methylcellulose (HPMC) polymer is able to produce micronized API crystals.[80–82] Unsurprisingly, increasing or decreasing the inhibitor concentration would lead to a decrease or increase in the particle size of the crystals respectively. Such direct-controlled crystallization can also be exploited through pH-dependent solubility of the APIs to obtain crystalline particles with varying crystal habits. Of late, researchers were able to produce needle-shaped hollow crystalline particles of the API for high-dose and carrier-free DPI formulations.[83] Moreover, these particles showed better aerosolization performance compared to the jet-milled crystals. Thus, predictably the majority of marketed products employ crystalline or microcrystalline APIs in the pulmonary drug delivery formulations due to some of these distinct advantages around high stability and purity composition. Also, as emphasized here, the benefits and significance of crystal habit modification through crystallization strategies cannot be understated for the aerodynamic behavior and pulmonary deposition. An example includes a widely prescribed DPI formulation containing a fixed-dose combination of microcrystalline fluticasone propionate and salmeterol xinafoate marketed as Advair® Diskus® (GlaxoSmithKline) for the treatment of asthma and chronic obstructive pulmonary disease (COPD).[84]

Recent advances in this field have led to the exploration of sound-assisted crystallization (Sonocrystallization) of APIs for particle size and crystal habit modification.[85] Recently, the sonocrystallization technique was applied to engineer needle-shaped salbutamol sulfate crystals with narrow particle size distribution.[86] The application of ultrasound generates highly localized temperature and pressure regions (cavitation), inducing a number of rapid primary nucleation sites growing into small size crystals.[87]

Co-crystallization is another approach that has been explored for particle growth and particle engineering.[88] Co-crystals are formed between the API and one or more co-formers bonded through hydrogen bonds or non-covalent forces.[89] This approach has become popular for improving the bioavailability of hydrophobic drugs by enhancing the solubility and dissolution of the crystalline APIs.[90] The benefits afforded by formulations for pulmonary delivery prepared from co-crystallization of the API and a co-former range from reduced drug toxicity in bronchial cells and increased drug absorption.[91] Also, co-crystallization approaches aided by the spray drying process produce particles with narrow size distribution and better powder flow compared to the co-crystals produced through other methods.[92] Moreover, the engineered particles with co-crystals formed by spray freeze-drying have been found to possess a larger specific surface area desired for the pulmonary delivery development.[93]

5.4.2 Novel Advanced Approaches

Advanced particle formation techniques, use of nanoparticles and surface engineering through dry coating techniques are being employed as novel approaches for targeted drug delivery to the lungs for the therapeutic treatment of several diseases, right from asthma, pneumonia, other respiratory diseases, cancer to, recently, even diabetes. Some of these cutting-edge approaches are discussed below.

5.4.2.1 Supercritical fluid technologies

In the last couple of decades, supercritical fluid (SCF) technology has garnered a lot of attention as a tool to generate and design particle properties for pharmaceutical applications. This also includes the production of respirable quality particles for aerosolized drug delivery applications.

Fundamentally, the SCF technology exploits the properties of the supercritical fluid for particle formation applications. A supercritical fluid is a thermodynamic state of a chemical substance that exhibits both liquid-like and gas-like properties above the critical temperature (Tc) and pressure (Pc). Carbon dioxide is the most widely used for SCF applications owing to its abundance, low cost, non-toxic nature and accessible critical pressure (Pc=7.38 MPa) and temperature (Tc=31.18°C) parameters.

Like the spray drying process, in SCF technology the particle formation is primarily controlled by the mass transfer kinetics. Based on the behavior of the supercritical fluid to act as a solvent and antisolvent, the SCF process is classified into two main categories as below.

Rapid expansion of supercritical solution (RESS): in this SCF process the supercritical fluid is used as a solvent. The solute material desired for particle conversion is dissolved in the supercritical fluid. The solution is then decompressed rapidly leading to a rapid drop in temperature and pressure to achieve adiabatic expansion. This is followed by spraying the expanded mixture through a nozzle to cause precipitation of particles. The RESS process is relatively simple and a commonly recognized SCF technology used to prepare organic solvent-free fine dry particles. However, it is limited by the solubility restrictions of the pharmaceutical organic solids in the non-polar supercritical solvent (CO_2).

Gas antisolvent (GAS): in the GAS SCF process, the supercritical fluid acts as an antisolvent to cause precipitation of fine particles or small droplets. This is carried out in the presence of an organic solvent like acetone, dichloromethane (DCM) and dimethyl sulfoxide (DMSO). During the process, the supercritical fluid acting as antisolvent is bubbled through the solution. The mixture expands with an increase in the pressure causing high supersaturation and rapid nucleation to obtain the final product in the form of precipitated crystals. Thus, the high mass transfer kinetics achieved in this case is owing to the low viscosity and high diffusivity of supercritical fluid. The GAS SCF process is preferred for the poorly water-soluble APIs. The order of addition of the solvent (organic solvent), antisolvent (supercritical fluid) and the solute (drug) composition is vital for the resultant product from this process. The choice of organic solvent is also critical.

There are other variations of the two major SCF approaches mentioned above. The Particles from Gas Saturated Solutions (PGSS) belongs to the first category SCF method. On the other hand, Supercritical Fluid Antisolvent (SAS), Precipitation with Compressed Antisolvent (PCA) and Solution Enhanced Dispersion by Supercritical Fluids (SEDS) methods adhere to the second category. In the SAS and PCA processes, the supercritical fluid penetrates the solute droplets, causing a decrease in its solubility followed by precipitation into particles. The SEDS method is based on the same antisolvent principle except that it employs a co-axial nozzle to flow the antisolvent and solute resulting in better mixing of these components.

Similar to the previously mentioned particle generation techniques, several process parameters and conditions need to be optimized to attain desired particle properties using the SCF process. Operating conditions and process parameters such as temperature, pressure, composition of the solute (drug), choice of solvent, antisolvent properties and flow rates are important factors that can affect the particle properties. Mechanistically, the mass transfer process determines particle formation, and a high mass transfer allows faster nucleation and results in smaller and less agglomerated particles.

The SCF method can produce particles in the micro- to the nano-scale range. The particles produced can be in the pure form or an encapsulated assembly form. With SCF technology, it is possible to obtain particles typically having homogeneous properties like particle size, narrow size distribution, shape, solid-state and surface texture compared to those obtained using the micronization method. These particle characteristics lead to less cohesivity or improved flow property allowing better aerosolization performance (high FPF). Recently, SCF technology has shown substantial promise in the preparation of macromolecule particles like proteins or genes for inhalation applications. Although having all the benefits of the previously discussed well-established techniques and the potential to become a single step particle generation and engineering process, SCF is still unable to achieve the necessary traction within the particle engineering community. The use of organic solvents presents toxicity issues of the solvents like DMSO. Moreover, the SCF process scale-up remains a challenge for exploiting the full potential of this technique.

5.4.2.2 Surface modification through dry coating

The most common formulation strategy during the development of the DPI delivery system is to employ a carrier-based powder composition. The carrier is a larger particle and acts as a host material for the micron-sized API guest particles. The generation of these highly interactive powder mixtures relies predominantly on the cohesive-adhesive interactions of the carrier and micronized API particles. Although this traditional approach in principle is a form of dry coating technique, the main difference arises in terms of the coating efficiency or drug loading achieved, providing overall better quality of the coating. In dry coating, the high adhesive interactions between the guest-host system are exploited by the application of high shearing forces during the mixing operation to achieve the dry coated particles.

Lately, an inclination toward environment-friendly and green technologies, like dry powder coating, over the conventional solvent-based approaches is observed. This is due to concerns for safety and the environment (zero-emission of volatile organic solvents), low energy consumption (required for drying or evaporation operations), moisture sensitivity of materials in aqueous coatings and overall lower investment and operating costs. Dry powder coating can be achieved by thermal adhesion, electrostatic attraction or liquid-assisted methods. With the exception of electrostatic methods, the coating is achieved in a mixer, in which the substrates are brought into intimate contact with the fine, coating powder, which may be multi-component, where shearing of the fine powder enables it to be spread over, and adhere to, the host surface. One such example would be a popular dry powder or particle coating method described by Pfeffer et al.[94] It involves mechanical treatment of the powders resulting in the coating of bigger-sized host particles with smaller-sized guest particles. Additionally, in some cases, these coated systems might be further cured (thermally or UV) to achieve the desired strength and properties of the coat, e.g., epoxy resin-based coatings. The dry powder coating techniques based on the interparticle forces involved are as follows:

1. van der Waals forces assisted coating
2. Electrostatic powder coating
3. Thermal adhesion. This includes UV, laser or electron beam-assisted coating.

The dry coating is the surface engineering technique gaining importance in the pharmaceutical industry mainly for powder flow improvement applications. However, it has shown applicability in the improvement of powder properties for inhalation applications. The surface modification through dry coating modifies the CAB between the carrier and API particles improving the drug delivery efficiency.[95–97] Other potential benefits include a reduction in the electrostatic charging in the dispersed micronized particles.[98] Table 5.6 reports some of the dry coating studies using different dry coating devices and guest-host combinations for aerosol-based drug delivery applications.

Mechanistically, there are two central stages involved in the dry coating process as depicted in Figure 5.6. The first step involves the dispersion and de-aggregation of coating material guiding the extent of interparticle collision interactions between the guest and host. This is followed by adhesion and spreading of the coating composite on the surface responsible for the strength of the coating.

The dry powder process is affected by the material properties and the process parameters. Size stands out the most, for example, particle A may coat particle B if ten times smaller, though may not if they are equally sized. Typically, a higher host-to-guest particle size ratio and higher energy input during mixing led to better coating strength.[99] Also, dry coating being a surface phenomenon, the interfacial properties of the interacting solids cannot be underestimated. Furthermore, the degree of the coating depends on the mechanics inside the mixer, i.e., the frequency and nature of collisions.

TABLE 5.6 Dry coating studies for pharmaceutical inhalation drug delivery applications from literature

NO.	DEVICE	HOST	HOST	COMMENTS	REF.
1	Mechanofusion	Salbutamol Sulphate (3.6 µm) Salmeterol xinafoate (1.0 µm) Triamcinolone acetonide (1.9 µm)	Magnesium stearate	Improvement in bulk densities of micronized powders, cohesion reduction and improved aerosolization indicated by higher FPF and smaller agglomerate sizes.	97
2	Mechanofusion	Lactose powders (L300–4µm and P450–20 µm)	Magnesium stearate (7.9 µm)	Lactose P450 grade showed most improved fluidization characteristics on coating. The aerosolization behavior defined by entrainment and de-agglomeration is related to powder properties.	96
3	Mechanofusion	Salbutamol sulphate, Lactose monohydrate	Leucine, lecithin, magnesium stearate	Selective modifications of API with force control agents led to better control over the cohesive-adhesive balance (CAB) and better blend uniformity, contrary to the that observed with the carrier particle modification.	102
4	Mechanofusion, high shear mixer (HSM)	Lactose monohydrate (103.4 µm)	Magnesium stearate	Both the coating processes suitable for carrier engineering and improved aerodynamic performance (FPF). HSM showed superior coating.	103
5	Magnetically assisted impaction coating (MAIC)	Ibu-110, Ibu-90 Ibu-50, APAP coarse and micronized ascorbic acid, ultrafine and crystalline Avicel PH101,102 and 105 grades crospovidone, celphere	Hydrophilic silica (20 nm)	The dry coated powders exhibited improved flow, packing and fluidization characteristics.	104
6	Turbula mixing	Lactose monohydrate	Magnesium stearate (6.9 µm)	Formulations with surface modified carrier with spray dried drug provided best in vitro lung deposition (FPF).	105

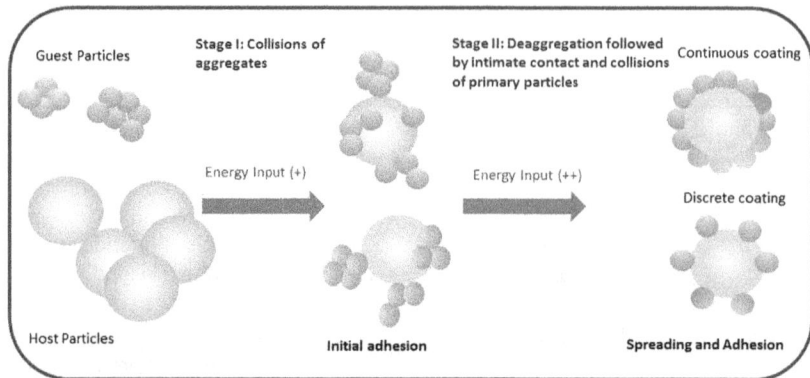

FIGURE 5.6   Stagewise depiction of the dry coating process.

As such the interparticle interactions between the guest (drug) and the carrier (host) can be significantly affected by the choice of the mixer or mixing technique.[100] Also, other extrinsic factors like temperature, humidity and the presence of any surface moisture affect the coating attained. The coating achieved can be discrete or continuous in nature conditional to the system and processing operation parameters like amount of guest concentration, properties of guest-host particles and energy input, type of coating device, etc. Recently, regarding the percentage of guest particles by weight to achieve a monolayer coverage on the host particle, Yang et al. provided the following relation:[101]

$$Gwt\% = \frac{\left(Nd^3 \rho_d\right)}{\left(D^3 \rho_D\right) + \left(Nd^3 \rho_d\right)} X100 \tag{15}$$

$$Here, N = \frac{4(D+d)^2}{d^2} \tag{16}$$

This relation for calculating the weight percentage of guest concentration to achieve a complete monolayer coverage assumes that: i) both the guest and host particles are spherical, ii) guest particles are of the same size and iii) there is no elastoplastic deformation in the particles during the coating process.

In quantitative terms, experimentally the quality of particle coating can be directly assessed by the surface area coverage (SAC) of the guest particles over the host surface. Considering the size range of the guest and hosts involved in this process, imaging techniques like scanning electron microscopy (SEM) coupled with image processing tools can provide us with an estimation of the percentage SAC coverage.

From a thermodynamic standpoint, the spreading of a liquid droplet can be predicted based on the surface energy of the individual components and their interaction. However, it is observed that such a straightforward approach is unreliable for powders, as it does not consider particle properties such as size, shape, density, roughness, etc. Also, importantly, the continuum nature of the liquid phase compared to the powder system is a decisive differentiating factor. In the dry coating process, the adhesion component of the process can be ascribed to the interparticle interaction force like vdW attraction between the smaller and larger particles assisted by impaction forces provided by different coating or mixing devices that help in the attachment of the guest particles onto the host surfaces. On the other hand, in the case of electrostatic powder coating (corona charging or tribocharging), the electrostatic attraction forces are the dominant driving force for the adhesion mechanism. Recently, it was suggested that the dry coating process is governed by two main parameters. The first parameter is referred to as the Stokes number expressed as the ratio of energy input to the strength of the guest particle agglomerates. This parameter can be said to influence the spreading of coating onto the host surface. The second parameter gives us the relationship between the relative cohesion and adhesion strength of the host and guest particles.[106]

Overall, engineering the particle surfaces with dry particle coating could help in tackling the influence of environmental factors, like humidity, in material handling and processing. Since the surface physicochemical nature is critical in guiding the bulk properties, the emphasis is on the development of technologies that would ensure that the alteration occurs only at the substrate surface level keeping intact the inherent bulk phase to avoid any unexpected consequences for the resultant product. Dry coating, being one such technique, has still immense untapped potential for powder-based formulation development aimed at targeted drug delivery to the lungs.

5.4.2.3 Nanotechnology approaches

The use of advanced drug delivery systems containing nanoparticles is commonplace in the pharmaceutical industry. These also include the use of nano drugs or nanocarriers for pulmonary delivery systems. The large surface-to-volume ratio accessible from the nanomaterials and the resulting dominance of the surface physical and chemical properties can be exploited for pulmonary drug delivery. This has found special applications in increasing solubility and dissolution, rapid absorption, improving bioavailability, precise drug targeting, extended or delayed drug release and enhancing drug safety.

Nanoparticles can be created by top-down approaches like particle comminution or through a bottom-up approach like the precipitation method. Thus, techniques described previously like milling, recrystallization, spray drying and supercritical fluid technologies are suitable for nanoparticle generation. The preparation or synthesis of nanoparticles is critical for pharmaceutical applications, since at the nano range the particle properties show significant differences from the bulk of the same bigger (micron size) particle. Therefore, vigilant monitoring and control of nanoparticle preparation processes as well as the physicochemical properties are vital. The increase in the surface area during the preparation approach increases the free surface energy of the particles often leading to problems like particle agglomeration. Hence, to develop a stable nanoparticle system, surface modifiers like surfactants, surface chemical functionality (silanization), etc., are used to decrease the free energy of the system.

The size of a nanoparticle, in particular, has a tendency to influence the pharmacokinetics, biodistribution and safety of the nanomedicines. Certain animal studies of the nanoparticle deposition in the nasopharyngeal and tracheobronchial region revealed that nanoparticles smaller than 100 nm size were able to penetrate the pulmonary mucus layer compared to its larger (>100 nm) counterparts.[107] Moreover, often the smaller size fraction of these nanoparticles are able to successfully cross the biological barriers. Likewise, as mentioned previously, the size of the nanoparticles has been found to play an imperative role in the efficient targeting and desired drug accumulation in tumor treatments.[108,109] The drug serum or plasma absorption and phagocytic uptake are also dependent on the nanoparticle properties like the size and attached functionality. Thus, in recent times a substantial effort has been put into developing 'stealth' nanoparticles that can evade the alveolar macrophages.[110,111] These 'stealth' particles can attain prolonged blood half-life, have selective accumulation in the tissues and have drug targeting specificity. A high curvature morphology of the particles and/or hydrophilic surface property is essential to reduce opsonization reactions and subsequent clearance by macrophages.[112]

In the nano-based drug delivery systems, the nanoparticle is used as a carrier (nanocarrier) for drug loading and efficient delivery to the lungs. Thus, during the formulation and development, the therapeutic agents are usually either dissolved, attached to, or entrapped in nanoparticles. The nanosystems typically used in the drug delivery to the lungs are liposomes, solid-lipid nanoparticles (SLNs), polymeric nanoparticles, protein nanocarriers, inorganic nanoparticles and dendrimers.

The polymeric nanocarrier fabrication methods applied to pulmonary drug delivery involve polyelectrolyte complex formation, double emulsion/solvent evaporation techniques, or emulsion polymerization techniques. Nanoparticle synthesis using polymerization and ionotropic gelation methods are commonly employed in pharmaceutical applications. In the polyelectrolyte complex formation technique, two oppositely charged polymers are mixed to entrap the drug into the polymer matrix of the nanocarrier. A closely linked technique called ionotropic gelation uses the ability of the polyelectrolytes to crosslink with the counterion to form a mesh network of the hydrogel. In the double emulsion/solvent evaporation technique, the emulsification of the dissolved drug and polymer such as poly(lactic-co-glycolide (PLGA) in the organic solvent is achieved in an aqueous media containing surfactants to form drug-loaded polymeric nanoparticles. PLGA has gained popularity as a polymeric excipient for drug delivery applications owing to its biodegradability and biocompatibility.

Usually, the nanocarriers are functionalized to achieve a selective affinity and cellular targeting. The attachment of ligands or molecules on these nanoparticle surfaces provides specific affinities toward biological molecules. Different functionalization techniques include peptide or amino acid conjugation, PEGylation, oligo nucleation, etc. PEGylation provides stability to a range of drugs (protein, peptides, small molecules) by providing pharmacokinetic advantages like protection against metabolism and immune response. Likewise, the attachment of a ligand on nanoparticles can also affect drug targeting.

Additionally, lipid-based delivery systems like liposomes and solid lipid nanoparticles (SLN) have also achieved a fair bit of admiration as a safe and well-tolerated drug delivery vehicle to the lungs due to the presence of the same lipids in the lungs as used in the preparation of liposome nanoparticles. Liposomes are synthesized by high shear mixing or homogenization of a drug in the suspension of dissolved lipids. The liposomal suspension can be freeze-dried or spray-dried to produce nanoparticle dry powder for inhalation. Recently, two of the approved messenger RNA (mRNA) Covid-19 vaccines from Pfizer-BioNTech and Moderna were administered as lipid nanoparticle formulation against the SARS-CoV-2 infection.[113] Such lipid nanoparticle-conjugated vaccines have been found to enhance immunogenic response compared to normal formulations.

Overall, these different techniques to generate and engineer nanoparticles with tight control over particle properties evidently demonstrate the immense potential and benefits of nanoparticle pulmonary drug delivery. However, a major challenge to the nanomedicine for targeted lung delivery application remains regarding concern around the inherent toxicity of nanoparticles. The migration of the inhaled nanoparticles from the alveolar cells to the systemic circulation may cause detrimental vascular effects. Also, the toxicity of additional materials (polymers, solvents, etc.) used in the nanoparticle synthesis may pose apprehension for a full-scale utilization of this particle engineering technology.

5.5 OUTLOOK AND FUTURE PERSPECTIVES

A better understanding begets better innovation. The formulation strategies aided with new particle engineering tools are a more pragmatic and promising approach for safe and efficient targeted drug delivery to the lungs over efforts directed towards the development of new delivery devices. Throughout this chapter, we have highlighted the immense significance of a range of particle properties in the development of functional products for pulmonary delivery. Also, it has been emphasized that in a majority of cases there exists a complex interplay between the properties that guide the particle and powder behavior. Thus, a comprehensive understanding and a holistic view of these properties would help in optimizing and predicting the final product performance. As described in this chapter, there is a range of targeted approaches that can be undertaken to achieve the desired control over different particle attributes for pulmonary drug delivery. However, a complete mechanistic understanding of these engineering approaches holds the key to a successful particle design strategy. To reiterate, safety and efficacy are of paramount importance, especially when administering potent low-dose therapeutics. Particle engineering techniques that could enhance these two parameters along with the specificity of drug targeting action are highly desired. Several modern and advanced techniques discussed have shown a massive potential to be developed into a scale-up platform technology providing a quick, cost-effective, safe and sustainable solution for tailoring particle properties.

Moreover, several new therapeutic modalities are being explored and developed to meet the rapidly changing needs of pulmonary drug therapy. These modalities attempt to achieve a step-change moving from small molecules to including macromolecules like proteins, peptides, nucleic acids and antibodies within the drug delivery landscape. There is a constant push to develop innovative technologies for converting promising therapeutic agents to successful pulmonary therapies. Recently, vaccine delivery applications through the pulmonary route have gained a lot of interest due to the advantages of ease of administration and non-invasive route of vaccine administration. Vaccines formulated as dry powders for inhalation applications can avoid some of the complexities inherent to the cold chain supply and linked to logistical challenges. In addition, vaccines administered through the pulmonary route have been shown to induce mucosal and systemic immunity. Spray freeze drying (SFD) technology has shown considerable potential for desired particle engineering intended for vaccine delivery. Also, continuous efforts are being invested into modifying the excipients suitable for the formulation and delivery of biopharmaceuticals. Commercially available excipients or carriers, like PulmoSphere® particles or Biohale®, with tailor-made particle properties that aid in stabilizing the biologics as well as enhancing the safety profile of biopharmaceutical formulations are being industrialized. Thus, as these particle engineering technologies continue to develop and mature, a new range of advanced and smart pulmonary drug delivery products is envisioned for consistent and efficient delivery of drugs.

REFERENCES

1. Zhou, Q. (Tony), Tang, P., Leung, S. S. Y., Chan, J. G. Y. & Chan, H.-K. Emerging inhalation aerosol devices and strategies: Where are we headed? *Adv. Drug Deliv. Rev.* 75, 3–17 (2014).
2. Dolovich, M. B. & Dhand, R. Aerosol drug delivery: Developments in device design and clinical use. *Lancet* 377(9770), 1032–1045 (2011).
3. Weers, J. G. & Miller, D. P. Formulation design of dry powders for inhalation. *J. Pharm. Sci.* 104(10), 3259–3288 (2015).
4. de Boer, A. H. *et al.* Dry powder inhalation: Past, present and future. *Expert Opin. Drug Deliv.* 14(4), 499–512 (2017).
5. Malcolmson, R. J. & Embleton, J. K. Dry powder formulations for pulmonary delivery. *Pharm. Sci. Technolo. Today* 1(9), 394–398 (1998).
6. Das, S., Tucker, I. & Stewart, P. Inhaled dry powder formulations for treating tuberculosis. *Curr. Drug Deliv.* 12(1), (2015).
7. Pietsch, W. Size enlargement by agglomeration. In *Hand book of powder science and technology* (eds. Fayed, M. E. & Otten, L.) 202–377. (Chapman and Hall, 1997).
8. Das, S., Larson, I., Young, P. & Stewart, P. Agglomerate properties and dispersibility changes of salmeterol xinafoate from powders for inhalation after storage at high relative humidity. *Eur. J. Pharm. Sci.* 37(3–4), 442–450 (2009).
9. Chaudhuri, B., Mehrotra, A., Muzzio, F. J. & Tomassone, M. S. Cohesive effects in powder mixing in a tumbling blender. *Powder Technol.* 165(2), 105–114 (2006).
10. Israelachvili, J. N. *Intermolecular and surface forces.* (Academic Press, 2015). https://doi.org/10.1016/C2011-0-05119-0.
11. Castellanos, A, The relationship between attractive interparticle forces and bulk behaviour in dry and uncharged fine powders. *Adv. Phys.* 54(4), 263–376 (2005).
12. Johnson, K. L. Mechanics of adhesion. *Tribol. Int.* 31(8), 413–418 (1998).
13. Derjaguin, B. V., Muller, V. M. & Toporov, Y. P. Effect of contact deformations on the adhesion of particles. *Prog. Surf. Sci.* 45(1–4), 131–143 (1994).
14. Butt, H. J. Capillary forces: Influence of roughness and heterogeneity. *Langmuir* 24(9), 4715–4721 (2008).
15. Young, P. M., Price, R., Tobyn, M. J., Buttrum, M. & Dey, F. Effect of humidity on aerosolization of micronized drugs. *Drug Dev. Ind. Pharm.* 29(9), 959–966 (2003).
16. Valverde, J. M. *Fluidization of fine powders: Cohesive versus dynamical aggregation.* (Springer Science & Business Media, 2013).

17. Rowley, G. & Mackin, L. A. The effect of moisture sorption on electrostatic charging of selected pharmaceutical excipient powders. *Powder Technol.* 135–136, 50–58 (2003).
18. Grosvenor, M. P. & Staniforth, J. N. The influence of water on electrostatic charge retention and dissipation in pharmaceutical compacts for powder coating. *Pharm. Res.* 13(11), 1725–1729 (1996).
19. Eilbeck, J., Rowley, G., Carter, P. A. & Fletcher, E. J. Effect of contamination of pharmaceutical equipment on powder triboelectrification. *Int. J. Pharm.* 195(1–2), 7–11 (2000).
20. Eilbeck, J., Rowley, G., Carter, P. A. & Fletcher, E. J. Effect of materials of construction of pharmaceutical processing equipment and drug delivery devices on the triboelectrification of size-fractionated lactose. *Pharm. Pharmacol. Commun.* 5(7), 429–433 (1999).
21. Podczeck, F., Newton, J. M. & James, M. B. Influence of relative humidity of storage air on the adhesion and autoadhesion of micronized particles to particulate and compacted powder surfaces. *J. Colloid Interface Sci.* 187(2), 484–491 (1997).
22. Lin, Y. W., Wong, J., Qu, L., Chan, H. K. & Zhou, Q. T. Powder production and particle engineering for dry powder inhaler formulations. *Curr. Pharm. Des.* 21(27), 3902–3916 (2015).
23. Zeng, X. M., Martin, G. P., Marriott, C. & Pritchard, J. The effects of carrier size and morphology on the dispersion of salbutamol sulphate after aerosolization at different flow rates. *J. Pharm. Pharmacol.* 52(10), 1211–1221 (2000).
24. Kaialy, W., Alhalaweh, A., Velaga, S. P. & Nokhodchi, A. Influence of lactose carrier particle size on the aerosol performance of budesonide from a dry powder inhaler. *Powder Technol.* 227, 74–85 (2012).
25. Ooi, J., Traini, D., Hoe, S., Wong, W. & Young, P. M. Does carrier size matter? A fundamental study of drug aerosolisation from carrier based dry powder inhalation systems. *Int. J. Pharm.* 413(1–2), 1–9 (2011).
26. Duddu, S. P. *et al.* Improved lung delivery from a passive dry powder inhaler using an engineered PulmoSphere® powder. *Pharm. Res.* 19(5), 689–695 (2002).
27. Mullins, M. E., Michaels, L. P., Menon, V., Locke, B. & Ranade, M. B. Effect of geometry on particle adhesion. *Aerosol Sci. Technol.* 17(2), 105–118 (1992).
28. Otsuka, M. & Kaneniwa, N. Effect of grinding on the crystallinity and chemical stability in the solid state of cephalothin sodium. *Int. J. Pharm.* 62, 65–73 (1990).
29. Otte, A., Zhang, Y., Carvajal, M. T. & Pinal, R. Milling induces disorder in crystalline griseofulvin and order in its amorphous counterpart. *Cryst. Eng. Comm.* 14(7), 2560–2570 (2012).
30. Trasi, N. S., Boerrigter, S. X. M. & Byrn, S. R. Investigation of the milling-induced thermal behavior of crystalline and amorphous griseofulvin. *Pharm. Res.* 27(7), 1377–1389 (2010).
31. Chang, R. Y. K., Chen, L., Chen, D. & Chan, H.-K. Overcoming challenges for development of amorphous powders for inhalation. *Expert Opin. Drug Deliv.* 17(11), 1583–1595 (2020).
32. Müller, T., Krehl, R., Schiewe, J., Weiler, C. & Steckel, H. Influence of small amorphous amounts in hydrophilic and hydrophobic APIs on storage stability of dry powder inhalation products. *Eur. J. Pharm. Biopharm.* 92, 130–138 (2015).
33. Descamps, M., Willart, J. F., Dudognon, E. & Caron, V. Transformation of pharmaceutical compounds upon milling and comilling: The role of Tg. *J. Pharm. Sci.* 96(5), 1398–1407 (2007).
34. De Gusseme, A., Neves, C., Willart, J. F., Rameau, A. & Descamps, M. Ordering and disordering of molecular solids upon mechanical milling: The case of fananserine. *J. Pharm. Sci.* 97(11), 5000–5012 (2008).
35. Willart, J. F., Dujardin, N., Dudognon, E., Danède, F. & Descamps, M. Amorphization of sugar hydrates upon milling. *Carbohydr. Res.* 345(11), 1613–1616 (2010).
36. Shah, U. V., Karde, V., Ghoroi, C. & Heng, J. Y. Y. Influence of particle properties on powder bulk behaviour and processability. *Int. J. Pharm.* 518(1–2), 138–154 (2017).

37. Shah, U. V. *et al.* Decoupling the contribution of surface energy and surface area on the cohesion of pharmaceutical powders. *Pharm. Res.* 32(1), 248–259 (2015).

38. Karde, V. & Ghoroi, C. Influence of surface modification on wettability and surface energy characteristics of pharmaceutical excipient powders. *Int. J. Pharm.* 475(1–2), 351–363 (2014).

39. Jong, T., Li, J., Morton, D. A. V., Zhou, Q. (Tony) & Larson, I. Investigation of the changes in aerosolization behavior between the jet-milled and spray-dried colistin powders through surface energy characterization. *J. Pharm. Sci.* 105(3), 1156–1163 (2016).

40. Ho, R. & Heng, J. Y. Y. A review of inverse gas chromatography and its development as a tool to characterize anisotropic surface properties of pharmaceutical solids. *KONA Powder Part. J.* 30, 164–180 (2012).

41. Traini, D., Rogueda, P., Young, P. & Price, R. Surface energy and interparticle forces correlations in model pMDI formulations. *Pharm. Res.* 22(5), 816–825 (2005).

42. Ho, R., Muresan, A. S., Hebbink, G. A. & Heng, J. Y. Y. Influence of fines on the surface energy heterogeneity of lactose for pulmonary drug delivery. *Int. J. Pharm.* 388(1–2), 88–94 (2010).

43. Das, S. C., Tucker, I. G. & Stewart, P. J. Surface energy determined by inverse gas chromatography as a tool to investigate particulate interactions in dry powder inhalers. *Curr. Pharm. Des.* 21(27), 3932–3944.

44. Saleem, I., Smyth, H. & Telko, M. Prediction of dry powder inhaler formulation performance from surface energetics and blending dynamics. *Drug Dev. Ind. Pharm.* 34(9), 1002–1010 (2008).

45. Schiavone, H., Palakodaty, S., Clark, A., York, P. & Tzannis, S. T. Evaluation of SCF-engineered particle-based lactose blends in passive dry powder inhalers. *Int. J. Pharm.* 281(1–2), 55–66 (2004).

46. Wagner, K. G., Dowe, U. & Zadnik, J. Highly loaded interactive mixtures for dry powder inhalers: Prediction of the adhesion capacity using surface energy and solubility parameters. *Die Pharm. Int. J. Pharm. Sci.* 60(5), 339–344.

47. Sethuraman, V. V. & Hickey, A. J. Powder properties and their influence on dry powder inhaler delivery of an antitubercular drug. *AAPS PharmSciTech* 3(4), 7 (2002).

48. Podczeck, F. The influence of particle size distribution and surface roughness of carrier particles on the in vitro properties of dry powder inhalations. *Aerosol Sci. Technol.* 31(4), 301–321 (1999).

49. Tan, B. M. J., Chan, L. W. & Heng, P. W. S. Improving dry powder inhaler performance by surface roughening of lactose carrier particles. *Pharm. Res.* 33(8), 1923–1935 (2016).

50. Flament, M. P., Leterme, P. & Gayot, A. The influence of carrier roughness on adhesion, content uniformity and the in vitro deposition of terbutaline sulphate from dry powder inhalers. *Int. J. Pharm.* 275(1–2), 201–209 (2004).

51. Adi, S. *et al.* Effects of mechanical impaction on aerosol performance of particles with different surface roughness. *Powder Technol.* 236, 164–170 (2013).

52. Ferrari, F. *et al.* The surface roughness of lactose particles can be modulated by wet-smoothing using a high-shear mixer. *AAPS PharmSciTech* 5(4), (2004).

53. Raula, J., Lähde, A. & Kauppinen, E. I. Aerosolization behavior of carrier-free l-leucine coated salbutamol sulphate powders. *Int. J. Pharm.* 365(1–2), 18–25 (2009).

54. Eilbeck, J., Rowley, G., Carter, P. A. & Fletcher, E. J. Powder triboelectrification. *Int. J. Pharm.* 195(1–2), 7–11 (2000).

55. Karner, S., Maier, M., Littringer, E. & Urbanetz, N. A. Surface roughness effects on the tribo-charging and mixing homogeneity of adhesive mixtures used in dry powder inhalers. *Powder Technol.* 264, 544–549 (2014).

56. Otsuka, M. & Ishii, M. Improvement of theophylline anhydrate stability at high humidity by surface-physicochemical modification. *Colloids Surf. B. Biointerfaces* 76(1), 158–163 (2010).

57. Shariare, M. H., Leusen, F. J. J., de Matas, M., York, P. & Anwar, J. Prediction of the mechanical behaviour of crystalline solids. *Pharm. Res.* 29(1), 319–331 (2012).

58. Sun, C. C. & Kiang, Y. H. On the identification of slip planes in organic crystals based on attachment energy calculation. *J. Pharm. Sci.* 97(8), 3456–3461 (2008).

59. Shah, U. V. *et al.* Effect of milling temperatures on surface area, surface energy and cohesion of pharmaceutical powders. *Int. J. Pharm.* 495(1), 234–240 (2015).

60. Chow, M. Y. T. *et al.* Inhaled powder formulation of naked siRNA using spray drying technology with l-leucine as dispersion enhancer. *Int. J. Pharm.* 530(1–2), 40–52 (2017).

61. Aquino, R. P. *et al.* Dry powder inhalers of gentamicin and leucine: Formulation parameters, aerosol performance and in vitro toxicity on CuFi1 cells. *Int. J. Pharm.* 426(1–2), 100–107 (2012).

62. Maa, Y.-F., Nguyen, P.-A., Sit, K. & Hsu, C. C. Spray-drying performance of a bench-top spray dryer for protein aerosol powder preparation. *Biotechnol. Bioeng.* 60(3), 301–309 (1998).

63. Vanbever, R. *et al.* Formulation and physical characterization of large porous particles for inhalation. *Pharm. Res.* 16(11), 1735–1742 (1999).

64. Vehring, R. Pharmaceutical particle engineering via spray drying. *Pharm. Res.* 25(5), 999–1022 (2008).

65. Dellamary, L. A. *et al.* Hollow porous particles in metered dose inhalers. *Pharm. Res.* 17(2), 168–174 (2000).

66. Ben-Jebria, A. *et al.* Large porous particles for sustained protection from carbachol-induced bronchoconstriction in guinea pigs. *Pharm. Res.* 16(4), 555–561 (1999).

67. Geller, D. E., Weers, J. & Heuerding, S. Development of an inhaled dry-powder formulation of tobramycin using PulmoSphere™ technology. *J. Aerosol Med. Pulm. Drug Deliv.* 24(4), 175–182 (2011).

68. Pham, D.-D., Fattal, E., Ghermani, N., Guiblin, N. & Tsapis, N. Formulation of pyrazinamide-loaded large porous particles for the pulmonary route: Avoiding crystal growth using excipients. *Int. J. Pharm.* 454(2), 668–677 (2013).

69. Vehring, R., Foss, W. R. & Lechuga-Ballesteros, D. Particle formation in spray drying. *J. Aerosol Sci.* 38(7), 728–746 (2007).

70. Vehring, R., Snyder, H. & Lechuga-Ballesteros, D. Spray drying. *Drying Technol. Biotechnol. Pharm. Appl.* 179–216 (2020). https://doi.org/10.1002/9783527802104.ch7.

71. Maas, S. G. *et al.* The impact of spray drying outlet temperature on the particle morphology of mannitol. *Powder Technol.* 213(1–3), 27–35 (2011).

72. Pilcer, G., Sebti, T. & Amighi, K. Formulation and characterization of lipid-coated tobramycin particles for dry powder inhalation. *Pharm. Res.* 23(5), 931–940 (2006).

73. Chernov, A. A. *Modern Crystallography III.* (Springer, 1984). https://doi.org/10.1007/978-3-642-81835-6.

74. Hadjittofis, E. *et al.* Influences of crystal anisotropy in pharmaceutical process development. *Pharm. Res.* 35(5), (2018).

75. Shah, U. V. *et al.* Effect of crystal habits on the surface energy and cohesion of crystalline powders. *Int. J. Pharm.* 472(1–2), 140–147 (2014).

76. Heng, J. Y. Y., Bismarck, A. & Williams, D. R. Anisotropic surface chemistry of crystalline pharmaceutical solids. *AAPS PharmSciTech* 7(4), (2006).

77. Heng, J. Y. Y., Bismarck, A., Lee, A. F., Wilson, K. & Williams, D. R. Anisotropic surface energetics and wettability of macroscopic form I paracetamol crystals. *Langmuir* 22(6), 2760–2769 (2006).

78. Roberts, K. J., Docherty, R. & Tamura, R. *Engineering crystallography: From molecule to crystal to functional form.* (Springer, 2017).

79. Croker, D. M. *et al.* Demonstrating the influence of solvent choice and crystallization conditions on phenacetin crystal habit and particle size distribution. *Org. Process Res. Dev.* 19(12), 1826–1836 (2015).

80. Steckel, H., Rasenack, N., Villax, P. & Müller, B. W. In vitro characterization of jet-milled and in-situ-micronized fluticasone-17-propionate. *Int. J. Pharm.* 258(1–2), 65–75 (2003).

81. Rasenack, N., Steckel, H. & Müller, B. W. Preparation of microcrystals by in situ micronization. *Powder Technol.* 143–144, 291–296 (2004).

82. Steckel, H., Rasenack, N. & Müller, B. W. In-situ-micronization of disodium cromoglycate for pulmonary delivery. *Eur. J. Pharm. Biopharm.* 55(2), 173–180 (2003).

83. Yazdi, A. K. & Smyth, H. D. C. Hollow crystalline straws of diclofenac for high-dose and carrier-free dry powder inhaler formulations. *Int. J. Pharm.* 502(1–2), 170–180 (2016).

84. Hanania, N. A. *et al.* The efficacy and safety of fluticasone propionate (250 µg)/salmeterol (50 µg) combined in the diskus inhaler for the treatment of COPD. *Chest* 124(3), 834–843 (2003).

85. Guo, Z., Zhang, M., Li, H., Wang, J. & Kougoulos, E. Effect of ultrasound on anti-solvent crystallization process. *J. Cryst. Growth* 273(3–4), 555–563 (2005).

86. Dhumal, R. S., Biradar, S. V., Paradkar, A. R. & York, P. Particle engineering using sono-crystallization: Salbutamol sulphate for pulmonary delivery. *Int. J. Pharm.* 368(1–2), 129–137 (2009).

87. Louhi-Kultanen, M., Karjalainen, M., Rantanen, J., Huhtanen, M. & Kallas, J. Crystallization of glycine with ultrasound. *Int. J. Pharm.* 320(1–2), 23–29 (2006).

88. Aakeröy, C. B. Crystal engineering: Strategies and architectures. *Acta Crystallogr. Sect. B.* 53(4), 569–586 (1997).

89. Desiraju, G. R. Crystal and co-crystal. *Cryst. Eng. Comm.* 5(82), 466–467 (2003).

90. Karashima, M. *et al.* Enhanced pulmonary absorption of poorly soluble itraconazole by micronized cocrystal dry powder formulations. *Eur. J. Pharm. Biopharm.* 115, 65–72 (2017).

91. do Amaral, L. H. *et al.* Development and characterization of dapsone cocrystal prepared by scalable production methods. *AAPS PharmSciTech* 19(6), 2687–2699 (2018).

92. Alhalaweh, A. *et al.* Theophylline cocrystals prepared by spray drying: Physicochemical properties and aerosolization performance. *AAPS PharmSciTech* 14(1), 265–276 (2013).

93. Tanaka, R., Hattori, Y., Otsuka, M. & Ashizawa, K. Application of spray freeze drying to theophylline-oxalic acid cocrystal engineering for inhaled dry powder technology. *Drug Dev. Ind. Pharm.* 46(2), 179–187 (2020).

94. Pfeffer, R., Dave, R. N., Wei, D. & Ramlakhan, M. Synthesis of engineered particulates with tailored properties using dry particle coating. *Powder Technol.* 117(1–2), 40–67 (2001).

95. Zhou, Q. T. & Morton, D. A. V. Drug-lactose binding aspects in adhesive mixtures: Controlling performance in dry powder inhaler formulations by altering lactose carrier surfaces. *Adv. Drug Deliv. Rev.* 64(3), 275–284 (2012).

96. Zhou, Q. T., Armstrong, B., Larson, I., Stewart, P. J. & Morton, D. A. V. Understanding the influence of powder flowability, fluidization and de-agglomeration characteristics on the aerosolization of pharmaceutical model powders. *Eur. J. Pharm. Sci.* 40(5), 412–421 (2010).

97. Zhou, Q. T., Qu, L., Larson, I., Stewart, P. J. & Morton, D. A. V. Improving aerosolization of drug powders by reducing powder intrinsic cohesion via a mechanical dry coating approach. *Int. J. Pharm.* 394(1–2), 50–59 (2010).

98. Jallo, L. J. & Dave, R. N. Explaining electrostatic charging and flow of surface-modified acetaminophen powders as a function of relative humidity through surface energetics. *J. Pharm. Sci.* 104(7), 2225–2232 (2015).

99. Otles, S., Lecoq, O. & Dodds, J. A. Dry particle high coating of biopowders: An energy approach. *Powder Technol.* 208(2), 378–382 (2011).

100. Jetzer, M. W., Schneider, M., Morrical, B. D. & Imanidis, G. Investigations on the mechanism of magnesium stearate to modify aerosol performance in dry powder inhaled formulations. *J. Pharm. Sci.* 107(4), 984–998 (2018).

101. Yang, J., Sliva, A., Banerjee, A., Dave, R. N. & Pfeffer, R. Dry particle coating for improving the flowability of cohesive powders. *Powder Technol.* 158(1–3), 21–33 (2005).

102. Begat, P., Price, R., Harris, H., Morton, D. A. V. & Staniforth, J. N. The influence of force control agents on the cohesive-adhesive balance in dry powder inhaler formulations. *KONA Powder Part. J.* 23, 109–121 (2005).

103. Bungert, N., Kobler, M. & Scherließ, R. In-depth comparison of dry particle coating processes used in DPI particle engineering. *Pharmaceutics* 13(4), (2021).

104. Ghoroi, C. *et al.* Dispersion of fine and ultrafine powders through surface modification and rapid expansion. *Chem. Eng. Sci.* 85, 11–24 (2013).

105. Benke, E., Farkas, Á., Szabó-Révész, P. & Ambrus, R. Development of an innovative, carrier-based dry powder inhalation formulation containing spray-dried meloxicam potassium to improve the in vitro and in silico aerodynamic properties. *Pharmaceutics* 12(6), (2020).

106. Tamadondar, M. R., de Martín, L., Thalberg, K., Björn, I. N. & Rasmuson, A. The influence of particle interfacial energies and mixing energy on the mixture quality of the dry-coating process. *Powder Technol.* 338, 313–324 (2018).

107. Murgia, X. *et al.* Size-limited penetration of nanoparticles into porcine respiratory mucus after aerosol deposition. *Biomacromolecules* 17(4), 1536–1542 (2016).

108. Gaumet, M., Vargas, A., Gurny, R. & Delie, F. Nanoparticles for drug delivery: The need for precision in reporting particle size parameters. *Eur. J. Pharm. Biopharm.* 69(1), 1–9 (2008).

109. Yuan, F. *et al.* Vascular permeability in a human tumor xenograft: Molecular size dependence and cutoff size. *Cancer Res.* 55(17), 3752–3756 (1995).

110. Fang, C. *et al.* In vivo tumor targeting of tumor necrosis factor-alpha-loaded stealth nanoparticles: Effect of MePEG molecular weight and particle size. *Eur. J. Pharm. Sci.* 27(1), 27–36 (2006).

111. Moreira, J. N., Hansen, C. B., Gaspar, R. & Allen, T. M. A growth factor antagonist as a targeting agent for sterically stabilized liposomes in human small cell lung cancer. *Biochim. Biophys. Acta Rev. Biomembr.* 1514(2), 303–317 (2001).

112. Brigger, I., Dubernet, C. & Couvreur, P. Nanoparticles in cancer therapy and diagnosis. *Adv. Drug Deliv. Rev.* 54(5), 631–651 (2002).

113. Abdellatif, A. A. H., Tawfeek, H. M., Abdelfattah, A., El-Saber Batiha, G. & Hetta, H. F. Recent updates in COVID-19 with emphasis on inhalation therapeutics: Nanostructured and targeting systems. *J. Drug Deliv. Sci. Technol.* 63, 102435 (2021).

Particle Architectonics for Pulmonary Drug Delivery

6

Kohsaku Kawakami

Contents

6.1 INTRODUCTION

The lung is an attractive portal for both systemic and local delivery of drugs (1–4). Pulmonary drug delivery is gaining increasing attention with an increase in the number of biopharmaceuticals, which are difficult to administer via the oral route. Drugs can be formulated in either the liquid or solid state for the pulmonary route. Representative delivery technologies include the use of nebulizers, pressured metered-dose inhalers, and dry powder inhalers (DPI). Although all of them have advantages and disadvantages, the DPI seems to be the most attractive type of the device because of high stability

DOI: 10.1201/9781003182566-8

and low volume of formulation. However, the design of the dry powder formulation for inhalation must be done carefully to achieve the desired performance of drugs.

Dry powders for pulmonary drug delivery must be introduced into the lungs only by the aspiration force of patients. The aerodynamic size of the particles is known to be a dominant factor in determining the deposition site of the drug in the lung. Simple reduction in the particle size generally increases the adhesion/cohesion energy between the particles, which may result in their aggregation. Thus, control of the density, morphology, and surface properties of the particles must be considered as well. To enable such "architectonics", spray-drying is the most common technology for manufacturing inhalation particles. This chapter discusses technologies for designing inhalable particles using spray-drying to maximize the therapeutic effect of drugs.

6.2 FATE OF DRUG PARTICLES IN THE LUNG

The aerodynamic size of the particles is one of the most important parameters that determine the deposition site of drugs in the lung (5–8). Several deposition models are available for estimating the efficacy of particle delivery as a function of their aerodynamic size. The most representative is the International Commission on Radiological Protection (ICRP) model (9), which was developed based on both experimental observations and model calculations by considering complicated lung structures. Figure 6.1 presents the efficiency of particle deposition after aspiration as a function of the aerodynamic diameter based on this model. The deposition site is determined by three factors: impaction, sedimentation, and Brownian diffusion of the particles. Particles smaller than 100 nm effectively reach the alveolar region where Brownian diffusion plays a dominant role. In addition, if particles are sufficiently small, they can escape mucociliary clearance after deposition in the lung (10). Moreover, macrophage clearance has been shown to be minimized (11). Rapid dissolution and permeation across biological membranes are also expected. Another benefit of nanoparticles is that a size reduction to below 200 nm enables sterile filtration during the manufacturing process. However, with current powder technologies, particles smaller than 100 nm are difficult to manufacture and handle. Therefore, particles of a few micrometers are regarded as the best practical option, which also exhibit good deposition owing to the appropriate balance of impaction and sedimentation forces. Commercially formulated inhalable particles are generally of this size.

Dry powder inhalation is a convenient option for pulmonary drug delivery because stabilization and administration of a large amount of drug can easily be achieved compared to other methods, including the use of metered-dose inhalers and nebulizers (10,12). Spray-drying is one of the most common manufacturing methods for inhalation particles, which allows the regulation of particle size by changing the solution and instrumental conditions (13–15). Moreover, particle morphology can be manipulated to various forms, such as hollow (16,17) or porous (18,19) particles, to decrease the aerodynamic size. In the following sections, the focus will be on the design of inhalable particles to control the size, density, and surface properties of spray-dried particles.

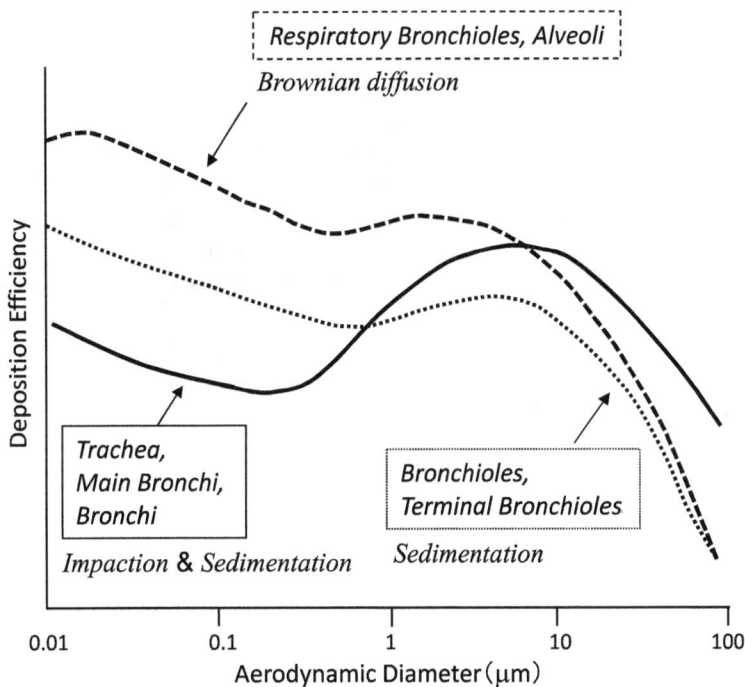

FIGURE 6.1 Deposition efficiency of inhaled particles as a function of their aerodynamic diameters. The deposition sites and the most influential factors for the deposition are described in the figure. (Adapted after modification from "ICRP Publication 66", Smith 1994 (9).)

6.3 DOWN-SIZING OF SOLID PARTICLES

Both top-down and bottom-up methodologies are available for controlling particle size. Milling is a simple top-down method for producing nano- to microparticles. However, it does not offer much flexibility for tuning particle properties, and the resultant particles are generally adhesive/cohesive. The aspiration force by patients during the administration is too weak to disintegrate the aggregated particles. Various efforts are possible to control the properties of the particles using bottom-up approaches, and spray-drying is the most common option. The selection of instrument parameters, such as nozzle diameter and atomizing pressure, enables the control of particle size (14,15). The concentration of the solution is the simplest parameter to affect particle size. Given that one particle is formed by drying one droplet, the diameter of the particle, d_p, can be calculated using the following equation:

$$d_p = d_d \left(\frac{\rho_d}{\rho_p} C \right)^{\frac{1}{3}},$$

(1)

where d_d is the diameter of the droplet, ρ_d and ρ_p are the densities of the droplet and particle, respectively, and C is the fraction of the solute in the droplet, that is, the concentration. It is obvious that smaller particles can be obtained by decreasing concentration of the solution. Decreasing droplet size is also an option to reduce particle size, with which the surface tension of the feed solution is expected to be correlated. One may expect a correlation between the equilibrium surface tension and the droplet size; however, the equilibrium surface tension cannot be obtained during the atomization process because the time required for the diffusion of the surfactant molecules to reach the droplet surface is not provided. Thus, the surface tension in a millisecond needs to be understood to determine its correlation with particle size.

Figure 6.2 shows the dynamic surface tensions of representative surfactant solutions up to 10 s (20). The equilibrium surface tension cannot be obtained even above the critical micellar concentration (CMC) at this timescale, except for sodium dodecyl sulfate (SDS) which has the smallest molecular weight, that is, the fastest diffusion rate.

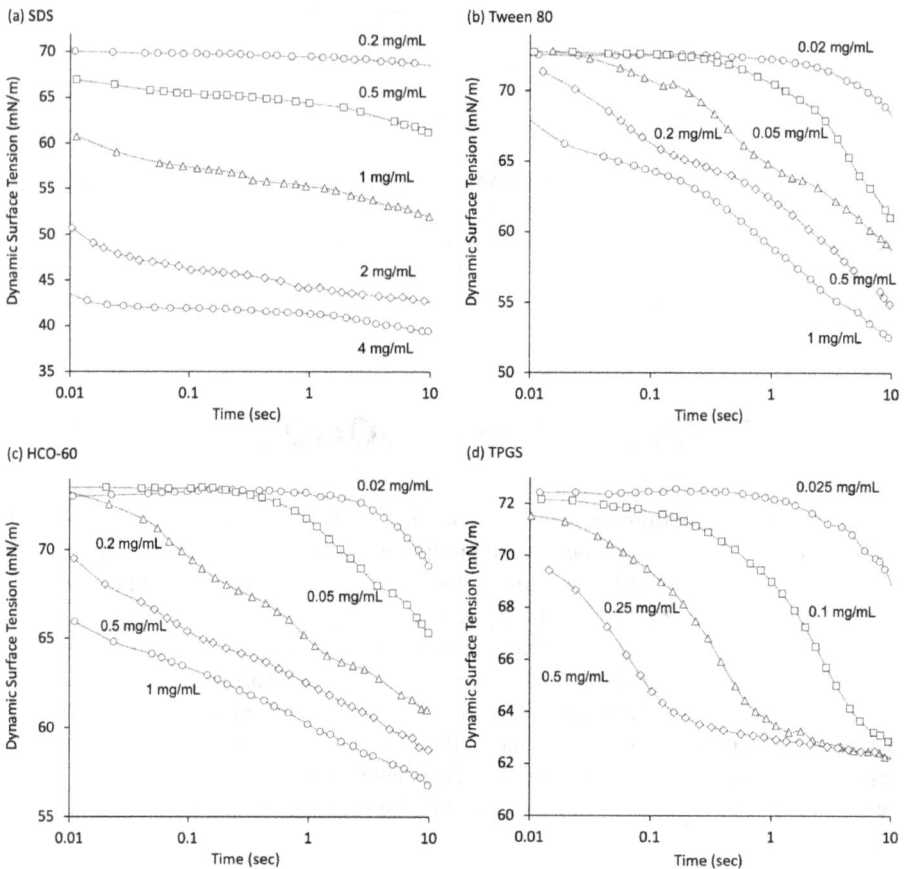

FIGURE 6.2   Dynamic surface tensions of surfactant solutions obtained by the bubble pressure method. The surfactant types are described in the figure. (Adapted from Kawakami et al. 2010 (20) with permission.)

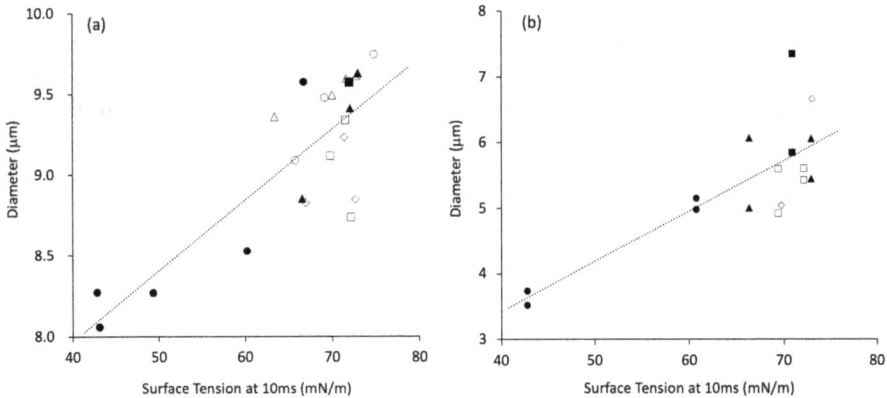

FIGURE 6.3 Relationship between (a) the size of sprayed droplet of surfactant solutions and their surface tension at 10 ms and (b) size of the spray-dried maltose particles in the presence of surfactants, and the surface tension of the surfactant solutions at 10 ms. Surfactant types: SDS (●), HCO-60 (○), TPGS (□), Gelucire (▲), C12E9 (△), and Tw80 (◇). Water (no surfactants) (■). (Adapted from Kawakami et al. 2010 (20) with permission.)

Spray-drying is expected to be completed within few seconds (20). Thus, the surface tension cannot be lowered as expected from the equilibrium surface tension values during spray-drying process. Figure 6.3(a) shows the correlation between the diameter of atomized droplets and surface tension at 10 ms after the creation of the surface. The acceptable correlation indicates that the surface tension in the millisecond timescale could be regarded as the dominant factor in determining the droplet size. Figure 6.3(b) shows the particle size which includes maltose as the main component as a function of the surface tension of the feed solution at 10 ms. Despite the decrease in goodness of fit, the observations suggest that surface tension is an important factor for controlling the particle size. The factors that violate this correlation include the loss of very small particles, different shapes and densities of the particles, and coalescence of both atomized droplets and dried particles. Nevertheless, in addition to the instrumental parameters, the solution parameters, which include the surface tension on a millisecond timescale and concentration, are important factors for determining the size of spray-dried particles.

6.4 MANIPULATION OF PARTICLE MORPHOLOGY

One of the typical problems of powder inhalation is the poor dispersion efficiency of drug particles because of their large surface area. The most common approach for overcoming this problem is the use of a carrier, such as lactose particles, on which the drug particles are adsorbed. Efficacy of this method can be enhanced by mixing lactose particles of different sizes (21–24). Because lactose particles are generally larger than drug particles by more than an order of magnitude, they do not reach deep into the lungs. Drug particles must be detached from the carrier during the inhalation; however, this process is difficult to control. Therefore, the use of excipients for controlling the surface properties of drug particles is another option for avoiding the aggregation problem of drug particles.

Aerodynamic size is defined as the size of a sphere with a standard density that has the same terminal settling velocity. Aerodynamic diameter, d_a, is related to geometric diameter, d_g, using the following equation, if the particles move in the continuum regime (25,26).

$$d_a = d_g \sqrt{\frac{1}{\chi} \frac{\rho_p}{\rho_o}}, \qquad (2)$$

where χ and ρ_o are the dynamic shape factor and standard density, respectively. χ is unity for spherical particles and larger than that for irregular ones (25), meaning that an increase in the irregularity of the particle shape decreases the aerodynamic size.

Psicose is a compound that cannot be spray-dried because of its low glass transition temperature (T_g). However, it becomes possible by using excipients. Figure 6.4 shows scanning electron microscope (SEM) images of spray-dried psicose particles prepared using aspartame, cluster dextrin (cDex), polyvinylpyrrolidone (PVP), and hydroxypropyl methylcellulose (HPMC) as additives (27). Aspartame particles are spherical in shape, whereas polymer particles possesses a wrinkled surface, which can be explained by the removal of solvent from the inside of the particles after the formation of polymer skin on the surface of the droplet (26). The wrinkled surface structure of the PVP particles disappears upon the addition of psicose, whereas the surface structure is retained for the cDex and HPMC particles.

Peclet number, Pe, is a convenient parameter for understanding the morphology of spray-dried particles. The mass transport of solutes and/or dispersed components in

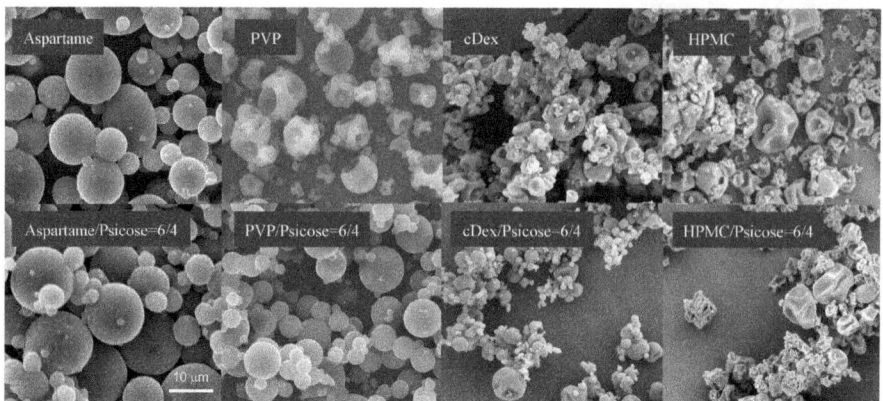

FIGURE 6.4 SEM images of spray-dried psicose and psicose/additive particles. Compositions are presented in the images. Magnification was the same for all the images.

droplets in the radial direction during the drying process can be comprehended using the following equation (26):

$$Pe = \frac{R_d{}^2}{\tau D_i} \tag{3}$$

where R_d and τ are the radius of the droplet and the drying time, respectively. D_i is the diffusion coefficient of the component i. A Pe smaller than unity is obtained for a component that can diffuse rapidly enough to catch up with the shrinkage of the droplets. In this case, a homogeneous distribution of the component in the particle is expected. However, if a certain component cannot catch up with the shrinkage of the droplets, Pe will have a much larger value than unity, which would result in its accumulation in the surface region of the particle. Polymeric additives are supposed to accumulate on the surface region because of their much larger molecular weight relative to that of drug molecules. Therefore, the surface properties of spray-dried particles greatly depend on the properties of the polymers added.

Particle properties/morphologies can be manipulated by using volatile components during spray-drying process. Perfluorooctyl bromide is used as a porogen in Pulmosphere™ technology, which will be discussed in more detail in Section 6.7. As another example, if ammonium bicarbonate (ABC) is contained in the spray-dried solution, it is immediately transformed into the gaseous components, carbon dioxide and ammonia, during the drying process. Figure 6.5 (a and b) shows the effect of ABC on spray-dried budesonide particles (28). Simple spray-drying provided spherical particles; however, a porous structure was obtained by adding ABC to the spray-drying solution. The bulk densities of these particles were 0.132 and 0.078 g/cm³, respectively. Thus, the density was reduced to almost half when ABC was used. Figure 6.5 (c and d) presents another example of the pore formation by ABC, where poly(lactide-co-glycolide acid) (PLGA) was used as the particle material (29). In this case, distinct pores are observed on the surface.

The evaporation of ABC during the spray-drying does not always add a porous structure to the particles. When it was applied to HPMC/psicose particles, the wrinkling of the surface was thinned and grew, likely caused by rapid vaporization of ABC, to form petaloid structures (Figure 6.5 (e and f)) (30). Growth of the petaloid structure was observed with an increase in inlet temperature up to 130°C, which is likely due to an increase in the velocity of the gaseous components removed from the droplets. A further increase in the drying temperature decreased the surface area because of the rubbering of the particles. Figure 6.6 shows the specific surface area and fine particle fraction (FPF) of petaloid particles obtained using Andersen cascade impactor analysis. A comparison with ABC-free particles indicated that the specific surface area increased dramatically upon the addition of ABC to spray-drying solutions. The surface area exhibited maximum values when the inlet temperature was 130 or 140°C. The increase in surface area with temperatures up to 130°C can be explained by the growth of the petaloid structure, whereas the decrease in the surface area above that temperature was due to the aggregation of the particles. FPF values exhibited a similar trend with the specific surface area, showing a maximum at 22.4% when the inlet temperature was 130°C. ABC can be completely removed from the particles during spray-drying. Use of volatile components is an effective way to improve the inhalation properties of spray-dried particles.

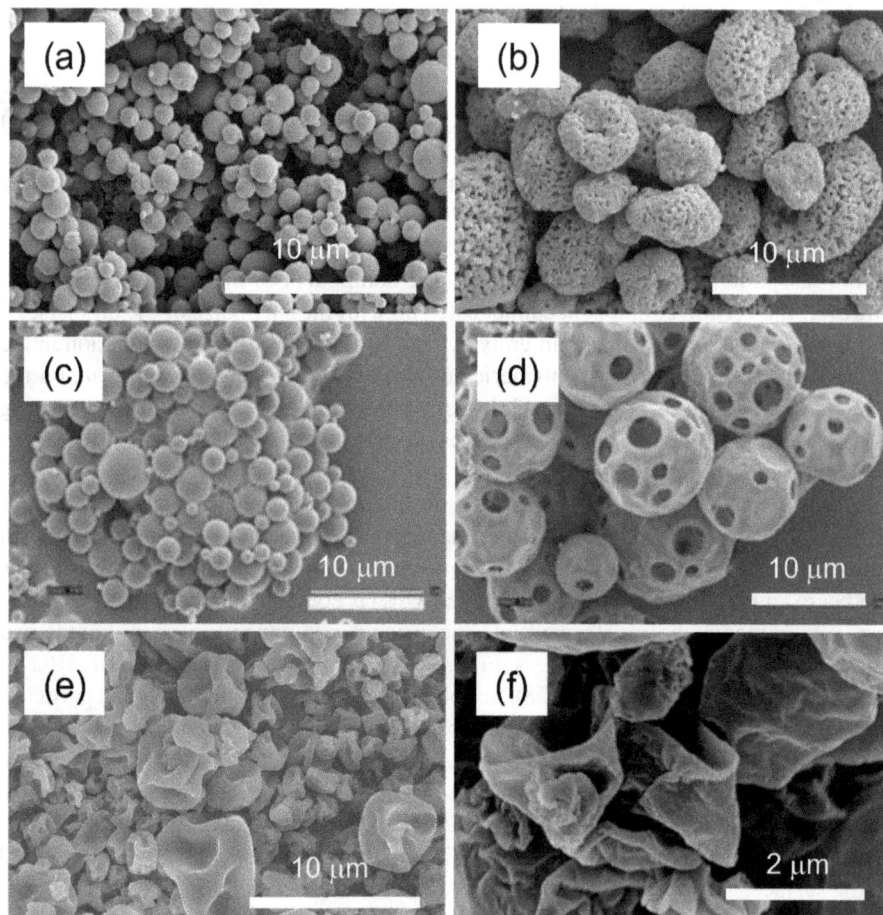

FIGURE 6.5 SEM images of spray-dried particles. (a) Budesonide particles produced from its ethanol/water=95/5 solution. (b) Budesonide particles produced from its ethanol/water=8/2 solution that contained ABC. The initial budesonide/ABC ratio was 85/15, but ABC was removed during the spray-drying. (c) PLGA particles produced from its dichloromethane solution. (d) PLGA particles produced from its dichloromethane solution containing ABC. The ABC/PLGA ratio was initially 2/5, but ABC was removed during the spray-drying. (e) HPMC/psicose=4/6 particles produced from its aqueous solution. (f) HPMC/psicose=4/6 particles produced from its aqueous solution that contained ABC. The equal amount of ABC with that of HPMC+psicose was added to the solution, but ABC was removed during the spray-drying. ((a) and (b) were adapted from Nolan et al. 2009 (28), (c) and (d) were from Yang et al. 2009 (29), and (e) and (f) were from Kawakami et al. 2014 (30))

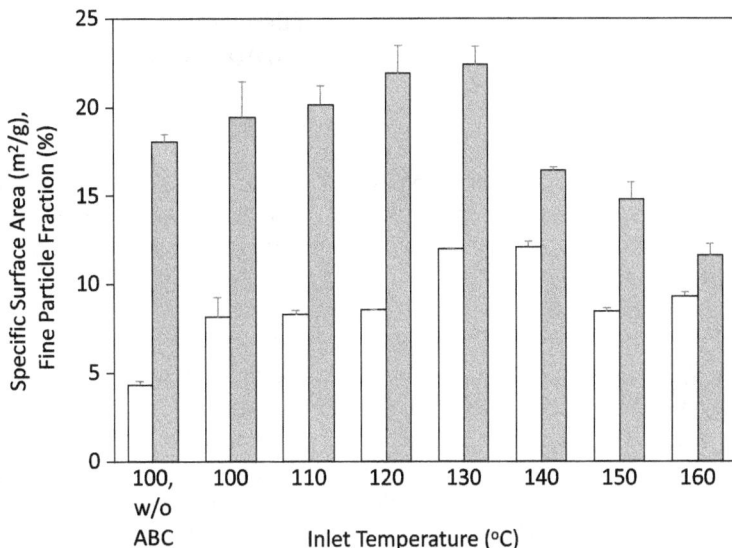

FIGURE 6.6 Specific surface area (white) and fine particle fraction (gray), which was obtained using Andersen cascade impactor analysis, of HPMC/psicose = 4/6 spray-dried particles as a function of inlet temperature. The equal amount of ABC as that of HPMC + psicose was added to the solution, except the sample indicating "w/o ABC"; however, ABC was removed during the spray-drying.

6.5 MISCIBILITY OF SPRAY-DRIED COMPONENTS

If multiple components are subjected to spray-drying and each of them retains the glass state, the thermodynamics of mixing will then be elucidated in terms of the mean-field approximation theory. The Gibbs energy of mixing two components, ΔG_i, can be expressed using the Flory-Huggins equation as follows:

$$\frac{\Delta G_i}{kT} = \frac{\varphi_1^i}{r_1} \ln \varphi_1^i + \frac{\varphi_2^i}{r_2} \ln \varphi_2^i + \chi \varphi_1^i \varphi_2^i, \tag{4}$$

where Φ_1^i, and Φ_2^i are the fractions of components 1 and 2 of phase i, respectively. k and T are the Boltzmann constant and temperature, respectively. r_1 and r_2 are the segment numbers of components 1 and 2, respectively. χ is a parameter that describes the interaction energy between the components. Because the mixing entropy (sum of the first and the second terms on the right-hand side of the equation) is always negative, molecular-level mixing is favored for negative χ. If the mixture is separated into phases rich in components 1 and 2, the overall Gibbs energy, ΔG, is calculated by

$$\Delta G = X_1 \Delta G_1 + X_2 \Delta G_2, \tag{5}$$

where subscripts 1 and 2 represent the phases rich in 1 and 2, respectively. X is the fraction of each phase. The equilibrium state can be determined by minimizing ΔG.

Practical formulations are not always in an equilibrium state because of the competition with dynamic factors during the manufacturing and slow dynamics after solidification (27). Figure 6.7 shows the DSC (differential scanning calorimetry) curves of psicose/PVP mixtures prepared by freeze-drying and spray-drying, where the presence of multiple T_gs indicate phase separation. When the mixture was prepared by freeze drying (Figure 6.7(a)), psicose was miscible with PVP when the PVP/psicose ratio was above 6/4, whereas phase separation was anticipated when the PVP/psicose ratio was below 5/5. Both T_gs were found at the same temperature when the PVP/ratio was smaller than this. One of them almost agreed with the T_g of the pure psicose. T_g of the mixed phase, $T_{g,\text{mix}}$, can be calculated using the Gordon-Taylor equation (31).

$$T_{g,mix} = \frac{w_1 T_{g1} + K w_2 T_{g2}}{w_1 + K w_2}, where\ K = \frac{\rho_1 \Delta\alpha_2}{\rho_2 \Delta\alpha_1} \tag{6}$$

where $T_{g,\text{mix}}$ and T_{gi} are the T_g of the mixture and that of component i, respectively. w_i, ρ_i, and $\Delta\alpha_i$ are the weight fraction, density, and thermal expansivity change at T_g, respectively. The solubility of psicose in the PVP carrier can be calculated as ca. 33% using this equation, regardless of the total mixing ratio. This calculation is reasonable because the pure psicose phase does not appear when the psicose amount is below 40%.

In contrast to the freeze-dried products, phase separation was observed for all the spray-dried mixtures (Figure 6.7(b)) because of the contribution of the dynamic factor, that is, phase separation due to the different diffusion rates of each component during spray-drying. Based on this observation, polymeric additives are always expected to cover spray-dried particles when low-molecular-weight drugs are sprayed together.

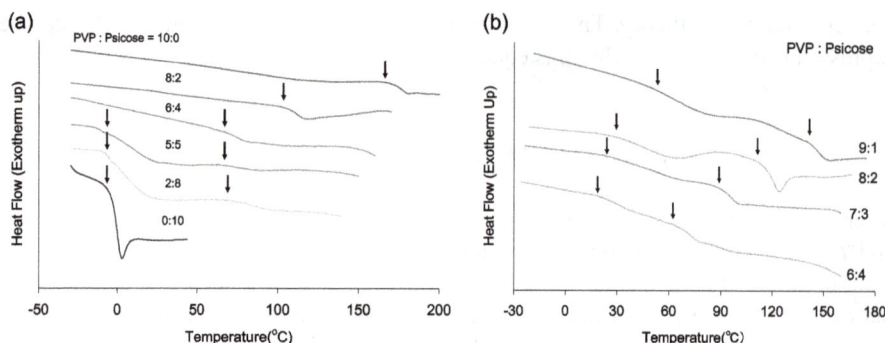

FIGURE 6.7 DSC curves of (a) freeze-dried and (b) spray-dried psicose/PVP formulations. The mixing ratios are presented in the figure. Arrows indicate glass transition temperatures. (Adapted from Kawakami et al. 2013 (27) with permission.)

In fact, when HPMC was used as an additive, spray-dried particles were obtained for HPMC/psicose ratio up to 2/8 in a reproducible manner, and even HPMC/psicose = 1/9 particles were occasionally obtained (30). This seemed to be due to the protection of psicose, which has a very low T_g, by HPMC as a low-hygroscopicity shell.

Surface composition of spray-dried particles can be confirmed by X-ray photoelectron spectroscopy (XPS). If the molecule for which surface accumulation is to be confirmed has a characteristic atom, it can be detected easily. Even if it is not the case, the surface composition can be assumed by ratio of carbon and oxygen atoms. When 0.5% of Gelucire 44/14 or tocopheryl polyethyleneglycol succinate was added to maltose, their proportions on spray-dried particle surface were determined to be ca. 90% and 82%, respectively, by the XPS analysis (20). It was calculated based on the difference in carbon/oxygen ratio of maltose and surfactant molecules.

6.6 NANOPARTICLE-BASED ARCHITECTONICS

Although nanoparticles have several advantages for pulmonary drug delivery, as introduced in Section 6.2 (10), their use is practically difficult because of the aggregation problem. Nevertheless, nanoparticles can be a building block for obtaining microparticles that offer good aerodynamic performance.

Aggregation of nanoparticles may result in low-density microparticles, which are advantageous for pulmonary drug delivery. One of the great achievements of this strategy is the Technosphere® technology, which was used for formulation of commercial inhalable insulin (Afrezza®). It employed aggregates of fumaryl diketopiperazine nanocrystals (32), on which insulin molecules are adsorbed, to form microparticles with an aerodynamic diameter of 2.5 μm. The insulin molecules are adsorbed in a monomeric form to achieve more rapid action (T_{max}: 12–14 min) than that of the injectable formulation (T_{max}: 45–60 min), in which insulin is dissolved in a hexameric form.

Yang et al. used nanoparticle-aggregate particles for the administration of octreotide acetate via the pulmonary route (33). The peptide drug was mixed with sodium deoxycholate to form a hydrophobic ion pair and was then transformed into nanoparticles using phospholipids and other additives. Spray freeze drying of the nanoparticle suspension provided nanoparticulate aggregates of ca. 5 μm in size. Table 6.1 shows the pharmacokinetic parameters of the animal study, where nanoparticle-aggregate formulation and solution of octreotide were administered to rats via the pulmonary route, in comparison with subcutaneous (s.c.) administration of the solution. Both pulmonary-administered formulations provided immediate absorption; however, the plasma concentration of the solution decreased quickly, whereas that for the nanoparticle aggregate decreased slowly. The area under the curve (AUC) for the nanoparticle aggregate was twice that of the solution and much higher than that of s.c. administration.

Nanoparticles may be aggregated in the form of hollow particles after spray-drying under certain operating conditions (16,34) because the diffusion of particles is assumed to be slow, as discussed in Section 6.3.1 This process is illustrated schematically in

TABLE 6.1   Pharmacokinetic parameters after administration of octreotide formulations to rats (0.5 mg/kg)

	NANOPARTICLE AGGREGATES (PULMONARY)	SOLUTION (PULMONARY)	SOLUTION (S.C.)
$t_{1/2}$ (h)	2.96±1.98	2.22±0.68	4.59±5.90
T_{max} (h)	0.30±0.10	0.15±0.08	1.00
C_{max} (ng/mL)	205±61	212±53	60.9±19.0
MRT (h)	2.23±0.51	1.50±0.29	2.66±0.35
AUC (ng/mL·h)	355±63	176±25	228±52

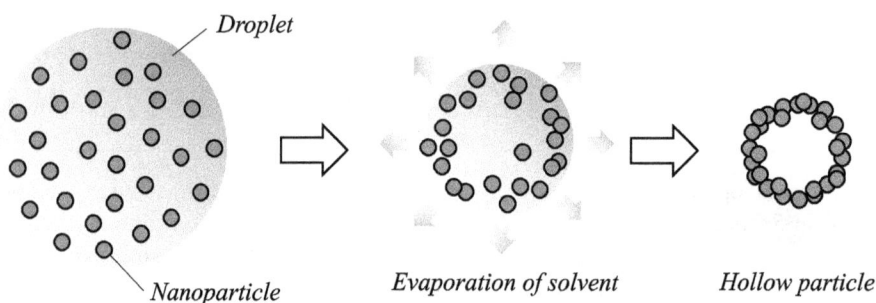

FIGURE 6.8   Mechanism of formation of nanoparticulate hollow particle.

Figure 6.8. Hollow particles may be suitable for pulmonary drug delivery because of their low density (35). Sung et al. encapsulated rifampicin into PLGA nanoparticles, followed by spray-drying to form nanoparticulate aggregated hollow particles (36). The pharmacokinetic parameters obtained after inhalation of the hollow particles were similar to those obtained for the solution. However, the drug concentrations in the lung tissue and bronchoalveolar lavage components were much higher than those for the solution.

The problem associated with the aggregation of nanoparticles may be overcome by entrapping them into a microparticulate matrix. In this case, the distribution of the particles in the lung after inhalation follows that of microparticles; however, other advantages specific to nanoparticles, such as avoidance of mucociliary clearance and efficient absorption after deposition, should be reserved. Ohashi et al. incorporated rifampicin-containing PLGA nanoparticles into mannitol particles using spray-drying (35). The uptake of rifampicin by macrophages was enhanced using the microparticles. Imaging studies showed that PLGA nanoparticles were effectively retained in the lung. In contrast, bare PLGA microparticles were rapidly eliminated from the lungs. Ungaro et al. entrapped tobramycin in PLGA-based nanoparticles, followed by encapsulation in lactose microparticles (36). In this study, the effect of modification of PLGA nanoparticles on the inhalation properties was observed. Poly(vinyl alcohol) (PVA)-modified alginate/PLGA nanoparticles reached deep in the lung, whereas PVA-modified chitosan/

PLGA nanoparticles were mainly located in the upper airways. Thus, the surface properties and size of nanoparticles remain important, even though they were encapsulated in the lactose microparticles.

6.7 LIPID-BASED ARCHITECTONICS

Lipids are promising excipients for pulmonary route because of their safety and unique amphiphilic properties for controlling particle morphology (37). The most representative platform of lipid-based inhalable particles is the Pulmosphere™ technology, where low-density microparticles are prepared by spray-drying lipid emulsions (38,39). The emulsion may accommodate fine drug crystals (39). During spray-drying, lipid emulsions accumulate on the surface region of the sprayed droplets to form hollow particles, the mechanism of which is the same as that for the formation of hollow nanoparticulate aggregates introduced in the previous section. Subsequently, the perfluorooctyl bromide in the lipid emulsion evaporates to form a porous shell. Examples of molecules/drugs that were successfully delivered to the lung using this technology include immunoglobulin (38), budesonide (40), and ciprofloxacin (41). Many review papers that introduce PulmoSphere™ technology in more detail are available (37,39).

We have established a technology to produce mesoporous phospholipid particles that utilize liquid-liquid phase separation for molding the particles in a spherical shape, followed by freeze drying to add a porous structure (Figure 6.9) (42). It has been shown to improve oral absorption of poorly soluble drugs (43). However, the properties of mesoporous phospholipid particles, including low density and high safety, indicate their potential as promising drug carriers for pulmonary drug delivery. Moreover, they can

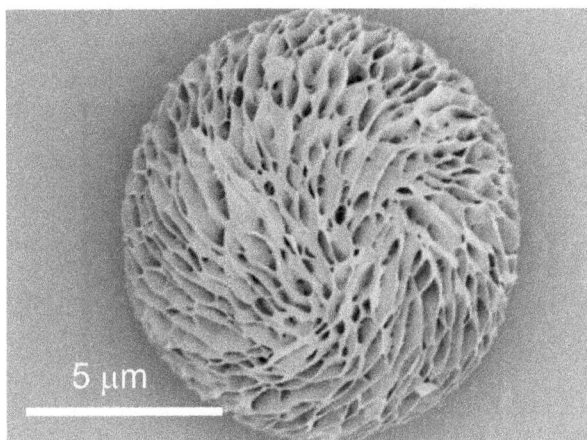

FIGURE 6.9 A SEM image of mesoporous phospholipid particle. (Adapted from Zhang et al. 2015 (42) with permission.)

TABLE 6.2   Excipients for inhalable products listed in FDA database

EXCIPIENTS	MAXIMUM DAILY EXPOSURE OR POTENCY
Sugars	
Lactose	90 mg
Mannitol	6 mg
Lipids/Surfactants and related compounds	
Benzalkonium chloride	0.02 w/w%
Cetylpyridinium chloride	
Cholesterol	1.57 w/v%
1,2-distearoyl-sn-glycero-3-phosphocholine	51 mg
Oleic acid	0.01 w/w%
Polysorbate 80	1 mg
Sodium lauryl sulfate	
Sorbitan trioleate	0.86 mg
Soybean lecithin	0.1 w/w%
Polymers	
Carrageenan	0.42 mg
Gelatin	100 mg
Hypromelose 2906 (4 mPa·s)	45.67 mg
Oils and organic solvents	
Glycerin	5 w/w%
Nutmeg oil	
Propylene glycol	25 w/w%
Turpentine oil	
Other small organics	
Glycine	2 mg
Menthol	0.02 w/w%
Methylparaben	0.03 w/w%
Nitric acid	0.86 w/w%
Propylparaben	0.01 w/w%
Saccharin (sodium)	0.05 w/w%
Thymol	0.01 w/w%
Inorganics	
Ferric oxide yellow	0.04 mg
Magnesium stearate	0.08 mg
Silicon dioxide	
Titanium dioxide	2 mg
Zinc oxide	3.11 w/v%

Buffer components are not listed

accommodate both hydrophilic and hydrophobic compounds because they are composed of a lipid bilayer. Studies to prove efficacy of mesoporous phospholipid particles for pulmonary drug delivery are in process.

6.8 EXCIPIENTS FOR PULMONARY ROUTE

The use of excipients provides a variety of options for controlling particle properties. However, the safety requirements for excipients used for the pulmonary route are much more stringent than those for oral formulations. As the lung is a closed system, unlike the gastrointestinal tract, all excipients must be decomposed to safe small compounds. Almost no mechanical stress and only a small amount of enzymes are available for the decomposition of the excipients. Administration frequency and period can also be factors to determine types and amount of excipients for the pulmonary route to avoid their accumulation in the lung.

The fact that the shape and size of the excipients can be a safety factor is a major feature of the pulmonary route. As discussed earlier, the deposition site of the particles is influenced by their aerodynamic size. In addition, the shape of the particles is also related to safety, as nanomaterials with high aspect ratio are known to cause stress to cells during internalization (44). Thus, if the dissolution rate of the excipient is slow, its shape can be an issue.

To date, only a limited number of excipients have been approved by the FDA for the pulmonary route (45). Table 6.2 shows a list of excipients for inhalable products in the FDA database and clearly indicates that the most approved excipients can only be used in trace amounts. Lactose can be used at a relatively large amount because it is a common carrier. The most important material in the list for designing sophisticated inhalable particles may be 1,2-distearoyl-sn-glycero-3-phosphocholine (distearoylphophatidylcholine). Other phospholipids are also expected to be building blocks of the pulmonary formulation because they are regarded to be safe and have the abilities to form various molecular assemblies. Unfortunately, common excipients for pulmonary delivery in the literature, which include PLGA, chitosan, and cyclodextrins, are not listed. Expanding the options of additives should lead to the evolution of particle architectonics for pulmonary drug delivery.

6.9 CONCLUDING REMARKS

Particle architectonics is essential for achieving effective pulmonary drug delivery. In this chapter, technologies to control the physicochemical properties of inhalable particles using spray-drying are described. Particle formation using spray-drying is a very rapid process, wherein the size, shape, and mixing state of multiple components are controlled, which is a competition of dynamic and thermodynamic factors.

Other novel methods for preparing inhalable particles, such as spray freeze drying and thin-film freezing, are also under development. However, the use of spray-drying technology still has advantages because large-scale production using these new technologies is still difficult. Although the number of approved excipients is still small, continuous efforts in this field would make inhalation a more common option for drug administration.

The pulmonary route is expected to be a promising portal for delivering biopharmaceuticals, which are difficult to administer orally. In fact, many inhalable biopharmaceuticals pipelines can be found in clinical trials (4). Two inhalable insulin products, Exbera® and Afrezza®, had limited success; however, the problem did not lie with the products but availability of other methods of administration, where custom of treatment would need to change. So far, the majority of research on the design of spray-dried particles were for small molecules. Different considerations are required for biopharmaceuticals because of their low stability during manufacturing and storage compared to small molecules, and their being in the lung. Further progress in this field should make contribution to more effective use of biopharmaceuticals.

REFERENCES

1. Patton, J.S. Mechanisms of macromolecule absorption by the lungs. *Adv. Drug Deliv. Rev.* 19(1), 3–36 (1996).
2. Patton, J.S., Fishburn, C.S. & Weers, J.G. The lungs as a portal of entry for systemic drug delivery. *Proc. Am. Thorac. Soc.* 1(4), 338–344 (2004).
3. Shoyele, S.A. & Slowey, A. Prospects of formulating proteins/peptides as aerosols for pulmonary drug delivery. *Int. J. Pharm.* 314(1), 1–8 (2006).
4. Fröhlich, E. & Salar-Behzadi, S. Oral inhalation for delivery of proteins and peptides to the lungs. *Eur. J. Pharm. Biopharm.* 163, 198–211 (2021).
5. Katz, I.M., Schroeter, J.D. & Martonen, T.B. Factor affecting the deposition of aerosolized insulin. *Diabetes Technol. Ther.* 3(3), 387–397 (2001).
6. Patton, J.S. & Byron, P.R. Inhaling medicines: Delivering drugs to the body through the lungs. *Nat. Rev. Drug Discov.* 6(1), 67–74 (2007).
7. Shekunov, B.Y., Chattopadhyay, P., Tong, H.H.Y. & Chow, A.H.L. Particle size analysis in pharmaceutics: Principles, methods and applications. *Pharm. Res.* 24(2), 203–227 (2007).
8. Park, S.S. & Wexler, A.S. Size-dependent deposition of particles in the human lung at steady-state breathing. *J. Aerosol Sci.* 39(3), 266–276 (2008).
9. Smith, H. *ICRP publication 66: Human respiratory tract model for radiological protection.* (New York: Pergamon, 1994).
10. Zhang, J., Wu, L., Chan, H.K. & Watanabe, W. Formation, characterization, and fate of inhaled drug nanoparticles. *Adv. Drug Deliv. Rev.* 63(6), 441–455 (2011).
11. Geiser, M. Update on macrophage clearance of inhaled micro- and nanoparticles. *J. Aerosol Med. Pulm. Drug Deliv.* 23(4), 207–217 (2010).
12. Sou, T. *et al.* New developments in dry powder pulmonary vaccine delivery. *Trends Biotechnol.* 29(4), 191–198 (2011).
13. Jones, M.D. *et al.* An investigation into the dispersion mechanisms of ternary dry powder inhaler formulations by the quantification of interparticulate forces. *Pharm. Res.* 25(2), 337–348 (2008).

14. Okuyama, K. & Lenggoro, I.W. Preparation of nanoparticles via spray route. *Chem. Eng. Sci.* 58(3–6), 537–547 (2003).
15. Chow, A.H.L., Tong, H.H.Y., Chattopadhyay, P. & Shekunov, B.Y. Particle engineering for pulmonary drug delivery. *Pharm. Res.* 24(3), 411–437 (2007).
16. Tsapis, N. *et al.* Trojan particles: Large porous carriers of nanoparticles for drug delivery. *Proc. Natl. Acad. Sci. U. S. A.* 99(19), 12001–12005 (2002).
17. Hadinoto, K., Phanapavudhikul, P., Kewu, Z. & Tan, R.B.H. Dry powder aerosol delivery of large hollow nanoparticulate aggregates as prospective carriers of nanoparticulate drugs: Effects of phospholipids. *Int. J. Pharm.* 333(1–2), 187–198 (2007).
18. Edwards, D.A. *et al.* Large porous particles for pulmonary drug delivery. *Science* 276(5320), 1868–1871 (1997).
19. Yang, Y. *et al.* Development of highly porous large PLGA microparticles for pulmonary drug delivery. *Biomaterials* 30(10), 1947–1953 (2009).
20. Kawakami, K. *et al.* Investigation of the dynamic process during spray-drying to improve aerodynamic performance of inhalation particles. *Int. J. Pharm.* 390(2), 250–259 (2010).
21. Zeng, X.M., Martin, G.P., Tee, S.K. & Marriott, C. The role of fine particle lactose on the dispersion and deaggregation of salbutamol sulfate in an air stream in vitro. *Int. J. Pharm.* 176(1), 99–110 (1998).
22. Jones, M.D. & Price, R. The influence of fine excipient particles on the performance of carrier-based dry powder inhalation formulations. *Pharm. Res.* 23(8), 1665–1674 (2006).
23. Adi, H., Larson, I. & Stewart, P.J. Adhesion and redistribution of salmeterol xinafoate particles in sugar-based mixtures for inhalation. *Int. J. Pharm.* 337(1–2), 229–238 (2007).
24. Jones, M.D. *et al.* An investigation into the dispersion mechanisms of ternary dry powder inhaler formulations by the quantification of interparticulate forces. *Pharm. Res.* 25(2), 337–348 (2008).
25. DeCarlo, P.F. *et al.* Particle morphology and density characterization by combined mobility and aerodynamic diameter measurements. Part 1: Theory. *Aerosol Sci. Tech.* 38, 1185–1205 (2004).
26. Vehring, R. Pharmaceutical particle engineering via spray drying. *Pharm. Res.* 25(5), 999–1022 (2008).
27. Kawakami, K. *et al.* Competition of thermodynamic and dynamic factors during formation of multi-component particles via spray-drying. *J. Pharm. Sci.* 102(2), 518–529 (2013).
28. Nolan, L.M. *et al.* Excipient-free nanoporous microparticles of budesonide for pulmonary delivery. *Eur. J. Pharm. Sci.* 37(5), 593–602 (2009).
29. Yang, Y. *et al.* Development of highly porous large PLGA microparticles for pulmonary drug delivery. *Biomaterials* 30(10), 1947–1953 (2009).
30. Kawakami, K. *et al.* Low-density microparticles with petaloid surface structure for pulmonary drug delivery. *J. Pharm. Sci.* 103(4), 1309–1313 (2014).
31. Hancock, B.C. & Zografi, G. The relationship between the glass transition temperature and the water content of amorphous pharmaceutical solids. *Pharm. Res.* 11(4), 471–477 (1994).
32. Kraft, K.S. & Grant, M. Preparation of macromolecule-containing dry powders for pulmonary delivery. In *Macromolecular drug delivery (Belting M Ed)* 165–174. (New York: Humana Press, 2009).
33. Yang, L. *et al.* Development of a pulmonary peptide delivery system using porous nanoparticle-aggregate particles for systemic application. *Int. J. Pharm.* 451(1–2), 104–111 (2013).
34. Hadinoto, K., Phanapavudhikul, P., Kewu, Z. & Tan, R.B.H. Novel formulation of large hollow nanoparticles aggregates as potential cariers in inhaled delivery of nanoparticulate drugs. *Ind. Eng. Chem. Res.* 45(10), 3697–3706 (2006).
35. Sung, J.C., Pulliam, B.L. & Edwards, D.A. Nanoparticles for drug delivery to the lungs. *Trends Biotechnol.* 25(12), 563–570 (2007).
36. Sung, J.C. *et al.* Formulation and pharmacokinetics of self-assembles rifampicin nanoparticle systems for pulmonary delivery. *Pharm. Res.* 26(8), 1847–1855 (2009).

37. Cipolla, D., Shekunov, B., Blanchard, J. & Hickey, A. Lipid-based carriers for pulmonary products: Preclinical development and case studies in humans. *Adv. Drug Deliv. Rev.* 75, 53–80 (2014).
38. Bot, A.I. *et al.* Novel lipid-based hollow-porous microparticles as a platform for immunoglobulin delivery to the respiratory tract. *Pharm. Res.* 17(3), 275–283 (2000).
39. Weers, J.G., Miller, D.P. & Tarara, T.E. Spray-dried PulmoSphere™ formulations for inhalation comprising crystalline drug particles. *AAPS PharmSciTech* 20(3), 103 (2019).
40. Duddu, S.P. *et al.* Improved lung delivery from passive dry powder inhaler using an engineered PulmoSphere powder. *Pharm. Res.* 19(5), 689–695 (2002).
41. McShane, P.J. *et al.* Ciprofloxacin dry powder for inhalation (ciprofloxacin DPI): Technical design and features of an efficient drug–device combination. *Pulm. Pharmacol. Ther.* 50, 72–79 (2018).
42. Zhang, S. *et al.* Totally phospholipidic mesoporous particles. *J. Phys. Chem. C.* 119(13), 7255–7263 (2015).
43. Kawakami, K. *et al.* Physicochemical properties of solid phospholipid particles as a drug delivery platform for improving oral absorption of poorly soluble drugs. *Pharm. Res.* 34(1), 208–216 (2017).
44. Sharifi, S. *et al.* Toxicity of nanomaterials. *Chem. Soc. Rev.* 41(6), 2323–2343 (2012).
45. Pilcer, G. & Amighi, K. Formulation strategy and use of excipients in pulmonary drug delivery. *Int. J. Pharm.* 392(1–2), 1–19 (2010).

Engineered Particles for Aerosolization and Lung Deposition

7

Rachel Yoon Kyung Chang and Hak Kim Chan

Contents

DOI: 10.1201/9781003182566-9

7.1 INTRODUCTION

During the 1980s, engineered particles were first explored by Igor Gonda and colleagues for improving aerodynamic behavior[1,2] and for water proofing to minimize hygroscopic growth of aerosols during transit in the humid environment of the respiratory tract.[3] Aerosols, particularly amorphous particles, absorb water from the surrounding environment and cause changes in their size, phase (amorphous to crystalline), morphology and chemical composition, which can all impact pharmacology of the drug. Driven by strong commercial interests in dry powder inhalation (DPI) products resulting from phasing out of CFC (Chlorofluorocarbon) propellants and development of inhaled therapeutic proteins[4-7] in the 1990s, engineered particles have continued to be explored for enhancing aerosol performance of DPI formulations. Table 7.1 shows the type of engineered particles (elongated, porous, wrinkled, spikey), method of production, characterization techniques, and physicochemical properties of the particles.

This chapter will cover particle engineering strategies for improving the aerosol performance and lung deposition of dry powder formulations. The influence of physical properties such as particle size and morphology, as well as chemically engineered particles through co-formulation with hydrophobic amino acids, metal stearates, or active pharmaceutical ingredients (APIs) will be covered. Production methods used in commercial inhalation products including milling and spray drying, and those that are used in inhalation powders under development such as spray freeze drying, controlled precipitations, particle replication in non-wetting templates technology, and thin film freeze drying will be included. Finally, characterization techniques for assessing particle morphology, roughness, chemical composition, and electrostatic charge will be covered, followed by the impact of particle engineering on lung deposition.

TABLE 7.1 Examples of studies exploring different particle types, method of production, and characterization techniques

PARTICLE MORPHOLOGY	DRUG	METHOD OF PREPARATION	CHARACTERIZATION TECHNIQUES	PHYSICOCHEMICAL PROPERTIES	REF
Elongated	Nedocromil	Crystallization	Polarizing microscopy, SEM, DSC, TGA, FTIR, XRD, moisture sorption isotherm determination	Length: 2–7 μm; width: <1 μm; MMAD: <1 μm	16
	Rifapentine	Precipitation followed by spray drying	LD, SEM, aerosol performance (MSLI), XRD, DVS, biological assay	Length: 4–7 μm; width: <0.3 μm; MMAD: 1.7 μm FPF_{loaded}: 83%	17
Porous	siRNA	Spray freeze drying	LD, SEM, aerosol performance (ACI), XRD, DVS, biological assay	VMD: 5.6 μm; MMAD: 1.2 μm; $FPF_{emitted}$: 64%	131
	Tobramycin	Spray drying	LD, SEM, XRD, DSC, XPS, SSA, specific pore volume, porosity, density, Raman spectroscopy	VMD: 2.5 μm; MMAD based on calculation: 1.6 μm	132
Wrinkled	Bovine serum albumin	Spray drying	LD, SEM, aerosol performance (MSLI), XRD, TGA, fractal dimension analysis	VMD: 3 μm; $FPF_{recovered}$: 27% and 41% for smooth and wrinkled particles, respectively	133
	Rifapentine	Spray drying	LD, SEM, aerosol performance (MSLI), XRD, DVS, biological assay	VMD: 2.0 μm; MMAD: 1.9 μm; FPF_{loaded}: 69%	17
Spikey	Hydroxyapatite	Precipitation	SEM, aerosol performance (ACI)	Particle diameter: 3.9–6.9 μm; FPF: 85%	28

Note: ACI, Andersen cascade impactor; DSC, Differential scanning calorimetry; DVS, dynamic vapor sorption; FPF, fine particle fraction; FTIR, Fourier-transform infrared; LD, laser diffraction; MMAD, mass median aerodynamic diameter; MSLI, multistage liquid impinger; SEM, scanning electron microscopy; SSA, specific surface area; TGA, thermal gravimetric analysis; VMD, volumetric median diameter; XRD, X-ray diffraction; XPS, X-ray photoelectron spectroscopy.

7.2 PARTICLE SIZE

Particle size is a crucial particulate property that influences aerosol performance. It can be expressed as the geometric diameter (physical diameter of the particle) or aerodynamic diameter, D_a. D_a is defined as diameter of a spherical particle with a unit density that settles at the same velocity as the particle of interest in air,

$$D_a = D_g \sqrt{\frac{1}{\chi} \cdot \frac{\rho}{\rho_o}} \tag{1}$$

where D_g is the geometric diameter, χ the dynamic shape factor, ρ the particle density, and ρ_o the unit density (1 g/cm^3). The desirable aerodynamic diameter that leads to lung deposition and distribution is often referred to as 1–5 μm.[8–10] Particles with a D_a smaller than 0.5 μm are more likely to be exhaled, while those greater than 5 μm tend to deposit in the oropharynx and upper respiratory tract.[10] Particles in the range of 1–2 μm are likely to deposit in the peripheral region (i.e., alveoli) of the lungs.[8] Particles with small D_a can be achieved by simply decreasing the geometric size (see Equation 1). However, particles with a small geometric diameter suffer from poor flowability and dispersibility due to strong inter-particulate forces in the powders.[8,11] To enhance aerosol performance, cohesion between fine particles can be partly overcome by increasing the shear force through increasing the air flow through the powder inhaler. This was exemplified in dispersion of mannitol powders with various median diameters and air flow rates.[12] Smaller mannitol powder with a mass median diameter of 2.7 μm exhibited poor dispersibility, but this was improved by increasing the air flow of the powder inhaler (i.e., from 30 L/min to 120 L/min).[12] Particle size can also affect bioactivity of drugs. For instance, the receptor for the β$_2$ agonist salbutamol is mostly concentrated in the alveolar wall, requiring peripheral delivery. In fact, the effectiveness of salbutamol was significantly greater with the finer aerosol (3.3 μm) as compared with 7.7 μm aerosol, highlighting the importance of strategic engineering of particle size for the drug of interest.[13] The optimal drug distribution in the airways is dependent on the precise location of target receptors (often localized) or site of infection (global).

7.3 MORPHOLOGICALLY ENGINEERED PARTICLES

Over the years, great effort has been devoted to morphological engineering of particles for improving the aerosol performance of powder at molecular, particulate, and aerosol levels. At the molecular level, different particle shapes (due to different crystal habits or polymorphs) of a given crystalline material will possess different chemical functional groups on the particle surfaces that will impact the surface energy, electrostatic interactions, hygroscopicity, and resulting capillary force. In turn, these differences will be manifested in the inter-particulate forces at the particulate level, making them cohesive and existing as agglomerates in a powder. The strength of the agglomerate (σ) is given by:

$$\sigma = 15.6\phi^4 \frac{W}{D} \tag{2}$$

where ϕ is the packing fraction, W is the non-equilibrium value of the work of adhesion, and D is the particle physical diameter.[14] Particle morphology determines the particle packing in an agglomerate as well as the specific surface area and friction that will influence powder flowability and emptying from an inhaler. On the other hand, particle morphology affects the aerodynamic diameter via the shape factor and density, where a large χ and small ρ would reduce D_a of a particle (from Equation 1).

7.3.1 Elongated Particles

Elongated particles have a smaller aerodynamic diameter than that of spherical particles with the same volume or mass. The aerodynamic diameter of elongated particles is determined by its width rather than by its length. For elongated particles, the ratio of the D_a to the physical diameter (D_f) initially increases with the aspect ratio (i.e., length/width), and then levels off at a D_a/D_f value of about 2 when the aspect ratio is great than 15–20 (Figure 7.1).[2] Chan and Gonda exploited this aerodynamic advantage to produce elongated particles of the anti-asthmatic drugs cromoglycic acid and nedocromil (Figure 7.2) that exhibited superior aerosol performance with mass median aerodynamic diameter (MMAD, diameter at which 50% of the particles by mass are larger and 50% are smaller) of 0.7 and 0.9 μm, respectively.[15,16] More recently, the application of elongated particles has been extended to inhaled antibiotics, where an inhalable form of crystalline rifapentine with a MMAD of 1.7 μm and a fine particle fraction (FPF) of 83% was produced for the intended treatment of tuberculosis infection.[17] Elongated

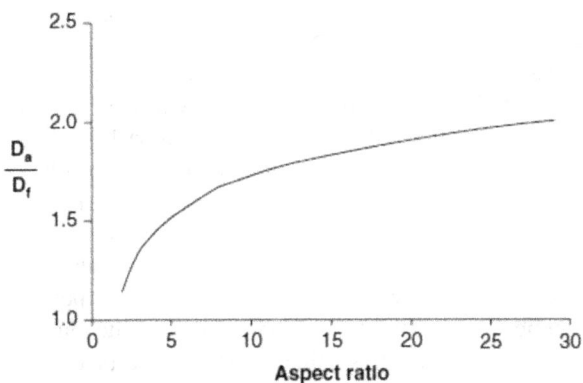

FIGURE 7.1   Relationship between the aspect ratio of elongated particles and the aerodynamic diameter. Reprinted from Ref. 14. Copyright 2008 with permission from Taylor & Francis.

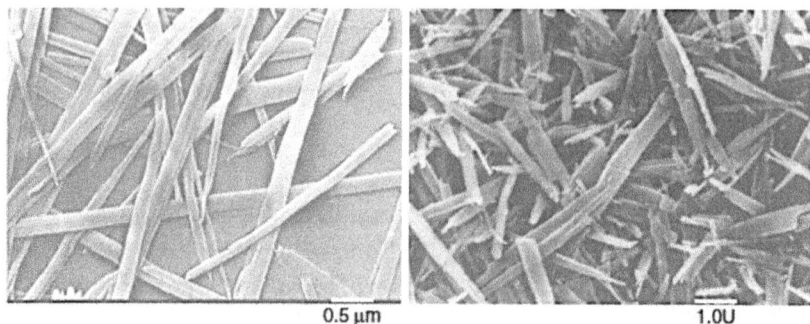

0.5 µm   1.0U

FIGURE 7.2   Scanning electron microscopy images of elongated particles of cromoglycic acid (left) and nedocromil (right). Reprinted from Ref.14. Copyright 2008 with permission from Taylor & Francis.

particles have been shown to have minimal device-dependent aerosolization performance. In fact, elongated rifampicin did not show any differences in the powder dispersibility when dispersed by two different inhalers, the Aeroliser and the Handihaler, giving FPF values of ~60% regardless of the device type or flow rate, while spherical particles exhibited varying respective FPF values of 51% and 37%, respectively.[18]

7.3.2 Porous and Wrinkled Particles

Porous and wrinkled particles have a low particle density (<0.5 g/cm^3), which leads to a low D_a (see Equation (1)). Additionally, porous particles have a large surface area (>50 m/g) to increase drag force, which further reduces the D_a. Particles with a high porosity and/or wrinkled surfaces have lower inter-particulate cohesive forces (van der Waals force) due to reduced particle mass and/or decreased area of contact between the particles, leading to less particle agglomeration and better lung delivery efficiency. These particles have been shown to improve peripheral lung deposition by reducing impaction in the extra-thoracic (i.e., mouth and throat) and tracheobronchial airways. Moreover, for porous particles, pulmonary delivery was found to be largely independent of the peak inspiratory flow rate of patients, which can help reduce dosing variability.[19,20] These traits make porous particles a desirable approach for inhaled drug delivery to the deep lung for treatment of pulmonary diseases (e.g., cystic fibrosis), and systemic delivery (e.g., insulin). One of the pioneering works by Edwards *et al.* demonstrated that large porous particles with geometric diameters of above 5 µm and a low density of 0.4 g/cm^3 could be inspired deep into the lungs and escape clearance by alveolar macrophages due to large geometric size.[21] In addition, inhaled larger porous insulin particles led to higher systemic bioavailability and suppressed systemic glucose levels for a longer period of time as compared with smaller non-porous particles. Examples of porous particles are the AIR® and PulmoSphere™ technologies that were developed for DPI formulation in the late 1990s. The AIR® technology involves spray drying of GRAS (generally recognized as safe) excipients, including lung surfactant (dipalmitoylphosphatidylcholine), albumin, and disaccharides (e.g., lactose) using a co-solvent system to produce large porous particles.[22] This AIR system was used to develop inhaled insulin powders, which allowed efficient drug delivery to the deep lung and exhibited similar efficacy as the standard subcutaneously injected insulin in clinical studies.[4] AIR® pulmonary drug delivery system was also applied for other drugs such as salbutamol sulfate[23] and levodopa.[24] PulmoSphere™ technology utilizes a pore forming agent (e.g., perfluorocyte bromide), surface modifier (e.g., calcium chloride), and lung surfactant (distearoylphosphatidylcholine). Compared to the AIR® technology, particles produced through PulmoSphere are generally smaller with geometric diameter of 1–5 μm and a foam-like morphology.[25] This technology has been applied for many different dry powder inhalation systems such as tobramycin,[26] budesonide,[19] and ciprofloxacin.[27]

7.3.3 Spikey (Pollen-like) Particles

Pollen-like particles with a spherical core and conical protrusions on the surface exhibit a larger physical diameter but retain a lower bulk density. These spiky particles can enhance the flowability, aerosolization, and deposition properties as compared with particles that have similar volumes and equivalent diameters.[28] Pollen-like particles were reported to exhibit better flowability, higher emitted dose, and higher FPF than sphere-, plate-, cube-, and needle-shaped particles in a similar size range.[29] The protruded dendritic surface features would increase the distance between two interacting particles and minimize inter-particulate forces and aggregation tendency.

7.3.4 Other Shaped Particles (PRINT Technology)

Particle replication in non-wetting templates (PRINT) technology has been used to produce various shapes of particles. Cylindrical particles containing BSA and lactose, pollen-like triangular shaped particles containing immunoglobulin G and lactose, and torus particles containing itraconazole (anti-fungal drug), zanamivir (influenza drug), DNase, or siRNA have been produced.[30] Torus particles of zanamivir exhibited an over three-fold improvement in aerosol performance as compared with conventional DPI Relenza (GlaxoSmithKline). Furthermore, aerosols of torus particles (containing lactose, albumin, and leucine) exhibited uniform lung deposition upon pulmonary delivery in a canine deposition model.[30]

7.4 CHEMICALLY ENGINEERED PARTICLES

7.4.1 Co-Formulation with Hydrophobic Amino Acids

Hydrophobic amino acids, L-leucine in particular, have been used to enhance the dispersibility of dry powder inhalation formulations.[31–33] The hydrophobic and surface-active properties of leucine help alter the surface morphology and surface energy of the particles during spray drying, thereby enhancing powder dispersibility. The dispersibility of spray dried powder formulation containing salbutamol sulfate and lactose was improved by adding 5–20% (w/w) leucine, resulting in a higher emitted dose of >95% as compared with the powder with no amino acid (70% emitted dose).[31] Furthermore, increasing the leucine mass fraction from 5% to 20% (w/w) increased the FPF from <50% to 78% of the total loaded powder. In addition, leucine was extensively studied for its protection of spray dried powders against moisture-induced deterioration of aerosol performance. Using formulations containing a wide range of leucine concentrations, Li *et al.* reported the relationship between the physicochemical nature of the API, water uptake properties, and stability of the powders at elevated relative humidity (RH).[33,34] The presence of leucine caused an upward trend in aerosol performance of disodium cromoglycate (DSCG) powders resulting from reduced device retention and increased deposition in the lower stages of the impactor. Even a small amount of leucine (2%, w/w) greatly improved the aerosolization performance with a higher $FPF_{recovered}$ value of 72% as compared with spray dried DSCG alone (58%). The aerosol performance of the powders plateaued at leucine concentrations beyond 10–20% (w/w), suggesting no further changes in the surface energies and/or cohesive forces of the particles. Indeed, X-ray photoelectron spectroscopy (XPS) showed that the maximum surface enrichment of leucine was reached at 60–70% (molar percent) when the concentration of leucine in the feed solution was 30–50% (molar percent), which is equivalent to 10–20% (w/w) (Figure 7.3). Storage of spray dried pure DSCG powders at 75% RH for 24 h drastically reduced the aerosol performance ($FPF_{recovered}$ dropped to 2%) with significant powder retention in the capsule after dispersion due to severe powder agglomeration caused by capillary forces at high RH. However, the presence of 10–20% (w/w) leucine prevented the deleterious effect of high RH on aerosol

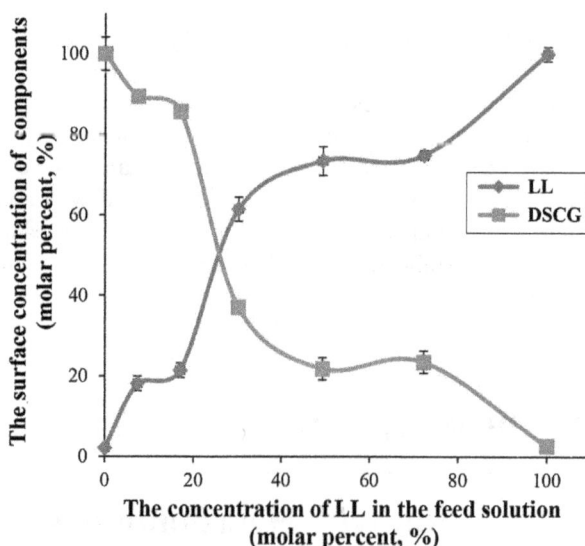

FIGURE 7.3 Relationship between feed concentration and surface concentration of L-leucine (LL) based on X-ray photoelectron spectroscopy. Reprinted from Ref. 33. Copyright 2016 with permission from Elsevier.

performance. Leucine imparted moisture protection likely by forming a crystalline shell on the surface of particles and better protection was observed with increasing leucine content. During spray drying, leucine is enriched on the particle surface due to its hydrophobicity and surface activity[35] compared with other APIs and excipients in the droplets. As leucine has a relatively low aqueous solubility (~22 mg/mL), it becomes supersaturated and precipitates on the surface of particles during drying. To confer moisture protection, leucine must exist in the crystalline form, which has very low water uptake propensity and reduces inter-particulate interaction caused by moisture. At the amorphous state, leucine recrystallizes when exposed to 60% RH, which causes deterioration of the aerosol performance. Hence, crystalline leucine should be considered in dry powder inhalation formulations over the amorphous form as it can reduce the hygroscopicity of the particle surface area, thereby providing moisture protection and limiting hydroscopic growth of aerosols in the airways. However, complete coverage of particle surface by crystalline hydrophobic amino acid may impede drug dissolution and impact bioavailability.

It is feasible to modulate the crystallinity and surface coverage of leucine on the particles using organic solvents that alter the supersaturation level of leucine in drying droplets.[36,37] Additionally, the drug can also modulate the crystallinity of leucine. When present at 5–20 wt.%, leucine was increasingly crystalline in co-spray dried DSCG powders but was amorphous when co-spray dried with salbutamol sulfate and only became crystalline at 40 wt.%. Besides leucine, other hydrophobic amino acids such as isoleucine, trileucine, methionine, and valine can also mitigate the damaging effect of moisture on dispersibility of dry powders.[38,39]

7.4.2 Co-Formulation with Metal Stearates

Magnesium stearate (MgSt) is a hydrophobic lubricant that is considered as a GRAS-type excipient for inhalation. It is approved for DPI products such as Foradil Certihaler, Seebri Breezhaler, and Incruse Ellipta. MgSt provides moisture protection and reduces cohesion and adhesion between particles, resulting in improved aerosolization performance.[40,41] The lubricating nature of MgSt caused greater de-agglomeration efficiency of co-milled API-lactose-MgSt blends and improved aerosol performance.[40] The fine particle dose of the API in lactose blends containing 5% (w/w) MgSt remained reasonably high even after storage at 75%/25°C RH for 15 days, while those without MgSt rapidly deteriorated. The poor solubility of MgSt in water and organic solvents has limited its application onto particle surfaces mainly by dry coating.[42–46] MgSt and sucrose stearate (1–5%) as coating materials are applied by mechanofusion, which improves the flowability and dispersibility of DPI powders.[42,47] In contrast, sodium stearate (NaSt) has a higher solubility in water and organic solvents (e.g., >10 mg/mL compared with <0.1 mg/mL of MgSt in 50% ethanol at 40°C[48]) and was applied for particle surface enrichment using spray drying.[49] Co-spray dried DSCG formulations containing 10% (w/w) NaSt exhibited a better aerosol performance (FPF value of 89%) than DSCG alone powder (68%), while further increasing the NaSt content did not show additional benefits.[48] Although the presence of hydrophobic stearates can protect hygroscopic powders against moisture-induced degradation during production and storage, excessive use will likely hinder drug dissolution in the lungs.

7.4.3 Co-Formulation of APIs

Inhalation powders can be co-formulated with another API component that is more resistant to water uptake to confer protection from moisture-induced powder degradation and subsequent loss of dispersibility. By co-spray drying hydrophilic colistin and hydrophobic rifapentine drugs (mass ratio of 1:1), the aerosol performance of the combination powder was still retained after exposure to a high RH of 75% for 24 h, whereas spray dried colistin showed a significant drop in the FPF.[50] Similarly, through surface enrichment of colistin particles by rifampicin, the combination powder exhibited a high aerosolization efficiency even after storage at 75% RH.[51] Interestingly, the moisture sorption isotherm of the co-formulation was simply the add-up of that of each of the API components (i.e., spray dried rifampicin and colistin alone). This suggests that hydrophobic API in the co-formulation does not prevent moisture uptake *per se*, but prevents fusion of colistin particles through the hydrophobic coating of rifampicin. In fact, the moisture sorption of the co-formulation was found to be reversible with no recrystallization event of the amorphous colistin. In a subsequent study, colistin was co-formulated with ciprofloxacin. The presence of colistin improved the dispersibility of the co-formulation with FPF values of 46%, 55%, and 67% when spray dried in the colistin: ciprofloxacin mass ratio of 1:9, 1:3, and 1:1, respectively.[52] Although ciprofloxacin alone formed amorphous and unstable particles, once spray dried and underwent recrystallization within an hour of exposure to 55% RH,[53] these co-spray dried powders remained relatively stable and dispersible when exposed to 55% RH for 60 days. In the co-formulation containing colistin and ciprofloxacin at a mass ratio of 1:1, no significant change in FPF was observed even after storage at 75% RH for one day, but a significant drop (from 72% to 19%) was detected after seven days of storage. However, incorporation of leucine to the co-formulation at a mass ratio of 1:1:1 protected the powder with no significant changes to the FPF values after seven days of storage at 75% RH. The improved stability was likely due to the presence of hydrophobic leucine on the particle surface as described above (Section 7.4.1) and/or interaction of leucine with ciprofloxacin through hydrogen bonding.[54]

In a follow-up study, colistin was co-spray dried with hydrophobic azithromycin to determine the amount of hydrophobic API needed to prevent moisture-induced decrease in aerosol performance.[55] Although 20% (w/w) azithromycin could not impart moisture protection, 50% by weight could protect the co-formulation against deterioration of the FPF when dispersed at 75% RH. Similarly, by co-spray drying with rifampicin at a weight ratio of 6:4, amorphous and unstable spray dried kanamycin could be made stable and dispersible even after one month of storage at 53% RH.[56] Again, the stability of the co-formulation was attributed to surface enrichment of hydrophobic rifampicin on kanamycin particles.

While surface coverage by hydrophobic APIs provides protection against moisture-induced impairment of aerosol performance, dissolution of the co-formulations may be affected. Indeed, the dissolution rate of colistin was reduced with increasing amount of hydrophobic azithromycin in the co-spray dried formulation.[57] On the other hand, the dissolution rate of colistin was unaffected when co-formulated with hydrophobic rifampicin, likely due to incomplete coating of the particle surface enabling ingress of the dissolution medium.[58]

7.5 PRODUCTION METHODS

7.5.1 Methods Used in Commercial Inhalation Products

7.5.1.1 Milling

Conventionally, inhalation powders have been produced by drug crystallization, followed by milling to achieve particles of inhalable size.[59,60] In general, drugs particles are broken down by impaction with milling balls or with one another in high-velocity air jets. In addition to conventional ball mills or the more efficient vibration mills, there are different types of jet mills, including fluid impact mills, opposed jet mills, spiral jet mills, over chamber jet mills, and fluidized bed opposed jet mills.[61] Dry milling produces micron-sized particles with high electrostatic charge[8] and surface activity,[62] rendering the powder to agglomeration, which affects the aerosol performance.[10] Moreover, milling creates local amorphous sites on the particle surface that could recrystallize during manufacture or storage, causing fusion or aggregation of particles which may be no longer inhalable.[63] The instability of micronized particles is more pronounced with increasing storage temperature and humidity.[64] This uncontrolled particle growth following micronization can be overcome through controlled recrystallization of the micronized powder by conditioning it at an elevated temperature and/or humidity for an extended period of time. Although this forms physically stable particles, the particle size post-conditioning may change, and the process can be time consuming and economically impractical.[64] Alternatively, drug particles can be milled whilst suspended in a suitable non-solvent (i.e., wet milling), which encourages recrystallization of any amorphous regions formed during milling. Compared with dry milling, wet milling is useful for handling temperature sensitive compounds (liquid slurry dissipates heat from the mill), has minimal yield loss, and can improve batch homogeneity. Furthermore, in-process conditioning with conditioning gas (e.g., nitrogen) and solvent vapors can eliminate amorphous regions and confer physical stability of the micronized powder.[65] Micronization of the active ingredient followed by blending with lactose monohydrate is commonly used in dry powder inhalation products such as Trelegy Ellipta, Airduo Respiclick, and Pulmicort Turbuhaler.

7.5.1.2 Spray drying

Spray drying is a well-established one-step process that is rapid, economical, and easy to scale-up.[66] Since the early 1990s, spray drying has been extensively studied for producing drugs for pulmonary delivery in dry powder inhalation systems, which has led to successful production of commercial therapeutics, including insulin (Exubera® by Pfizer), tobramycin (TOBI®, Noartis), colismethate (Colobreathe, Teva UK), and mannitol (Bronchitol® and Aridol®, Pharmaxis).

In spray drying, a drug solution or suspension is atomized to fine droplets that are rapidly evaporated in a current of warm air to form dry particles, which are then separated *via* a cyclone or filter and collected. Particles produced by spray drying are relatively uniform in size and shape and have physical diameters suitable for inhalation delivery. One of the major challenges associated with spray drying is the amorphous nature of spray dried particles that are vulnerable to moisture-induced degradation. To overcome this stability issue, various process and formulation strategies have been proposed, such as increasing the outlet temperature to induce glass transition by insulating the drying chamber,[67] the use of drug suspension over solution,[68] and the use of surface active hydrophobic excipients and/or APIs.[69] Another limitation of spray drying is the unsuitability of materials that are sensitive to mechanical shear stress of atomization.[70] Moreover, drugs that may decompose by oxidation at liquid-air interface should be avoided, but the impact could be minimized by using an inert gas over air.[66] Production of inhalation powders containing microencapsulated drugs has been feasible by coupling multifluid nozzles with spray drying. Using a three-fluid nozzle with two concentric channels (drug-containing feed in the core and coat-forming on the outer stream), polymers such as chitosan and PLGA have been successfully used for drug encapsulation.[71–73] More recently, the Nano Spray Dryer that can capture nanoparticles by electrostatic collection has been introduced. It utilizes a piezoelectrically driven vibrating mesh atomizer to produce finer droplets with a narrow span.[74] This technology has been applied for producing inhalable powder formulations of model drugs, excipients, proteins, and enzymes.[74–77] For biologics, stabilizers such as disaccharides (e.g., trehalose, sucrose) are routinely used to preserve the integrity of proteins in spray dried powders.[78] Sugars are known to stabilize proteins in solid state by (i) restricting molecular mobility in an amorphous matrix to prevent conformational changes and/or (ii) by hydroxyl groups of sugar forming hydrogen bonds with the protein to maintain protein native structure.[79] However, these amorphous sugars are prone to crystallization particularly in the presence of surrounding moisture, which is detrimental to the stability of proteins. Moreover, during spray drying, biologics are exposed to sheer and thermal stresses that could cause protein degradation and ultimately, loss of bioactivity. Hence, hydrophobic amino acids (Section 7.4.1) are commonly used in combination with disaccharides, low inlet temperature is utilized in spray drying, and the resulting powders are often stored at a low RH to circumvent these issues. There is no doubt spray drying has been shown to be a promising powder production and particle engineering strategy for dry powder inhalation systems.

7.5.2 Methods Used in Inhalation Powders under Development

7.5.2.1 Spray freeze drying

Freeze drying, or lyophilization, is the gold standard method for drying thermosensitive substances, especially those that undergo rapid degradation in solutions (e.g., biopharmaceutics such as insulin). Spray freeze drying is another method of drying heat labile compounds, which is a two-step process involving (i) atomization of the feedstock into a freezing medium that turns fine spray into frozen droplets, followed by (ii) lyophilization to remove ice through sublimation resulting in a dry powder. Spray freeze drying has a high yield (almost 100%) when conducted as a batch process, and it produces spherical and highly porous particles with a low density[80] that may enhance aerosol performance by decreasing the particle density and packing density (see Equations 1 and 2).[5,81,82] When the same atomization but different drying process were used to produce protein powders, spray freeze drying produced larger, porous particles than spray drying (small, dense particles) with significantly higher FPF.[83] Owing to its high surface area, spray freeze dried particles can improve bioavailability of compounds that have low water solubility. Additionally, spray freeze drying allows processing of thermosensitive drugs and excipients that may be degraded in spray drying.

Spray freeze dried powders of nucleic acids,[84] insulin,[85] bovine serum albumin,[86] liposomal ciprofloxacin,[87] and vaccine(s)[88] have been successfully produced for inhalation delivery. Although spray freeze drying produces high-quality dehydrated products, as a batch process it is difficult to scale up and is energy intensive, thus a very expensive particle production process. In 1991, atmospheric spray freeze drying was invented to enable commercialization of spray freeze drying,[89] and later studies further improved the setup.[90,91] In general, atmospheric spray freeze drying involves drying of frozen droplets by a steam of dry cold gas inside an insulated stainless-steel gas vessel. Through improved mass and heat transfer rates, the drying time is reduced, and the resulting powder is free-flowing with larger surface area and high solubility.[89]

In principle, once the spray freeze dried powders are produced, they can be processed further by filling directly into the capsules, blisters, or a reservoir inside the DPI device. In practice, there can be challenges in handling these low-density porous particles as the fill weight may be more difficult to control accurately and reproducibly; also these particles tend to be fragile and easier to fragment.

7.5.2.2 Other methods

Supercritical fluid technology was first applied to particle engineering more than two decades ago and different variations have since been attempted in the pharmaceutical industry, with (i) rapid expansion of supercritical solution and (ii) antisolvent precipitation being the most common and simple methods.[92] Method (i) involves an extractor to solubilize drugs in the supercritical carbon dioxide that is then passed through a nozzle, allowing for precipitation of the drug through rapid expansion for supercritical fluid in the expansion vessel. In method (ii), the drug is dissolved in an organic solvent (e.g., ethanol) and the solution comes into contact with supercritical carbon dioxide with causes the precipitation of the dissolved drug as fine particles. The technology has not been commercialized for the pharmaceutical industry, as scale-up of the high-pressure pressure as a reproducible particle production method is challenging. Supercritical precipitation fluid extraction of emulsion has been used for particle precipitation of nanoparticle encapsulating proteins and genes. The method enables the use of aqueous suspensions and the organic solvent residual in the powder is low, which is highly favorable for inhaled therapeutics.

High gravity controlled precipitation technology is a nanoprecipitation technique that is available at the commercial production scale. It involves high-gravity micro-mixing to control the nucleation and crystallization of drug particles.[93] Two liquid streams (drug solution and anti-solvent) are fed into the device and mixed into the center of a packed bed containing wire mesh packing materials, which is rotated at a high speed and subjected to high gravity due to centrifugal force. Flowing through the rotating packing, the liquids are influenced by the high gravitational force to spreading and splitting into thin films, threads, and very fine droplets for enhanced mixing. In the anti-solvent mode, drug solution and an anti-solvent are mixed, causing precipitation of the drug as small particles, whereas in the reactive mode two streams containing respective reactants will undergo chemical reaction to produce the particles.

Confined liquid impinging jets have been used to produce inhalable particles through flash precipitation.[94,95] A jet of drug solution and a jet of anti-solvent directly opposing each other are rigorously mixed together, resulting in drug precipitation. As the two liquid jets are facing each other, the velocity of the streams needs to be precisely controlled to prevent unbalanced flow and mixing. On the other hand, the use of multi-inlet vortex mixer allows mixing of streams of reactants at unequal volumetric flows.[96] As a result, supersaturation and solvent composition can be controlled by adjusting the content and velocity of individual streams.

7.5.2.3 Newer technologies

Particle replication in non-wetting templates (PRINT) is a particle molding technology that enables fabrication of monodisperse, non-spherical particles of predefined shape and size. It utilizes low surface energy polymeric molds with micro- and nano-cavities that can be filled with drugs and/or excipients, followed by extraction of the particles out of the molds for particle collection. PRINT technology has been utilized in producing inhalable particles containing small molecule drugs and biologic macromolecules such as BSA, immunoglobulin G, DNase, siRNA, zanamivir, and itraconazole.[30]. This method has reached the cGMP-scale manufacture for preclinical and clinical production[97] and may facilitate advancement in particle engineering for improved pulmonary drug delivery.

Thin-film freeze drying (TFFD) is a new cryogenic technique that has recently been utilized in preparing highly porous and brittle powder matrices that are suitable for inhalation delivery.[98] In TFFD, liquid cryogen is filled in a rotating metal drum and a liquid solution or suspension is added dropwise into the drum. When the droplets (2–4 mm in diameter) impact on the drum, they spread to form thin films (100–400 µm thick) that freeze, which are then collected using a metal blade.[99] The collected films are lyophilized for solvent removal by sublimation. TFFD can partially alleviate gas-liquid interface and shear stress that is associated with spray freeze drying which can contribute to protein aggregation.[100] TFFD technology has been utilized in producing inhalable dry powder formulations of remdesivir,[101] tacrolimus,[102] and siRNA-encapsulated lipid nanoparticles.[103]

7.6 CHARACTERIZATION TECHNIQUES

7.6.1 Particle Morphology and Roughness

7.6.1.1 Specific surface area (SSA)

Specific surface area (SSA) is the total surface area per unit of mass of a powder. SSA of inhalation powders is a valuable metric as it is related to changes in physical properties of the formulation such as particle size distribution, surface roughness, and porosity.

SSA of powders can be characterized by physical adsorption of a gas (e.g., nitrogen) on the surface of the sample at –196°C. The volume of gas adsorbed as a monolayer over the particle surface is determined using the Brunauer–Emmett–Teller (BET) equation, and the SSA is calculated based on the molar volume of the gas and the average area occupied by the gas molecules. BET analysis involves lengthy experimental times and has poor resolution for powders with SSA below 0.5 m/g (using nitrogen). As SSA is closely associated with particle roughness and porosity, it can provide an indirect indication of the particle shape; irregularly shaped and porous particles have higher SSA.

7.6.1.2 Fractal dimension analysis

Fractal dimension analysis is a useful means for describing the shape properties of irregular-shaped particles, and those with a high degree of particle surface roughness or higher angularity have higher fractal dimensions.[104] Furthermore, it can be used to predict the aerodynamic diameter of particles with rough surfaces, with a trend in decreasing diameter with increasing surface roughness.[105] Surface fractal dimension can be obtained by gas adsorption, light scattering, or image analysis. Determining the fractal dimension by image analysis is very tedious and requires numerous images of well dispersed particles to be collected and analyzed. As such, light scattering and gas adsorption have been more commonly utilized. Tang et al. used both light scattering and gas adsorption to determine the surface fractal dimensions of smooth and corrugated bovine serum albumin (BSA) particles.[106] Fractal dimensions obtained from the two methods corroborated well when the number of gas-adsorbed layers on the particles were between one and ten for corrugated particles, and one and two for smooth particles.

7.6.1.3 Scanning electron microscopy (SEM)

Scanning electron microscopy (SEM) is routinely used to visually inspect the particle size, shape, and texture of inhalation powders at high resolutions after production and over storage to detect any physical changes to the particles (e.g., formation of solid bridges, agglomerates) that may impact dispersibility of the inhalation powder formulations.[68,107–109] For example, Ke et al. used SEM analysis to show that budesonide-lactose powders obtained from spray dried solution contained deformed, crystallized, or caked particles after a one-day storage at 25°C/60% RH or 40°C/75% RH, while those obtained from spray drying of suspension remained physically stable.[68] Quantitative assessment of particle morphological features requires representative samples to be taken followed by image acquisition at various areas of the samples to provide sufficient counting statistics to show an accurate description of the bulk powder.

7.6.1.4 Laser diffraction

While SEM provides information on particle size, the particle size distribution of inhaled powder formulations is commonly measured by laser diffraction. Laser diffraction measures the angular variation in intensity of scattered light as a beam passes through dispersed powder samples. Particle size is reported as a volume equivalent sphere diameter (i.e., volume mean diameter, VMD) and assumes that measured particles are spherical.

7.6.1.5 Atomic force microscopy (AFM)

Particle size, morphology, and roughness can be measured by SEM and atomic force microscopy (AFM). It is an excellent technique for visualizing particles with sizes ranging between 1 nm and 10 µm, and allows quantitative particle size measurement.[110] AFM relies on the physical interaction between a sensing probe on a cantilever and the sample surface. AFM topographical imaging can capture subtle features of particles that are likely to be lost in the SEM. Acquisition of an AFM height map can provide information on the surface morphology of the particles, as well as other quantitative measurements such as depth, length, volume, and surface area of individual particles. A study by Adi *et al.* showed that AFM topographic images of smooth and corrugated spray dried powders of BSA were similar to that observed by SEM, and the root mean square roughness (which characterizes surface roughness) was substantially higher for the corrugated particles.[111] Furthermore, a direct relationship between the root mean square roughness, particle adhesion, and *in vitro* aerosol performance had been reported; as the extent of corrugation increased, particle adhesion was reduced, which subsequently led to an increase in FPF.[112] The study highlighted the potential role of AFM in predicting aerosolization performance of particles for inhalation.

7.6.1.6 White-light interferometry

Scanning white-light interferometry offers a rapid and reliable method of quantitatively analyzing the surface roughness of particles. The sample is scanned through the z-axis in noncontact mode using white light to generate 3D models of the surface height. The technique enables rapid collection of 3D topographical data without the risk of damaging the samples and has sub-nanometer vertical resolution with lateral spatial resolution of 150 nm. White-light interferometry was applied to assess the surface morphology of spray dried powder formulations containing BSA and lactose prepared at varying degrees of surface roughness.[113] Root mean square roughness was quantified by white-light optical profilometry, which showed increasing values as the surface roughness of the particles increased, and the data corroborated with the AFM-derived values.

Table 7.2 lists characterization techniques commonly used for analyzing powder formulations. There is no single 'best' method that is suitable in all applications, as each has its advantages and limitations. Although the optimal method would depend on the objective of the study, there are some key considerations in designing the study: (i) Is the aim to obtain data on the whole powder (bulk) or individual particles? (ii) Is 2D data sufficient or is 3D data required? (iii) Is the resolution of the method sufficient? (iv) Does the method provide only indirect rather than direct measurement? These considerations would impact the amount of time and effort spent on the characterization. For example, measurement of the SSA can indirectly provide information on the particle surface roughness of the bulk powder at a low resolution without taking the particle shape into account. In contrast, AFM enables direct measurement of the surface roughness of individual particles at a high resolution, but it is impossible to measure the bulk

TABLE 7.2   Commonly used techniques for characterizing physical, chemical, and charge properties of powder formulations

TECHNIQUES	INFORMATION DERIVED	PRINCIPLE	KEY APPLICATION
Specific surface area	Surface area of particles	Measures the gas volume adsorbed on the particle surface	Indirectly provides information on particle shape
Fractal dimension analysis	Particle morphology	Photos of well dispersed individual particles are collected followed by image analysis	Shape properties of irregular-shaped particles can be determined
Scanning electron microscopy	Particle size, morphology, and texture	Well dispersed individual particles are imaged at high resolutions	Assessment of morphological changes to powders during storage
Laser diffraction	Particle size distribution	The angle and intensity of light scattering from the dispersed particles are measured as a laser beam passes through a dispersed sample	Assessment of particle size distribution of powders comprised of spherical particles
Atomic force microscopy	Particle size, morphology, and texture	A surface sensing probe is used to image the particle by raster scanning	Topographical imaging and other quantitative measurements such as depth, length, volume, and surface area of individual particles
Atomic force microscopy-infrared spectroscopy	Molecular composition and structure as well as particle size, morphology, and texture	Cantilever motion detects sample thermal expansion caused by infrared radiation and spectra are simultaneously collected	Study of drug-excipient interactions at nanoscale; monitor chemical changes during production and storage
White-light interferometry	Particle surface texture	Sample is scanned (z-axis) in noncontact model using white light	Builds 3D models of surface height; assessment of surface roughness
X-ray photon spectroscopy	Quantitative atomic composition and chemistry	Photoelectron emission is characterized upon irradiation of sample using X-ray	Study of chemical composition and distribution of drug and of excipients on particle surface

(Continued)

TABLE 7.2 (CONTINUED) Commonly used techniques for characterizing physical, chemical, and charge properties of powder formulations

TECHNIQUES	INFORMATION DERIVED	PRINCIPLE	KEY APPLICATION
Time-of-flight secondary ion mass spectrometry	Isotopic, elemental and molecular information from the particle surface	An ion beam is irradiated on sample causing mass separation of the emitted ions from the surface	Visualizes particle structures and chemical residues
Fourier transform infrared spectroscopy	Molecular composition and structure of bulk powder	Infrared radiation is applied to the sample, and the absorbance is measured	Study of drug-drug and drug-excipient interaction
Electrical low-pressure impaction	Electrostatic charge or aerosols	Electrically insulated impactor collects particles according to size and concurrently measures charge with electrometers	Assessment of aerosol charge profiles
Bipolar charge analyzer	Electrostatic charge or aerosols	Separates and measures positively and negatively charged particles according to aerodynamic particle size fractions	Assessment of aerosol charge profiles

powder sample. Hence, the robustness, practicality, skill level required, speed, cost, type of sample, and data required should all be considered when assessing the suitability of a method.

7.6.2 Chemical Composition and Distribution

7.6.2.1 X-ray photoelectron spectroscopy (XPS)

Compositional and chemical state information of the surface of a particle can be characterized using X-Ray spectroscopy (XPS). This technique is highly surface sensitive with depth analysis of 0–10 nm and uses X-ray irradiation to identify the chemistry and functional groups on the particle. Chemical composition of spray dried powder that contained different ratios of DSCG and leucine was analyzed using XPS.[33] Those that contained more leucine, a surface-active excipient, exhibited a higher surface enrichment of this hydrophobic amino acid (Figure 7.3). However, the surface concentration of leucine plateaued at 73% (molar percent) as the molar percentage of leucine was increased to approximately 50% in the liquid feed for spray drying. Similarly, the XPS analysis of spray dried powders that contained different ratios of colistin and rifampicin showed surface enrichment but not complete coverage of rifampicin on the particle surface.[58] This XPS data could be used to explain why the surface enrichment of rifampicin did not retard the dissolution rate of colistin in the co-spray dried formulation. In another study, XPS measurement showed that 50% by weight of azithromycin provided a near complete coating (97% molar percent) on the colistin containing particle's surface, which was sufficient to prevent moisture-induced deterioration of powder dispersibility.[55] It is worth noting that although the surface composition of the two components should theoretically add up to 100%, the sum of the actual values can range between 95% and 108%[33] due to uncertainties in the quantitative analysis of XPS data.

7.6.2.2 Time-of-flight secondary ion mass spectrometry (ToF-SIMS)

Like XPS, time-of-flight secondary ion mass spectrometry (ToF-SIMS) provides elemental, chemical state, and molecular information about the surface of the particles. ToF-SIMS probes chemical composition at an average depth of 1–2 nm and has a spatial resolution of <0.1 µm. An advantage of ToF-SIMS is that the 3D chemical characterization derived from *in-situ* focused ion beam section with high mass resolution and high spatial resolution imaging. With ToF-SIMS analysis, it is feasible to visualize the distribution of drug and excipient on the particle's surface, which can be used to detect uniformity of drug distribution. DSCG and leucine were co-spray dried using various molar or weight ratios and then analyzed using ToF-SIMS. The measurement showed a major step increment of surface concentration of leucine when the molar percent in the feed solution was increased from 18% to 30% (i.e., 5% to 10% (w/w)), followed by a more gradual increase in the particle surface coverage of leucine.[33] Overall, the ToF-SIMS data corroborated well with the XPS data, indicating that 10% (w/w) leucine in the formulation composition was a key percentage that enriched the particle surface concentration of leucine, with 20–40% (w/w) providing the most effective, yet incomplete surface coverage to impart desirable particle properties of better dispersibility and moisture protection (Figure 7.4). Likewise, ToF-SIMS analysis of colistin co-spray dried with azithromycin[55] or rifampicin[58] revealed surface enrichment of the hydrophobic drugs.

7.6.2.3 AFM-based techniques

In addition to topographical imaging described in Section 7.6.1.4, AFM allows for the characterization of surface chemistry and surface energy. The surface energies of drug particles, lactose carriers, and packaging material can be used to predict the interaction strength between each pair of these components and determine their compatibility in the formulation. Berard *et al.* used AFM to measure the surface energy between lactose carriers and zanamivir drug crystals after exposure to various RH conditions.[114] They showed that the adhesion forces between the carrier and the drug gradually increased with the RH.

Owing to the high-resolution of AFM, surface structures and textures can be assessed at an atomic level, enabling differentiation between the crystalline and amorphous regions within a particle. This feature of AFM is particularly useful when analyzing milled powders. As discussed in Section 7.5.1, high-energy milling process can create amorphous regions that can elicit changes to aerosol performance on storage. These amorphous regions

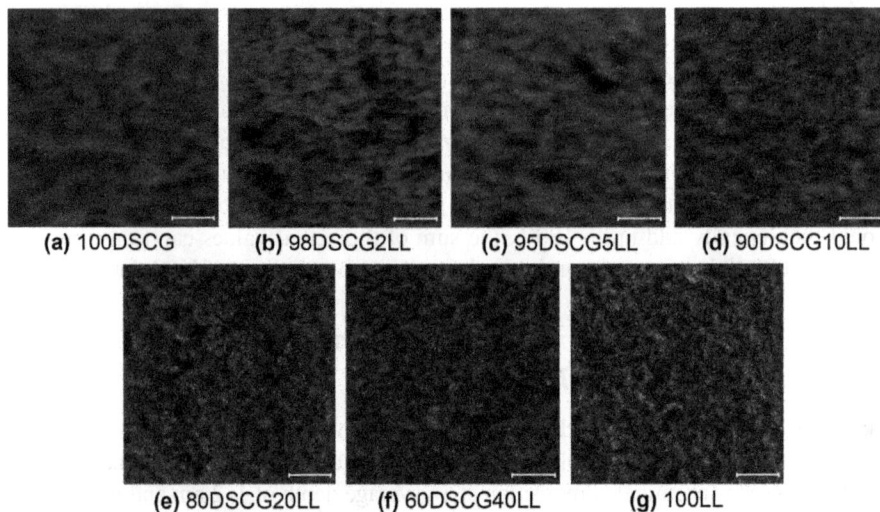

FIGURE 7.4 Distribution of DSCG (red) and leucine (green) on the surface of particles measured by ToF-SIMS. The scale bar represents 10 μm. Reprinted from Ref. 33. Copyright 2016 with permission from Elsevier.

are often unstable and prone to revert to a more stable crystalline state, particularly in the presence of moisture, causing neighboring particles to fuse and agglomerate. In fact, AFM surface analysis of milled salbutamol sulphate powders showed a higher degree of amorphous regions as compared with pre-micronization powders, with the former exhibiting increased moisture uptake.[115] In addition to amorphous regions, AFM can also distinguish different polymorphic forms, which are highly relevant in pharmaceutical applications as they may have different physicochemical properties that affect powder dispersion, dissolution, solubility, and storage stability.[116] Hence, AFM assessment can potentially be applied as a research and quality control tool to identify any surface irregularities, crystalline defects, or impurities that could lead to instability of the powder formulations.

More recently, advanced spectroscopic techniques such as AFM-infrared spectroscopy (AFM-IR) have been applied to outperform conventional IR spectroscopic techniques that were unable to detect subtle changes in particles due to the limited spatial resolution (1.5–10 μm).[117] The spatial resolution of AFM-IR ranges from 0.5 nm to 50 nm[117] and is deemed suitable for investigating drug-excipient interactions at nanoscale and monitoring any chemical changes during manufacture and storage.[78] Using AFM-IR, the distribution of drugs (fluticasone propionate and salmeterol xinafoate) and excipient (lactose) were assessed in individual aerosol particles of the commercial inhalation product Seretide.[118] Such advanced spectroscopic chemical analysis can help study the effect of drug distribution on the aerosol performance of the powders and the consistency of their dose uniformity. AFM-IR has also been applied to study the stability of biologics (bacteriophage) in inhalation powders.[119] As the bacteriophage powder was hygroscopic, the formulation was embedded in resin for measurement, demonstrating the feasibility of chemically analyzing moisture-sensitive powders containing nano-sized virus particles.

7.6.2.4 Fourier transform infrared spectroscopy (FTIR)

Fourier transform infrared spectroscopy (FTIR) can be used to study drug-drug and drug-excipient interactions in the powder formulations.[120] FTIR has also been utilized in studying secondary structure of proteins in powder formulations, which can provide indication about structural integrity of the proteins in solid state.[121] Protein powder samples are mixed with spectroscopy-grade potassium bromide and then pressed into a pellet for analysis. Preliminary studies are needed to ensure that the compression pressure does not damage the proteins.[122]

7.6.3 Electrostatic Charge

7.6.3.1 Electrical low-pressure impaction (ELPI)

Electrostatic charge profiles of aerosols can be assessed using a modified electrical low-pressure impactor (ELPI) system.[123,124] All 13 impactor stages are electrically insulated from each other, with the last 12 stages individually connected to electrometers with sensitivity at femtoampere levels (Figure 7.5). Aerosol particles are deposited on the stages according to their aerodynamic diameters while their charges are measured by the electrometers. Inhaled pharmaceutical aerosols from metered dose inhalers such as Ventolin, Flixotide, Tilade, and QVAR[123,124] were analyzed using this ELPI system. In general, these different commercial inhalers had different aerosol charge profiles, which may have implications on deposition of the inhaled particles in the respiratory tract and regulatory aspects of generic aerosol products. The ELPI system has also been utilized in studying the effect of RH on powder inhaler aerosols.[125,126] Micronized salbutamol particles had an electronegative charge when aerosolized from lactose blends at a low RH, while those stored at a higher storage RH showed a reduction in the net charge-to-mass ratio.[126] Another study demonstrated the effect of RH (during dispersion) on the charge of aerosols from Pulmicort and Bricanyl Turbuhalers using ELPI, where the charging behavior was shown to be inhaler-dependent.[125] As dry powder inhalers may exhibit drug-specific response to particle charging at different surrounding and storage RHs, these factors may need to be taken into account when designing inhalation products.

7.6.3.2 Bipolar charge analyzer

Bipolar charge analyzer (BOLAR) is the first commercially available instrument that can separate and measure positively and negatively charged particles according to their aerodynamic particle size fractions (Figure 7.6). BOLAR has been used to study the influence of modifying an Aerolizer inhaler design on bipolar charge of mannitol powder aerosols.[127] The charge-to-mass profiles showed that the charging of the aerosols was related to the mass distributions, although the bipolar charge nature of the aerosols remained qualitatively similar regardless of the modified inhaler designs. However, the magnitude of charge could be decreased by either increasing the grid voidage or reducing the air inlet size of the inhaler.[127] In contrast, changing the length of

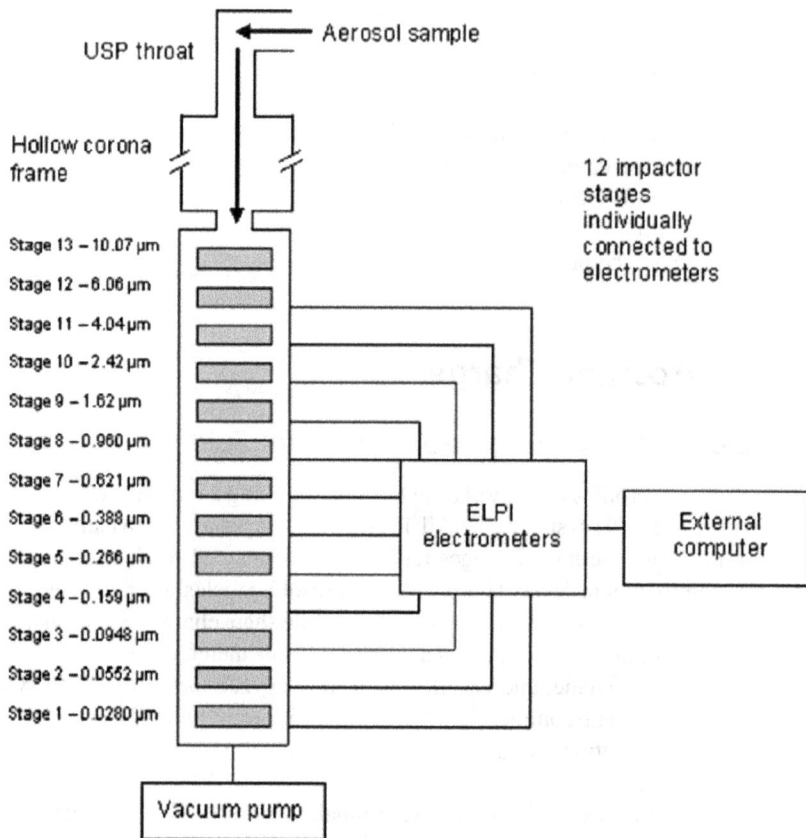

FIGURE 7.5   Schematic diagram of the EPLI instrument setup. Reprinted from Ref. 124. Copyright 2005 with permission from Elsevier.

the mouthpiece or the material of the inhaler did not have obvious effect on the bipolar charge. Currently, the effect of electrostatic charge on aerosol deposition in the lungs has been underexplored due to the scarcity of human data.

7.6.4 Other Commonly Used Bulk Characterization Methods

Physical properties such as crystallinity, melting, phase transition, and residual solvent content can be assessed by thermal analyses such as thermogravimetric analysis (TGA) and differential scanning calorimetry (DSC). The crystallinity and crystal structures are usually confirmed by X-ray diffraction (XRD). Residual solvent in the powder can be characterized by the loss of powder weight on drying, Karl-Fischer titration, and other spectroscopic methods. Moisture sorption profiles of the bulk powder can be studied using dynamic vapor sorption (DVS).

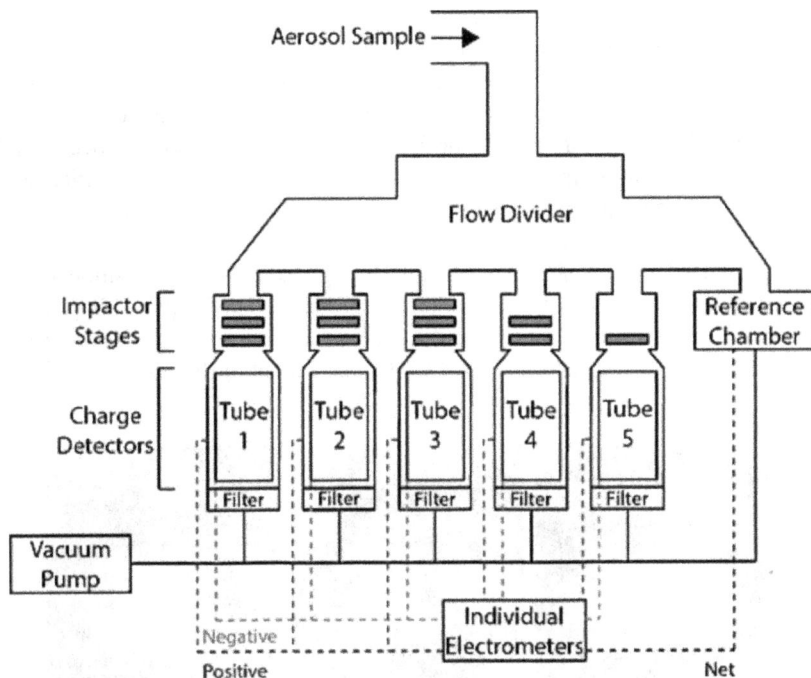

FIGURE 7.6 Schematic diagram of the BOLAR. Reprinted from Ref. 134. Copyright 2015 with permission from American Chemical Society.

7.7 EFFECT ON LUNG DEPOSITION

Although information regarding aerosol deposition in the lungs can be obtained *indirectly* by pharmacokinetic measurement of the drug concentration in the blood, imaging using gamma scintigraphy or positron emission tomography provides direct measurement of both total dose and regional distribution of aerosols in the lungs. However, there have been very limited imaging studies on lung deposition of particles with engineered particle size and porosity.

It is well known that the particle size of inhaled particles affects lung deposition, but most of the human data supporting this has come from comparative studies on commercial products, instead of fundamental studies focusing on establishing the relationship between size and deposition. In asthmatic subjects, inhalation of monodisperse aerosols of albuterol with an MMAD of 1.5, 3, and 6 μm each produced a total lung deposition of 56, 50, and 46%, with corresponding penetration index values of 0.79, 0.60, and 0.36, respectively, indicating that decreasing aerosol particle size improved lung penetration and deposition.[128] However, these aerosols were monodispersed and generated from a spinning-disk aerosol generator for inhalation, and these conditions bear little resemblance to the inhalation of aerosols through a powder inhaler device. The first study on the effect of particle size of a dry powder inhaled through a DPI was reported by Glover *et al.*[129] Spray dried powders with a volume median diameter of 2, 3, and 4 µm were dispersed using an Aeroliser to produce aerosols with an aerodynamic diameter of 2.7, 3.6, and 5.4 µm (geometric standard deviation 2.4–2.7), respectively. When inhaled by healthy subjects, the lung deposition of the 5.4 µm aerosol was 21%, which was doubled to 45 and 39% for the 2.7 µm and 3.6 µm aerosols, respectively. The corresponding penetration index increased from 0.52 to 0.63 and 0.60, which showed that aerosols with smaller particles deposit better in the smaller airways and alveoli relative to the large airways (Figure 7.7).

Porous particles have shown some interesting and unique deposition behavior. Porous particles of budesonide PulmoSphere inhaled from Eclipse DPI produced a mean total lung deposition of 58% in healthy subjects with a relatively low inter-subject variation (coefficient of variation of 11–13 %), independent of the inspiratory flowrates

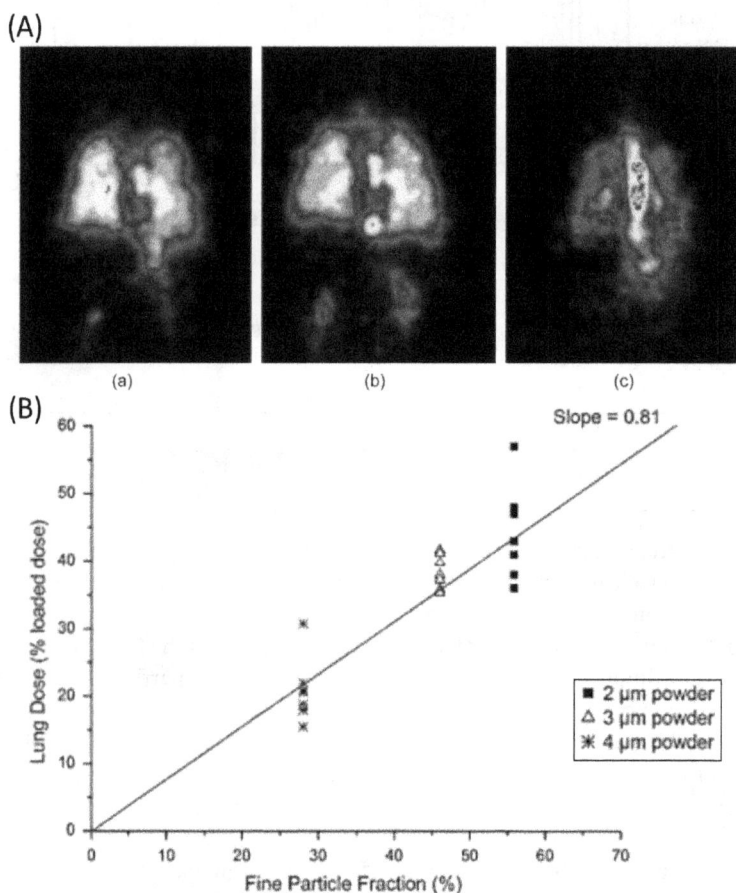

FIGURE 7.7   Coronal slices from the SPECT images obtained after inhaled administration of radiolabeled mannitol powders in three different subjects (A). Lung dose plotted as a function of fine particle fraction for three powders, with the regression line fitted with the intercept forced through the origin (B). Reprinted from Ref. 129. Copyright 2008 with permission from Elsevier.

of 25 or 50 L/min.[19] The flow independent deposition suggested that the impaction parameter (i.e., the square of the aerodynamic diameter multiplied by the air flow rate), that dictates impaction loss at the upper airways, remains fairly constant at the two different flowrates for these porous particles. These results were in stark contrast to non-porous micronized API carrier-based formulations. Regional deposition of these porous particles as expressed by the ratio of peripheral to central deposition was 1.1–1.2, showing a relatively even distribution of the particles in the lung.

To date, no imaging studies on the effects of particle electrostatic charge or elongated shape can be found. Historically, most of the lung deposition data on elongated particles was obtained from post-mortem human lung samples showing lodging of mineral fibers in the alveoli,[130] showing the small aerodynamic diameter of these particles. There is a clear gap in the research on the lung deposition of engineered particles described in this chapter, which may be filled in the future.

REFERENCES

1. Chan, H.-K. & Gonda, I. Aerodynamic properties of elongated particles of cromoglycic acid. *J Aerosol Sci* 20(2), 157–168 (1989). https://doi.org/10.1016/0021-8502(89)90041-4.
2. Gonda, I. & Abd El Khalik, A.F. On the calculation of aerodynamic diameters of fibers. *Aerosol Sci Technol* 4(2), 233–238 (1985). https://doi.org/10.1080/02786828508959051.
3. Hickey, A.J., Gonda, I., Irwin, W.J. & Fildes, F.J.T. Effect of hydrophobic coating on the behavior of a hygroscopic aerosol powder in an environment of controlled temperature and relative humidity. *J Pharm Sci* 79(11), 1009–1014 (1990). https://doi.org/10.1002/jps.2600791113.
4. Rosenstock, J., Muchmore, D., Swanson, D. & Schmitke, J. AIR inhaled insulin system: A novel insulin-delivery system for patients with diabetes. *Expert Rev Med Devices* 4(5), 683–692 (2007). https://doi.org/10.1586/17434440.4.5.683.
5. Maa, Y.F., Nguyen, P.A., Sweeney, T., Shire, S.J. & Hsu, C.C. Protein inhalation powders: Spray drying vs spray freeze drying. *Pharm Res* 16(2), 249–254 (1999). https://doi.org/10.1023/a:1018828425184.
6. Bosquillon, C., Préat, V. & Vanbever, R. Pulmonary delivery of growth hormone using dry powders and visualization of its local fate in rats. *J Control Release* 96(2), 233–244 (2004). https://doi.org/10.1016/j.jconrel.2004.01.027.
7. Andya, J.D. *et al.* The effect of formulation excipients on protein stability and aerosol performance of spray-dried powders of a recombinant humanized anti-IgE monoclonal antibody. *Pharm Res* 16(3), 350–358 (1999). https://doi.org/10.1023/a:1018805232453.
8. Chow, A.H., Tong, H.H., Chattopadhyay, P. & Shekunov, B.Y. Particle engineering for pulmonary drug delivery. *Pharm Res* 24(3), 411–437 (2007). https://doi.org/10.1007/s11095-006-9174-3.
9. Newman, S.P. & Clarke, S.W. Therapeutic aerosols 1–Physical and practical considerations. *Thorax* 38(12), 881–886 (1983). https://doi.org/10.1136/thx.38.12.881.
10. Malcolmson, R.J. & Embleton, J.K. Dry powder formulations for pulmonary delivery. *Pharm Sci Technol Today* 1(9), 394–398 (1998). https://doi.org/10.1016/S1461-5347(98)00099-6.
11. Yang, M.Y., Chan, J.G. & Chan, H.K. Pulmonary drug delivery by powder aerosols. *J Control Release* 193, 228–240 (2014). https://doi.org/10.1016/j.jconrel.2014.04.055.

12. Chew, N.Y. & Chan, H.K. Influence of particle size, air flow, and inhaler device on the dispersion of mannitol powders as aerosols. *Pharm Res* 16(7), 1098–1103 (1999). https://doi.org/10.1023/a:1018952203687.

13. Johnson, M.A., Newman, S.P., Bloom, R., Talaee, N. & Clarke, S.W. Delivery of albuterol and ipratropium bromide from two nebulizer systems in chronic stable asthma. Efficacy and pulmonary deposition. *Chest* 96(1), 6–10 (1989). https://doi.org/10.1378/chest.96.1.6.

14. Chan, H.-K. What is the role of particle morphology in pharmaceutical powder aerosols? *Expert Opin Drug Deliv* 5(8), 909–914 (2008). https://doi.org/10.1517/17425247.5.8.909.

15. Chan, H.K. & Gonda, I. Respirable form of crystals of cromoglycic acid. *J Pharm Sci* 78(2), 176–180 (1989). https://doi.org/10.1002/jps.2600780221.

16. Chan, H.K. & Gonda, I. Physicochemical characterization of a new respirable form of nedocromil. *J Pharm Sci* 84(6), 692–696 (1995). https://doi.org/10.1002/jps.2600840606.

17. Chan, J.G. et al. A novel inhalable form of rifapentine. *J Pharm Sci* 103(5), 1411–1421 (2014). https://doi.org/10.1002/jps.23911.

18. Son, Y.J. & McConville, J.T. A new respirable form of rifampicin. *Eur J Pharm Biopharm* 78(3), 366–376 (2011). https://doi.org/10.1016/j.ejpb.2011.02.004.

19. Duddu, S.P. et al. Improved lung delivery from a passive dry powder inhaler using an engineered PulmoSphere powder. *Pharm Res* 19(5), 689–695 (2002). https://doi.org/10.1023/a:1015322616613.

20. Weers, J.G. et al. Pulmonary formulations: What remains to be done? *J Aerosol Med Pulm Drug Deliv* 23(Suppl 2), S5–S23 (2010). https://doi.org/10.1089/jamp.2010.0838.

21. Edwards, D.A. et al. Large porous particles for pulmonary drug delivery. *Science* 276(5320), 1868–1871 (1997). https://doi.org/10.1126/science.276.5320.1868.

22. Vanbever, R. et al. Formulation and physical characterization of large porous particles for inhalation. *Pharm Res* 16(11), 1735–1742 (1999). https://doi.org/10.1023/a:1018910200420.

23. Ben-Jebria, A. et al. Large porous particles for sustained protection from carbachol-induced bronchoconstriction in guinea pigs. *Pharm Res* 16(4), 555–561 (1999). https://doi.org/10.1023/a:1018879331061.

24. Bartus, R.T. et al. A pulmonary formulation of L-dopa enhances its effectiveness in a rat model of Parkinson's disease. *J Pharmacol Exp Ther* 310(2), 828–835 (2004). https://doi.org/10.1124/jpet.103.064121.

25. Weers, J., Tarara, T. & Clark, A. US20040105820A1 Phospholipid-based powders for inhalation, Google Patents, (2004).

26. Newhouse, M.T. et al. Inhalation of a dry powder tobramycin PulmoSphere formulation in healthy volunteers. *Chest* 124(1), 360–366 (2003). https://doi.org/10.1378/chest.124.1.360.

27. Stass, H. et al. Inhalation of a dry powder ciprofloxacin formulation in healthy subjects: A phase I study. *Clin Drug Investig* 33(6), 419–427 (2013). https://doi.org/10.1007/s40261-013-0082-0.

28. Hassan, M.S. & Lau, R. *In 13th international conference on biomedical engineering.* (eds. C.T. Lim & J.C.H. Goh) 1434–1437 (Berlin, Heidelberg: Springer Berlin Heidelberg, 2009).

29. Hassan, M.S. & Lau, R.W. Effect of particle shape on dry particle inhalation: Study of flowability, aerosolization, and deposition properties. *AAPS PharmSciTech* 10(4), 1252–1262 (2009). https://doi.org/10.1208/s12249-009-9313-3.

30. Garcia, A. et al. Microfabricated engineered particle systems for respiratory drug delivery and other pharmaceutical applications. *J Drug Deliv* 2012, 941243 (2012). https://doi.org/10.1155/2012/941243.

31. Seville, P.C., Learoyd, T.P., Li, H.Y., Williamson, I.J. & Birchall, J.C. Amino acid-modified spray-dried powders with enhanced aerosolisation properties for pulmonary drug delivery. *Powder Technol* 178(1), 40–50 (2007). https://doi.org/10.1016/j.powtec.2007.03.046.

32. Feng, A.L. et al. Mechanistic models facilitate efficient development of leucine containing microparticles for pulmonary drug delivery. *Int J Pharm* 409(1–2), 156–163 (2011). https://doi.org/10.1016/j.ijpharm.2011.02.049.

33. Li, L. *et al*. L-leucine as an excipient against moisture on in vitro aerosolization performances of highly hygroscopic spray-dried powders. *Eur J Pharm Biopharm* 102, 132–141 (2016). https://doi.org/10.1016/j.ejpb.2016.02.010.

34. Li, L. *et al*. Investigation of L-leucine in reducing the moisture-induced deterioration of spray-dried salbutamol sulfate power for inhalation. *Int J Pharm* 530(1–2), 30–39 (2017). https://doi.org/10.1016/j.ijpharm.2017.07.033.

35. Gliński, J., Chavepeyer, G. & Platten, J.K. Surface properties of aqueous solutions of L-leucine. *Biophys Chem* 84(2), 99–103 (2000). https://doi.org/10.1016/s0301-4622(99)00150-7.

36. Boraey, M.A. *et al*. Improvement of the dispersibility of spray-dried budesonide powders using leucine in an ethanol–water cosolvent system. *Powder Technol* 236, 171–178 (2013). https://doi.org/10.1016/j.powtec.2012.02.047.

37. Rabbani, N.R. & Seville, P.C. The influence of formulation components on the aerosolisation properties of spray-dried powders. *J Control Release* 110(1), 130–140 (2005). https://doi.org/10.1016/j.jconrel.2005.09.004.

38. Lechuga-Ballesteros, D. *et al*. Trileucine improves aerosol performance and stability of spray-dried powders for inhalation. *J Pharm Sci* 97(1), 287–302 (2008). https://doi.org/10.1002/jps.21078.

39. Yu, J., Chan, H.K., Gengenbach, T. & Denman, J.A. Protection of hydrophobic amino acids against moisture-induced deterioration in the aerosolization performance of highly hygroscopic spray-dried powders. *Eur J Pharm Biopharm* 119, 224–234 (2017). https://doi.org/10.1016/j.ejpb.2017.06.023.

40. Lau, M., Young, P.M. & Traini, D. Co-milled API-lactose systems for inhalation therapy: Impact of magnesium stearate on physico-chemical stability and aerosolization performance. *Drug Dev Ind Pharm* 43(6), 980–988 (2017). https://doi.org/10.1080/03639045.2017.1287719.

41. Young, P.M. *et al*. Characterization of a surface modified dry powder inhalation carrier prepared by "particle smoothing". *J Pharm Pharmacol* 54(10), 1339–1344 (2002). https://doi.org/10.1211/002235702760345400.

42. Kumon, M. *et al*. Application and mechanism of inhalation profile improvement of DPI formulations by mechanofusion with magnesium stearate. *Chem Pharm Bull (Tokyo)* 56(5), 617–625 (2008). https://doi.org/10.1248/cpb.56.617.

43. Zhou, Q.T. *et al*. Characterization of the surface properties of a model pharmaceutical fine powder modified with a pharmaceutical lubricant to improve flow via a mechanical dry coating approach. *J Pharm Sci* 100(8), 3421–3430 (2011). https://doi.org/10.1002/jps.22547.

44. Zhou, Q.T. *et al*. Investigation of the extent of surface coating via mechanofusion with varying additive levels and the influences on bulk powder flow properties. *Int J Pharm* 413(1–2), 36–43 (2011). https://doi.org/10.1016/j.ijpharm.2011.04.014.

45. Zhou, Q.T. *et al*. Effect of surface coating with magnesium stearate via mechanical dry powder coating approach on the aerosol performance of micronized drug powders from dry powder inhalers. *AAPS PharmSciTech* 14(1), 38–44 (2013). https://doi.org/10.1208/s12249-012-9895-z.

46. Zhou, Q.T., Qu, L., Larson, I., Stewart, P.J. & Morton, D.A. Improving aerosolization of drug powders by reducing powder intrinsic cohesion via a mechanical dry coating approach. *Int J Pharm* 394(1–2), 50–59 (2010). https://doi.org/10.1016/j.ijpharm.2010.04.032.

47. Iida, K., Hayakawa, Y., Okamoto, H., Danjo, K. & Luenberger, H. Effect of surface layering time of lactose carrier particles on dry powder inhalation properties of salbutamol sulfate. *Chem Pharm Bull (Tokyo)* 52(3), 350–353 (2004). https://doi.org/10.1248/cpb.52.350.

48. Yu, J., Romeo, M.C., Cavallaro, A.A. & Chan, H.K. Protective effect of sodium stearate on the moisture-induced deterioration of hygroscopic spray-dried powders. *Int J Pharm* 541(1–2), 11–18 (2018). https://doi.org/10.1016/j.ijpharm.2018.02.018.

49. Parlati, C. *et al.* Pulmonary spray dried powders of tobramycin containing sodium stearate to improve aerosolization efficiency. *Pharm Res* 26(5), 1084–1092 (2009). https://doi.org/10.1007/s11095-009-9825-2.

50. Zhou, Q.T. *et al.* Novel inhaled combination powder containing amorphous colistin and crystalline rifapentine with enhanced antimicrobial activities against planktonic cells and biofilm of pseudomonas aeruginosa for respiratory infections. *Mol Pharm* 12(8), 2594–2603 (2015). https://doi.org/10.1021/mp500586p.

51. Zhou, Q.T. *et al.* Synergistic antibiotic combination powders of colistin and rifampicin provide high aerosolization efficiency and moisture protection. *AAPS J* 16(1), 37–47 (2014). https://doi.org/10.1208/s12248-013-9537-8.

52. Shetty, N. *et al.* Improved physical stability and aerosolization of inhalable amorphous ciprofloxacin powder formulations by incorporating synergistic colistin. *Mol Pharm* 15(9), 4004–4020 (2018). https://doi.org/10.1021/acs.molpharmaceut.8b00445.

53. Shetty, N. *et al.* Effects of moisture-induced crystallization on the aerosol performance of spray dried amorphous ciprofloxacin powder formulations. *Pharm Res* 35(1), 7 (2018). https://doi.org/10.1007/s11095-017-2281-5.

54. Shetty, N. *et al.* Influence of excipients on physical and aerosolization stability of spray dried high-dose powder formulations for inhalation. *Int J Pharm* 544(1), 222–234 (2018). https://doi.org/10.1016/j.ijpharm.2018.04.034.

55. Zhou, Q.T. *et al.* How much surface coating of hydrophobic azithromycin is sufficient to prevent moisture-induced decrease in aerosolisation of hygroscopic amorphous colistin powder? *Aaps J* 18(5), 1213–1224 (2016). https://doi.org/10.1208/s12248-016-9934-x.

56. Momin, M.A.M. *et al.* Co-spray drying of hygroscopic kanamycin with the hydrophobic drug rifampicin to improve the aerosolization of kanamycin powder for treating respiratory infections. *Int J Pharm* 541(1–2), 26–36 (2018). https://doi.org/10.1016/j.ijpharm.2018.02.026.

57. Mangal, S. *et al.* Understanding the impacts of surface compositions on the in-vitro dissolution and aerosolization of co-spray-dried composite powder formulations for inhalation. *Pharm Res* 36(1), 6 (2018). https://doi.org/10.1007/s11095-018-2527-x.

58. Wang, W. *et al.* Effects of surface composition on the aerosolisation and dissolution of inhaled antibiotic combination powders consisting of colistin and rifampicin. *AAPS J* 18(2), 372–384 (2016). https://doi.org/10.1208/s12248-015-9848-z.

59. Pilcer, G. & Amighi, K. Formulation strategy and use of excipients in pulmonary drug delivery. *Int J Pharm* 392(1–2), 1–19 (2010). https://doi.org/10.1016/j.ijpharm.2010.03.017.

60. Shoyele, S.A. & Cawthorne, S. Particle engineering techniques for inhaled biopharmaceuticals. *Adv Drug Deliv Rev* 58(9–10), 1009–1029 (2006). https://doi.org/10.1016/j.addr.2006.07.010.

61. Nakach, M., Authelin, J.-R., Chamayou, A. & Dodds, J. Comparison of various milling technologies for grinding pharmaceutical powders. *Int J Miner Process* 74, S173–S181 (2004). https://doi.org/10.1016/j.minpro.2004.07.039.

62. Feeley, J.C., York, P., Sumby, B.S. & Dicks, H. Determination of surface properties and flow characteristics of salbutamol sulphate, before and after micronisation. *Int J Pharm* 172(1–2), 89–96 (1998). https://doi.org/10.1016/S0378-5173(98)00179-3.

63. Chikhalia, V., Forbes, R.T., Storey, R.A. & Ticehurst, M. The effect of crystal morphology and mill type on milling induced crystal disorder. *Eur J Pharm Sci* 27(1), 19–26 (2006). https://doi.org/10.1016/j.ejps.2005.08.013.

64. Ng, W.K., Kwek, J.W. & Tan, R.B. Anomalous particle size shift during post-milling storage. *Pharm Res* 25(5), 1175–1185 (2008). https://doi.org/10.1007/s11095-007-9497-8.

65. Kazmi, A. *et al.* WO2014144894A1 Methods and systems for conditioning of particulate crystalline materials, Google Patents, (2018).

66. Chan, H.K. & Kwok, P.C. Production methods for nanodrug particles using the bottom-up approach. *Adv Drug Deliv Rev* 63(6), 406–416 (2011). https://doi.org/10.1016/j.addr.2011.03.011.

67. Islam, M.I.U. & Langrish, T.A.G. An investigation into lactose crystallization under high temperature conditions during spray drying. *Food Res Int* 43(1), 46–56 (2010). https://doi .org/10.1016/j.foodres.2009.08.010.

68. Ke, W.R., Kwok, P.C.L., Khanal, D., Chang, R.Y.K. & Chan, H.K. Co-spray dried hydrophobic drug formulations with crystalline lactose for inhalation aerosol delivery. *Int J Pharm* 602, 120608 (2021). https://doi.org/10.1016/j.ijpharm.2021.120608.

69. Chang, R.Y.K., Chen, L., Chen, D. & Chan, H.K. Overcoming challenges for development of amorphous powders for inhalation. *Expert Opin Drug Deliv* 17(11), 1583–1595 (2020). https://doi.org/10.1080/17425247.2020.1813105.

70. Maa, Y.F. & Prestrelski, S.J. Biopharmaceutical powders: Particle formation and formulation considerations. *Curr Pharm Biotechnol* 1(3), 283–302 (2000). https://doi.org/10.2174 /1389201003378898.

71. Wan, F. *et al.* Modulating protein release profiles by incorporating hyaluronic acid into PLGA microparticles via a spray dryer equipped with a 3-fluid nozzle. *Pharm Res* 31(11), 2940–2951 (2014). https://doi.org/10.1007/s11095-014-1387-2.

72. Kašpar, O., Jakubec, M. & Štěpánek, F. Characterization of spray dried chitosan–TPP microparticles formed by two- and three-fluid nozzles. *Powder Technol* 240, 31–40 (2013). https://doi.org/10.1016/j.powtec.2012.07.010.

73. Wan, F. *et al.* One-step production of protein-loaded PLGA microparticles via spray drying using 3-fluid nozzle. *Pharm Res* 31(8), 1967–1977 (2014). https://doi.org/10.1007/ s11095-014-1299-1.

74. Schmid, K., Arpagaus, C. & Friess, W. Evaluation of the nano spray dryer B-90 for pharmaceutical applications. *Pharm Dev Technol* 16(4), 287–294 (2011). https://doi.org/10.3109 /10837450.2010.485320.

75. Heng, D., Lee, S.H., Ng, W.K. & Tan, R.B. The nano spray dryer B-90. *Expert Opin Drug Deliv* 8(7), 965–972 (2011). https://doi.org/10.1517/17425247.2011.588206.

76. Li, X., Anton, N., Arpagaus, C., Belleteix, F. & Vandamme, T.F. Nanoparticles by spray drying using innovative new technology: The Büchi nano spray dryer B-90. *J Control Release* 147(2), 304–310 (2010). https://doi.org/10.1016/j.jconrel.2010.07.113.

77. Lin, Y.W., Wong, J., Qu, L., Chan, H.K. & Zhou, Q.T. Powder production and particle engineering for dry powder inhaler formulations. *Curr Pharm Des* 21(27), 3902–3916 (2015). https://doi.org/10.2174/1381612821666150820111134.

78. Chang, R.Y.K., Chow, M.Y.T., Khanal, D., Chen, D. & Chan, H.K. Dry powder pharmaceutical biologics for inhalation therapy. *Adv Drug Deliv Rev* 172, 64–79 (2021). https://doi .org/10.1016/j.addr.2021.02.017.

79. Chang, R.Y.K. *et al.* Inhalable bacteriophage powders: Glass transition temperature and bioactivity stabilization. *Bioeng Transl Med* 5(2), e10159 (2020). https://doi.org/10.1002/ btm2.10159.

80. Qian, L. & Zhang, H. Controlled freezing and freeze drying: A versatile route for porous and micro-/nano-structured materials. *J Chem Technol Biotechnol* 86(2), 172–184 (2011). https://doi.org/https://doi.org/10.1002/jctb.2495.

81. D'Addio, S.M. *et al.* Aerosol delivery of nanoparticles in uniform mannitol carriers formulated by ultrasonic spray freeze drying. *Pharm Res* 30(11), 2891–2901 (2013). https://doi .org/10.1007/s11095-013-1120-6.

82. Wang, Y., Kho, K., Cheow, W.S. & Hadinoto, K. A comparison between spray drying and spray freeze drying for dry powder inhaler formulation of drug-loaded lipid-polymer hybrid nanoparticles. *Int J Pharm* 424(1–2), 98–106 (2012). https://doi.org/10.1016/j .ijpharm.2011.12.045.

83. Maa, Y.-F., Nguyen, P.-A., Sweeney, T., Shire, S.J. & Hsu, C.C. Protein inhalation powders: Spray drying vs spray freeze drying. *Pharm Res* 16(2), 249–254 (1999). https://doi.org/10 .1023/A:1018828425184.

84. Liang, W. *et al.* Using two-fluid nozzle for spray freeze drying to produce porous powder formulation of naked siRNA for inhalation. *Int J Pharm* 552(1–2), 67–75 (2018). https://doi .org/10.1016/j.ijpharm.2018.09.045.

85. Ali, M.E. & Lamprecht, A. Spray freeze drying for dry powder inhalation of nanoparticles. *Eur J Pharm Biopharm* 87(3), 510–517 (2014). https://doi.org/10.1016/j.ejpb.2014 .03.009.

86. Yu, Z., Garcia, A.S., Johnston, K.P. & Williams, R.O., 3rd Spray freezing into liquid nitrogen for highly stable protein nanostructured microparticles. *Eur J Pharm Biopharm* 58(3), 529–537 (2004). https://doi.org/10.1016/j.ejpb.2004.04.018.

87. Sweeney, L.G. *et al.* Spray-freeze-dried liposomal ciprofloxacin powder for inhaled aerosol drug delivery. *Int J Pharm* 305(1–2), 180–185 (2005). https://doi.org/10.1016/j.ijpharm .2005.09.010.

88. Amorij, J.P. *et al.* Pulmonary delivery of an inulin-stabilized influenza subunit vaccine prepared by spray-freeze drying induces systemic, mucosal humoral as well as cell-mediated immune responses in BALB/c mice. *Vaccine* 25(52), 8707–8717 (2007). https://doi .org/10.1016/j.vaccine.2007.10.035.

89. Mumenthaler, M. & Leuenberger, H. Atmospheric spray-freeze drying: A suitable alternative in freeze-drying technology. *Int J Pharm* 72(2), 97–110 (1991). https://doi.org/10.1016 /0378-5173(91)90047-R.

90. Wang, Z.L., Finlay, W.H., Peppler, M.S. & Sweeney, L.G. Powder formation by atmospheric spray-freeze-drying. *Powder Technol* 170(1), 45–52 (2006). https://doi.org/10.1016 /j.powtec.2006.08.019.

91. Rogers, T.L. *et al.* Enhanced aqueous dissolution of a poorly water soluble drug by novel particle engineering technology: Spray-freezing into liquid with atmospheric freeze-drying. *Pharm Res* 20(3), 485–493 (2003). https://doi.org/10.1023/a:1022628826404.

92. Reverchon, E., De Marco, I. & Torino, E. Nanoparticles production by supercritical anti-solvent precipitation: A general interpretation. *J Supercrit Fluids* 43(1), 126–138 (2007). https://doi.org/10.1016/j.supflu.2007.04.013.

93. Hu, T.-T., Wang, J.-X., Shen, Z.-G. & Chen, J.-F. Engineering of drug nanoparticles by HGCP for pharmaceutical applications. *Particuology* 6(4), 239–251 (2008). https://doi.org /10.1016/j.partic.2008.04.001.

94. Bénet, N., Muhr, H., Plasari, E. & Rousseaux, J.M. New technologies for the precipitation of solid particles with controlled properties. *Powder Technol* 128(2–3), 93–98 (2002). https://doi.org/10.1016/S0032-5910(02)00175-4.

95. Johnson, B.K. & Prud'homme, R.K. Flash nanoprecipitation of organic actives and block copolymers using a confined impinging jets mixer. *Aust J Chem* 56(10), 1021–1024 (2003). https://doi.org/10.1071/CH03115.

96. Liu, Y., Cheng, C., Liu, Y., Prud'homme, R.K. & Fox, R.O. Mixing in a multi-inlet vortex mixer (MIVM) for flash nano-precipitation. *Chem Eng Sci* 63(11), 2829–2842 (2008). https://doi.org/10.1016/j.ces.2007.10.020.

97. Hoppentocht, M., Hagedoorn, P., Frijlink, H.W. & de Boer, A.H. Technological and practical challenges of dry powder inhalers and formulations. *Adv Drug Deliv Rev* 75, 18–31 (2014). https://doi.org/10.1016/j.addr.2014.04.004.

98. Overhoff, K.A. *et al.* Novel ultra-rapid freezing particle engineering process for enhancement of dissolution rates of poorly water-soluble drugs. *Eur J Pharm Biopharm* 65(1), 57–67 (2007). https://doi.org/10.1016/j.ejpb.2006.07.012.

99. Overhoff, K.A., Johnston, K.P., Tam, J., Engstrom, J. & Williams, R.O. Use of thin film freezing to enable drug delivery: A review. *J Drug Deliv Sci Technol* 19(2), 89–98 (2009). https://doi.org/10.1016/S1773-2247(09)50016-0.

100. Engstrom, J.D. *et al.* Formation of stable submicron protein particles by thin film freezing. *Pharm Res* 25(6), 1334–1346 (2008). https://doi.org/10.1007/s11095-008-9540-4.

101. Sahakijpijarn, S., Moon, C., Koleng, J.J., Christensen, D.J. & Williams Iii, R.O. Development of remdesivir as a dry powder for inhalation by thin film freezing. *Pharmaceutics* 12(11), (2020). https://doi.org/10.3390/pharmaceutics12111002.

102. Sahakijpijarn, S. *et al.* Using thin film freezing to minimize excipients in inhalable tacrolimus dry powder formulations. *Int J Pharm* 586, 119490 (2020). https://doi.org/10.1016/j.ijpharm.2020.119490.

103. Wang, J.L. *et al.* Aerosolizable siRNA-encapsulated solid lipid nanoparticles prepared by thin-film freeze-drying for potential pulmonary delivery. *Int J Pharm* 596, 120215 (2021). https://doi.org/10.1016/j.ijpharm.2021.120215.

104. Arasan, S., Akbulut, S. & Hasiloglu, A.S. The relationship between the fractal dimension and shape properties of particles. *KSCE J Civ Eng* 15(7), 1219 (2011). https://doi.org/10.1007/s12205-011-1310-x.

105. Tang, P., Chan, H.K. & Raper, J.A. Prediction of aerodynamic diameter of particles with rough surfaces. *Powder Technol* 147(1–3), 64–78 (2004). https://doi.org/10.1016/j.powtec.2004.09.036.

106. Tang, P., Chew, N.Y.K., Chan, H.-K. & Raper, J.A. Limitation of determination of surface fractal dimension using N2 adsorption isotherms and modified Frenkel–Halsey–Hill theory. *Langmuir* 19(7), 2632–2638 (2003). https://doi.org/10.1021/la0263716.

107. Chang, R.Y.K. *et al.* Storage stability of inhalable phage powders containing lactose at ambient conditions. *Int J Pharm* 560, 11–18 (2019). https://doi.org/10.1016/j.ijpharm.2019.01.050.

108. Chang, R.Y.K. *et al.* Production of highly stable spray dried phage formulations for treatment of *Pseudomonas aeruginosa* lung infection. *Eur J Pharm Biopharm* 121, 1–13 (2017). https://doi.org/10.1016/j.ejpb.2017.09.002.

109. Lin, Y. *et al.* Storage stability of phage-ciprofloxacin combination powders against Pseudomonas aeruginosa respiratory infections. *Int J Pharm* 591, 119952 (2020). https://doi.org/10.1016/j.ijpharm.2020.119952.

110. Eaton, P. & West, P. *Atomic force microscopy.* (Oxford: Oxford University Press, 2010).

111. Adi, H., Traini, D., Chan, H.K. & Young, P.M. The influence of drug morphology on aerosolisation efficiency of dry powder inhaler formulations. *J Pharm Sci* 97(7), 2780–2788 (2008). https://doi.org/10.1002/jps.21195.

112. Adi, S. *et al.* Micro-particle corrugation, adhesion and inhalation aerosol efficiency. *Eur J Pharm Sci* 35(1–2), 12–18 (2008). https://doi.org/10.1016/j.ejps.2008.05.009.

113. Adi, S. *et al.* Scanning white-light interferometry as a novel technique to quantify the surface roughness of micron-sized particles for inhalation. *Langmuir* 24(19), 11307–11312 (2008). https://doi.org/10.1021/la8016062.

114. Bérard, V. *et al.* Affinity scale between a carrier and a drug in DPI studied by atomic force microscopy. *Int J Pharm* 247(1–2), 127–137 (2002). https://doi.org/10.1016/s0378-5173(02)00400-3.

115. Begat, P., Young, P.M., Edge, S., Kaerger, J.S. & Price, R. The effect of mechanical processing on surface stability of pharmaceutical powders: Visualization by atomic force microscopy. *J Pharm Sci* 92(3), 611–620 (2003). https://doi.org/10.1002/jps.10320.

116. Yip, C.M. & Ward, M.D. Atomic force microscopy of insulin single crystals: Direct visualization of molecules and crystal growth. *Biophys J* 71(2), 1071–1078 (1996). https://doi.org/10.1016/s0006-3495(96)79307-4.

117. Kurouski, D., Dazzi, A., Zenobi, R. & Centrone, A. Infrared and Raman chemical imaging and spectroscopy at the nanoscale. *Chem Soc Rev* 49(11), 3315–3347 (2020). https://doi.org/10.1039/c8cs00916c.

118. Khanal, D., Zhang, J., Ke, W.R., Banaszak Holl, M.M. & Chan, H.K. Bulk to nanometer-scale infrared spectroscopy of pharmaceutical dry powder aerosols. *Anal Chem* 92(12), 8323–8332 (2020). https://doi.org/10.1021/acs.analchem.0c00729.

119. Khanal, D., Chang, R.Y.K., Morales, S., Chan, H.-K. & Chrzanowski, W. High resolution nanoscale probing of bacteriophages in an inhalable dry powder formulation for pulmonary infections. *Anal Chem* 91(20), 12760–12767 (2019). https://doi.org/10.1021/acs.analchem.9b02282.

120. Mangal, S. *et al.* Understanding the impacts of surface compositions on the in-vitro dissolution and aerosolization of co-spray-dried composite powder formulations for inhalation. *Pharm Res* 36(1), 6 (2018). https://doi.org/10.1007/s11095-018-2527-x.

121. Yang, M. *et al.* Characterisation of salmon calcitonin in spray-dried powder for inhalation: Effect of chitosan. *Int J Pharm* 331(2), 176–181 (2007). https://doi.org/10.1016/j.ijpharm.2006.10.030.

122. Chan, H.K., Ongpipattanakul, B. & Au-Yeung, J. Aggregation of rhDNase occurred during the compression of KBr pellets used for FTIR spectroscopy. *Pharm Res* 13(2), 238–242 (1996). https://doi.org/10.1023/a:1016091030928.

123. Glover, W. & Chan, H.-K. Electrostatic charge characterization of pharmaceutical aerosols using electrical low-pressure impaction (ELPI). *J Aerosol Sci* 35(6), 755–764 (2004). https://doi.org/10.1016/j.jaerosci.2003.12.003.

124. Kwok, P.C., Glover, W. & Chan, H.K. Electrostatic charge characteristics of aerosols produced from metered dose inhalers. *J Pharm Sci* 94(12), 2789–2799 (2005). https://doi.org/10.1002/jps.20395.

125. Kwok, P.C. & Chan, H.K. Effect of relative humidity on the electrostatic charge properties of dry powder inhaler aerosols. *Pharm Res* 25(2), 277–288 (2008). https://doi.org/10.1007/s11095-007-9377-2.

126. Young, P.M. *et al.* Influence of humidity on the electrostatic charge and aerosol performance of dry powder inhaler carrier based systems. *Pharm Res* 24(5), 963–970 (2007). https://doi.org/10.1007/s11095-006-9218-8.

127. Wong, J. *et al.* Bipolar electrostatic charge and mass distributions of powder aerosols – Effects of inhaler design and inhaler material. *J Aerosol Sci* 95, 104–117 (2016). https://doi.org/10.1016/j.jaerosci.2016.02.003.

128. Usmani, O.S., Biddiscombe, M.F. & Barnes, P.J. Regional lung deposition and bronchodilator response as a function of beta2-agonist particle size. *Am J Respir Crit Care Med* 172, 1497–1504 (2005). https://doi: 10.1164/rccm.200410-1414OC.

129. Glover, W., Chan, H.-K., Eberl, S., Daviskas, E. & Verschuer, J. Effect of particle size of dry powder mannitol on the lung deposition in healthy volunteers. *Int J Pharm* 349(1–2), 314–322 (2008). https://doi.org/10.1016/j.ijpharm.2007.08.013.

130. Timbrell, V. *In inhaled particles V.* (ed. W.H. Walton) 347–369. (Oxford: Pergamon, 1982).

131. Okuda, T. *et al.* Development of spray-freeze-dried siRNA/PEI powder for inhalation with high aerosol performance and strong pulmonary gene silencing activity. *J Control Release* 279, 99–113 (2018). https://doi.org/10.1016/j.jconrel.2018.04.003.

132. Miller, D.P. *et al.* Physical characterization of tobramycin inhalation powder: I. Rational design of a stable engineered-particle formulation for delivery to the lungs. *Mol Pharm* 12(8), 2582–2593 (2015). https://doi.org/10.1021/acs.molpharmaceut.5b00147.

133. Chew, N.Y., Tang, P., Chan, H.K. & Raper, J.A. How much particle surface corrugation is sufficient to improve aerosol performance of powders? *Pharm Res* 22(1), 148–152 (2005). https://doi.org/10.1007/s11095-004-9020-4.

134. Wong, J. *et al.* Measuring bipolar charge and mass distributions of powder aerosols by a novel tool (BOLAR). *Mol Pharm* 12(9), 3433–3440 (2015). https://doi.org/10.1021/acs.molpharmaceut.5b00443.

SECTION III

Novel Technologies

Recent Advances in Inhalable Nanomedicine for Lung Cancer Therapy

8

Hadeer M. Abdelaziz,
Mohamed Teleb Sherine N. Khattab,
Adnan A. Bekhit, Kadria A. Elkhodairy,
and Ahmed O. Elzoghby

Contents

DOI: 10.1201/9781003182566-11

8.1 CANCER EPIDEMIOLOGY

Lung cancer remains a major threat terrifying the world. According to the American Cancer Society in 2021, it's responsible for 235,760 new cases and about 131,880 deaths in both men and women representing 25% of total cancer deaths. All international efforts are collaborating to achieve optimum cancer control in an attempt to lessen the global burden in both more developed and less developed countries.

There are several risk factors which potentiate lung cancer development including smoking, radon gas, secondhand smoke, occupational exposure, and air pollution [1]. There is a direct link between smoking and lung cancer, in which smoking contributes to 80–90% of lung cancer cases and accounts for 160,000 deaths per year. Unfortunately, secondhand smoking is considered as the third leading cause for lung cancer, accounting for more than 3,000 deaths per year [2,3]. Pathogenesis of lung cancer is initiated upon exposure to a carcinogen which either activate oncogenes or inactivates tumor suppressor genes, resulting in abnormal dividing and rapidly growing lung cells [4,5]. Lung cancer is classified into two major types: non-small cell lung carcinoma (NSCLC) and small cell lung carcinoma (SCLC). This classification is based on the origin of abnormal lung cells as well as the smoking status of the patient. NSCLC is the most common and aggressive type of lung cancer representing 80–85% of all cases. NSCLC is subdivided into three types; adenocarcinoma, squamous cell (epidermoid) carcinoma, and large cell carcinoma. Adenocarcinoma represents 40% of all lung cancers in which it originates in outer parts of lung and is predominant in smokers as well as non-smokers. Squamous cell accounts for 25–30% of lung cancer cases in which it occurs in the center of the lungs mainly in cells lining the passage of respiratory tract, and it is a common type in smokers. Large cell carcinoma is responsible for 10–15% of lung cancer cases and is characterized by undifferentiated rapidly growing cells which possibly originate anywhere in the lungs. On the other hand, SCLC represents 10–15% of all cases in which it originates in the bronchi almost near the center of the chest. Compared to NSCLC, SCLC grow and spread rapidly which usually occurs in smokers rather than non-smokers [6,7]. There is an obvious difference in the histology of lung cells among various types of lung cancers.

8.2 TREATMENT STRATEGIES

Lung cancer is a silent disease which is unfortunately diagnosed when symptoms appear at advanced and late stages [8]. Even when symptoms appear they are confusing and misinterpreted with infections or long-term effects from smoking [9]. Such delay in diagnosis has resulted in poor prognosis and reduces the chances of chemotherapeutic agents to succeed which in turn convert the treatment goals from curative to palliative. In such cases chemotherapeutics are considered as palliative care, which only aim to reduce patients' suffering and ameliorate their quality of life rather than to prolong survival life [4]. The standard treatment protocols, including surgery, radiotherapy, chemotherapy, or a combination of all three, are based on the type of lung carcinoma as well as its stage [4,7]. Surgical resection of tumor is considered as first line of choice mainly for NSCLC at their early stages including (0, I, II, IIIA). However, the role of surgery is limited at stages IIIB and IV due to wide dissemination of tumor in which it becomes difficult to completely remove the tumor. In most cases it is recommended to use chemotherapy, radiotherapy, or combination of both after surgical resection in order to shrink and control any residual cancerous cells. On the other hand, chemotherapy is first line of choice for SCLC as well as advanced stages of NSCLC mainly at stage IV [7,10].

The most common protocols for NSCLC are based on platinum chemotherapy including cisplatin or carboplatin in addition to at least one of the following chemotherapeutic agents: vinorelbine, etoposide, gemcitabine, docetaxel, and pemetrexed. These combinations hold great promise against lung cancer [11,12]. However, the low aqueous solubility, extensive first pass metabolism, and lack of both selectivity and targetability of systemically administered anticancer drugs remain the major obstacles which impede their success. Moreover, they affect the rapidly growing tumor cells as well as healthy cells [13,14]. Therefore, to achieve a therapeutic level, it is required to deliver anticancer drugs in very high doses which in turn is associated with several toxic side effects [13].

Despite the great effort exerted by researchers to improve the standards of life for lung cancer patients, the five-year survival rate still less than 15% for NSCLC and 5% for SCLC. This could be attributed to multidrug resistance (MDR) in which most lung cells become insensitive to cytotoxic activity of chemotherapeutic agents and develop resistance to their action [15]. In lung cancer, NSCLC cells are intrinsically resistant to certain anticancer drugs due to genetic and epigenetic heterogeneity, while SCLC cells acquire resistance due to frequent administration of chemotherapeutic agents [15].

Based on the above mentioned limitations of conventional chemotherapy, experts are trying to explore other alternatives to maximize therapeutic effects with the least possible side effects. The pulmonary route has gained great interest in its ability to deliver a drug directly to lungs either for localized or systemic treatment [16,17]. This approach is based on the unique characteristics of lungs, which provide large surface area, thin alveolar epithelium, high vascularization, high bioavailability, great capacity for solute exchange, in addition to great tendency in evading the first pass effect [18,19]. Direct delivery of chemotherapeutic agents via inhalation is considered a potential platform for lung cancer treatment in which localized (regional) delivery of anticancer agents increase the chances of their accumulation within tumor cells so that they could exert their killing effect on tumor cells rather than normal cells [20]. Therefore, inhalable chemotherapeutic agents escape from systemic dilution and exert their cytotoxic activity at doses lower than those required during systemic delivery, which in turn minimizes dose limiting toxicities. Moreover, this needle-free approach could possibly improve the patients compliance and upgrade their quality of life as well as their survival rates [20].

8.3 CHALLENGES FACING LOCALIZED DRUG DELIVERY

Inhalable chemotherapeutic agents should be properly delivered deeply into lungs to exert their therapeutic activity [20]. However, there are major obstacles facing their effective delivery during their journey along respiratory tract including particle size and pulmonary clearance mechanism (Figure 8.1) [19–23].

Deposition of particles within lungs relies on three different mechanisms including impaction, sedimentation, and diffusion. During inhalation, fine particles in nanorange whose particle size < 1μm are liable to be exhaled prior reaching deep lung sites, whereas larger particles whose particle size is > 5μm will deposit at oropharynx as well as upper respiratory tract via impaction. Therefore, adjusting particles size in range 1–5 μm could guarantee lung deposition in which particles will sediment via gravitational force. Apart from impaction and sedimentation, Brownian motion plays a crucial role for deep alveolar deposition. This was achieved via dissolution of inhalable particles when they become in direct contact with alveolar fluids as well as concentration gradient influence diffusion [19,20].

Besides adjusting particle size, the inhalable particles should overcome various pulmonary clearance mechanisms in order to meet the criteria for appropriate delivery to tumor site. Normally, upper ways of lungs possess a mucociliary escalator system in which they are lined with ciliated columnar epithelial globet cells along with submucosal glands that secrete mucus forming a bilayer of mucus blanket over the ciliated epithelium. This mechanism eliminates most of deposited insoluble particles with sizes greater than 6 μm in which they are trapped within mucus bilayer, moved toward the pharynx and swept away [20,22,23]. On the other hand, smaller particles rapidly deposit

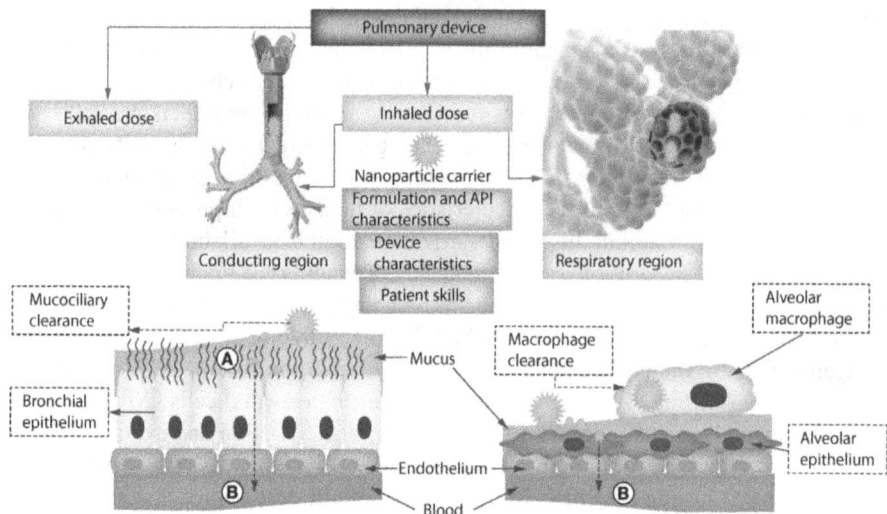

FIGURE 8.1 Schematic illustration for the fate of inhalable drug delivery [24].

in alveolar region and escape from the mucociliary escalator. However, these insoluble particles are phagocytosed via alveolar macrophages and subsequently cleared either by lymphatic system or moved towards the ciliated airways along currents in alveolar fluid which are then cleared via the mucociliary escalator [23]. The normal healthy lungs of non-smokers possess an effective balance in mucociliary escalator between ciliated and mucus-producing cells in addition to five to seven alveolar macrophages per alveolus to keep alveolar region free from any foreign particles. However, during inflammation and infection of lungs, the mucociliary escalator balance is disturbed which results in accelerated clearance of inhalable payloads and minimizes their retention time as well as their effectiveness. Moreover, phagocytosis reduces half-life of inhalable drugs to a few hours, which in turn requires frequent dose administration [23].

Although inhalable particles should have suitable particle size in micro-range (1–5 μm), these microparticles are liable to phagocytosis by alveolar macrophages. Several approaches were adopted to reach a compromise between adjusting particle size and escaping from clearance mechanism to guarantee effective delivery of therapeutic payloads with controlled release deeply into lungs [20].

8.4 AEROSOL DRUG DELIVERY DEVICES

To date, four clinically promising aerosol pulmonary delivery systems to deliver therapeutic agents into lungs based on type of device are dry powder inhalers (DPI), nebulizers, pressurized metered dose inhalers (pMDI), and soft-mist inhalers [25,26]. Liquid-based drug delivery systems are classified into pMDI and nebulizer. Pulmonary drug delivery via nebulization provides several advantages over pMDI in which they are propellant free, produce large amount of aerosolized drug droplets from suspension or drug solution over long period of time with least patient collaboration and suitable for children (under 2 years) and elderly especially in chronic disorders such as lung cancer. The efficiency of nebulized aerosol is highly influenced by PH, viscosity, surface tension, drug concentration, and osmolarity. However, many obstacles face their wide use including long administration time, poor stability, tendency of drug leakage before reaching site of action, and frequent administration [27]. On the other hand, dry powder inhalers (DPIs) as a solid-based delivery system are designed to overcome problems encountered with nebulizers as well as pMDI by offering several benefits (e.g., non-invasive, propellant free, easy to handle, easy to operate, long term stability, maintain sterility, sustained release profile and suitable for hydrophobic drugs) [28]. DPI formulations must undergo additional formulating steps to ensure efficient delivery of therapeutic agents. In most cases active drugs either alone or loaded within nanocarriers are blended with non-respirable water soluble excipients/carriers such as lactose, mannitol, glucose, sorbitol, sucrose and maltitol. Lactose is the only FDA-approved carrier [27]. However, a due care is required during using lactose with protein-based active ingredients to avoid possible Schiff's base reaction [29].

Recently, soft-mist inhalers were developed to overcome the limitations associated with pMDI, DPI, and nebulizers. The soft-mist inhalers are capable of utilizing mechanical energy generated from spring to acutate-metered drug solution in addition to producing an optimal aerosol independent of inspiratory flow rate. The resultant aerosols possess higher fine particle fraction (FPF) compared to other inhaler devices which guarantee high lung deposition [25].

8.5 APPLICATIONS OF INHALABLE NANOPARTICLE-BASED DRUG FOR LUNG CANCER

Nanoparticle-based drug delivery systems are a promising method to overcome the problems associated with the conventional chemotherapy. They offer many advantages including ability to enhance bioavailability of poorly water soluble drugs, minimize dose frequency, incorporate hydrophilic and lipophilic bioactives, reduce systemic toxicities, control drug release, and have high selectivity. Moreover, they can help in the improvement in drug localization at site of action via both passive and active targeting [20,30]. Passive targeting was achieved via enhanced permeation and retention (EPR) in which nanoparticles utilize tumor cell abnormalities including hyper vascularization and poor lymphatic drainage, while active targeting was achieved via receptor mediated endocytosis where targeting ligands decorating surface of nanoparticles were directed to overexpressed receptors in malignant cells [20,31].

Several nanocarriers are used for the delivery of bioactive chemotherapeutic agents for treatment of lung cancer. These nanocarriers classified into lipid based and non-lipid based. Most commonly used lipid-based nanocarriers include solid lipid nanoparticles, liposomes, micelles, lipid nanocapsule, while non-lipid nanocarriers include polymeric nanoparticles, dendrimers, mesoporous nanoparticles, and metallic nanoparticles [20].

Several attempts have been carried out to improve the therapeutic delivery to lung tissues via inhalation. Most approaches are based on combining the merits of both micro- and nanoparticles.

8.5.1 Inhalable Nebulized Nanosuspension

Nebulization of drug-loaded nanoparticle suspension enables generation of high yield of aerosolized droplets over long periods of time, which can improve compliance of lung cancer patients [20]. However, the small density of nanocarriers impedes their effective deposition in deep lung tissues because of their easy exhalation. Therefore, particular devices e.g., nebulizers are used to generate micro-size droplets that could readily deposit in lung tissues. Nebulization of gemcitabine (GEM)-loaded gelatin nanoparticle suspension (150–200 nm) has generated aerosolized droplets of median aerodynamic diameter (MMAD) of 2 μm, and fine particle fraction (FPF) of 76% resulted in effective lung deposition and increased GEM accumulation in lung cancer cells (Table 8.1) [32]. Inhalational nanoencapsulation of GEM can overcome its short half-life and chemical

TABLE 8.1 Examples of inhalable nanosuspension and nanocomposites DPI

DDS	DRUG	TYPES OF NANOCARRIERS	MODE OF INHALATION	CARRIER IF PRESENT	KEY OUTCOME	REF
GNCs	GEM	Polymeric	Nebulized nanosuspension		Genipin crosslinkers managed to sustain release of GEM up to 30% for 24 h	[32]
HAS	ETP BER	Protein	DPI nanocomposites	Mannitol	Improved aerosolization performance with MMAD 2.11 μm and FPF 77.8%	[33]
LF-CS	DOX EA	Electrostatic complex	DPI nanocomposites	Mannitol	LF and CS facilitated active targeting to Tf and CD44 receptors which improved intracellular uptake of co-loaded drugs	[34]
SLNs	BER RAP	Lipid	DPI nanocomposites	Mannitol: Maltodextrin: leucine	RAP-phospholipid complex bilayer not only improve release of hydrophobic RAP but also minimize alveolar surface tension	[35]
LCNPs	PMS RSV	Lipid	DPI nanocomposites	Mannitol: inulin: leucine	This multicarrier displayed MMAD 2.41 μm and FPF of 61.6%	[36]
TPGS1K and TPGS5K	PTX	Mixed polymeric micelles	DPI nanocomposites	Lactose	Controlled release of PTX only 30% for 72 h	[37]

GEM: Gemcitabine, GNCs: Gelatin nanoparticles, DPIs: Dry powder inhalers, HAS: Human Serum Albumin, ETP: Etoposide, BER: Berberine, LF: Lactoferrin, CS: Chondroitin Sulphate, DOX: Doxorubicin, EA:Ellagic acid, RAP: Rapamycin, SLN: Solid Lipid Nanoparticles, LCNPs: Liquid Crystalline Nanoparticles, PMS: Pemetrexed, RSV: Resveratrol, TPGS: α-tocopheryl succinate-polyethylene glycol.

instability and reduce its systemic toxicity. Crosslinking of gelatin nanoparticles with genipin resulted in sustained release of the water soluble GEM in simulated lung fluid with about 30% released after 24 hr.

8.5.2 Inhalable Protein Nanocomposites

Dry powder inhalers (DPIs) in the form of spray-dried nanocomposites are unique systems for pulmonary delivery of anti-cancer drugs (Table 8.1) [20]. On one hand, they are superior to nebulized liquid nanosuspension in terms of longer stability time, shorter administration time, less drug leakage and easier handling. On the other hand, being composed of microencapsulated nanoparticles, they combine the merits of both nano-carriers (improved tumor targeting and enhanced cellular uptake) and microparticles (deep lung deposition). Albumin nanoparticles are known by their enhanced accumulation in tumor cells via binding to Albondin and SPARC receptors overexpressed by cancer cells [33]. Therefore, localized co-delivery of etoposide nanocrystals and berberine to lung cancer cells was enabled by loading into albumin nanocomposites. The dual drug-loaded albumin nanoparticles were spray-dried in presence of mannitol resulting in inhalable nanocomposites with proper MMAD (2.112 μm) and high FPF (77.86%) revealing deep lung deposition. The nanocomposites were readily reconstituted (redispersibility index, RI = 1) where mannitol dissolves in alveolar fluid releasing the drug-loaded nanoparticles to be internalized by lung cancer cells. In mice bearing lung tumor, the inhaled particles showed powerful anti-tumor efficacy with 2.8 fold reduction in lung weights, 3.6 fold reduction in vascular endothelial growth factor (VEGF) expression level, and 16% reduction in Ki67-expression compared to systemic therapy.

In addition to albumin, nanocomposites based on the electrostatic complex of cationic protein lactoferrin and polyanionic polysaccharide chondroitin sulfate displayed favorable aerosolization performance [34]. The spray-dried mannitol-based nanocomposites demonstrated MMAD of 2.68 μm and FPF of 89.5%. Co-encapsulation of doxorubicin and ellagic acid nanocrystals into this nanocomplex enhanced their efficacy against lung cancer cells via binding to Tf and CD44 receptors overexpressed by lung cancer cells. The inhalable nanocomposites showed better antitumor efficacy with higher Caspase-3 levels (6.99 ng/g tissue) rather than systemic nanocarriers and inhaled free drugs (2.79 and 3.79 ng/g tissue, respectively).

8.5.3 Inhalable Lipid Nanocomposites

The pulmonary deposition of lipid nanocarriers could be enhanced by spray drying with inert carriers (Table 8.1). Microencapsulation of glyceryl monostearate lipid nanoparticles loaded with berberine into a carrier mixture of mannitol:maltodextrin:leucine resulted in nanocomposites with FPF of 62.9% [35]. Prior to microencapsulation, coating the surface of berberine lipid NPs with rapamycin-phospholipid complex bilayer was found to significantly reduce the FPF of nanocomposites from 65.6% to 55.5% and MMAD to 3.28 μm. However, the complex enhanced the release of the extremely hydrophobic rapamycin to help the synergistic antitumor efficacy of berberine/

rapamycin combined therapy. In addition, the phospholipid corona acted as lung sur-factant by reducing the alveolar surface tension and decreasing the friction in lung tissue. The inhaled nanocomposites demonstrated significant suppression of tumor growth and reduction of number and diameter of metastatic lung foci in lung cancer animal models.

In addition to solid lipid nanoparticles, Abdelaziz et al. [36] fabricated inhalable monoolein-based liquid crystalline nanoparticles (LCNPs) for co-delivery of synergis-tic combination of pemetrexed (PMS) and resveratrol (RSV). Surface functionalization of LCNPs via chondroitin sulphate (CS) and lactoferrin (LF) guarantee active target-ing and improve cellular uptake. The optimized LF/CS-coated PEM-RES-LCNPs were incorporated into a mixture of mannitol:inulin:leucine at ratio of 1:3 w/w via spray dry-ing. The resulted dry powder nanocomposites possessed MMAD of 2.41 µm and FPF of 61.6% which allow deep lung deposition and managed to improve antitumor efficacy in lung cancer-bearing mice as supported by the in vivo bioimaging. Moreover, the optimized inhalable nanocomposites managed to upgrade the survival rate of treated mice up to 60% compared to only 30% treated with inhalable free powder of PMX/RSV mixture.

Different nanocarriers including liposomes, solid lipid nanoparticles, and polymeric nanoparticles were adopted to overcome the regional toxicity facing clinical applica-tion of inhalable solution of lipophilic antineoplastic agents (e.g., paclitaxel, PTX) for combating primary or metastatic lung cancer [37]. However, these nanocarriers were intratracheally administered thus handicapping their wide clinical trials. Therefore, inhalable dry powder of PTX was formulated in the form of mixed polymeric micelles based on α-tocopheryl succinate-polyethylene glycol 1000 and 5000 Da (TPGS1K and TPGS5K) then embedded in lactose matrix via spray drying [37]. Different molar ratios of mixed TPGS5K and TPGS1K were screened until reaching the lowest CMC values (16.33 and 17.89 µM) corresponding to the combinational molar ratio of 5:5 and 7:3, respectively. The formulated system offered controlled release of PTX with only 30% released after 72 h, improved cytotoxic activity and remarkable in vitro deposition into lungs with high FPF of 60%.

8.5.4 Inhalable Drug-Polymer Nano-Conjugates

In addition to proteins and lipids, dry powder inhalers were successfully fabricated from polymer-drug conjugates (**Table 8.2**). Among polymers, poly(amidoamine) PAMAM dendrimers can offer precisely tailored particle size and reproducible pharmacokinet-ics. Acid-sensitive conjugate of DOX was obtained by coupling with generation 4 (G4), carboxylated PAMAM dendrimer (G4-12DOX) via pH-labile hydrazone bond [38]. Therefore, the drug was only released at the acidic intracellular tumor pH which in turn hampered systemic and local toxicity. Moreover, high drug loading of 27.2% w/w could be achieved by coupling to the available surface groups. Co-spray drying of the nano-sized drug conjugate (9.9 nm) with mannitol carrier resulted in microparticles. Notably, increasing the content of G4-12DOX conjugate resulted in a significant drop in FPF and emitted dose (ED). However, all the resulted DPIs were still in the acceptable range with ED up to 82%, FPF up to 63%, and MMAD up to 4.5 µm which were higher than

TABLE 8.2 Examples of inhalable drug-polymer nanoconjugate

DDS	DRUG	TYPES OF NANOCARRIERS	MODE OF INHALATION	CARRIER IF PRESENT	KEY OUTCOME	REF
G4 PAMAM dendrimer	DOX	Drug-polymer nanoconjugate	DPI nanocomposites	Mannitol	Site specific DOX release due to pH-labile hydrazone bond that only respond to intracellular pH drop at tumor cells	[38]
PEG1000-PAMAM	DOX	Drug-polymer nanoconjugate	pMDIs		PEGylation decreased mucus trapping and facilitate transport of DOX across pulmonary epithelium pMDIs using minimal amount of cosolvent (ethanol; <0.4%; v/v) could enable deep lung deposition with high FPF up to 80%	[39]
LA46-EO23-LA46-PAMAM	DOX	Drug-polymer nanoconjugate	pMDIs		Triblock copolymer excipient was used to obtain cosolvent-free pMDIs with similar aerodynamic performance	[40]
HA	Pt	Drug-polymer nanoconjugate	Intratracheal aerosol		Trehalose (2.5%wt) was used as cryoprotectant during lyophilization	[41]

PTX: Paclitaxel, PAMAM: poly(amidoamine), G4: Generation 4 carboxylated PAMAM dendrimer, PEG: Polyethylene glycol, pMDIs: Pressurized metered-dose inhalers, LA46-EO23-LA46: polylactide-PEG-polylactide, HA-Pt: hyaluronan-cisplatin conjugates.

those of commercial products. After deep lung deposition, mannitol quickly dissolves to release the drug nanoconjugtes thus escaping macrophage phagocytosis [38].

Consequent PEGylation (PEG1000) of PAMAM dendrimers remarkably increased the transport of DOX across pulmonary epithelium. PEGylation decreased mucus trapping and transiently interact with intercellular tight junctions which in turn facilitate the transpithelial transport of DOX. A pseudo-solution formulation of PEGylated PAMAM-DOX conjugates could be prepared in pressurized metered-dose inhalers (pMDIs) using minimal amount of cosolvent (ethanol; <0.4%; v/v) and demonstrated high FPF up to 80% indicating deep lung deposition [39]. However, the presence of cosolvents not only increased the aerodynamic size but also was associated with additional toxicity. Therefore, another approach was adopted to formulate a cosolvent-free pMDIs containing conjugates via a melting process that managed to display similar aerodynamic performance [40]. Notably, introducing the biodegradable triblock copolymer excipient polylactide-PEG-polylactide to formulations could potentially modify the aerodynamic particle size of PAMAM-DOX conjugates thus tuning lung deposition of aerosol according to tumor site on respiratory tract.

Another interesting example of inhalable polymer-drug nanoconjugates is hyaluronan-cisplatin conjugates, HylaPlat™ (HA-Pt) [41]. Intratracheal aerosol administration of the conjugate remarkably suppressed the tumor growth of Lewis lung carcinoma (LLC) mouse orthotopic allograft model without causing side effects. Thus, the aerosolized nanoconjugate was effective at a dose of 7.5 mg/kg, which is less than half the systemic dose of cisplatin. The enhanced cytotoxic efficacy of the nanoconjugate could be correlated to the interaction of HA with CD44 receptors overexpressed by cisplatin-resistant lung cancer cells. The highly water-soluble lyophilized HA-Pt conjugate dissolved quickly after lung deposition by virtue of trehalose (2.5%wt) used as a cryoprotectant and then degraded via endogenous hyaluronidase enzyme thus facilitating release of cisplatin.

8.5.5 Inhalable Nano-in-Porous Microparticles

Dry powder inhaler microparticles (DPI MPs) have been extensively studied for pulmonary delivery due to their tendency to achieve deep lung deposition (Figure 8.2). However, their cohesiveness and opsonization via alveolar macrophages handicap their appropriate aerosolization performance. Therefore, large porous microparticles (LPMP) were adopted as possible novel inhalable approaches to overcome these limitations. They combine the merits of both nano- and microparticles. Thanks to their low density (<0.4 g/cm3), high geometric diameter (D_g) up to 30 μm and mass median aerodynamic diameter (MMAD) (1–3 μm) guarantee their proper delivery into deep parts of lungs with longer residence time.

The high porosity of the light LPMP was mainly based on the choice of suitable porogen. Among the widely used porogens during development of LPMP were gasforming porogens (ammonium bicarbonate). Their superiority over extractable (pluronics) and osmogen (cyclodextrins) porogens was attributed to their high tendency in preventing drug leaching out and enhancing encapsulation efficiency. The synthesis of inhalable highly porous microparticles in the presence of ammonium bicarbonate (AB)

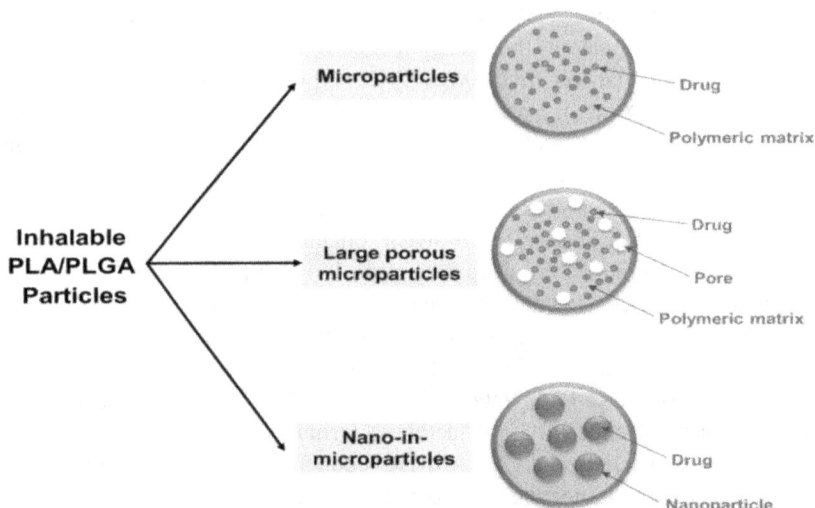

FIGURE 8.2 Schematic illustration displaying the difference between various types of inhalable polymeric carriers [49].

could be achieved via various techniques such as double emulsion-solvent evaporation technique, supercritical anti-solvent (SAS), and electrospraying technique (Table 8.3).

Kim et al. [42] managed to prepare inhalable highly porous microspheres for the delivery of doxorubicin (DOX) using the biocompatible and biodegradable polymer PLGA. He adopted double emulsion-solvent evaporation technique followed by freeze drying. The optimized microspheres displayed high aerosolization performance with D_g (14 um) and MMAD (3.6 μm). The proposed system managed to sustain the release of DOX up to two weeks thus reducing frequency of inhalation and minimizing undesirable toxic side effects associated with DOX. The surface of DOX-PLGA microspheres could be decorated with active targeting ligand such as TRAIL (tumor necrosis factor (TNF)-related apoptosis inducing ligand) to ensure selectivity and specificity to tumor cells rather than normal cells [43]. The TRAIL/DOX PLGA microspheres potentiate apoptosis in lung cancer-bearing mice. The synergistic cytotoxicity was reflected in remarkable reduction in lung weight by 1.7 fold decrease as compared to DOX-PLGA microspheres. In another study, W. Li et al. [44] introduced poly(cyclohexane-1,4-diyl acetone dimethylene ketal) (PCADK) to PLGA in ratio 2:8 to prepare porous mixed matrix microspheres for delivery of DOX. The resulted porous microspheres displayed a promising aerodynamic profile with MMAD (2.48 μm), high encapsulation efficiency (77%), and improved drug release up to 64% compared to only 46% from PLGA microspheres. The significant upgrade in DOX release could be explained by presence of PH-sensitive biocompatible and biodegradable PCADK. This was strongly reflected in the results of the in vivo evaluations which manifested higher antiproliferation and stronger anticancer effects compared to PLGA microspheres. In an attempt to overcome multidrug resistance (MDR), DOX was co-delivered with microRNAs (miR-519c) into inhalable PLGA microspheres with adaptive MMAD < 10 μm [45]. The miR-519c was responsible for down-regulation of the overexpressed ATP Binding Cassette Subfamily

TABLE 8.3 Examples of inhalable nano-in-porous microparticles (LPMPs) and nanoaggregates

DDS	DRUG	TYPES OF NANOCARRIERS	MODE OF INHALATION	PREPARATION TECHNIQUE	KEY OUTCOME	REF
DOX-PLGA	DOX	Polymeric	DPI LPMPs	Double emulsion solvent evaporation/ freeze drying	High aerosolization performance with D_g (14 um) and MMAD (3.6 μm)	[42]
TRAIL/ DOX PLGA	DOX	Polymeric	DPI LPMPs	Double emulsion solvent evaporation/ freeze drying	TRAIL improve selectivity and specificity to tumor cells rather than normal cells	[43]
PCADK/ PLGA	DOX	Polymeric	DPI LPMPs	Double emulsion solvent evaporation/ freeze drying	The PH-sensitive PCADK significantly upgrade DOX release	[44]
PLGA	Oridonin	Polymeric	DPI LPMPs	Double emulsion solvent evaporation/ freeze drying	The fast release of oridonin within 1 hr guarantee its preferential accumulation within tumor site without suffering from alveolar phagocytosis	[46]
PLGA	Oridonin	Polymeric	DPI LPMPs	Electrospraying	Electrospraying overcome the traditional tedious preparation process without affecting aerosolization performance	[47]
CHT-in-PLLA PMs	siRNA DOX	Polymeric	DPI LPMPs	Supercritical anti-solvent	This system displayed favorable aerodynamic profile and maintained the stability of siRNA	[48]
	PTX CIS		DPI Nanoaggregates	Spray Drying	The destabilizer L-leucine triggered NPs assembly to improve the flowability of inhalable dry powder	[50]

(Continued)

TABLE 8.3 (CONTINUED) Examples of inhalable nano-in-porous microparticles (LPMPs) and nanoaggregates

DDS	DRUG	TYPES OF NANOCARRIERS	MODE OF INHALATION	PREPARATION TECHNIQUE	KEY OUTCOME	REF
Soya lecithin and oleic acid	PTX DOX	NLPs	DPI Nanoaggregates	Solvent evaporation/ Spray drying	Compared to Tween 80 & Tween 20, cremophor EL successfully reversed drug resistance and potentiate chemotherapeutic efficacy of drugs	[52]
Stearic acid	9-Br-Nos	NLPs	DPI Nanoaggregates	Nanoemulsion/spray drying	Effervescent technique overcomes lipid-based nanoaggregates that may affect size and inadequately release primary NPs in lungs excipients	[51,53]
SPIONs		Magnetic NPs	DPI Trojan MPs	Chemical precipitation	Cubic magnetic nano-aggregates exhibited high in vitro aerosol deposition with FPF of 67% upon exposing to external magnetic field	[54]
SPIONs		Magnetic NPs	DPI Trojan MPs	Spray drying	PEG and HPβCD potentiated the adherence of SPIONs to form outer crust of the nanoaggregates Ammonium carbonate and magnesium stearate improve aerosolization performance of inhalable trojan MPs	[55]

CHT: Chitosan, PLLA PMs: poly-L-lactide porous microparticles, SAS: Supercritical anti-solvent, AB: Ammonium bicarbonate, PCADK: poly(cyclohexane-1,4-diyl acetone dimethylene ketal), 9-Br-Nos: 9-Bromo-noscapine, NLS: Nanostructured lipid particles, SPIONs: Superparamagnetic iron oxide nanoparticles, HPβCD: hydroxypropyl-β-cyclodextrin

G Member 2 (ABCG2) thus preventing outflux of DOX and potentiating its preferential accumulation in the tumor site. Therefore, the proposed synergistic combination successfully induced cellular apoptosis and cell cycle arrest at S phase.

Similarly, the double emulsion solvent evaporation technique followed by freeze drying was used to fabricate inhalable porous PLGA microspheres for delivery of oridonin [46]. The resulted porous microarchitecture possessed D_g~10 μm, MMAD (2.72 μm) and FPF (30%) thus facilitating deep lung deposition. The fast release of oridonin within 1 hr by virtue of diffusion and erosion of PLGA could guarantee its preferential accumulation within tumor site without suffering from alveolar phagocytosis. The in vivo evaluations in NSCLC rat models confirmed the potentiated antiangiogenic and apoptotic activity of inhalable oridonin-loaded LPMP compared to free oridonin powder and gemcitabine. Worth mentioning is that inhalable oridonin microspheres could be prepared by another technique. Zhu et al. [47] introduced the electrospraying technique as an easy and rapid method for preparation of inhalable porous PLGA microspheres to overcome the traditional tedious and complicated preparation procedures. The electrospraying porous microspheres (EPMs) displayed FPF 19% adequate for pulmonary delivery to deep sites of lungs. In vitro release manifested the release of oridonin from EPMs along 20 h depending on diffusion and erosion of PLGA. EPMs proved their potency against lung cancer in rat models by preventing angiogenesis and promoting apoptosis.

Xu et al. [48] introduced another preparation technique based on ion gelation followed by supercritical anti-solvent (SAS) technique during synthesis of inhalable porous microspheres. Herein siRNA-loaded chitosan nanoparticles (siRNA-CHT) were embedded with DOX in the vicinity of poly-L-lactide porous microparticles. The optimized system exhibited an excellent adaptive aerosolization performance with $D_g > 10$ μm, low aerodynamic density (0.4 g/cm^3), MMAD (1–5 μm) and FPF > 50% which guarantee deep alveolar deposition. Notably, there were no significant changes in both MMAD and geometric diameter (D_g) with increasing the amount of loaded Dox. The inhalable nano-embedded porous microparticles (NEPMs) not only maintained the stability of siRNA after its release in the lungs due to reduced nuclease activity in the airways but also sustained release of both siRNA (~60% in 24 hr) and DOX (60%–80% for 60 hr) from these porous architectures in drug-resistant H69AR human small cell lung cancer cells without causing tissue damage.

8.5.6 Inhalable Flocculated Nano-Agglomerates

Inhalable hollow nano-agglomerates (nanoaggregates or Trojan particles) are inhalable hybrid microparticles (MPs) which merge the drug release and delivery properties of nanoparticles (NPs) with the enhanced aerosolization performance of large porous microparticles (LPMP) [20]. Short spray drying time is an essential prerequisite for development of hollow nanoagglomerates in which NPs were held together via van der Waal forces and self-assemble forming a shell, leaving behind hollow particles in the center [20]. These nanoaggregates should be highly dispersible so that upon exposing to lung fluids they should redisperse and dissolve resulting in the initial NPs. Therefore some excipients could be added (e.g., lactose, trehalose, mannitol, L-leucine and hydroxypropyl β-cyclodextrin) to prevent cohesiveness of NPs and guarantee their redispersibility (Table 8.3). It was reported that L-leucine served as a destabilizer that disrupts the electrostatic double layer provided by surfactant thus inducing NPs assembly [50]. L-leucine improved the flowability and reduced surface energy of inhalable dry powder thus ensuring deep lung deposition of chemotherapeutic payloads including paclitaxel (PTX) and cisplatin (CIS).

Lipid-based nanoparticles could be loaded within this inhalable microstructure. Various drying approaches could be used during the preparation process such as spray drying, freeze drying, supercritical and electrospraying [51]. In this study, inhalable nanoaggregates were developed via solvent evaporation method followed by spray drying in which lipid-based NPs were successfully co-loaded with PTX and DOX in the presence of surfactant [52]. The effect of different surfactants such as cremophor EL, Tween 80 and Tween 20 on antitumor activity of PTX and DOX was screened. The particle size of cremophor EL-based inhalable nanoaggregates was 394.1 nm whereas Tween 80 and Tween 20 possessed particle sizes 575.6 nm and 460.7 nm, respectively. The in vivo evaluations showed that using cremophor EL as surfactant could reverse drug resistance and potentiate chemotherapeutic efficacy of drugs.

Unfortunately, lipid-based nanoaggregates may suffer from size-related problems and inadequate release of primary NPs in lungs. Therefore effervescent technology could be a potential approach to overcome the problems associated with traditional methods [51,53]. The lipid-based NPs were co-sprayed with effervescent matrix including sodium carbonate, citric acid, and ammonium hydroxide. A study compared effervescent and non-effervescent lipid-based inhalable nanoaggregates. The results indicated the superiority of effervescent-based inhalable dry powders over non-effervescent inhalable dry powder. The effervescent technique manifested high aerosolization performance with MMAD 2.3 μm, improved in vitro cytotoxicity, enhanced cellular uptake in A549 lung cancer cells, and improved pharmacokinetic parameters as well as bio-distribution in albino mice.

Superparamagnetic iron oxide nanoparticle (SPIONs) loaded Trojan particles also known as superparamagnetic iron oxide nanoaggregates were proposed as a promising inhalable dry powder. In this study, the surface of SPIONs was functionalized with polytroxane [54]. The concentration of coating polymer polytroxane used highly influenced the crystal size and shape of nanoaggregates. Low concentration resulted in cubic magnetic nanoaggregates, whereas high concentration resulted in rhombic dodecahedron magnetic nanoaggregates. Notably, cubic magnetic nanoaggregates exhibited high in vitro aerosol deposition with FPF of 67% upon exposing to external magnetic field even at low inhalation flow rates (15 and 30 L/min). In another study SPIONs were spray dried with PEG and hydroxypropyl-β-cyclodextrin (HPβCD) [55]. PEG potentiated the adherence of SPIONs together forming the outer crust of the nanoaggregates. However, large aggregates may hinder aerosolization. Therefore excipients such as ammonium carbonate and magnesium stearate were added during the formulation in an attempt to improve aerosolization performance of inhalable trojan microparticles in which MMAD was remarkably improved from 10.2 μm to 2.2 μm. These SPIONs loaded Trojan microparticles were sensitive to magnetic field in which particles deposited on stages of next-generation impactor (NGI) were increased by four-fold upon exposure to external magnetism.

8.5.7 Inhalable Mucoadhesive Nanoparticles

The bioadhesive nanoparticles that adhere to biological mucus membranes are known as mucoadhesive nanoparticles. Such adherence to lung mucosa prolongs drug release and thus reduces dose frequency. Moreover, owing to the positive charge of mucoadhesive polymers, they could disrupt intercellular tight junctions thus increasing cellular uptake and drug absorption [56].

Chitosan (CHT) serves as a promising excipient during synthesis of inhalable spray dry powders mainly due to its mucoadhesiveness and enhancement of drug absorption in lungs (Table 8.4) [57]. At the acidic medium of tumor (< pH 6.5), the primary amines of CHT will be protonated which mediate its interaction with the negatively charged sialic acid of mucins, thus overcoming the mucociliary clearance and prolonging its residence time within the lungs. Notably, HTCC derivatives avoid PH dependence in solubilizing CHT. This could be attributed to chitosan quaternization by introducing quaternary ammonium group to CHT structure thus improving the solubility of CHT by virtue of permanent positive charge regardless pH of medium [58]. In this aspect, the surface of inhalable solid lipid nanoparticles (SLNs) was modified with folate-grafted copolymer of PEG and chitosan derivative (N-[(2-hydroxy-3-trimethylammonium)propyl] chitosan chloride, HTCC). The endotracheal administration of paclitaxel-loaded F-PEG-HTCC-coated lipid nanoparticles enabled selective delivery of PTX within lungs regardless blood vessels. The enhanced efficacy could be attributed to both active targeting achieved via folate-mediated endocytosis in addition to prolonged residence of PTX up to 6 h owing to the mucoadhesive nature of CHT. Notably, inhalable F-PEG-HTCC-coated lipid nanoparticles significantly increase PTX concentration after 6 h by 32 fold compared to inhalable free taxol.

8.5.8 Inhalable Hierarchical Multi-Stage Target Nanoparticles

The hierarchical structured particles are a multi-stage targeted system in which each stage in the hierarchy consists of selected material for a specific function, thus overcoming the multiple obstacles facing localized drug delivery [59]. They hold great promise due to their wide applications in drug delivery, controlled release, and protecting environmentally sensitive therapeutic payloads. They load, preserve, transport, and release the drug locally at tumor site thus improving therapeutic efficiency and minimizing systemic undesirable side effects.

Chen et al. [60] successfully developed a novel inhalable DPI of yuanhuacine-loaded RGDfk–histidine–PLGA multifunctional nanoparticles (MNPs) (yuanhuacine/MNPs) in the presence of lactose mixture to trigger sequential multistage targeting (Figure 8.3). The nanoparticles were prepared via emulsion solvent evaporation technique. Then NPs were mixed with rough lactose to prepare DPI. Rough lactose was mainly added to improve flowability of powder, and fine lactose enhanced the tendency of yuanhuacine separation from powder (Table 8.4). Optimizing lactose mixture with a ratio of 10:1 (rough: fine lactose) facilitated delivery of inhalable yuanhuacine/MNPs

TABLE 8.4 Examples of inhalable mucoadhesive, hierarchical multi-stage target and lung surfactant nanoparticles

DDS	DRUG	TYPES OF NANOCARRIERS	MODE OF INHALATION	CARRIER IF PRESENT	KEY OUTCOME	REF
SLNs-F-PEG-HTCC	PTX	Lipid modified copolymer	Endotracheal		HTCC derivative avoids PH dependence in solubilizing CHT Folate provided receptor mediated endocytosis that guarantees optimum delivery of PTX with prolonged residence up to 6 h	[57]
RGDfk–histidine– PLGA MNPs	yuanhuacine	Inorganic nanoparticles	DPI nanocomposites	Lactose	The hierarchal sequential multistage targeting resulted in better in vitro and in vivo evaluations compared to yuanhuacine/PLGA-NPs	[60]
DPPC and DPPE-PEG	PTX	Lipopolymer	DPI		The mucopenetrating DPPE-PEG provided longer residence in lungs PEG chain length highly influence aerosolization performance	[62]

HTCC: N-[(2-hydroxy-3-trimethylammonium)propyl] chitosan chloride, F: Folate, MNP: Magnetic nanoparticles, DPPC: dipalmitoylphosphatidylcholine, DPPE-PEG: dipalmitoyl phosphatidyl ethanolamine methoxy (polyethyleneglycol), DPPG: dipalmitoylphosphatidylglycerol.

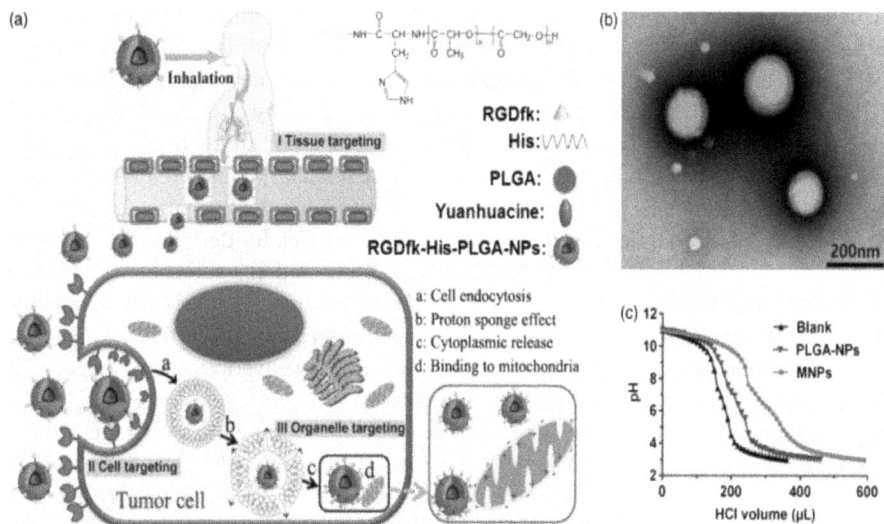

FIGURE 8.3 Schematic fabrication of inhalable intelligent hierarchical multi-stage RGDfk–histidine–PLGA-NPs for mitochondrial-targeted drug delivery [60].

deeply into **lungs tissue targeting level** (Stage I). The surface of PLGA was chemically grafted with RGDfk (Arginine-Glycine-Aspartic Acid, f: phenyl alanine, k: lysine) ligands to actively target integrin avb3 receptors on lung-resident cancer cells through receptor-mediated endocytosis, which guarantees **cellular targeting level** (Stage II). At acidic pH of endosomes (pH 5.5) and lysosomes (pH 4.5), the chemically grafted histidine groups of PLGA and the guanidino groups of RGDfk conferred high positivity to MNPs which triggered the escape of smart MNPs from intracellular endosomal/lysosomal pathway via proton sponge effect. Moreover, this phenomenon facilitated the interaction of positively charged MNPs with negatively charged mitochondrial membrane, which opened the frontier for **organelle targeting level** (Stage III) to potentiate the mitochondrial-related apoptosis.

The in vitro cellular uptake of yuanhuacine/MNPs manifested a 1.54-fold increase in drug concentration compared to yuanhuacine/PLGA-NPs. This could be attributed to the RGDkf graft that triggered receptor endocytosis. In vivo evaluations confirmed the superiority of yuanhuacine/MNPs by inducing 33% apoptotic rate compared to 25% of yuanhuacine/PLGA-NPs and 18.5% of free yuanhuacine.

8.5.9 Inhalable Lung Surfactant-Mimic Nanocarriers

Inhalable microparticles based on the synthetic phospholipids that mimic lung surfactants were very promising approach for drug delivery. They are characterized by their biocompatibility, biodegradability, high transition temperature above that of body, controlled drug release profile and minimize associated drug toxicity. Moreover, they reduce the surface tension of particles and potentiate the migration and delivery of inhalable particles to peripheral parts of lungs. Among the extensively studied phospholipid lung surfactants are dipalmitoylphosphatidylcholine (DPPC), dipalmitoylphosphatidylglycerol (DPPG) and dipalmitoyl phosphatidyl ethanolamine methoxy(polyethyleneglycol) (DPPE-PEG) [61]. Respirable dry powder could be obtained by co-spray drying (co-SD) phospholipids mimic surfactants along with organic solution in a closed-mode system [62,63]. Herein, SD technique was selected to reduce residual water and upgrade the stability of phospholipids by rendering them into thermodynamically stable dry powder.

Meenach et al. [62] developed inhalable microparticles for delivery of PTX-based lipopolymer in which phospholipid surfactants (DPPC) represented the core, whereas PEGylated phospholipid surfactant (DPPE-PEG) represented the outer shell (**Table 8.4**). Thanks to the mucopenetrating DPPE-PEG that confered stealth effect to guarantee longer residence in lungs by preventing opsonization by alveolar macrophages. The chain length of PEG highly influenced the aerosolization performance. PEG 2k chain length could facilitate deep lung deposition based on appropriate MMAD 4 µm and FPF 64% unlike PEG 5k which resulted in poor aerosolization with MMAD 6.8 µm and FPF 55.4%. Besides the safety profile of lung mimic-based DPIs, they remarkably managed to improve PTX loading, sustained PTX in vitro release over weeks and upgrade PTX cytotoxic chemotherapeutic outcomes.

8.5.10 Inhalable Gene Nanocarriers

Tremendous progress has been witnessed in the development of novel innovative approaches that could synergistically conquer multidrug resistance MDR. Genes delivery (e.g., short-interfering RNA (siRNA) and microRNAs (miRNA)) play a potential role in silencing genetic expression of oncogenes in cells and restoring natural tumor suppressor genes, respectively which in turn improve cellular internalization of co-administered chemotherapy and upgrade their intended therapeutic outcomes (Table 8.5) [48]. However, naked genes are highly liable to rapid degradation and renal clearance which minimize their bioactivity. Therefore, the delivery of genes specifically for lung cancer treatment are highly challenging which require special tailoring of inhalable gene nanocarriers to guarantee their efficient accumulation within tumor site via passive and active targeting and subsequently maximize drug concentration and devastate MDR [48,64].

Polymeric nanocarriers (polyplexes) including (poly(lactic-co-glycolic) acid (PLGA), poly-L-lactide (PLLA), polyethyleneimine (PEI), polyesters) are promising nonviral gene vectors characterized by their low toxicity, non-immunogenicity, highly stability during storage which facilitate their wide scale production [48,64,65].

Among polymers, polyethyleneimine (PEI) could be tailored to develop drug-polymer conjugate served as a promising carrier for co-delivery of gene and chemotherapy. Briefly, DOX was conjugated to PEI via pH-sensitive linkers either hydrazone (PEI-HZ-DOX) or cis-aconitic anhydride (CA) then complexed with Bcl2 siRNA to form PEI-HZ-DOX/siRNA or PEI-CA-DOX/siRNA, respectively [66]. This complex was directly delivered to lungs via microsprayer which resulted in enhanced deposition of DOX and siRNA in lungs thus upgrading cellular apoptosis and antitumor efficacy relative to mono-delivery of DOX or siRNA (Figure 8.4). In addition to PEI, functional polyesters

TABLE 8.5   Examples of inhalable gene carriers

DDS	DRUG	TYPES OF NANOCARRIERS	MODE OF INHALATION	KEY OUTCOME	REF
PEI	DOX Bcl2 siRNA	Drug-polymer conjugate (Polyplexes)	Microsprayer	pH-sensitive linkers either hydrazine or cis-aconitic anhydride quickly responded to sudden drop in intracellular pH guaranteed site specific deposition of DOX and siRNA	[66]
PE4K-A13- and PE4K-A13-NPs	siRNA	Amino-thiol polyesters	Micropump nebulizer	Modification using PEG 2000 DMG lipid or amphiphilic Pluronic F-127 reduced surface charge of NPs and improved serum stability Longer hydrophobic alkyl chains potentiated intracellular uptake of NPs	[64,65]
dTAT	pDNA	Cell-penetrating peptides	Intratracheal	Calcium chloride improved the stability of dTAT-pDNA, in vitro gene expression, and transfection efficiency	[67]

PEI: Polyethyleneimine, CA: cis-aconitic anhydride, C6-SH: 1-hexanethiol, C10-SH: 1-decanethiol, dTAT: dimerized TAT peptide, pDNA: plasmid DNA

are among selective polyplex nanoparticles (NPs) that managed to preferentially deliver siRNA to lung tumor cells rather than normal cells [64,65]. Amino-thiol polyesters nanoparticles with Mw = 4,200 g/mol (PE4K) were modified with A13 and 1-hexane-thiol (C6-SH)/1-decanethiol (C10-SH) then PE4K-A13-0.33C6 and PE4K-A13-0.33C10 NPs were further modified using PEG 2000 DMG lipid or amphiphilic Pluronic block copolymers (Pluronic F-127) to decrease surface charge of NPs, minimize non-specific

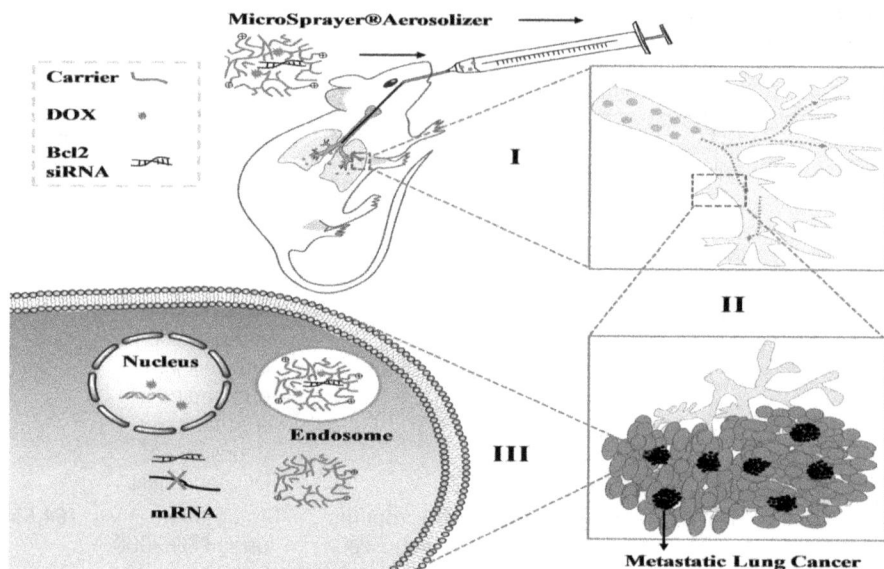

FIGURE 8.4 Schematic illustration for inhalable codelivery of DOX and siRNA to the lung cancer cells [68].

protein interactions and increase serum stability [64]. Functionalized polyesters were able to bind to siRNA under the complexation conditions (pH 4.2, 10 mM, and polymer/siRNA weight ratio of 30:1). Confocal microscopy manifested the stronger fluorescence signal and faster cellular internatization of C10-Cy5.5-siRNA NPs within A549-Luc cells rather than C6-Cy5.5-siRNA NPs. This could be attributed to longer hydrophobic alkyl chains that potentiate fusion of NPs with cellular membrane. In vivo evaluations of inhalable NPs via micropump nebulizer (total NP volume of 400 μL) emphasized that changing route of administration from intravenous to aerosol inhalation could significantly overcome siRNA biodistribution challenge by re-directing accumulation of NPs from liver to lungs which in turn guarantee proper gene silencing (~65% knockdown of luciferase expression) in the A549 orthotopic lung tumors. These functional polyester NPs were extended in another study to evaluate how different cells could respond differently using matched tumor/normal lung cell line pair (HCC4017/HBEC30-KT) [65]. Herein, no cell-specific targeting ligands were required in which the selectivity of NPs based mainly on their physicochemical properties so that they were preferentially accumulated into HCC4017 tumor cells rather than HBEC30-KT normal cells. Therefore, siRNA targeting ubiquitin B (siUBB) was selectively delivered to HCC4017 resulted in enhanced siUBB-mediated apoptosis and remarkable tumor growth suppression. Notably, selective NPs displayed extended retension in tumor tissues for over 1 week in which they were capable of mediating gene silencing in both xenograft and orthotopic lung tumors via intravenous injection and aerosol inhalation, respectively.

Besides polymers (polyplexes), cell-penetrating peptides (CPPs) play a potential role in gene delivery. Herein, dimerized TAT peptide (dTAT) derived from HIV-1 TAT peptide was evaluated for delivery of plasmid DNA (pDNA) [67]. However dTAT-pDNA complexes displayed low transfection efficiency. Therefore, calcium chloride was added to complex to form (dTAT-pDNA-Ca^{2+} complex) in an attempt to improve stability, in vitro gene expression and transfection efficiency. The intratracheal administration of dTAT-pAT2R-Ca^{2+} remarkably attenuated the growth of Lewis lung carcinoma (LLC) allografts in mouse lungs which confirmed the efficient delivery of apoptosis-inducer gene, angiotensin II type 2 receptor (AT2R).

8.5.11 Inhalable Nano-Theranostics

Nano-theranostics, theragnostics, are novel multifunctional nanosystems which integrate therapeutic and diagnostic features into one system thus enabling early diagnosis and treatment [69–71]. Functionalized gold nanoparticles (GNPs, AuNPs) have been extensively studied for theragnosis of lung cancer (Table 8.6) [70]. However, their nano-size make them liable to exhalation or mucociliary clearance which handicap their appropriate delivery into deep lung tissues. Therefore, Silva et al. [70] developed a novel respirable nano-in-microparticles (NIMs) (CHT-AuNPs) in which POxylated AuNPs were incorporated into chitosan matrix (CHT) via supercritical CO_2-assisted spray drying (SASD) technique to overcome the nanosystem limitations. The resulted ultrafine dry powder formulations displayed excellent aerodynamic profile with MMAD 3.2–3.8 μm, FPF 47% that guarantee deep lung deposition. Herein, theragnostic approach was achieved via surface functionalization of AuNPs with the biocompatible optically stable always-on fluorescent oligo(2-oxazoline) and laminin peptide (YIGSR) for active targeting of lung cancer. Notably, the addition of peptide YIGSR along with oligomer played a crucial role in improving the encapsulation of AuNPs within micropowders and upgrading FPF of powder.

Besides multifunctional POxylated AuNPs, superparamagnetic iron oxide nanoparticles (SPIONs) 20% (w/w) and either 2.8% (w/w) doxorubicin (DOX) or 10% (w/w) fluorescent nanospheres were efficiently incorporated into lactose matrix (2.5% w/v total feed concentration) via spray drying technique [69]. In vitro aerosolization performance of dry powder using next generation impaction manifested MMAD 3.27 μm, FPF > 90% and GSD ± 1.69. Worth mentioning that endotracheal administration of dry powder of fluorescently labeled NIMs in healthy mice displayed superior magnetic-field-dependent targeting with significant upgrade in fluorescent intensity and total iron content in left magnetized lung relative to inhalable liquid aerosol. This reduced targeting during liquid aerosol administration could be attributed to dissociation of SPIONs and fluorescent nanospheres. Notably, DOX maintained its therapeutic cytotoxicity in dry powder NIMs even after spray drying. Therefore, this system managed to achieve localized targeting to specific magnetized lung regions with minimal toxicity to healthy tissues.

In addition to their targeting modality, inhalable MNPs have great tendency to uniquely induce loco-regional hyperthermia in the presence of alternating magnetic field (AMF) [72]. This phenomenon guarantee preferential killing of malignant cells either in primary and metastatic lung cancers via thermal sensitization and/or ablation at the malignant/ metastatic site. In this study, iron oxide MNPs were spray dried with D-mannitol to develop magnetic nanocomposite microparticles (MnMs) for the thermal management of aggressive recurrent triple negative breast cancer (TNBC) that

TABLE 8.6 Examples of inhalable nano-theranostics

DDS	DRUG	TYPES OF NANOCARRIERS	MODE OF INHALATION	CARRIER IF PRESENT	KEY OUTCOME	REF
CHT-AuNPs		Inorganic nanoparticles	Nano-in-microparticles		Laminin peptide (YIGSR) improved the encapsulation of AuNPs within micropowders, increased FPF of powder and allowed active targeting to lung cancer	[70]
SPIONs	DOX or fluorescent nanospheres	Magnetic nanoparticles	Endotracheal	Lactose	Endotracheal administration of dry powder displayed superior magnetic-field-dependent targeting and total iron content in left magnetized lung relative to inhalable liquid aerosol	[69]
Iron oxide MNPs		Magnetic nanoparticles	Nanocomposite microparticles	D-mannitol	Inhalable MNPs induced loco-regional hyperthermia with significant cellular damage in the presence of alternating magnetic field (AMF)	[72]
USRPs	Gd	Inorganic nanoparticles	Intrapulmonary nebulization		Single dose of 10 Gy conventional radiation one day after inhalation of USRPs were adequate to induce radiosensitizing effects and potentiate radiotherapeutic efficacy without systemic adverse effects	[71]

AuNPs: Gold nanoparticles, USRPs: Gadolinium-based ultra-small rigid platforms, Gd: Gadolinium primarily infiltrates the lungs. The respirable DPI possessed MMAD <5 μm that facilitated proper deposition throughout the lungs. This study adopted screening the impact of inhalable MnMs in inducing hyperthermia at low (0.1 mg/ mL) and high (1 mg/ mL) dose of MNPs with or without AMF exposure using in vitro 3D tumor tissue analogs (TTA) physiologically relevant metastatic TNBC model. The results indicated that incubation of TTA with high concentration of MNPs in the presence of AMF were sufficient to induce magnetic hyperthermia associated with increased cellular death/ damage. However, no noticeable adverse effects were reported in the absence of AMF.

In addition to thermal sensitization manifested by inhalable magnetic nanotheranostics, radiosensitization could be achieved via multifunctional theranostic gadolinium-based ultra-small rigid platforms (USRPs) [71]. These particles comprised of a polysiloxane matrix and DOTA (1,4,7,10-tetraazacyclododecane-1,4,7,10 -tetraacetic acid) as a chelating agent covalently grafted on the inorganic surface (Gd-DOTA). The loco-regional deposition of high Z-elements nanoparticles (e.g., gold, platinum, or gadolinium) on the tumors located in the lung, highly radio-sensitive organ, could maximize the effects of X-rays. The results indicated that exposing mice to single dose of 10 Gy conventional radiation one day after inhalation of USRPs (50 μL of ~20 mM [Gd $^{3+}$]) were adequate to induce radiosensitizing effects and potentiate radiotherapeutic efficacy without systemic adverse effects. Notably, they successfully improved mean survival time up to 112 days compared to 77 days for irradiated mice without receiving USRPs. Therefore, this system played a crucial role in overcoming radiotherapeutic failure resulted from the resistance of lung tumors. Moreover, USRPs also served as imaging probes based on the fluorescence Cyanine 5.5 (Cy5.5) covalently grafted on the nanoparticles (USRPs-Cy5.5) that could be non-invasively detected within lungs after intrapulmonary nebulization in healthy mice with bioluminescent orthotopic lung cancer of luciferase-modified human NSCLC H358 cells (H358-Luc).

8.6 CHALLENGES AND LIMITATIONS

Despite the tremendous improvement in pulmonary delivery of chemotherapy, there are several technological challenges that handicap successful clinical trials. The current devices used for delivery of inhalable formulations during clinical trials require special tailoring to overcome clearance mechanisms (e.g., mucociliary escalator and alveolar macrophages) in addition to guarantee sustained release of chemotherapeutic payloads in the respiratory tract thus flattening the local concentration peaks of chemotherapy and ensuring their effective delivery for adequate period of time throughout the lung tumor site [20,57]. Despite the promising outcomes of phase I/II study during clinical human evaluations of inhalable doxorubicin (DOX) along with systemic platinum-based therapy in NSCLC patients, few patients still suffered from dose limiting pulmonary-toxicity [69]. In an attempt to minimize toxicity to whole lungs, Dames and his coworkers managed to target therapeutic payload using iron oxide nanoparticles to specific lung lobe in mice in the presence of external magnetic field [73]. However, the dissociation of nanoparticles and drug during liquid aerosol administration reduced the chances of efficient therapeutic delivery to magnetized lung lobe. Up till now there is a missing link during development of aerosol chemotherapy. Researchers pay a great attention to understand long-term adverse effects to the lung to guarantee safety and efficacy in comparison to conventional systemic delivery [32].

8.7 CONCLUSION AND FUTURE DIRECTIONS

Some nanomedicines are showing great progress in clinical trials. In the future, pre-clinical research of inhalable nanomedicine aims to find its way in clinical translation through addressing the challenges, conquering the limitations of overcoming drug resistance, improving therapeutic outcomes, and focusing on the preferential accumulation of inhalable drugs to lung cancer cells rather than healthy cells. Worth mentioning is that the production of nanomedicine is very sophisticated and is a multistage process, thus limiting the scale-up production and reproducibility of the nanomedicine. Moreover, further tailoring of nanomedicine parameters is required (e.g., loading efficiency, organ biodistribution, and pharmacokinetics).

8.8 FINANCIAL AND COMPETING INTEREST DISCLOSURE

The authors have no other relevant affiliations or financial involvement with any organization or entity with a financial interest in or financial conflict with the subject matter or materials discussed in the manuscript apart from those disclosed. No writing assistance was utilized in the production of this manuscript.

REFERENCES

1. Alberg AJ, Brock MV, Ford JG, Samet JM, Spivack SD. Epidemiology of lung cancer: Diagnosis and management of lung cancer, 3rd ed: American college of chest physicians evidence-based clinical practice guidelines. *Chest* 2013;143:e1S–e29S.
2. Eldridge L. *What are the leading causes of lung cancer?* Verywell; 2017.
3. Centers for Disease Control and Prevention. *What are the risk factors for lung cancer?* Centers for Disease Control and Prevention; 2017.
4. Wu K, Wong E, and Chaudhry S. Lung cancer pathogenesis. *McMaster Pathophysiology Review* 2012.
5. Murthy SV. *Medical school pathology review.* In slide share; 2013.

6. American Cancer Society. *What is non-small cell lung cancer?* Atlanta, GA: American Cancer Society; 2016.

7. Zappa C, Mousa SA. Non-small cell lung cancer: Current treatment and future advances. *Translational Lung Cancer Research* 2016;5(3):288–300.

8. Midthun DE. Early detection of lung cancer. *F1000Research* 2016;5:1–11.

9. Ellis PM, Vandermeer R. Delays in the diagnosis of lung cancer. *Journal of Thoracic Disease* 2011;3(3):183–8.

10. American Cancer Society. *Treatment choices for non-small cell lung cancer, by stage.* Atlanta, GA: American Cancer Society; 2017.

11. American Cancer Society. *Chemotherapy for non-small cell lung cancer.* Atlanta, GA: American Cancer Society; 2017.

12. Einhorn LH. First-line chemotherapy for non–small-cell lung cancer: Is there a superior regimen based on histology? *Journal of Clinical Oncology* 2008;26(21):3485–6.

13. Chidambaram M, Manavalan R, Kathiresan K. Nanotherapeutics to overcome conventional cancer chemotherapy limitations. *Journal of Pharmacy & Pharmaceutical Sciences* 2011;14(1):67–77.

14. UKEssays. Chemotherapy And Selective Toxicity [Internet]. November 2013. [Accessed 23 March 2015]; Available from: https://www.ukessays.com/essays/biology/chemotherapy-and-selective-toxicity-biology-essay.php?vref=1.

15. Shanker M, Willcutts D, Roth JA, Ramesh R. Drug resistance in lung cancer. *Lung Cancer: Targets and Therapy* 2010;1:23–36.

16. Patil JS, Sarasija S. Pulmonary drug delivery strategies: A concise, systematic review. *Lung India: Official Organ of Indian Chest Society* 2012;29(1):44–9.

17. Sana S, Khwaja O, Qazi Mohammad Sajid J, Mohammad Amjad K, Usman S, Khan MKA, Mohd. Haris S, Salman A. Advances and implications in nanotechnology for lung cancer management. *Current Drug Metabolism* 2017;18:30–8.

18. Agu RU, Ugwoke MI, Armand M, Kinget R, Verbeke N. The lung as a route for systemic delivery of therapeutic proteins and peptides. *Respiratory Research* 2001;2(4):198–209.

19. Paranjpe M, Müller-Goymann CC. Nanoparticle-mediated pulmonary drug delivery: A review. *International Journal of Molecular Sciences* 2014;15(4):5852–73.

20. Abdelaziz HM, Gaber M, Abd-Elwakil MM, Mabrouk MT, Elgohary MM, Kamel NM, Kabary DM, Freag MS, Samaha MW, Mortada SM, Elkhodairy KA, Fang J-Y, Elzoghby AO. Inhalable particulate drug delivery systems for lung cancer therapy: Nanoparticles, microparticles, nanocomposites and nanoaggregates. *Journal of Controlled Release* 2018;269:374–92.

21. Sou T, Meeusen EN, de Veer M, Morton DAV, Kaminskas LM, McIntosh MP. New developments in dry powder pulmonary vaccine delivery. *Trends in Biotechnology* 2011;29(4):191–8.

22. Zarogoulidis P, Chatzaki E, Porpodis K, Domvri K, Hohenforst-Schmidt W, Goldberg EP, Karamanos N, Zarogoulidis K. Inhaled chemotherapy in lung cancer: Future concept of nanomedicine. *International Journal of Nanomedicine* 2012;7:1551–72.

23. El-Sherbiny IM, El-Baz NM, Yacoub MH. Inhaled Nano- and microparticles for drug delivery. *Global Cardiology Science and Practice* 2015;2015(1):2. https://doi.org/10.5339/GCSP.2015.2.

24. Bardoliwala D, Javia A, Ghosh S, Misra A, Sawant K. Formulation and clinical perspectives of inhalation-based nanocarrier delivery: A new archetype in lung cancer treatment. *Therapeutic Delivery* 2021;12(5):397–418.

25. Ibrahim M, Verma R, Garcia-Contreras L. Inhalation drug delivery devices: Technology update. *Medical Devices (Auckland, NZ)* 2015;8:131–9.

26. Moreno-Sastre M, Pastor M, Salomon CJ, Esquisabel A, Pedraz JL. Pulmonary drug delivery: A review on nanocarriers for antibacterial chemotherapy. *Journal of Antimicrobial Chemotherapy* 2015;70(11):2945–55.

27. Lee W-H, Loo C-Y, Traini D, Young PM. Inhalation of nanoparticle-based drug for lung cancer treatment: Advantages and challenges. *Asian Journal of Pharmaceutical Sciences* 2015;10(6):481–9.

28. Goel A, Baboota S, Sahni JK, Ali J. Exploring targeted pulmonary delivery for treatment of lung cancer. *International Journal of Pharmaceutical Investigation* 2013;3(1):8–14.

29. Finot P-A, Bujard E, Mottu F, Mauron J. Availability of the true Schiff's bases of lysine. Chemical evaluation of the Schiff's base between lysine and lactose in milk. In: Friedman M, editor. *Protein crosslinking: Nutritional and medical consequences.* Boston, MA: Springer US; 1977, pp. 343–65.

30. Ahmad J, Akhter S, Rizwanullah M, Amin S, Rahman M, Ahmad MZ, Rizvi MA, Kamal MA, Ahmad FJ. Nanotechnology-based inhalation treatments for lung cancer: State of the art. *Nanotechnology, Science and Applications* 2015;8:55–66.

31. Jun Yan Chan E, Hui W. Introduction for design of nanoparticle based drug delivery systems. *Current Pharmaceutical Design* 2017;23(14):2108–12.

32. Youngren-Ortiz SR, Hill DB, Hoffmann PR, Morris KR, Barrett EG, Forest MG, Chougule MB. Development of optimized, inhalable, gemcitabine-loaded gelatin nanocarriers for lung cancer. *Journal of Aerosol Medicine and Pulmonary Drug Delivery* 2017;30(5):299–321.

33. Elgohary MM, Helmy MW, Abdelfattah E-ZA, Ragab DM, Mortada SM, Fang J-Y, Elzoghby AO. Targeting sialic acid residues on lung cancer cells by inhalable boronic acid-decorated albumin nanocomposites for combined chemo/herbal therapy. *Journal of Controlled Release: Official Journal of the Controlled Release Society* 2018;285:230–43.

34. Abd Elwakil MM, Mabrouk MT, Helmy MW, Abdelfattah EA, Khiste SK, Elkhodairy KA, Elzoghby AO. Inhalable lactoferrin-chondroitin nanocomposites for combined delivery of doxorubicin and ellagic acid to lung carcinoma. *Nanomedicine* 2018;13:2015–35.

35. Kabary DM, Helmy MW, Abdelfattah EA, Fang JY, Elkhodairy KA, Elzoghby AO. Inhalable multi-compartmental phospholipid enveloped lipid core nanocomposites for localized mTOR inhibitor/herbal combined therapy of lung carcinoma. *European Journal of Pharmaceutics and Biopharmaceutics: Official Journal of Arbeitsgemeinschaft fur Pharmazeutische Verfahrenstechnik Ev* 2018;130:152–64.

36. Abdelaziz HM, Elzoghby AO, Helmy MW, Abdelfattah E-ZA, Fang J-Y, Samaha MW, Freag MS. Inhalable lactoferrin/chondroitin-functionalized monoolein nanocomposites for localized lung cancer targeting. *ACS Biomaterials Science and Engineering* 2020;6(2):1030–42.

37. Rezazadeh M, Davatsaz Z, Emami J, Hasanzadeh F, Jahanian-Najafabadi A. Preparation and characterization of spray-dried inhalable powders containing polymeric micelles for pulmonary delivery of paclitaxel in lung cancer. *Journal of Pharmacy & Pharmaceutical Sciences* 2018;21(1s):200s–14s.

38. Zhong Q. Co-spray dried mannitol/poly(amidoamine)-doxorubicin dry-powder inhaler formulations for lung adenocarcinoma: Morphology, in vitro evaluation, and aerodynamic performance. *AAPS PharmSciTech* 2018;19(2):531–40.

39. Zhong Q, da Rocha SR. Poly(amidoamine) dendrimer-doxorubicin conjugates: In vitro characteristics and pseudosolution formulation in pressurized metered-dose inhalers. *Molecular Pharmaceutics* 2016;13(3):1058–72.

40. Zhong Q, Humia BV, Punjabi AR, Padilha FF, da Rocha SRP. The interaction of dendrimer-doxorubicin conjugates with a model pulmonary epithelium and their cosolvent-free, pseudo-solution formulations in pressurized metered-dose inhalers. *European Journal of Pharmaceutical Sciences: Official Journal of the European Federation for Pharmaceutical Sciences* 2017;109:86–95.

41. Ishiguro S, Cai S, Uppalapati D, Turner K, Zhang T, Forrest WC, Forrest ML, Tamura M. Intratracheal administration of hyaluronan-cisplatin conjugate nanoparticles significantly attenuates lung cancer growth in mice. *Pharmaceutical Research* 2016;33(10):2517–29.

42. Kim I, Byeon HJ, Kim TH, Lee ES, Oh KT, Shin BS, Lee KC, Youn YS. Doxorubicin-loaded highly porous large PLGA microparticles as a sustained- release inhalation system for the treatment of metastatic lung cancer. *Biomaterials* 2012;33(22):5574–83.

43. Kim I, Byeon HJ, Kim TH, Lee ES, Oh KT, Shin BS, Lee KC, Youn YS. Doxorubicin-loaded porous PLGA microparticles with surface attached TRAIL for the inhalation treatment of metastatic lung cancer. *Biomaterials* 2013;34(27):6444–53.

44. Li W, Chen S-Q, Zhang L, Zhang Y, Yang X, Xie B, Guo J, He Y, Wang C. Inhalable functional mixed-polymer microspheres to enhance doxorubicin release behavior for lung cancer treatment. *Colloids and Surfaces B, Biointerfaces* 2020;196:111350.

45. Wu D, Wang C, Yang J, Wang H, Han H, Zhang A, Yang Y, Li Q. Improving the intracellular drug concentration in lung cancer treatment through the codelivery of doxorubicin and miR-519c mediated by porous PLGA microparticle. *Molecular Pharmaceutics* 2016;13(11):3925–33.

46. Zhu L, Li M, Liu X, Du L, Jin Y. Inhalable oridonin-loaded poly(lactic-co-glycolic)acid large porous microparticles for in situ treatment of primary non-small cell lung cancer. *Acta Pharmacologica Sinica B* 2017;7(1):80–90.

47. Zhu L, Li M, Liu X, Jin Y. Drug-loaded PLGA electrospraying porous microspheres for the local therapy of primary lung cancer via pulmonary delivery. *ACS Omega* 2017;2(5):2273–9.

48. Xu PY, Kankala RK, Pan YJ, Yuan H, Wang SB, Chen AZ. Overcoming multidrug resistance through inhalable siRNA nanoparticles-decorated porous microparticles based on supercritical fluid technology. *International Journal of Nanomedicine* 2018;13:4685–98.

49. Emami F, Mostafavi Yazdi SJ, Na DH. Poly(lactic acid)/poly(lactic-co-glycolic acid) particulate carriers for pulmonary drug delivery. *Journal of Pharmaceutical Investigation* 2019;49(4):427–42.

50. El-Gendy N, Berkland C. Combination chemotherapeutic dry powder aerosols via controlled nanoparticle agglomeration. *Pharmaceutical Research* 2009;26(7):1752–63.

51. Abdulbaqi IM, Assi RA, Yaghmur A, Darwis Y, Mohtar N, Parumasivam T, Saqallah FG, Wahab HA. Pulmonary delivery of anticancer drugs via lipid-based nanocarriers for the treatment of lung cancer: An update. *Pharmaceuticals* 2021;14(8):725.

52. Kaur P, Mishra V, Shunmugaperumal T, Goyal AK, Ghosh G, Rath G. Inhalable spray dried lipidnanoparticles for the co-delivery of paclitaxel and doxorubicin in lung cancer. *Journal of Drug Delivery Science and Technology* 2020;56:101502.

53. Jyoti K, Kaur K, Pandey RS, Jain UK, Chandra R, Madan J. Inhalable nanostructured lipid particles of 9-bromo-noscapine, a tubulin-binding cytotoxic agent: In vitro and in vivo studies. *Journal of Colloid and Interface Science* 2015;445:219–30.

54. Ragab DM, Rohani S. Cubic magnetically guided nanoaggregates for inhalable drug delivery: In vitro magnetic aerosol deposition study. *AAPS PharmSciTech* 2013;14(3):977–93.

55. Tewes F, Ehrhardt C, Healy AM. Superparamagnetic iron oxide nanoparticles (SPIONs)-loaded Trojan microparticles for targeted aerosol delivery to the lung. *European Journal of Pharmaceutics and Biopharmaceutics* 2014;86:98–104.

56. Mohammed MA, Syeda JTM, Wasan KM, Wasan EK. An overview of chitosan nanoparticles and its application in non-parenteral drug delivery. *Pharmaceutics* 2017;9(4):53.

57. Rosiere R, Van Woensel M, Gelbcke M, Mathieu V, Hecq J, Mathivet T, Vermeersch M, Van Antwerpen P, Amighi K, Wauthoz N. New folate-grafted chitosan derivative to improve delivery of paclitaxel-loaded solid lipid nanoparticles for lung tumor therapy by inhalation. *Molecular Pharmaceutics* 2018;15(3):899–910.

58. Freitas ED, Moura CF, Jr., Kerwald J, Beppu MM. An overview of current knowledge on the properties, synthesis and applications of quaternary chitosan derivatives. *Polymers (Basel)* 2020;12(12):2878.

59. Li W, Li Y, Liu Z, Kerdsakundee N, Zhang M, Zhang F, Liu X, Bauleth-Ramos T, Lian W, Mäkilä E, Kemell M, Ding Y, Sarmento B, Wiwattanapatapee R, Salonen J, Zhang H, Hirvonen JT, Liu D, Deng X, Santos HA. Hierarchical structured and programmed vehicles deliver drugs locally to inflamed sites of intestine. *Biomaterials* 2018;185: 322–32.

60. Chen R, Xu L, Fan Q, Li M, Wang J, Wu L, Li W, Duan J, Chen Z. Hierarchical pulmonary target nanoparticles via inhaled administration for anticancer drug delivery. *Drug Delivery* 2017;24(1):1191–203.

61. Gomez AI, Acosta MF, Muralidharan P, Yuan JX, Black SM, Hayes D, Jr., Mansour HM. Advanced spray dried proliposomes of amphotericin B lung surfactant-mimic phospholipid microparticles/nanoparticles as dry powder inhalers for targeted pulmonary drug delivery. *Pulmonary Pharmacology and Therapeutics* 2020;64:101975.

62. Meenach SA, Anderson KW, Zach Hilt J, McGarry RC, Mansour HM. Characterization and aerosol dispersion performance of advanced spray-dried chemotherapeutic pegylated phospholipid particles for dry powder inhalation delivery in lung cancer. *European Journal of Pharmaceutical Sciences: Official Journal of the European Federation for Pharmaceutical Sciences* 2013;49(4):699–711.

63. Meenach SA, Anderson KW, Hilt JZ, McGarry RC, Mansour HM. High-performing dry powder inhalers of paclitaxel DPPC/DPPG lung surfactant-mimic multifunctional particles in lung cancer: Physicochemical characterization, in vitro aerosol dispersion, and cellular studies. *AAPS PharmSciTech* 2014;15(6):1574–87.

64. Yan Y, Zhou K, Xiong H, Miller JB, Motea EA, Boothman DA, Liu L, Siegwart DJ. Aerosol delivery of stabilized polyester-siRNA nanoparticles to silence gene expression in orthotopic lung tumors. *Biomaterials* 2017;118:84–93.

65. Yan Y, Liu L, Xiong H, Miller JB, Zhou K, Kos P, Huffman KE, Elkassih S, Norman JW, Carstens R, Kim J, Minna JD, Siegwart DJ. Functional polyesters enable selective siRNA delivery to lung cancer over matched normal cells. *Proceedings of the National Academy of Sciences of the United States of America* 2016;113(39):E5702–E10.

66. Xu C, Tian H, Sun H, Jiao Z, Zhang Y, Chen X. A pH sensitive co-delivery system of siRNA and doxorubicin for pulmonary administration to B16F10 metastatic lung cancer. *RSC Advances* 2015;5(125):103380–5.

67. Ishiguro S, Alhakamy NA, Uppalapati D, Delzeit J, Berkland CJ, Tamura M. Combined local pulmonary and systemic delivery of AT2R gene by modified TAT peptide nanoparticles attenuates both murine and human lung carcinoma xenografts in mice. *Journal of Pharmaceutical Sciences* 2017;106(1):385–94.

68. Xu C, Wang P, Zhang J, Tian H, Park K, Chen X. Pulmonary codelivery of doxorubicin and siRNA by pH-sensitive nanoparticles for therapy of metastatic lung cancer. *Small* 2015;11(34):4321–33.

69. Price DN, Stromberg LR, Kunda NK, Muttil P. In vivo pulmonary delivery and magnetic-targeting of dry powder nano-in-microparticles. *Molecular Pharmaceutics* 2017;14(12):4741–50.

70. Silva AS, Sousa AM, Cabral RP, Silva MC, Costa C, Miguel SP, Bonifacio VDB, Casimiro T, Correia IJ, Aguiar-Ricardo A. Aerosolizable gold nano-in-micro dry powder formulations for theragnosis and lung delivery. *International Journal of Pharmaceutics* 2017;519(1–2):240–9.

71. Dufort S, Bianchi A, Henry M, Lux F, Le Duc G, Josserand V, Louis C, Perriat P, Cremillieux Y, Tillement O, Coll JL. Nebulized gadolinium-based nanoparticles: A theranostic approach for lung tumor imaging and radiosensitization. *Small (Weinheim an der Bergstrasse, Germany)* 2015;11(2):215–21.

72. Stocke NA, Sethi P, Jyoti A, Chan R, Arnold SM, Hilt JZ, Upreti M. Toxicity evaluation of magnetic hyperthermia induced by remote actuation of magnetic nanoparticles in 3D micrometastasic tumor tissue analogs for triple negative breast cancer. *Biomaterials* 2017;120:115–25.

73. Dames P, Gleich B, Flemmer A, Hajek K, Seidl N, Wiekhorst F, Eberbeck D, Bittmann I, Bergemann C, Weyh T, Trahms L, Rosenecker J, Rudolph C. Targeted delivery of magnetic aerosol droplets to the lung. *Nature Nanotechnology* 2007;2(8):495–9.

Thin-Film Freeze-Drying Process for Versatile Particles for Inhalation Drug Delivery

9

Chaeho Moon, Sawittree Sahakijpijarn, and Robert O. Williams III[1]

Contents

DOI: 10.1201/9781003182566-12

9.1 INTRODUCTION

Inhalation drug delivery has multiple advantages, including effective targeted administration to the lungs, fast absorption, and the prevention of first-pass metabolism.[1] However, until recently, several challenges for inhalation drug delivery have remained. Inhalation drug delivery has been limited to the treatment of certain lung diseases (e.g., asthma or chronic obstructive pulmonary disease (COPD). In addition, the efficacy of these treatments was decreased by poor and variable drug deposition in the lungs, as well as high deposition in the oropharynx region.[2–4] These challenges were overcome as technologies advanced. Newly developed devices in pressurized metered dose inhalers (pMDI), dry powder inhalers (DPI), nebulizers, soft-mist inhalers, as well as smart inhalers enhanced delivered dose levels, enhanced dose consistency, and improved patient compliance. Therefore, these developments allowed for more efficient and effective delivery of inhaled drugs.[5]

In addition to device technology, formulation technology has also advanced greatly in the last decade. Newly developed formulation technologies – e.g., PulmoSphere®, Technosphere®, iSPERSE™ (inhaled small particles easily respirable and emitted), or PRINT® (particle replication in non-wetting templates) – allow for higher drug loading in dry powders, enhance consistency through DPI and pMDI, enhance aerosolization, and allow for new types of inhaled drugs.[5] Inhalation drug delivery has become more advantageous as a result.

Thin-film freeze-drying (TFFD) is a particle engineering technology (i.e., another formulation technology advancement) that can be applied to the development of diverse drugs not only for oral or injectable dosages but also for inhalation. TFFD has been applied to various types of poorly water-soluble, small molecule drugs to enhance their solubility and aerosolization.[6-10] TFFD has also been applied to macromolecules to formulate them as dry powders to enhance their stability.[11-14]

TFFD utilizes a high degree of supercooling associated with ultra-rapid freezing, with rates up to 10^4 K/s.[13] In this process, solutions that contain drugs and excipients are applied (generally through syringes or tubes) onto a hollow, rotating, stainless steel drum. This drum is cooled using liquid nitrogen that flows into the drum. The temperature of the cooled drum can be as low as -190 °C, while typical processing temperatures are controlled between -40 °C and -160 °C, depending on the specific application.

The processing temperatures of TFFD are closely related to the desired degree of supercooling, which in turn affects the number of solvent crystals and the growth rate.[15] In TFFD, higher processing temperatures are associated with less supercooling, while lower processing temperatures are associated with more supercooling. Such extreme supercooling increases the nucleation of frozen solvent particles and hinders particle growth in the frozen solvent.[15] Once the freezing process begins, the solute in the unfrozen solvent domains is supersaturated and thus forced to precipitate. This supercooling also minimizes particle growth in the unfrozen domains, which occurs through Ostwald ripening. As described in Figure 9.1, the high degree of supercooling at lower

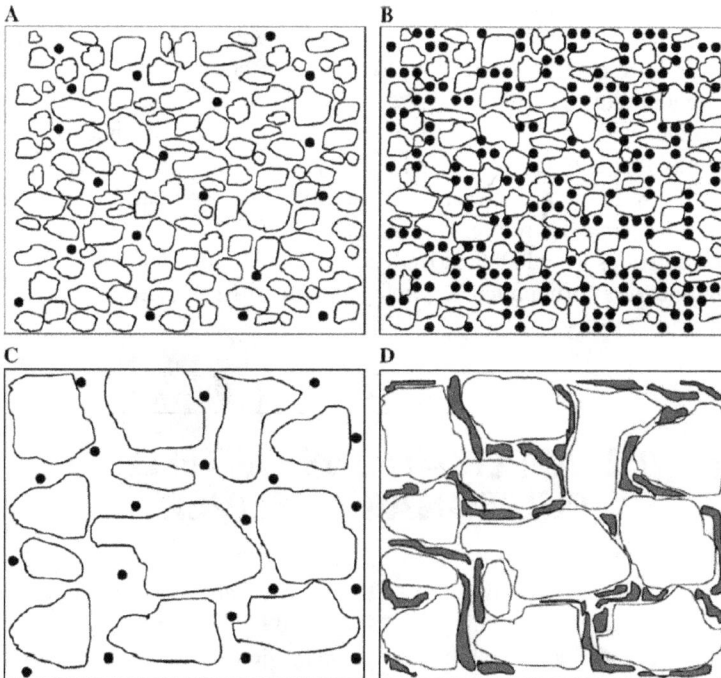

FIGURE 9.1 Frozen morphologies of dilute solution with high supercooling (A), concentrated solution with high supercooling (B), dilute solution with low supercooling (C), and concentrated solution with low supercooling (D). Amorphous ice particles are represented as white domains, and solute precipitate is represented by solid dots or gray regions.[16] Reproduced with permission from Elsevier.

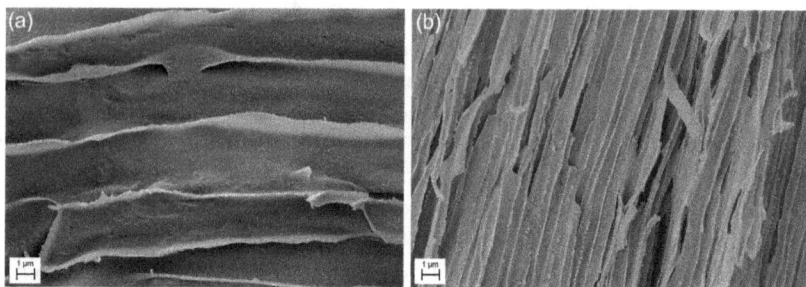

FIGURE 9.2   SEM images of TFFD mannitol–lysozyme (50/50 w/w) processed at -50 °C (A) and -120 °C (B).

processing temperatures generates thinner frozen solvent domains and the formation of more nuclei and more solid particles. The scanning electron microscope (SEM) images in Figure 9.2 show that the lower processing temperature (-120 °C) of TFFD mannitol–lysozyme (50/50 w/w) at 10% w/v solid loading produced smaller ice channels than the higher processing temperature (-50 °C).

Amorphous materials can be produced if the degree of supercooling is high enough to fully prevent the nucleation of crystals due to vitrification of the solution.[17] TFFD was initially applied to overcome the poor water solubility of drugs by forming amorphous solid dispersions (ASDs) of the drug. Several poorly water-soluble drugs (e.g., danazol,[18] fenofibrate,[19] repaglinide,[20] itraconazole[21]) have been successfully formulated as ASDs to enhance their solubility. However, TFFD produces nanoparticles of drugs and excipients that are suitable for delivery by inhalation. This is due to the unique characteristics of TFFD that prevent particle growth through ultra-rapid freezing with extreme supercooling. Therefore, the applications of TFFD was expanded to the production formulations for inhalation. In this chapter, TFFD is discussed as an advanced powder engineering formulation technology that can be utilized in several ways for inhalation drug delivery.

9.2 APPLICATIONS OF TFFD TO PULMONARY DELIVERY

The powder formulations produced by TFFD can be applied to pulmonary delivery in a few different ways via nebulizers, pMDIs, and DPIs. To evaluate if these powder formulations are suitable for pulmonary delivery, aerosolization of the formulations should be assessed. The Next Generation Pharmaceutical Impactor (NGI) is a cascade impactor to measure the aerosol performance of the formulations *in vitro*.[22] It is connected to a flow controller and a vacuum and intended to operate at an inlet flow rate between 30 and 100 L/min with a single vacuum connected. Different size ranges of aerosols can be deposited on seven different stages of collection cups and a micro-orifice collector (MOC) of the NGI, and the particle size distribution of the formulation

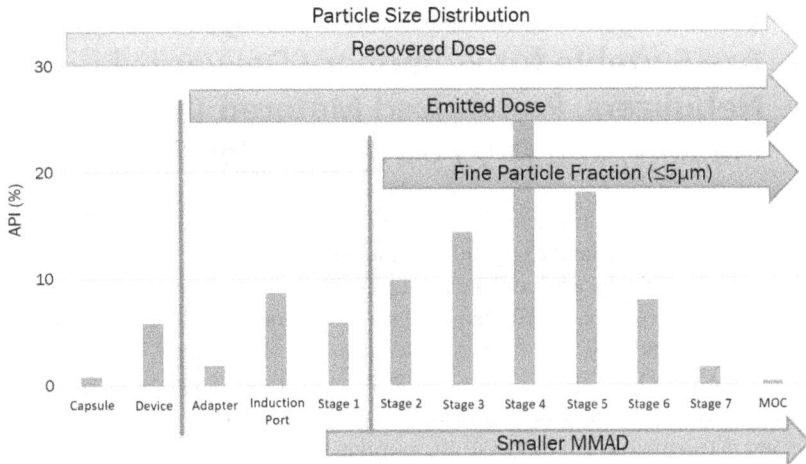

FIGURE 9.3 Description of parameters for aerosol performance based on NGI data. (MOC is micro-orifice collector; API is active pharmaceutical ingredient, MMAD is mass median aerodynamic diameter.)

can be calculated after drug recovery from capsule, device, adaptor, induction port, and each stage of NGI as shown in Figure 9.3. The larger particles deposit on stage 1, and the smaller particles deposit on MOC. At the inlet flow rate of 60 L/min, a portion of particles on stage 2 and the rest of smaller particles are a size range below 5 μm of mass median aerodynamic diameter (MMAD), which is considered the fine particle fraction (FPF). Table 9.1 summarizes the definition of typical parameters used to describe the aerosol performance of an inhaled product. These parameters are used to describe the aerosol performance of the formulations described in this chapter.

TABLE 9.1 Definition of parameters used to describe the aerosol performance of an inhaled product

PARAMETERS	DEFINITION	REFERENCE
MMAD	The mass median aerodynamic diameter (MMAD) divides the aerosol size distribution in half. It is the diameter at which 50% of the particles of an aerosol by mass are larger and 50% are smaller.	[1]
GSD	The geometric standard deviation (GSD) measures the dispersion of particle diameter and is defined as the ratio of the median diameter to the diameter at ±1 standard deviation from the median diameter.	[1]
FPF	The fine particle fraction (FPF) is the mass percentage of the drug particles below 5 μm in aerodynamic diameter	[23]
ED	The emitted dose (ED) is the mass of the drug emitted per actuation that is actually available for inhalation at the mouth	[1]

9.2.1 Brittle-Matrix Powders Made by TFFD Are Suitable for Pulmonary Delivery via Nebulizers, Pressurized Metered Dose Inhalers, and Dry Powder Inhalers

As described above, the ultra-rapid freezing of the drug and excipient solution produces nanoparticles of the drug and excipients. These nanoparticles are linked as nanostructured aggregates, and they agglomerate as micron-size particles in a brittle-matrix powder.[8,24] Figure 9.4 shows that TFFD can produce brittle-matrix powders from both small molecules (e.g., remdesivir) and macromolecules (e.g., lysozymes).[13,25] Brittle-matrix powders made by TFFD have unique physical properties, including large geometric particle size, high porosity, and high surface area.[8,24] These properties provide benefits on the aerodynamic properties of the powder, rendering it suitable for pulmonary drug delivery.[8,24] Several studies have demonstrated the feasibility of delivering brittle-matrix powders through various pulmonary delivery systems, including nebulizers, pressurized metered-dose inhalers, and dry powder inhalers.

9.2.1.1 Inhaled drug delivery via nebulizers

Aqueous-based formulations are often developed in the early stages of inhaled product development. Compared to solid dosage forms, liquid formulations are simpler and can be manufactured faster because they do not require additional processes (e.g., drying). Liquid formulations also avoid particle size reductions that can affect the stability of some compounds, especially biologics. However, some compounds, such as poorly water-soluble drugs, cannot be developed as solutions for nebulization due to their physical instability in aqueous conditions.

By employing ultra-rapid freezing, TFFD has been used to prepare dry powders for reconstitution and nebulization as brittle-matrix powders. Brittle-matrix powders produced using TFFD can enhance the solubility and dispersibility of drugs in an aqueous diluent.[26] Sinswat et al. used TFFD to develop a pulmonary delivery system for

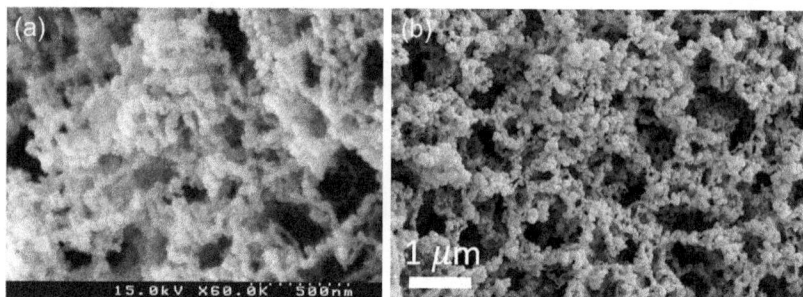

FIGURE 9.4 Brittle-matrix particle morphology of TFFD lysozyme (5 mg/mL) (A), reproduced with permission from Springer Nature, and TFFD remdesivir–Captisol® (20/80 w/w) (B). Reproduced from MDPI (open access).

tacrolimus.[26] Tacrolimus is an immunosuppressant widely used for the treatment of organ rejection after transplantation.[27] Oral formulations of tacrolimus have shown low and erratic bioavailability due to their inefficient absorption in the gastrointestinal tract and due to first-pass metabolism.[28] The long-term survival rate after lung transplant rejection has remained low.[29] This results from poor penetration of the drug in the lung following oral administration.[30]

A TFFD formulation of tacrolimus was prepared as a nanostructured brittle-matrix powder consisting of amorphous tacrolimus and lactose. This formulation could disperse easily in water at 10 mg/mL for nebulization.[26] In general, formulations containing nanoparticles are not thermodynamically stable because nanoparticles tend to reduce free energy through the growth and aggregation of particles.[31] The presence of surfactants and stabilizing polymers typically help minimize particle interactions by providing steric or ionic hindrance. Such stabilizers can cause alveolar epithelial damage, and they have not been proven safe for pulmonary drug delivery. Therefore, this study did not incorporate a stabilizer in the formulation.[31]

The physical stability of tacrolimus nanoparticles was investigated over the course of 30 min after dispersion. Particle size analysis using laser scattering measurements demonstrated that the tacrolimus dispersion exhibited a monodisperse distribution with a mean particle diameter of 239.2 nm at 5 min after dispersion. However, the analysis also showed a bimodal dispersion with a larger particle diameter of 240–352 nm at 30 min after dispersion.[31] To avoid any particle size change during nebulization, the formulation was administrated within 15 min after dispersion.[31] *In vitro* aerosolization testing using a NGI demonstrated that the nebulization of an aqueous TFFD tacrolimus dispersion (via an Aeroneb® Pro vibrating mesh nebulizer) exhibited acceptable aerosol performance (i.e., 4.06 μm MMAD, 2.7 GSD, 46.1% FPF, and 50.5% ED).[31]

In vitro dissolution tests showed that the formulation reached supersaturation in simulated lung fluid, which is 11 times higher than the equilibrium solubility of the crystalline form. Moreover, the stability of TFFD tacrolimus powder for reconstitution was investigated after storage under ambient conditions. The formulation was chemically stable with no change in drug potency. The TFFD tacrolimus also maintained its physical stability, remained amorphous, and could achieve supersaturation in simulated lung fluid, which contained magnesium chloride, sodium chloride, potassium chloride, sodium phosphate, sodium sulphate, calcium chloride, sodium acetate, sodium bicarbonate and sodium citrate dihydrate, protein, L-α-phosphatidylcholine,[32] throughout the period of three months.[33]

In vivo pharmacokinetic studies in mice showed that, compared to crystalline formulations, the TFFD amorphous tacrolimus dispersion exhibited lower T_{max} and higher C_{max} in both lung tissue and blood after a single dose through pulmonary administration via an Aeroneb® Pro and a four-port nose-only dosing chamber. The increases in solubility, wettability, and the dissolution rate of the amorphous nanoparticulate TFFD tacrolimus formulation provided superior drug bioavailability to the lung epithelial layer and a faster absorption rate compared to the crystalline formulation. However, there was no significant difference in drug absorption in lung tissue and in systemic circulation. One possible explanation that was provided for this observation is that the supersaturation occurs only briefly during the absorption phase before the elimination phase began.

The pharmacokinetic profile of the TFFD tacrolimus formulation was further investigated in both transplant and non-transplant rat models. The previous study from Ide et al. reported that in an allografted lung, a tacrolimus concentration of 270 ng/g is required to provide sufficient immunosuppression to prevent transplant rejection. Watts et al. reported no difference in overall lung deposition, blood, and lung levels between transplant and non-transplant rats.[31] Single-dose pulmonary administration of a tacrolimus dispersion can achieve a mean peak transplanted lung concentration of 399.8 ± 29.2 ng/g and a mean peak blood concentration of 4.88 ± 1.6 ng/mL (Figure 9.11A).[31] The drug levels in lung tissue were qualified using liquid chromatography/mass spectrometry (LC/MS) after a liquid extraction procedure (Figure 9.11B), while the systemic drug concentrations were analyzed by a Pro-Trac™ II FK506 Enzyme/linked Immunosorbent Assay (ELISA) kit (Diasorin Inc., Stillwater, MN).[31] Pulmonary drug delivery reduced systemic drug levels, with a lung-to-blood ratio of 55:1 in non-transplant rats and 59:1 in transplant rats.[31] A low systemic level of tacrolimus in the rat study minimizes the potential for adverse side effects. This is a promising strategy to increase patient compliance and improve clinical outcomes for the maintenance use of tacrolimus.

The safety and systemic elimination of TFFD tacrolimus were also investigated after pulmonary administration of a nebulized tacrolimus dispersion once daily for 28 consecutive days in Sprague Dawley (SD) rats. A complete blood count (CBC) and serum chemistry analysis demonstrated no clinically significant difference in liver and kidney function both one day and one week after the final pulmonary administration of normal saline and a tacrolimus colloidal dispersion via a nebulizer.[33] Likewise, histological analysis showed no evidence of inflammation, cell lysis, or histologic lesions in the lung, liver, spleen, or kidney tissues. Pulmonary administration of TFFD tacrolimus caused minimal or no pulmonary irritation, and no significant change in macrophage, monocyte, or mucus production was observed compared to the control group.[33] Tacrolimus is lipophilic by nature. Therefore, compared to a single dose, multiple dosing through pulmonary administration showed a significant increase in drug levels in the lung, and the systemic levels measured at trough were still lower than the trough after oral dosing.[33]

Recently, Das et al. compared the efficacy of a nebulized TFFD tacrolimus dispersion to the intramuscular injection of tacrolimus for the prevention of acute allograft rejection in an allogenic rodent lung transplant model.[34] Histological analysis revealed that rats treated by intramuscular injection and rats treated with a nebulized TFFD tacrolimus dispersion showed similar histological grades of rejection (mean scores of 3.4 ± 0.6 and 4.6 ± 0.9, respectively). These rejection levels are lower than the inhaled lactose group (a mean score of 11.38 ± 0.5, $p = .07$).[34] Therefore, pulmonary delivery of the TFFD tacrolimus dispersion showed similar efficacy in preventing acute rejection in addition to lower trough levels of tacrolimus in both blood and kidney tissues compared to the intramuscular injection of tacrolimus (29.2 vs. 118.6 ng/g, $p < .001$ in the kidney; 1.5 vs. 4.8 ng/mL, $p = .01$ in the blood).[34]

Another study by Yang et al. also showed the feasibility of using TFFD to develop nebulized formulations of poorly water-soluble drugs.[35] TFFD was used to prepare an itraconazole powder for reconstitution without the addition of a synthetic polymer or surfactant. Safety concerns arose because a surface-active excipient in an inhaled formulation may affect the function of the cell lipid bilayer membrane.[36]

Itraconazole was combined with mannitol and lecithin (in a 1:0.5:0.2 weight ratio, respectively) to prepare nanostructured aggregates in an amorphous solid solution.[35]

After reconstitution, a colloidal dispersion of itraconazole was delivered to the lung via an Aeroneb® Pro. The nebulization of the itraconazole colloidal dispersion exhibited optimal aerosol performance (2.38 μm MMAD, 2.56 GSD, and 66.96% FPF of the delivered dose). These nanostructured aggregates also wetted and dissolved rapidly in simulated lung fluid, and they subsequently produced a supersaturation level (27-times higher than its crystalline solubility) within 15 min.

A single-dose pharmacokinetic study in mice showed that the TFFD formulation exhibited high lung deposition and high systemic absorption, with a C_{max} of 1.6 g/mL in 2 h. This fast absorption rate and improved bioavailability are attributed to the formulation's small colloidal particle size, the large surface area of the TFFD nanostructured aggregates, and the high supersaturation level of the itraconazole solid solution.[35]

9.2.1.2 Inhaled drug delivery via pressurized metered dose inhalers (pMDI)

In pMDI systems, drugs are formulated either in solution or in suspension with a high pressure propellant. In general, drugs that are slightly soluble in hydrofluoroalkane (HFA) propellant are prepared as solutions with the addition of a co-solvent such as ethanol. Drugs that exhibit negligible solubility in HFA–ethanol co-solvent mixtures are prepared as micron-sized suspensions in HFA. To deliver drug particles to the deep lung, aerosols generated by the pMDI must fall within the range of respirable size (i.e., 1–5 μm MMAD). However, due to the small size of the drug particles, it is well known that pMDI suspensions have the propensity to exhibit physical stability problems such as particle growth (Ostwald-ripening), agglomeration upon settling, flocculation, and sediment compaction. These physical instabilities can cause inconsistent aerosol performance and variation in the emitted dose.[37] Moreover, mass loading in a pMDI formulation is limited because it affects the aerosol performance of the formulation. It was reported that a mass loading of up to 5% w/v caused an increase beyond the optimal range of the aerodynamic diameter.

Particle engineering techniques have been used to modify particle morphology to improve the colloidal stability of the primary particles without the addition of surfactants.[37,38] Engstrom et al. developed a new concept for dispersing flocculating nanorods in propellant to prepare stable suspensions for pMDI delivery. Engstrom et al. also compared the stability of a bovine serum albumin suspension generated from milling, spray drying, and TFFD.[39] TFFD produced low-density BSA nanorods measuring 50–100 nm in diameter, and these nanorods were linked together as a web structure. Meanwhile, wet milling produced cubic particles with diameters of 400–600 nm, and spray drying produced spheres with diameters of 3–6 μm with corrugated surfaces.

Due to the rapid and sticky attractive collision of nanorods, the dispersion of TFFD nanorods in HFA propellants produced low-density flocs with high free volume, which can stack together to fill the entire solvent volume and subsequently prevent settling and subsequent formation of a dense cake that cannot be redispersed readily. In contrast, the dispersion of cubes or spheres produced by wet milling and spray drying in HFA produced denser flocs with less space-filling volume, which flocculated and sedimented within a short period of time. The flocculated nanorods that contained BSA in 10 mM potassium phosphate buffer were produced by TFFD. It was found that the flocculated BSA nanorods that were suspended in the PFA propellant were stable against

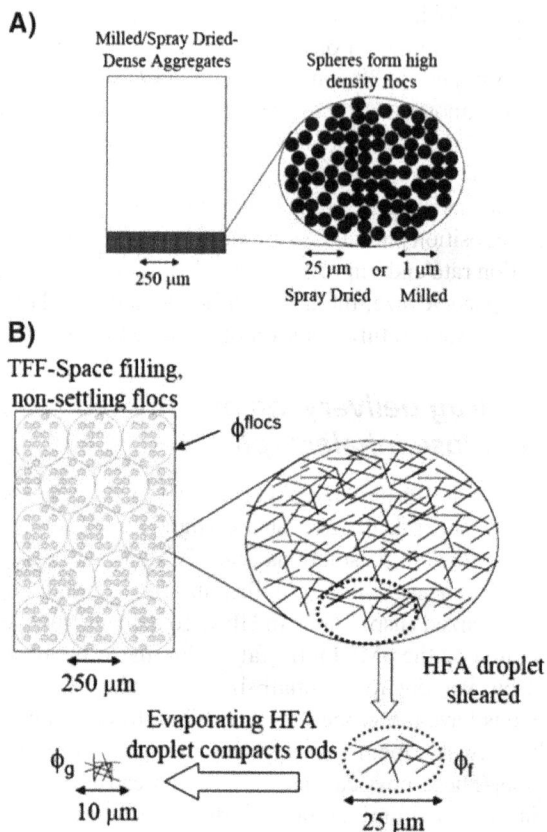

FIGURE 9.5 Suspensions of particles in HFA propellants: milled or spray-dried particles (A) and TFFD rod particles (B). Reproduced with permission from Springer Nature.[39]

sedimentation for up to 1 year at 25 °C without the addition of surfactants.[39] After actuation, the atomized HFA droplets can break apart and evaporate. Consequently, the templated flocs of nanorods were compressed and shrunk by capillary forces to produce porous and respirable particles (Figure 9.5A). *In vitro* aerodynamic testing using an Anderson cascade impactor (ACI) demonstrated that the open flocs containing TFFD nanorods exhibited an optimal high fine particle fraction (38–47%) with an emitted dose of 0.7 mg per actuation (Figure 9.5B).[39]

9.2.1.3 Inhaled drug delivery via dry powder inhalers (DPI)

Due to the unique properties of engineered particles prepared by TFFD, brittle-matrix powders have been introduced as a new platform for dry powders for inhalation. The brittle-matrix powder has a large geometric particle size and high porosity, which can be sheared apart by a passive DPI device to create smaller low-density microparticles (Figures 9.6 and 9.7).[8,24] This chapter includes the development of small-molecule drugs for pulmonary drug delivery, which is described case-by-case below.

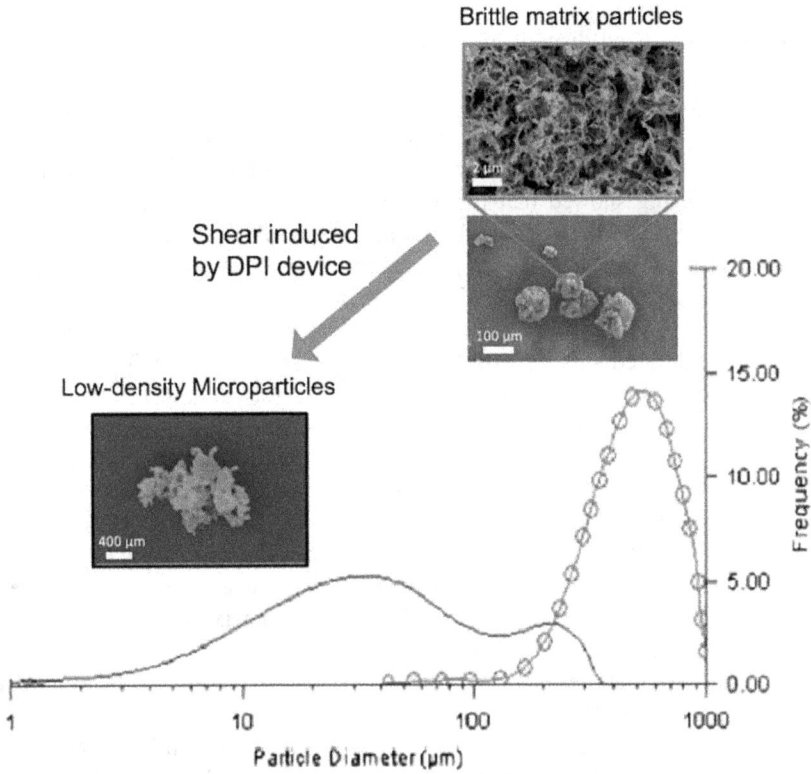

FIGURE 9.6   Geometric particle size distribution and surface particle morphology of a bulk powder (line with circles) and an aerosolized powder emitted from a DPI device (solid line). Modified and reproduced with permission from RDD Europe 2015, Virginia Commonwealth University.[24]

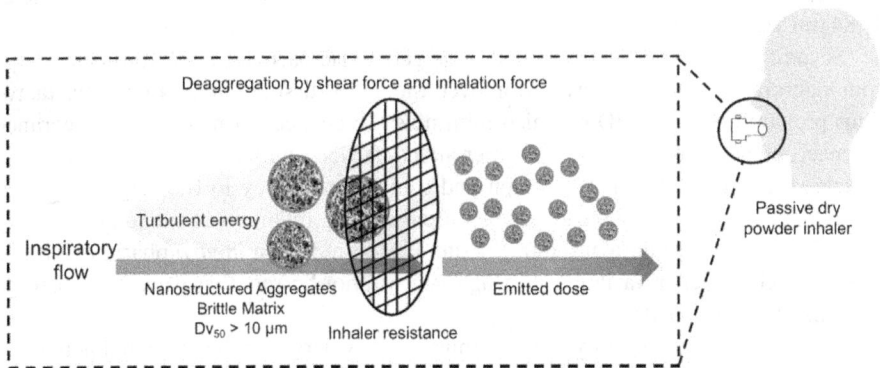

FIGURE 9.7   Passive inhaler inhalation of a nanostructured aggregate brittle-matrix dry powder made using TFFD. Reprinted with permission from Elsevier.[8]

9.2.1.3.1 Tacrolimus

In addition to nebulized dispersions, tacrolimus was also further developed as a dry powder for inhalation using TFFD. The drug loading of tacrolimus ranged from 50–100% w/w and various types of sugars (e.g., lactose, mannitol, trehalose, raffinose) in the formulation were optimized based on the aerodynamic properties.[8,24] The various types of sugar affected the physical and aerodynamic properties of the formulations.[24] Aerodynamic testing showed that the drug itself was aerosolizable, and it exhibited more than 50% FPF of the recovered dose and respirable particle size. However, the small amount of excipients (e.g., lactose, mannitol, or trehalose) helped improve the aerosol performance of the formulations. The in vitro aerodynamic testing by NGI and a Plastiape® high resistance RS01 inhaler demonstrated that TFFD tacrolimus–lactose (95:5) exhibited smaller MMAD and higher FPF than TFFD neat tacrolimus (2.61 ± 0.25 μm vs. 3.58 ± 0.36 μm, and 69.31 ± 3.45% vs. 54.21 ± 3.90%, respectively).[8] TFFD can produce an amorphous form of tacrolimus, which can increase its solubility, dissolution rate, and extent of absorption. Lactose in the formulation did not function as a stabilizer by intermolecular interaction, as 1D and 2D ^{13}C ssNMR spectra demonstrated no detectable interaction between lactose and tacrolimus.[8] Despite this, the formulation that contained 95% tacrolimus was chemically and physically stable after six months of storage at both 25 °C and 40 °C. With moisture protection, the aerosol performance of TFFD tacrolimus–lactose (95:5) brittle matrix powder was maintained after six months of storage at 25 °C and 60% RH.[8]

The pharmacokinetic profiles of TFFD tacrolimus and jet-milled tacrolimus were compared in a study by Wang.[40] The TFFD formulation contained 50% tacrolimus and 50% mannitol, while the micronized tacrolimus formulation with the same composition was prepared using wet-ball milling followed by a size reduction using jet milling. It was demonstrated that the TFFD formulations exhibited higher area under the curve (AUC) in the lung than the micronized formulation (1,707.47 ng·h/g vs. 729.53 ng·h/g, respectively). This indicates that the TFFD formulation exhibited higher lung bioavailability. Additionally, the lung clearance of the TFFD formulation was slower than the micronized formulation (2.64 h^{-1} vs. 0.56 h^{-1}, respectively). The slower lung clearance of the TFFD powder is possibly related to the larger geometric particle size of the TFFD particles (present as nanostructured aggregates) compared to the micronized particles (17.84 μm vs. 1.92 μm).

Several studies have reported that large geometric particles (> 10 μm) can escape from macrophage phagocytosis.[41] Moreover, the faster dissolution of amorphous tacrolimus prepared using TFFD can also minimize the chances of mucociliary clearance and macrophage uptake. In contrast, micronized particles with much smaller geometric particle size have a slower dissolution and a higher tendency to be phagocytized by macrophages. Slower lung clearance can prolong drug retention in the lung, allowing more of the drug to remain at the target site. Furthermore, an in vivo pharmacokinetic study showed a higher variation in drug concentration in rats that were administered micronized tacrolimus.[40]

The safety and tolerability of tacrolimus dry powders for inhalation and nebulized dispersions was further investigated in healthy subjects. A 3 mg dose of tacrolimus was administered via oral inhalation as either a dry powder or a nebulized colloidal dispersion. It was reported that both dosage forms showed low systemic adsorption, and they were well tolerated with no significant changes in CBC, liver, kidney, or lung function.[42]

TFFD tacrolimus is used clinically to target prophylaxis of organ rejection in patients receiving lung transplants. Phase 1 clinical trial for TFFD tacrolimus inhalation powder was completed in 2021, and phase 2 clinical study is scheduled in 2022.

9.2.1.3.2 Remdesivir

Remdesivir, an antiviral drug, was initially developed as injectable solution for the treatment of Ebola virus diseases. Later, the U.S. Food and Drug Administration (FDA) granted Emergency Use Authorization (EUA) to remdesivir for the treatment of COVID-19.[43] To improve the accessibility of the drug for outpatients who do not have access to the injectable administration of remdesivir, other dosage forms have been considered and investigated. The inhalation dosage form is one of the alternative routes that not only improves accessibility but also improves the efficiency of drug delivery to the lungs, which is a target site for this disease. Sahakijpijarn et al. reformulated remdesivir as a dry powder for inhalation using TFFD. Remdesivir was combined with different excipients (e.g., lactose, mannitol, sulfobutylether-β-cyclodextrin (Captisol®), or leucine) at various drug levels.[25] Similar to tacrolimus, the combination of remdesivir and excipients was formed as a low-density, highly porous brittle-matrix powder after TFFD.[25] The drug loading of formulations can be increased up to 80%, while the formulations exhibited excellent aerodynamic properties (> 70% FPF, < 2 µm MMAD).[25]

A single-dose 24-hour pharmacokinetic profile of TFFD remdesivir–leucine (80/20 w/w) and TFFD remdesivir–Captisol® (80/20 w/w) was compared in rats and Syrian hamsters.[25] The small animal models were selected in the PK studies because they have been reported as useful mammalian models for the study of pathogenesis, treatment, and vaccination against SAR-CoV-2.[44,45] Moreover, it was reported that the SAR-CoV-2 replication was efficient in the respiratory tract of Syrian hamsters, thereby developing mild lung disease similar to that found in early-stage COVID-19 patients.[44] Both pharmacokinetic evaluations in rats and hamsters showed that dry powder inhalation can deliver the drug to the lungs.[25,46] Captisol®, a solubilizer, appeared to affect the systemic absorption of remdesivir, since both studies demonstrated that TFFD remdesivir–Captisol® (80/20 w/w) demonstrated faster and higher systemic uptake, while TFFD remdesivir–leucine was slowly absorbed into systemic circulation.[25] A pharmacokinetic evaluation in hamsters showed that remdesivir can be converted to GS-441524, a parent nucleoside analogue core of remdesivir, both in the lungs and in plasma.[46] The plasma levels of remdesivir and GS-441524 were higher than the reported EC_{50}s of both remdesivir and GS-441524 (in human epithelial cells) over 20 h following a single-dose inhalation of TFFD remdesivir powder.[46]

Despite the fact that TFFD remdesivir–leucine (80/20 w/w) exhibited slower and lower absorption of remdesivir and GS-4412524 in the lungs, it showed a greater C_{max}, shorter T_{max}, and lower AUC of GS-441524 compared to TFFD remdesivir–Captisol® (80/20 w/w).[46] These results indicate that a lower total drug exposure is required to achieve a high and effective concentration against SAR-CoV-2.[46] Based on aerosol performance and pharmacokinetic profiles, the remdesivir dry powder for inhalation made using TFFD is a promising alternative dosage form for the treatment of patients with COVID-19 on an outpatient basis and earlier in the course of the disease.

9.2.1.3.3 Rapamycin

Rapamycin, or sirolimus, is an immunosuppressant that has been approved and is currently commercialized as an oral solution (Rapamune®) for the prevention of kidney allograft rejection. Rapamycin has also been used as an alternative drug for lung transplantation. Rapamycin is a hydrophobic and lipophilic drug that is insoluble in water (2.6 µg/mL).[47] The relatively low oral bioavailability of rapamycin (14–20%) requires a higher oral dose to reach the desired therapeutic window,[48] which increases the potential for adverse effects.

Carvalho et al. developed a rapamycin dry powder for inhalation for the treatment of both systemic and local diseases. The amorphous formulation containing rapamycin and lactose in a 1:1 weight ratio was prepared using TFFD. In the TFFD formulation, lactose was used as a matrix excipient to improve aerosolization. The crystalline formulation containing micronized rapamycin, micronized lactose, and coarse lactose in a weight ratio of 0.5:0.5:19, respectively, was prepared using wet-ball milling. The TFFD rapamycin dry powder exhibited higher aerosol performance than the crystalline physical mixture (72.11% FPF and 2.1 µm MMAD vs. 61.29% FPF and 2.43 µm MMAD, respectively). The single-dose pharmacokinetic profiles of amorphous and crystalline formulations after inhalation of the aerosol mist in a nose-only apparatus were compared in Sprague Dawley rats.

The crystalline formulation exhibited higher lung deposition than the amorphous formulation; however, both formulations were retained in the lungs for the same period of time.[9] Additionally, the amorphous formulation showed more of the drug in systemic circulation (8.6 ng•h/mL vs. 2.4 ng•h/mL AUC_{0-24}, respectively). This indicates that the amorphous form of the drug can improve solubility and increase the dissolution rate, thereby exhibiting higher *in vivo* systemic bioavailability.[9]

9.2.1.3.4 Niclosamide

Niclosamide, an FDA-approved anti-helminthic drug, has been investigated as an anti-cancer drug. Recently, several studies have reported the antiviral activity of niclosamide against severe acute respiratory syndrome coronavirus 2 (SARS-CoV-2).[49–51] The low water solubility of the drug results in the low and erratic bioavailability of niclosamide. More recently, a niclosamide inhalable dry powder was developed using TFFD as a potential therapeutic for COVID-19. This formulation consisted of 22% w/w niclosamide, 73% w/w mannitol, and 5% w/w leucine, and it exhibited desirable aerosol performance (86.0% FPF, 1.11 µm MMAD).[52]

Histopathology analysis showed that the liver, kidneys, and spleen of the rats were normal after three days of daily dosing with a high dose of inhaled niclosamide (~ 827.2 µg/kg of niclosamide). Mild signs of inflammation were observed in lung tissue due to the relatively high doses of niclosamide, but the air space and interstitial space appeared normal. Hence, the inhaled formulation was safe and tolerable after three days of multi-dose administration. The pharmacokinetic study in a Syrian hamster model demonstrated that the inhalation of TFFD niclosamide was able to achieve lung concentrations above the required IC_{90} levels for at least 24 h after a single administration.

Phase 1 clinical trial of the inhaled dry powder formulation of TFFD niclosamide was begun in 2021. The inhaled TFFD niclosamide dry powder is used clinically as an antiviral treatment with potential to address SARS-CoV-2 and other viral infections.

9.2.1.3.5 Voriconazole

Voriconazole is a second-generation triazole antifungal agent that has shown more potency and broader antifungal activity than first-generation triazole. Voriconazole is used for the treatment of invasive pulmonary aspergillosis (IPA) because it has shown improved clinical outcomes in immunocompromised subjects with IPA.[53] Voriconazole was developed as a dry powder for inhalation using TFFD. Voriconazole is classified as a glass-forming ability type 1, which has a high crystallization tendency. Using TFFD, the voriconazole was formed as a microstructured crystalline formulation.[6,54] The addition of a polymer with a high glass transition temperature, such as povidone K25 (PVP; voriconazole:PVP K25 in a 1:3 weight ratio), resulted in nanostructured amorphous formulation after the TFFD process.[54]

In vitro dissolution testing showed that the nanostructured amorphous formulation exhibited a faster dissolution rate than the microstructured crystalline formulation. This indicates that PVP K25 and the amorphous form of voriconazole contributed to an increased dissolution rate.[54] This faster dissolution was also translated into the *in vivo* pharmacokinetic profile of formulations. The pharmacokinetic profile of amorphous voriconazole and crystalline voriconazole was compared in rats. Following a single dose of 10 mg/kg voriconazole intratracheal insufflation using a DP-4 insufflator, TFFD voriconazole-PVP K25 (1:3) appeared to have a faster absorption rate, a faster elimination rate, and a shorter lung retention time than the microstructured crystalline voriconazole. This is possibly due to the higher solubility of amorphous voriconazole and the smaller surface area of TFFD voriconazole–PVP K25. The longer lung retention of the microstructured crystalline voriconazole provide a larger reservoir of voriconazole in the lung and more time to interact with fungal pathogens.

Inhaled TFFD voriconazole dry powder is used clinically for acute and chronic treatment of invasive pulmonary aspergillosis (IPA) and allergic bronchopulmonary aspergillosis (ABPA) and prophylaxis of IPA. Phase 1b clinical study of the inhaled dry powder of TFFD voriconazole was completed in 2021, and phase 2 clinical study is scheduled in 2022.

9.2.2 Surface Texture Modification to Improve Aerosolization by Nanocrystalline Aggregates

In addition to brittle-matrix particles, in some cases, drugs are formed as nanostructured crystalline nanoaggregates using the TFFD process. As mentioned earlier, voriconazole is classified as a glass-forming ability type 1 compound, which has a high crystallization tendency. Using TFFD, voriconazole was formulated to contain microstructured crystalline nanoaggregates. The large proportion of polymer in the voriconazole dry powders helped the voriconazole remain an amorphous, brittle-matrix nanostructured

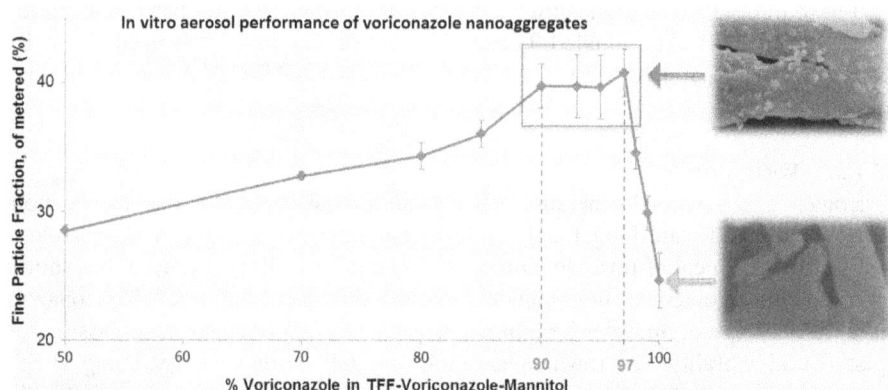

FIGURE 9.8   SEM figures of voriconazole formulations and the relationship between the percentage of voriconazole in the formulation and the fine particle fraction of voriconazole. Reprinted with permission from ACS Publications.

powder.[54] On the other hand, some excipients (e.g., mannitol) do not function as a crystallization inhibitor, hence voriconazole was formulated as micron-size crystalline nanoaggregates.[7]

In the study by Moon et al., atomic force microscopy and SEM/EDX analysis demonstrated that these voriconazole nanoaggregates have relatively smooth surfaces.[7] It was found that the addition of a small quantity of mannitol (< 10% w/w) in the formulation helps improve the aerosolization of voriconazole nanoaggregates. Figure 9.8 shows the relationship between FPF and the percentage of voriconazole in the formulation. The TFFD dry powder that contained only voriconazole showed poor aerosol performance (24.6% FPF of recovered dose) compared to other dry powder formulations. Using TFFD, submicron mannitol particles were produced and deposited onto the voriconazole nanoaggregates (Figure 9.9). These submicron mannitol particles modified the surface texture of the voriconazole nanoaggregates. The rough surface of the particles can decrease the contact area between the particles. As a consequence, the interparticulate forces are decreased, thereby improving the aerosolization of the voriconazole nanoaggregates (Figure 9.9).

Interestingly, the mannitol content served as a surface-modifying agent that affected the functionality and aerosol performance of voriconazole. Instead of adhering to the surface of the voriconazole nanoaggregates, the high amount of mannitol included in the TFFD voriconazole dry powder resulted in larger porous mannitol matrices surrounding the voriconazole nanoaggregates. This large, porous mannitol matrix did not function as a surface modifier because voriconazole nanoaggregates and mannitol matrices were agglomerated and did not separate during aerosolization. As shown in Figure 9.8, the formulations containing large proportions of mannitol (10–50% mannitol) showed poorer aerosol performance than the formulations that contained small proportions of mannitol (3–10%). This study demonstrated that a minimum amount of mannitol modifies the surface texture when using TFFD. This strategy would be a promising way to formulate a high–drug loading dry powder for inhalation.[7]

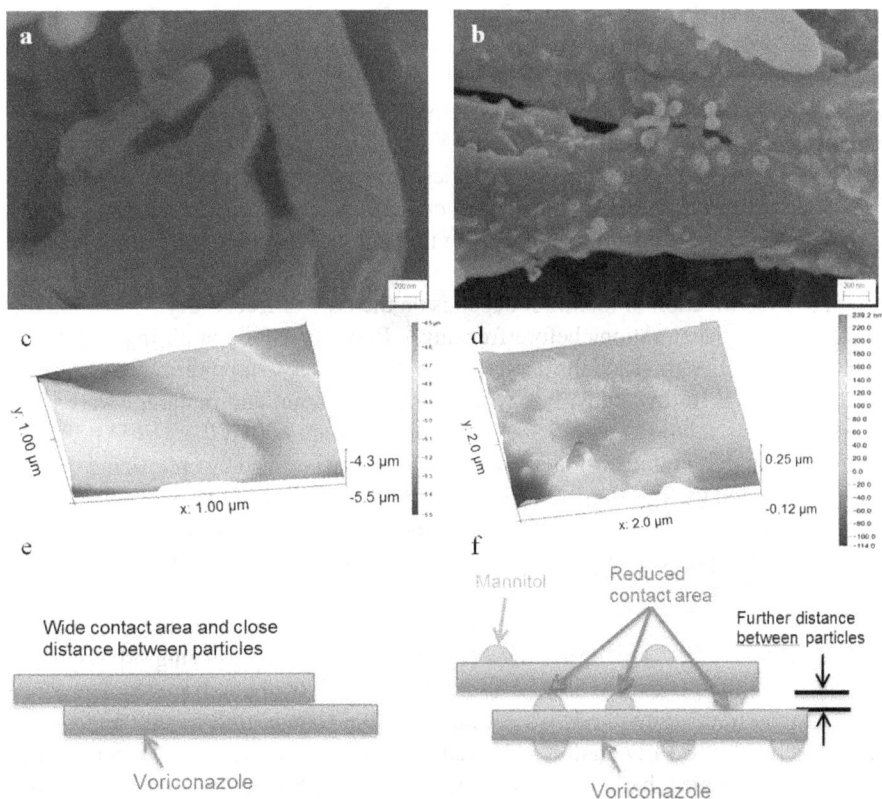

FIGURE 9.9 SEM images of TFFD voriconazole formulations: TFFD voriconazole (a) and TFFD voriconazole–mannitol (95:5 w/w) (b). Three-dimensional topography image of TFFD voriconazole formulations: TFFD voriconazole (c) and TFFD voriconazole–mannitol (95:5 w/w) (d). Illustration of the contact area and distance between particles of TFFD voriconazole formulations: TFFD voriconazole (e) and TFFD voriconazole–mannitol (95:5 w/w) (f). Reprinted with permission from ACS Publications.[7]

9.2.3 TFFD Production of Homogeneous Drug Particles in Powder

The ultra-rapid freezing rate of drug and excipient solutions on a cryogenic surface can minimize the mobility of the drug and the excipient in solutions at the molecular level. This prevents the segregation and heterogeneity of the solute, thus forming a homogeneous powder containing the drug and excipient. Solid-state nuclear magnetic resonance (ssNMR) was applied to compare the miscibility and domain sizes of the drug and the excipient in the formulations.[8] 1H spin–lattice relaxation time in a laboratory frame (T_1) and a rotating frame ($T_1\rho$) (obtained from ssNMR analysis) was used to calculate domain size using the spin diffusion equation.[55,56] Sahakijpijarn et al. revealed that a brittle-matrix powder that contained tacrolimus and lactose (50:50 w/w) showed good miscibility at a domain size of ~ 100 nm, which would indicate a required high level of homogeneity between the drug and excipient.[8]

The study by Moon et al. also showed that TFFD technology can produce a homogeneous and amorphous form of mannitol.[57] Mannitol is a bulking agent that is widely used in dry powder formulations of biologics. However, mannitol has a very low glass transition temperature, and this results in crystallization during freeze-drying. It has been reported that the stabilizing effect of mannitol for biologics decreases when mannitol crystallinity increases.[58]

The crystallization of mannitol depends on the type of freeze-drying method used and the solute concentrations before freezing.[58] Recently, Moon et al. investigated the effect of freezing methods on the crystallinity, homogeneity, and morphology of freeze-dried mannitol.[57] In this study, lysozyme (a model protein) and mannitol were mixed and prepared as solutions with a 10% w/v concentration before the TFFD process. It was found that the crystallization of mannitol can be minimized by optimizing the lysozyme content and the freezing rate. Using the liquid quench method, 70% w/w or higher lysozyme content was required to preserve amorphous mannitol during lyophilization, while the TFFD process required less lysozyme (50% w/w) to prevent crystallization during lyophilization.

TFFD has a faster freezing rate than liquid quench methods while also avoiding the Leidenfrost effect. This minimizes crystal growth during freezing. Moreover, the polymorphous homogeneity of freeze-dried mannitol (without lysozyme) produced using various freezing methods was evaluated using Raman microscopy analysis and eight scan points.[57] TFFD mannitol showed no spectrum differences between the eight points. This indicates that the ratio between α-, β-, and δ-mannitol are identical at all eight tested points, while samples prepared using other methods (i.e., liquid quench, vial quench, and shelf freezing) showed some significant differences in mannitol spectra from different scan points. This indicates that the α-, β-, and δ-mannitol are all heterogeneous. This result demonstrates that compared to other freezing methods, TFFD can produce more homogeneous polymorphs of mannitol throughout the sample.

As previously reported, TFFD can produce homogeneous powders, which would be required for dry powder inhalation. Homogeneous powder provides some benefits because it can improve dose uniformity and minimize lung dose variation. The advantage of TFFD when producing homogeneous powders has been applied to produce dry powders of drug combinations for inhalation.[59]

Watts et al. developed two different TFFD brittle matrix fixed-dose combinations: a dual combination of salmeterol xinafoate and mometasone furoate for asthma, and a triple combination of formoterol fumarate (LABA), tiotropium bromide (LAMA), and budesonide (ICS) for the treatment of COPD.[59] This study compared the aerosol performance of fixed-dose combinations and combination powder blends of two or three drugs. *In vitro* aerodynamic testing using the NGI and either Monodose® or Handihaler® dry powder inhaler (Figure 9.10A,B) devices at 4kPa pressure drop across the device demonstrated no significant difference in aerodynamic particle size distribution between individual drugs in the TFFD fixed-dose combinations (Table 9.2 and Figure 9.10).

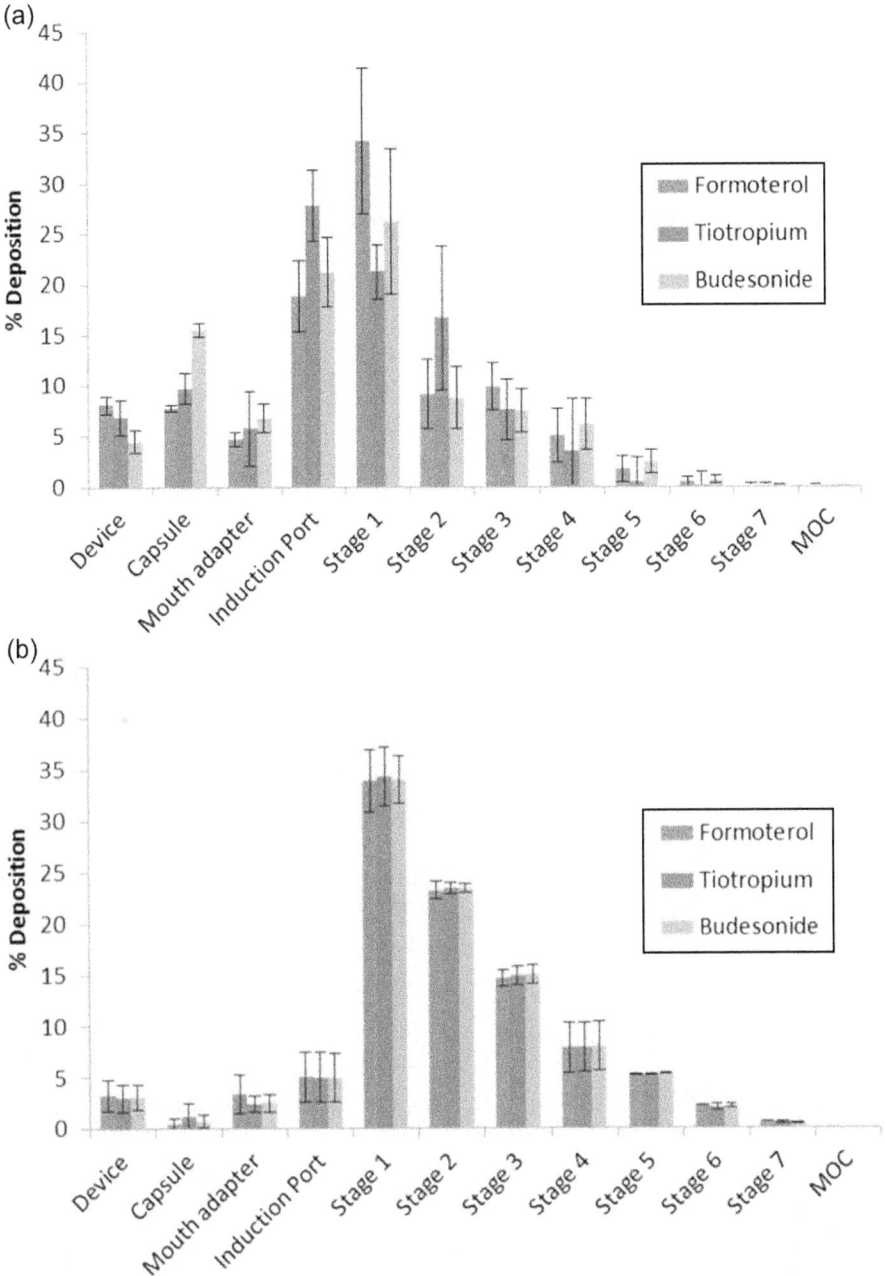

FIGURE 9.10   Aerodynamic particle size distribution delivered by Handihaler®: micronized (A), TFFD brittle matrix powder formulations (B). Reproduced with permission from RDD Europe 2015, Virginia Commonwealth University.[59]

TABLE 9.2 Aerodynamic properties of salmeterol xinafoate (SX) and mometasone furoate (MF) combination brittle matrix powder (BMP) formulations and micronized formulations delivered by a Monodose® inhaler.

FORMULATION	FPF (% OF DELIVERED)	FPF (% OF LOADED)	MMAD (MM)	GSD	TOTAL EMITTED DOSE (%)
Neat BMP SX/MF					
SX	55.52±4.78	52.90±4.18	3.58±0.32	3.55±1.12	95.31±1.13
MF	52.08±4.40	48.91±4.16	3.69±0.26	3.33±0.63	93.91±1.27
BMP Mannitol SX/MF					
SX	44.60±4.78	47.24±3.22	4.45±0.46	3.67±1.29	95.92±2.07
MF	43.91±3.37	41.06±3.47	4.43±0.36	3.86±1.53	93.49±1.70
Neat Micronized SX/MF					
SX	59.51±7.07	40.98±6.77	3.30±0.62	1.91±0.06	68.59±3.57
MF	34.29±5.78	24.50±4.91	4.45±0.96	2.01±0.02	71.18±3.12
Micronized Mannitol SX/MF					
SX	57.52±7.91	44.74±6.82	3.41±0.65	1.94±0.07	77.67±1.66
MF	30.07±6.20	23.84±5.05	4.84±0.92	1.94±0.02	79.20±0.57
Micronized Lactose SX/MF					
SX	56.15±9.58	41.39±8.60	3.65±0.58	1.00±0.01	73.88±1.14
MF	27.27±6.01	21.09±4.37	4.84±0.81	1.90±0.04	77.49±3.46

Reproduced with permission from RDD Europe 2015, Virginia Commonwealth University[59]

The TFFD dual combination powder prepared with or without mannitol did not show significant differences in FPF (% of delivered) (55.52 ± 4.78% for salmeterol, 52.08 ± 4.40% for mometasone without mannitol, 44.6 ± 4.78% for salmeterol, 43.91 ± 3.37% for mometasone with mannitol) and MMAD (3.58 ± 0.32 μm for salmeterol, 3.69 ± 0.26 μm for mometasone without mannitol, 4.45 ± 0.46 μm for salmeterol, 4.43 ± 0.36 μm for mometasone with mannitol). Likewise, there was no difference in the aerodynamic particle size distribution of triple combination aerosol.

In contrast, the combination powder blends showed differences in their aerodynamic particle size distributions of individual drugs. The dual combination powder blend of salmeterol xinafoate and mometasone without excipients, with micronized lactose, or with micronized mannitol exhibited FPFs of mometasone are significantly different and lower than salmeterol. Also, the aerodynamic particle size distribution of the triple combination blend presented that each drug was not identically aerosolized.

This study highlighted another application of TFFD to produce a fixed-dose therapy in powder form in which all drugs are homogeneous in a porous brittle-matrix powder. This results in improved content uniformity, homogeneity of powder dispersion upon aerosolization, co-deposition, and co-location of drugs at the target site of action.

9.2.4 Enhancement of Drug Absorption and Bioavailability in the Lungs Using TFFD Amorphous Drug Powders

Approximately 30% of drugs on the market and 60–70% of compounds under development are classified as BCS Class II drugs,[60] which have low solubility, but high permeability. For pulmonary drug delivery, the therapeutic efficacy of inhaled drug powder is limited by rapid clearance from the lungs. The slow dissolution of crystalline particles can result in extensive elimination, while the rapid dissolution of drugs in the lung fluid can facilitate the drug's penetration through the lung epithelium and thus minimizing mucociliary clearance and alveolar macrophage phagocytosis. This maximizes the local effective therapeutic concentration in the lungs.[61]

The use of ASDs is one of the most promising strategies for improving the solubility of poorly water-soluble drugs. The solubility of the amorphous form of a drug is generally higher than its crystalline form. The higher apparent solubility of amorphous drugs can enhance the dissolution rate of poorly water-soluble drugs in the alveolar aqueous mucus layer.[61]

Several studies have shown that TFFD can produce ASDs of poorly water-soluble drugs when the drug is combined with excipients in the optimal ratios.[21,35,62] In the study by Yang, leucine, which contains mainly dipalmitoylphosphatidylcholine (DPPC), the primary component of endogenous human lung surfactant, was used as a crystallization inhibitor to prepare itraconazole amorphous solid solution nanostructured aggregates.[35] One glass transition temperature was observed in the itraconazole–mannitol–lecithin formulation (1:0.5:0.2 w/w), indicating that a single-phase or solid solution was formed by the immobilization of molecularly dispersed itraconazole and excipients.[35] In contrast, the itraconazole–mannitol (1:0.5 w/w) mixture was partially crystalline, as it showed some sharp peaks on the XRD diffractogram. It was reported that a TFFD itraconazole–mannitol–lecithin formulation exhibited a concentration of dissolved itraconazole ((C) versus C_{eq} (C/C_{eq})) that was 22-times higher at 5 min in simulated lung fluid. The highest value was 27-times higher at 15 min.[35] Although the supersaturation decreased slowly to 7-times at 3 h, the C/C_{eq} of the formulation remained higher than the crystalline form throughout the dissolution study. The high supersaturation resulted in a high absorption rate of itraconazole from the lungs to the blood, as it exhibited a C_{max} of 1.64 µg/mL 2 h after administration by a nebulizer.[35]

Another study by Wang et al. also showed the benefits of the amorphous form of the drug on lung absorption and clearance.[40] Tacrolimus was formulated with mannitol at a 50:50 weight ratio and prepared as a dry powder using TFFD.[40] XRD diffractograms revealed that tacrolimus was amorphous, while mannitol was crystalline after the TFFD process.[40] Tacrolimus and mannitol were phase-separated, but compared to the micronized tacrolimus particles, the TFFD formulation showed more lung bioavailability and lower systemic absorption, as it demonstrated about 2.3 times higher AUC_{0-24h} in the lungs and less tacrolimus in the systemic (1–5 ng/mL) over 24 h after dry powder inhalation.[40] Moreover, TFFD powders exhibited slower lung clearance and longer lung retention time than micronized particles, which is likely due to their ability to avoid mucociliary clearance and macrophage uptake. On the other hand, the TFFD powders achieved the lower systemic absorption by reduced clearance and oral absorption.[40]

Therefore, this study supports the capacity of TFFD to modify the physical morphology of the drug, which can subsequently maximize therapeutic drug levels in the lungs while minimizing systemic drug levels.

9.2.5 TFFD Application for Biologics as Dry Powders for Inhalation

The feasibility of TFFD to prepare stable biological compounds as dry powders has been reported in several studies.[11,13,63] Since TFFD does not require atomization, the level of air–liquid interface and shear stress is lower than spray drying and spray freeze-drying (SFD). It has been reported that the activity of lactate dehydrogenase was preserved at 100% after the TFFD process, while SFD powders showed a 15–25% loss in protein activity.[13]

TFFD was recently applied to prepare vaccines as a dry powder. In a study by Thakkar, a TFFD ovalbumin-absorbed aluminum hydroxide dry powder containing 2% w/v trehalose was found to be stable after the TFFD process. Although slight particle aggregation was observed after three months of storage at 40 °C, this was not observed at other storage temperatures. Additionally, there was no significant difference in the anti-ovalbumin IgG levels among mice that were immunized with the ovalbumin–aluminum hydroxide vaccine, which was reconstituted from a dry powder stored at room temperature, 30 °C, and 40 °C for one month or three months.[63]

Another study from Xu et al. showed that TFFD could successfully convert liquid suspensions of the norovirus bivalent vaccine that contained norovirus strain GI.1 Norwalk virus like particles (VLP) and strain GII.4 Consensus VLP adsorbed on aluminum (oxy)hydroxide to a dry powder form.[11] With the optimal amount of cryoprotectants (e.g., trehalose or sucrose), the norovirus vaccine candidate dry powders prepared using TFFD showed no antigen loss or particle aggregation, and it preserved the relative potency of the antigens within a specified acceptable range. Moreover, the potency of the antigens in the TFFD formulation that contained 5.55% w/v sucrose was maintained in the specified acceptable range after eight weeks of storage at 40 °C and 75% RH.[11]

More recently, Wang et al. investigated the feasibility of inhalable dry powders for lipid nanoparticles prepared using TFFD.[14] Solid lipid nanoparticles (SLNs) are alternative carriers for the systemic delivery of inhaled biologics. The active compound is dissolved or dispersed in a solid lipid core, which is stabilized by a surfactant.[64] It has been reported that SLNs can improve the stability of biologics, increase bioavailability, prolong drug release in the lungs, enhance drug absorption, and improve cell uptake of macromolecule drugs.[65,66]

siRNA-SLNs containing lecithin, cholesterol, and a lipid–polyethylene glycol conjugate were prepared using solvent evaporation followed by TFFD, spray drying, and conventional shelf freeze-drying. *In vitro* aerodynamic testing demonstrated that SLNs made using TFFD showed smaller MMAD and higher FPF than SLNs made using spray drying (3.96 μm ± 0.97 μm vs. 5.97 μm ± 1.73 μm, and 37.01% ± 4.52% vs. 22.42% ± 12.88%, respectively). The analysis found no difference in the particle size, polydispersity index, or zeta potential of the siRNA-SLNs before and after the TFFD process and reconstitution. TFFD did not affect the function or the ability of SLNs to down-regulate TNF-α release from macrophages, because TNF-α siRNA-SLNs reconstituted from the TFFD powder and TNF-α siRNA-SLNs before TFFD showed a similar effect in reducing TNF-α release by the J774A.1 cells. This study highlighted another application of TFFD to prepare dry powders of biologics-encapsulated SLNs for pulmonary delivery by inhalation.[14]

9.3 PROCESSING DESIGN SPACES OF TFFD PROCESS INFLUENCE THE PROPERTIES OF THE FORMULATIONS

Like formulations processed using other technologies, the physicochemical and aerodynamic properties of the TFFD formulations vary by processing design spaces. These spaces of TFFD processing include excipients, solid loading, drug loading, processing temperature, and solvents.

9.3.1 Effect of Excipients on Physicochemical and Aerodynamic Properties of TFFD Powders

The excipient is one of the most remarkable processing design spaces for TFFD. For the last two decades, most DPI formulations (except the TOBI® Podhaler®) consist of lactose as an inactive ingredient.[5] During this era, DPI formulations were typically developed by blending micronized drugs with coarse lactose. However, in TFFD, the excipients (including lactose) are generally dissolved in a solvent system and processed by bottom-up, and they greatly affect the physicochemical and aerodynamic properties of the formulations.

9.3.1.1 Lactose

Lactose has been used in DPI formulations for many years, and it is considered a safe ingredient.[67] It is also a popular inactive ingredient used for TFFD. When lactose mono-hydrate, a stable form of lactose, is processed using TFFD, it is typically produced as amorphous lactose. This TFFD amorphous lactose is a nanostructured brittle matrix consisting of particles as small as 50 nm in powder formulations. While the amorphous form is physically less stable than the crystalline form, the amorphous lactose produced using TFFD has been shown to be stable for six months at 40 °C due to its relatively high T_g of 117 °C.[8] However, one should exercise caution about the storage conditions of TFFD powder formulations containing amorphous lactose. Amorphous lactose can be plasticized by water, and its T_g can be reduced significantly.[68] In the case of TFFD tacrolimus, amorphous lactose recrystallized at 25 °C with RH > 60%.[8]

Many formulations containing lactose have been produced using TFFD: rapamycin by Carvalho et al.,[9] remdesivir by Sahakijpijarn et al.,[25] and tacrolimus by Watts et al.,[31] Sinswat et al.,[26] and Sahakijpijarn et al.[8] All of these were formulated with amorphous lactose. As a result, these formulations were brittle-matrix powders. Brittle-matrix pow-ders containing amorphous lactose are highly aerosolizable. TFFD remdesivir contain-ing 20% w/w lactose resulted in a FPF of 87% and an MMAD of 1.28 μm.[25] Also, the aerosol properties of TFFD tacrolimus containing lactose surpassed TFFD tacrolimus containing mannitol, or trehalose (FPF 69.3 vs. 58.9 vs. 62.2%, respectively; MMAD 2.61 vs. 3.40 vs. 2.90 μm, respectively).[8] In addition to enhanced FPF and MMAD val-ues, TFFD tacrolimus with lactose has a higher SSA (73.6 m^2/g) than formulations con-taining mannitol (55.8 m^2/g) or trehalose (57.2 m^2/g), possibly as a result of generating smaller particles. Similar to TFFD tacrolimus, TFFD rapamycin with lactose resulted in a FPF of 72%, an MMAD of 2.1 μm, and an SSA of 85.7 m2/g.[9]

9.3.1.2 Mannitol

Mannitol is another popular excipient used in TFFD to produce powder formulations for DPIs. However, unlike lactose, mannitol is generally produced in crystalline forms using TFFD due to its relatively low T_g of 13 °C.[69] Mannitol has three crystalline forms: α, β, and δ forms. Usually, TFFD mannitol is itself a mixture of these three crystalline forms.[57] However, when mannitol is used as an inactive ingredient with other drugs, it typically assumes the δ-form, but the α-form has also been reported.[14] Since crystalline mannitol is formed using TFFD, the powder formulations containing mannitol are usu-ally physically stable and not hygroscopic unless other ingredients in the formulations are highly hygroscopic. Mannitol also produces brittle-matrix powders using TFFD.

Several drugs, including tacrolimus,[8,24,40] remdesivir,[25] voriconazole,[7,70] and itra-conazole,[35] were formulated as dry powders using TFFD. In addition to these small-molecule drugs, siRNA-encapsulated solid lipid nanoparticles were also formulated with mannitol to produce highly aerosolizable dry powders.[14]

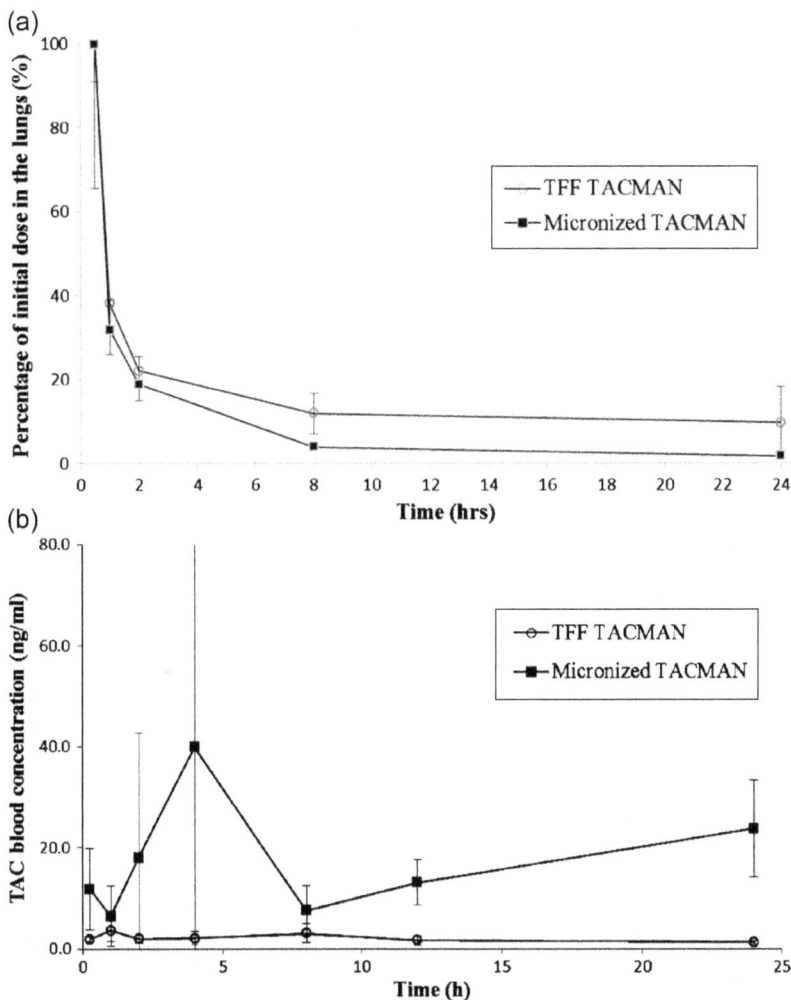

FIGURE 9.11 Tacrolimus concentration in rat lungs (A) and in the whole blood (B) after a single dry powder administration of TFFD and micronized tacrolimus formulations from a rotating brush generator. Modified and reprinted with permission from Springer Nature.[40]

In the case of TFFD remdesivir[25] and TFFD tacrolimus,[40] crystalline mannitol was formed in the powder formulations that consisted of amorphous drugs. Additionally, TFFD rhodamine B with mannitol also includes amorphous rhodamine B and crystalline mannitol.[71] Due to the low T_g of voriconazole (1 °C),[6] TFFD voriconazole containing mannitol is crystalline, and the crystalline mannitol was phase-separated from the crystalline voriconazole.[7] One interesting aspect of TFFD voriconazole when formulated with mannitol is that mannitol acts as a surface texture–modifying agent,[7] as described previously. When a low level of mannitol is used as an excipient for TFFD voriconazole, the crystalline mannitol particles (<200 nm) have existed on the crystalline voriconazole nanoaggregates (Figure 9.9). This reduces the cohesive and adhesive energies between the voriconazole particles and thus enhances aerosol performance.[7]

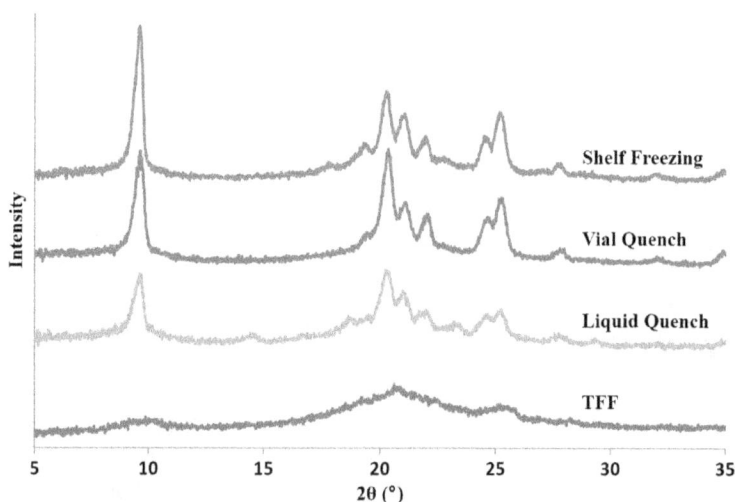

FIGURE 9.12 XRD of mannitol–lysozyme (% mannitol:% lysozyme) dried powder using various freezing methods. Reproduced with permission from Respiratory Drug Delivery 2016, Virginia Commonwealth University.[57]

The low T_g of mannitol causes difficulties when producing amorphous mannitol. However, TFFD itraconazole with mannitol (33% w/w) was produced in its amorphous form, and it was physically stable at 25 °C for 12 months.[35] The TFFD itraconazole dry powder presented only a single T_g of 44.5 °C, which falls between the glass transition temperatures of mannitol and itraconazole. Moon et al. reported another example of producing amorphous mannitol.[57] When lysozyme (50% w/w) was processed together with mannitol using TFFD, amorphous mannitol was produced, as illustrated in Figure 9.12. This amorphous mannitol was produced only when using TFFD, unlike other freezing methods. This suggests that the ultra-rapid freezing rate of TFFD can prevent the crystallization of mannitol if desired.[57]

When mannitol is used as an inactive ingredient for TFFD dry powder formulations, the addition of disaccharides (e.g., lactose, sucrose, or trehalose) is not recommended. Mannitol can work as a plasticizer for other saccharides when mixed together, and this significantly decreases their glass transition temperatures, thus inducing physical instability.[69]

9.3.1.3 Trehalose

Although trehalose has been used for TFFD tacrolimus dry powders for inhalation,[8] it was formulated mainly with large molecules and biologics using TFFD, such as vaccines,[11,63,72,73] proteins,[13] peptides, monoclonal antibodies, mRNA, siRNA, plasmid DNA, or bacteriophages.[74] The T_g of trehalose is relatively high (107 °C), similar to lactose.[69] Therefore, TFFD trehalose can be expected to be amorphous. In the case of TFFD tacrolimus–trehalose (95:5 w/w), trehalose was amorphous.[8]

For pulmonary delivery of TFFD powders that consist of small molecules as active ingredients, lactose and mannitol are more favorable due to its inferior aerodynamic properties of TFFD trehalose. So far, the only small molecule formulated and reported with trehalose is tacrolimus. However, as presented in the previous session, when tested using NGI tacrolimus with lactose resulted in better aerodynamic properties than tacrolimus with trehalose. Trehalose continues to be studied as a bulking agent for inhaled dry powder formulations of small molecules using TFFD, as well as a cryoprotectant for large molecules as a nonreducing disaccharide.

9.3.1.4 Sucrose

Similar to trehalose, sucrose is studied as an excipient used for TFFD dry powders for inhalation, especially for small-molecule drugs. Sucrose is hygroscopic after TFFD and must be stored in a dry environment. Still, it is a crucial excipient when macromolecules are formulated as TFFD dry powders because sucrose is very effective in preserving the activity of macromolecules.[75]

In an accelerated stability study, Xu et al. used sucrose as an excipient to produce a stable TFFD bivalent norovirus vaccine powder.[11] This TFFD vaccine powder was not intended to produce powder formulations for inhalation, but it demonstrated that sucrose is a suitable excipient that can be used to formulate macromolecules to maintain their activity. Therefore, future studies related to TFFD macromolecule powders, which are intended for any type of inhalation, can consider sucrose an applicable excipient.

9.3.1.5 Leucine

Leucine has not yet been used as an excipient for FDA-approved inhaled products, but several inhaled products consisting of leucine are in clinical trial stages.[76] Leucine is a dispersion-enhancing excipient, which enhances the aerosolization of dry powders because it reduces surface energy.[77,78]

Leucine has been used to produce TFFD remdesivir dry powders for inhalation.[25] When compared with other excipients (e.g., lactose, mannitol, or Captisol®) at the same drug loading levels, the TFFD remdesivir with leucine presented significantly lower MMAD and higher FPF. One possible reason is that leucine not only reduces surface energy but also forms a very fine brittle-matrix powder using TFFD. The TFFD remdesivir dry powders that consisted of more than 50% w/w leucine presented < 1 μm MMAD and $> 85\%$ FPF. Therefore, leucine can be considered a favorable excipient to make TFFD dry powder formulations that are highly aerosolizable.

However, two factors should be recognized when leucine is used to formulate TFFD dry powders. First, the water solubility of leucine is lower than other TFFD excipients such as lactose or mannitol, hence the solid loadings are studied and optimized when a high level of leucine is included in the feeding solution of TFFD. In the case of TFFD remdesivir at 20% drug loadings, TFFD remdesivir–leucine (80:20) was processed at 0.75% w/v solid loading, while other TFFD remdesivir powders containing lactose, mannitol, or Captisol were processed at 1.0% solid loadings.[25] Also, the interaction between leucine and drugs should be considered. Leucine can interact with drugs.[79,80] In some cases, this interaction is beneficial and can help stabilize dry powder formulations both physically and chemically. On the other hand, it may also cause physicochemical stability problems in dry powders when there is a strong interaction between leucine and drugs, and this must be studied during development of formulations by TFFD.

9.3.2 Solid Loading and Aerodynamic Properties of TFFD Formulations

For TFFD dry powder formulations, the solid loading of the feed solution or suspension affects its bulk density and aerodynamic properties. In addition to these properties, solid loading can affect the capacity of the manufacturing process because higher solid loading can produce more dry powder formulations in the same manufacture cycle. Therefore, solid loading is studied and optimized during development of TFFD formulations.

The effect of the bulk density and aerodynamic properties of voriconazole TFFD dry powder with different solid loadings is well described by Beinborn et al.[6] and Moon et al.[70] Typically, a lower solid loading results in lower bulk density and better aerodynamic properties. When voriconazole was processed using TFFD with no excipient and the same solvent system (i.e., 1,4-dioxane), the bulk density of the crystalline voriconazole dry powder, processed at 10% w/v, was about twice that of the bulk density of powders processed at 1% w/v (0.075 vs. 0.034 g/cm^3, respectively).[6] In this case, the aerodynamic properties of 1% w/v were better than those with 10% w/v, thus producing a TFFD voriconazole with higher FPF and lower MMAD. The same pattern was observed with TFFD voriconazole consisting of PVP K30 (67% w/w) processed in a water–1,4-dioxane (50:50 v/v) solvent system. While processing at 10% w/v, the solid loading produced a higher bulk density than processing at 1% w/v (0.070 vs. 0.014 g/cm^3, respectively), it resulted in lower FPF (4.8 vs. 20.2%, respectively).[6]

The surface texture–modified TFFD voriconazole nanoaggregates also demonstrated that lower solid loading enhanced aerodynamic properties when tested using NGI. When the feed solution was 1% w/v, the FPF increased to 67.5% compared to 2% (FPF 60.9%) and 3% (FPF 48.5%) solid loadings.[70]

Interestingly, when TFFD voriconazole dry powders without excipients were compared, the FPF was higher with 1% w/v solid loading than 0.1% w/v (37.8% vs. 28.6%, respectively), and the MMAD was lower, with 1% w/v compared to 0.1% w/v (4.2 μm vs. 5.1 μm, respectively).[6] TFFD remdesivir without excipients also demonstrated that powders processed with the higher solid loading aerosolize better.[25] The FPF of the recovered dose (< 5 μm) was considerably higher at 1% w/v than 0.5% and 0.25% (84.25 vs. 81.66 vs. 65.80%, respectively), and the MMAD was smaller (1.42 μm vs. 1.53 μm vs. 2.09 μm, respectively). This pattern persisted when 20% w/w of excipients (e.g., Captisol®, mannitol, lactose, or leucine) were included in the TFFD remdesivir dry powder formulations.

This result can be explained by the Brownian motion that affects the primary structure of TFFD voriconazole particles.[6] When the solid loading is very low (e.g., 0.1% w/v), the molecules in the frozen samples are far apart. Therefore, these particles cannot be suitably bridged. This induces heterogeneous primary particle size and irregular crystal growth.[6] On the other hand, when the solid loading is very high (e.g., 10% w/v), more particle bridging occurs. This aggregates particles and decreases brittleness, which adversely affects the aerodynamic properties of the formulation.

In some cases, the change in solid loadings does not affect aerodynamic properties of the TFFD powders. The amorphous TFFD tacrolimus brittle matrix, either with 50% or 95% w/w of lactose, at 0.75% and 2.5% w/w solid loadings, resulted in a very similar FPF and MMAD.[8]

9.3.3 Drug Loading Affects Particle Morphology and Aerosolization

Until recently, the development of inhaled pulmonary drugs focused on the treatment of COPD or asthma, which require small quantities of drug substances. As technologies developed, however, the drug substances delivered through the pulmonary route diversified. For instance, the TOBI® Podhaler® is a DPI that delivers tobramycin directly to the lung to treat cystic fibrosis. Afrezza® is another DPI that delivers inhaled insulin to the lung to treat diabetes. However, unlike COPD or asthma, these medical conditions often require high doses of drug substances. In the case of the TOBI Podhaler, a total of 112 mg of tobramycin is delivered with four inhalations.[81]

New DPI devices in development can deliver large amounts of dry powder to the lungs, but highly aerosolizable engineered dry powders (which can be formulated for high drug loading) can still reduce the burden of the amount of total dry powder loaded in the device. TFFD is one of the particle engineering technologies that can deliver dry powders to the lungs with very high drug loadings (e.g., >70% w/w drug contained in the powder). The influence of drug loading on the aerodynamic properties of TFFD dry powders is discussed in this section.

The drug loadings of TFFD dry powders containing voriconazole, tacrolimus, or remdesivir have been thoroughly studied. In the case of surface texture–modified TFFD voriconazole nanoaggregates, optimum aerodynamic properties were obtained at a drug loading between 90% and 97% w/w with phase-separated mannitol as a single excipient.[7] With higher drug loading and lower mannitol loading, phase-separated crystalline mannitol acts as a surface texture–modifying agent on the surface of the crystalline voriconazole nanoaggregates, where it reduces cohesive adhesive energy, resulting in the enhanced aerosolization of voriconazole nanoaggregates.[7] As the drug loading decreases, mannitol no longer acts as a surface texture–modifying agent, and the aerodynamic properties of the voriconazole nanoaggregates are degraded.

When PVP K30 was used as the single excipient, TFFD produced nanostructured, amorphous, aggregated voriconazole particles. Beinborn et al. studied the relationship between drug loadings and aerodynamic properties when voriconazole was formulated with PVP K30. They found that a lower drug loading (25% w/w) had a significantly higher SSA and exhibited better aerodynamic properties with higher FPF compared to a drug loading of 33% w/w.[6] Therefore, the relationship between drug loadings and the aerodynamic properties of TFFD voriconazole depends on the excipients, which can influence the particle morphology and crystallinity of TFFD powders.

Unlike amorphous TFFD voriconazole, amorphous TFFD remdesivir dry powders formulated with high drug loadings showed enhanced aerodynamic properties.[25] When remdesivir was formulated with Captisol®, lactose, or mannitol, the aerosol performance of TFFD remdesivir increased as the drug loading was increased up to 100%. This trend, however, was not observed with leucine. When the drug loading of leucine was between 20% and 80% w/w, the FPFs of these TFFD remdesivir dry powders were comparable to the TFFD remdesivir dry powder that lacked excipients. This indicates that amorphous TFFD remdesivir dry powder aerosolizes very well on its own, and the enhancement of aerosolization by leucine is minimized.

In case of TFFD tacrolimus with lactose, the highest drug loading (100% w/w) resulted in the lowest FPF and the largest MMAD compared to the drug loadings of 50–95% w/w,[8] at solid loadings of 0.75% w/v, with processing temperatures of either -70 °C and -130 °C. When compared to the 50–95% drug loadings, the formulation with 95% drug loading showed better aerosol performance at various processing temperatures (between -70 °C and -130 °C) and various solid loadings (between 0.75% and 2.50% w/v). Thus, TFFD was used to formulate a highly aerosolizable tacrolimus dry powder with excipient content as low as 5% w/w.

Based on each example above, it appears that even the same drug could result in different trends of particle morphology and aerosolization depending on the excipient used. Therefore, the effect of drug loading on particle morphology and aerosolization can vary depending on the combination of drug substance and excipients used in the TFFD process.

9.3.4 Processing Temperature and Supercooling

The degree of supercooling relates to nucleation and particle growth during the freezing process. A fast-freezing rate leads to extreme supercooling. Therefore, nucleation occurs quickly and with more nuclei, reducing the size of the solute particles generated. On the other hand, a slower freezing rate dramatically reduces supercooling, increasing the size of the solute particles generated. The processing temperature during the TFFD process influences the degree of supercooling and thus the size of particles.

The effect of the processing temperature on crystalline TFFD voriconazole nanoaggregates was previously evaluated at two temperatures: -60 °C and -150 °C.[70] By processing at the lower temperature of -150°C, smaller nanoparticles (200 nm vs. 500 nm) were generated due to the prevention of particle growth during the TFFD process. Also, nucleation at -150 °C was faster than the nucleation observed at -60°C. The smaller nanoparticles, which were confirmed by AFM and SEM, enhanced the aerosol performance on NGI with higher FPF (46.7% vs. 37.9% of recovered FPF).

Wang et al. also evaluated the effect of processing temperature on the aerosol performance of TFFD formulations.[71] In the study, a TFFD formulation containing rhodamine B-mannitol was processed at -50 °C and -140 °C. The result indicates that the lower processing temperature accelerated the cooling rate and improved aerosol performance with higher FPF and smaller MMAD. Additionally, the geometric particle size distribution of aerosolized TFFD rhodamine B-mannitol powders processed at lower temperatures showed a smaller particles with a narrower size distribution.

On the other hand, in the case of the tacrolimus–lactose TFFD, the processing temperature did not have a strong influence on the aerosol performance of the powder with solid loadings in the TFFD liquid feed solution of 0.75% and 2.50% w/v. The study evaluated the aerosol performance of two types of TFFD formulations of tacrolimus–lactose at two processing temperatures: -70 °C and -130 °C. One group of formulations had drug loadings from 50–100% w/w with solid loadings of 0.75% w/v. The other formulation had a drug loading in the TFFD powder of 95% with a solid loading of 2.50% w/v.[8] The higher temperature increased the SSAs of the powders, but the FPF and MMAD were not significantly different between the two temperatures.

9.3.5 Effect of Solvents on Morphology and Aerosol Properties

Some of the solvents used in the TFFD process are acetonitrile; 1,4-dioxane; t-butanol; and water. This is because they have relatively higher freezing points and relatively lower boiling points, which means these solvents can remain frozen during the lyophilization process. In many cases, the solvent systems for the TFFD process are chosen based on the solubility of the solutes (e.g., drugs and excipients),[15] but the choice of solvent system can also affect the properties of TFFD powders.

The morphology and aerodynamic properties of the surface texture–modified TFFD voriconazole nanoaggregates with various solvent systems were assessed.[70] During the study, TFFD voriconazole–mannitol (95:5 w/w) at 1% w/v solid loading was processed at -60 °C with binary solvent systems of water and acetonitrile (30, 50, and 70% v/v). While the crystallinity of the powders processed with three different solvent systems was the same, the aerosol performance of the powders was notably different. The TFFD voriconazole–mannitol processed with the higher portion of water (water–acetonitrile 70:30 v/v) resulted in the best aerosol performance, showing the highest FPF and the smallest MMAD. On the contrary, the binary solvent system with the lowest proportion of water (water–acetonitrile 30:70 v/v) resulted in the smallest FPF and the largest MMAD. In addition to the poorest aerosol performance, the SEM image confirmed that mannitol did not act as a surface-modifying agent on the surface of the voriconazole nanoaggregates. Instead, they became microscopic particles themselves when processed with water–acetonitrile (30:70 v/v). This result could be due to viscosity and cryophase separation of the binary solvent systems. Each solvent system must be selected based on properties of the drug, excipients and desired powder characteristics.

As the proportion of water increases in a binary solvent system of water–acetonitrile, the viscosity increases. When 30% (v/v) of acetonitrile is included in the water–acetonitrile, the viscosity is even higher than pure water alone.[82] The viscosity of the solvent plays a significant role in molecular movements during the freezing process.[70] In a solvent with high viscosity, the movement of molecules is disrupted while freezing, and particle growth can be interrupted. When the viscosity is low, however, the molecular movements are more tolerated, and the chances of particle growth are higher. Therefore, larger nanoparticles can be produced.

In addition, the binary solvent system of water–acetonitrile is phase-separated during the freezing process if the portion of acetonitrile is between 35% and 88% v/v.[83] Once the phase-separated, 88% (v/v) acetonitrile with water phase exists on the top layer, and 65% (v/v) water with acetonitrile is on the bottom as unfrozen. The large mannitol particles observed in TFFD voriconazole–mannitol (95:5) processed in water–acetonitrile (30:70 v/v) did not act as surface texture–modifying agent due to cryophase separation, and the powder exhibited poorer aerosol performance.[70]

In the binary solvent system of 1,4-dioxane–water, the viscosity influenced the aerosol performance of TFFD voriconazole–PVP K12.[6] Two binary solvent systems of 1,4-dioxane–water were evaluated on aerosol performance, and the higher viscous solvent system, 1,4-dioxane–water (20:80 v/v), produced higher FPF, compared to 1,4-dioxane–water (50:50 v/v). However, when 100% 1,4-dioxane was used as the solvent system, TFFD voriconazole–PVP K12 showed an even higher FPF. It was also amorphous, while the binary solvent system produced crystalline. This difference in crystallinity is explained by the recrystallization of voriconazole caused by residual water and the increased hygroscopicity of TFFD voriconazole–PVP K12 powders produced in 1,4-dioxane–water binary solvent systems.

9.4 DELIVERY OF TFFD POWDERS TO THE LUNG AS DPI RELIES ON LOADING DOSE, DEVICE, AND FLOW RATES

Several processing design spaces of the TFFD process that involve physicochemical and aerodynamic properties of TFFD dry powders, but some variables also stand for the aerosolization of the powder when delivered to the lungs.

9.4.1 Loading Dose

The amount of the TFFD powder loaded in the capsule can be a variable in the delivery of TFFD powders by DPI. TFFD voriconazole–mannitol (95:5) was tested for aerosol performance with different loading doses.[70] The bulk density of the conditioned TFFD voriconazole nanoaggregates was around 60 mg/cm³. Since the volume of the #3 capsule, which is used with Plastiape RS00 and RS01 devices, is 0.3 mL, the maximum powder loading for voriconazole nanoaggregates per #3 capsule is approximately 20 mg.[70] Therefore, the aerosol performance of the loading doses of 10 mg, 15 mg, and 20 mg per capsule was achieved. With a high-resistance RS00 device with a flow rate of 60 L/min, the TFFD voriconazole nanoaggregates did not show significant differences in FPF or MMAD, demonstrating that filling the powder full in the capsule did not influence aerosolization. However, using a high-resistance RS01 device with a flow rate of 60 L/min, the FPF was decreased and the MMAD was increased at the loading dose of 20 mg compared to 10 mg.

9.4.2 Device and Flow Rates

Even though the tested dry powder formulations are the same, different devices can result in different aerodynamic properties of the powder.[84] As described in the previous section, the aerosolization of the TFFD dry powders also differs depending on the devices.

High- and low-resistance RS00 and RS01 devices were used to assess the aerosol performance of the TFFD voriconazole nanoaggregates.[70] The test results show that the high-resistance RS00 device exhibited similar aerosolization between flow rates of 30 L/min and 60 L/min, indicating inhalation flow rate independence. On the contrary, the high-resistance RS01 achieved decreased FPF and larger MMAD at a flow rate of 30 L/min compared to 60 L/min. The low-resistance RS00 resulted in enhanced aerosol performance with a higher FPF and a smaller MMAD than the high-resistance RS00 at 60 L/min and 90 L/min; however, inhalation flow rate independence was not obtained. Similarly, the low-resistance RS01 also showed better aerosol performance than the high-resistance RS01 at 60 L/min and 90 L/min, but inhalation flow rate independence was not achieved. Overall, the high-resistance RS00 device seemed to perform best with TFFD voriconazole nanoaggregates due to its flow rate independence and enhanced aerosolization.

9.5 CONCLUSION

TFFD is an advanced formulation technology that is suitable to produce dry powders for inhalation drug delivery. The dry powders are suitable to be delivered to the lungs via nebulizer, pMDI, and DPI. By enhancing water solubility of the drugs, TFFD provides the dry powders of drugs that can be readily reconstituted for nebulization at point of administration to the patient. Low density flocs of protein formulation for pMDI can be also produced using TFFD that is stable against sedimentation. When the thin-film freeze-dried powders are used for DPI, the powders containing high levels of drugs are highly aerosolizable with high FPF and low MMAD, and consistent aerosolization is expected even with commercially available devices. Therefore, by producing versatile powders that can be used via different types of pulmonary delivery devices, the TFFD is an advanced powder engineering technology for developing formulations for inhalation.

CONFLICTS OF INTEREST

Williams reports a relationship with TFF Pharmaceuticals, Inc. that includes consulting or advising, equity or stocks, and funding grants. Moon reports a relationship with TFF Pharmaceuticals Inc. that includes consulting or advising. Moon, Sahakijpijarn, and Williams are coinventors on IP related to TFFD technology that is licensed to TFF Pharmaceuticals, Inc.

REFERENCES

1. Laube, B.L. *et al.* What the pulmonary specialist should know about the new inhalation therapies. *The European Respiratory Journal* 37(6), 1308–1331 (2011).
2. Depreter, F., Pilcer, G. & Amighi, K. Inhaled proteins: Challenges and perspectives. *International Journal of Pharmaceutics* 447(1–2), 251–280 (2013).
3. Hansel, T.T. & Barnes, P.J. *New drugs for asthma, allergy, and COPD.* (Basel and New York: Karger, 2001).
4. Hoppentocht, M., Hagedoorn, P., Frijlink, H.W. & de Boer, A.H. Developments and strategies for inhaled antibiotic drugs in tuberculosis therapy: A critical evaluation. *European Journal of Pharmaceutics and Biopharmaceutics: Official Journal of Arbeitsgemeinschaft fur Pharmazeutische Verfahrenstechnik e V* 86, 23–30 (2014).
5. Moon, C., Smyth, H.D.C., Watts, A.B. & Williams, R.O., 3rd Delivery technologies for orally inhaled products: An update. *AAPS PharmSciTech* 20(3), 117 (2019).
6. Beinborn, N.A., Lirola, H.L. & Williams, R.O., 3rd Effect of process variables on morphology and aerodynamic properties of voriconazole formulations produced by thin film freezing. *International Journal of Pharmacy* 429(1–2), 46–57 (2012).
7. Moon, C., Watts, A.B., Lu, X., Su, Y. & Williams III, R.O. Enhanced aerosolization of high potency nanoaggregates of voriconazole by dry powder inhalation. *Molecular Pharmaceutics* 16(5), 1799–1812 (2019).
8. Sahakijpijarn, S. *et al.* Using thin film freezing to minimize excipients in inhalable tacrolimus dry powder formulations. *International Journal of Pharmacy* 586, 119490 (2020).
9. Carvalho, S.R. *et al.* Characterization and pharmacokinetic analysis of crystalline versus amorphous rapamycin dry powder via pulmonary administration in rats. *European Journal of Pharmaceutics and Biopharmaceutics* 88(1), 136–147 (2014).
10. Yang, W., Johnston, K.P. & Williams, R.O., 3rd Comparison of bioavailability of amorphous versus crystalline itraconazole nanoparticles via pulmonary administration in rats. *European Journal of Pharmaceutics and Biopharmaceutics: Official Journal of Arbeitsgemeinschaft fur Pharmazeutische Verfahrenstechnik e V* 75, 33–41 (2010).
11. Xu, H. *et al.* Thin-film freeze-drying of a bivalent norovirus vaccine while maintaining the potency of both antigens. *International Journal of Pharmacy* 609, 121126 (2021).
12. AboulFotouh, K. et al. Formulation of dry powders of vaccines containing MF59 or AddaVax by thin-film freeze-drying: Towards a dry powder universal flu vaccine. *International Journal of Pharmaceutics* 624, 122021 (2022).
13. Engstrom, J.D. *et al.* Formation of stable submicron protein particles by thin film freezing. *Pharmaceutical Research* 25(6), 1334–1346 (2008).
14. Wang, J.L. *et al.* Aerosolizable siRNA-encapsulated solid lipid nanoparticles prepared by thin-film freeze-drying for potential pulmonary delivery. *International Journal of Pharmacy* 596, 120215 (2021).
15. Overhoff, K.A., Johnston, K.P., Tam, J., Engstrom, J. & Williams III, R.O. Use of thin film freezing to enable drug delivery: A review. *Journal of Drug Delivery Science and Technology* 19(2), 89–98 (2009).
16. Engstrom, J.D., Simpson, D.T., Lai, E.S., Williams, R.O., 3rd & Johnston, K.P. Morphology of protein particles produced by spray freezing of concentrated solutions. *European Journal of Pharmaceutics and Biopharmaceutics* 65(2), 149–162 (2007).
17. Yu, L. Amorphous pharmaceutical solids: Preparation, characterization and stabilization. *Advanced Drug Delivery Reviews* 48(1), 27–42 (2001).
18. Overhoff, K.A. *et al.* Novel ultra-rapid freezing particle engineering process for enhancement of dissolution rates of poorly water-soluble drugs. *European Journal of Pharmaceutics*

and *Biopharmaceutics: Official Journal of Arbeitsgemeinschaft fur Pharmazeutische Verfahrenstechnik e V* 65, 57–67 (2007).

19. Zhang, M. *et al.* Formulation and delivery of improved amorphous fenofibrate solid dispersions prepared by thin film freezing. *European Journal of Pharmaceutics and Biopharmaceutics: Official Journal of Arbeitsgemeinschaft fur Pharmazeutische Verfahrenstechnik e V* 82, 534–544 (2012).

20. Purvis, T., Mattucci, M.E., Crisp, M.T., Johnston, K.P. & Williams, R.O., 3rd Rapidly dissolving repaglinide powders produced by the ultra-rapid freezing process. *AAPS PharmSciTech* 8(3), E58 (2007).

21. Overhoff, K.A., Moreno, A., Miller, D.A., Johnston, K.P. & Williams, R.O., 3rd Solid dispersions of itraconazole and enteric polymers made by ultra-rapid freezing. *International Journal of Pharmacy* 336(1), 122–132 (2007).

22. Marple, V.A. *et al.* Next generation pharmaceutical impactor (a new impactor for pharmaceutical inhaler testing). Part I: Design. *Journal of Aerosol Medicine* 16(3), 283–299 (2003).

23. Paclawski, A., Szlek, J., Lau, R., Jachowicz, R. & Mendyk, A. Empirical modeling of the fine particle fraction for carrier-based pulmonary delivery formulations. *International Journal of Nanomedicine* 10, 801–810 (2015).

24. Watts, A.B., Wang, Y.-B., Johnston, K.P. & Williams, R.O., 3rd Respirable low-density microparticles formed in situ from aerosolized brittle matrices. *Pharmaceutical Research* 30(3), 813–825 (2013).

25. Sahakijpijarn, S., Moon, C., Koleng, J.J., Christensen, D.J. & Williams III, R.O. Development of remdesivir as a dry powder for inhalation by thin film freezing. *Pharmaceutics* 12(11), (2020).

26. Sinswat, P., Overhoff, K.A., McConville, J.T., Johnston, K.P. & Williams, R.O., 3rd Nebulization of nanoparticulate amorphous or crystalline tacrolimus–Single-dose pharmacokinetics study in mice. *European Journal of Pharmaceutics and Biopharmaceutics: Official Journal of Arbeitsgemeinschaft fur Pharmazeutische Verfahrenstechnik e V* 69, 1057–1066 (2008).

27. Scalea, J.R., Levi, S.T., Ally, W. & Brayman, K.L. Tacrolimus for the prevention and treatment of rejection of solid organ transplants. *Expert Review of Clinical Immunology* 12(3), 333–342 (2016).

28. Raman, V. *et al.* Clinical utility of monitoring tacrolimus blood concentrations in liver transplant patients. *Journal of Clinical Pharmacology* 41(5), 542–551 (2001).

29. Hayes, D., Jr., Zwischenberger, J.B. & Mansour, H.M. Aerosolized tacrolimus: A case report in a lung transplant recipient. *Transplantation Proceedings* 42(9), 3876–3879 (2010).

30. Martinet, Y. *et al.* Evaluation of the in vitro and in vivo effects of cyclosporine on the lung T-lymphocyte alveolitis of active pulmonary sarcoidosis. *American Review of Respiratory Disease* 138(5), 1242–1248 (1988).

31. Watts, A.B. *et al.* Characterization and pharmacokinetic analysis of tacrolimus dispersion for nebulization in a lung transplanted rodent model. *International Journal of Pharmaceutics* 384(1–2), 46–52 (2010).

32. Davies, N.M. & Feddah, M.R. A novel method for assessing dissolution of aerosol inhaler products. *International Journal of Pharmacy* 255(1–2), 175–187 (2003).

33. Watts, A.B. *et al.* Preclinical evaluation of tacrolimus colloidal dispersion for inhalation. *European Journal of Pharmaceutics and Biopharmaceutics* 77(2), 207–215 (2011).

34. Das, N.A. *et al.* The efficacy of inhaled nanoparticle tacrolimus in preventing rejection in an orthotopic rat lung transplant model. *Journal of Thoracic and Cardiovascular Surgery* 154(6), 2144–2151.e1 (2017).

35. Yang, W. *et al.* High bioavailability from nebulized itraconazole nanoparticle dispersions with biocompatible stabilizers. *International Journal of Pharmaceutics* 361(1–2), 177–188 (2008).

36. Morales, J.O., Peters, J.I. & Williams, R.O. Surfactants: Their critical role in enhancing drug delivery to the lungs. *Therapeutic Delivery* 2(5), 623–641 (2011).

37. Dellamary, L.A. *et al.* Hollow porous particles in metered dose inhalers. *Pharmaceutical Research* 17(2), 168–174 (2000).

38. Rogueda, P. Novel hydrofluoroalkane suspension formulations for respiratory drug delivery. *Expert Opinion on Drug Delivery* 2(4), 625–638 (2005).

39. Engstrom, J.D., Tam, J.M., Miller, M.A., Williams, R.O., 3rd & Johnston, K.P. Templated open flocs of nanorods for enhanced pulmonary delivery with pressurized metered dose inhalers. *Pharmaceutical Research* 26(1), 101–117 (2009).

40. Wang, Y.B. *et al.* In vitro and in vivo performance of dry powder inhalation formulations: Comparison of particles prepared by thin film freezing and micronization. *AAPS PharmSciTech* 15(4), 981–993 (2014).

41. Geiser, M. Update on macrophage clearance of inhaled micro- and nanoparticles. *Journal of Aerosol Medicine and Pulmonary Drug Delivery* 23(4), 207–217 (2010).

42. Sahakijpijarn, S., Beg, M., Levine, S.M., Peters, J.I. & Williams, R.O., 3rd A safety and tolerability study of thin film freeze-dried tacrolimus for local pulmonary drug delivery in human subjects. *Pharmaceutics* 13(5), (2021).

43. U.S. Food and Drug Administration. (2020, October 22). FDA Approves First Treatment for COVID-19 [Press release]. https://www.fda.gov/news-events/press-announcements/fda-approves-first-treatment-covid-19.

44. Chan, J.F. *et al.* Simulation of the clinical and pathological manifestations of coronavirus disease 2019 (COVID-19) in a golden Syrian hamster model: Implications for disease pathogenesis and transmissibility. *Clinical Infectious Diseases* 71, 2428–2446 (2020).

45. Imai, M. *et al.* Syrian hamsters as a small animal model for SARS-CoV-2 infection and countermeasure development. *Proceedings of the National Academy of Sciences* 117(28), 16587–16595 (2020).

46. Sahakijpijarn, S. *et al.* In vivo pharmacokinetic study of remdesivir dry powder for inhalation in hamsters. *International Journal of Pharmaceutics: X* 3, 100073 (2021).

47. Simamora, P., Alvarez, J.M. & Yalkowsky, S.H. Solubilization of rapamycin. *International Journal of Pharmaceutics* 213(1–2), 25–29 (2001).

48. MacDonald, A., Scarola, J., Burke, J.T. & Zimmerman, J.J. Clinical pharmacokinetics and therapeutic drug monitoring of sirolimus. *Clinical Therapeutics* 22(Suppl B), B101–B121 (2000).

49. Xu, J., Shi, P.Y., Li, H. & Zhou, J. Broad spectrum antiviral agent niclosamide and its therapeutic potential. *ACS Infectious Diseases* 6(5), 909–915 (2020).

50. Jeon, S. *et al.* Identification of antiviral drug candidates against SARS-CoV-2 from FDA-approved drugs. *Antimicrobial Agents and Chemotherapy* 64(7), (2020).

51. Pindiprolu, S. & Pindiprolu, S.H. Plausible mechanisms of niclosamide as an antiviral agent against COVID-19. *Medical Hypotheses* 140, 109765 (2020).

52. Jara, M.O. *et al.* Niclosamide inhalation powder made by thin-film freezing: Multi-dose tolerability and exposure in rats and pharmacokinetics in hamsters. *International Journal of Pharmacy* 603, 120701 (2021).

53. Sahakijpijarn, S., Peters, J.I. & Williams, R.O. *In inhalation aerosols 167–185* (CRC Press, 2019).

54. Beinborn, N.A., Du, J., Wiederhold, N.P., Smyth, H.D. & Williams, R.O., 3rd Dry powder insufflation of crystalline and amorphous voriconazole formulations produced by thin film freezing to mice. *European Journal of Pharmaceutics and Biopharmaceutics* 81(3), 600–608 (2012).

55. Lu, X. *et al.* Molecular interactions in posaconazole amorphous solid dispersions from two-dimensional solid-state NMR spectroscopy. *Molecular Pharmaceutics* 16(6), 2579–2589 (2019).

56. Hanada, M., Jermain, S.V., Lu, X., Su, Y. & Williams, R.O., 3rd Predicting physical stability of ternary amorphous solid dispersions using specific mechanical energy in a hot melt extrusion process. *International Journal of Pharmacy* 548(1), 571–585 (2018).

57. Moon, C., Watts, A.B. & Williams III, R.O. Thin film freezing for production of an amorphous mannitol/lysozyme formulation for inhalation: A comparison of freezing techniques. *Respiratory Drug Delivery* 3, 611–616 (2016).

58. Izutsu, K.-I., Yoshioka, S. & Terao, T. Decreased protein-stabilizing effects of cryoprotectants due to crystallization. *Pharmaceutical Research* 10(8), 1232–1237 (1993).

59. Watts, A.B., Carvalho, S.R., Liu, S., Peters, J.I. & Williams III, R.O. Brittle matrices as a DPI platform for combination therapies. *Respiratory Drug Delivery* 2, 517–522 (2015).

60. Nikolakakis, I. & Partheniadis, I. Self-emulsifying granules and pellets: Composition and formation mechanisms for instant or controlled release. *Pharmaceutics* 9(4), (2017).

61. AboulFotouh, K., Zhang, Y., Maniruzzaman, M., Williams, R.O., 3rd & Cui, Z. Amorphous solid dispersion dry powder for pulmonary drug delivery: Advantages and challenges. *International Journal of Pharmacy* 587, 119711 (2020).

62. Overhoff, K.A. *et al.* Effect of stabilizer on the maximum degree and extent of supersaturation and oral absorption of tacrolimus made by ultra-rapid freezing. *Pharmaceutical Research* 25(1), 167–175 (2008).

63. Thakkar, S.G., Ruwona, T.B., Williams, R.O., 3rd & Cui, Z. The immunogenicity of thin-film freeze-dried, aluminum salt-adjuvanted vaccine when exposed to different temperatures. *Human Vaccines and Immunotherapeutics* 13(4), 936–946 (2017).

64. Almeida, A.J. & Souto, E. Solid lipid nanoparticles as a drug delivery system for peptides and proteins. *Advanced Drug Delivery Reviews* 59(6), 478–490 (2007).

65. Liu, J. *et al.* Solid lipid nanoparticles for pulmonary delivery of insulin. *International Journal of Pharmacy* 356(1–2), 333–344 (2008).

66. Niu, M. *et al.* Biodistribution and in vivo activities of tumor-associated macrophage-targeting nanoparticles incorporated with doxorubicin. *Molecular Pharmaceutics* 11(12), 4425–4436 (2014).

67. Baldrick, P. & Bamford, D.G. A toxicological review of lactose to support clinical administration by inhalation. *Food and Chemical Toxicology* 35(7), 719–733 (1997).

68. Huppertz, T. & Gazi, I. Lactose in dairy ingredients: Effect on processing and storage stability. *Journal of Dairy Science* 99(8), 6842–6851 (2016).

69. Kim, A.I., Akers, M.J. & Nail, S.L. The physical state of mannitol after freeze-drying: Effects of mannitol concentration, freezing rate, and a noncrystallizing cosolute. *Journal of Pharmaceutical Sciences* 87(8), 931–935 (1998).

70. Moon, C., Sahakijpijarn, S., Koleng, J.J. & Williams III, R.O. Processing design space is critical for voriconazole nanoaggregates for dry powder inhalation produced by thin film freezing. *Journal of Drug Delivery Science and Technology* 54, 101295 (2019).

71. Wang, Y.B., Watts, A.B. & Williams, R.O. Effect of processing parameters on the physicochemical and aerodynamic properties of respirable brittle matrix powders. *Journal of Drug Delivery Science and Technology* 24(4), 390–396 (2014).

72. Li, X., Thakkar, S.G., Ruwona, T.B., Williams, R.O., 3rd & Cui, Z. A method of lyophilizing vaccines containing aluminum salts into a dry powder without causing particle aggregation or decreasing the immunogenicity following reconstitution. *Journal of Controlled Release* 204, 38–50 (2015).

73. Thakkar, S.G. *et al.* Intranasal immunization with aluminum salt-adjuvanted dry powder vaccine. *Journal of Controlled Release* 292, 111–118 (2018).

74. Zhang, Y., Soto, M., Ghosh, D. & Williams, R.O., 3rd Manufacturing stable bacteriophage powders by including buffer system in formulations and using thin film freeze-drying technology. *Pharmaceutical Research* 38(10), 1793–1804 (2021).

75. Chen, D. & Kristensen, D. Opportunities and challenges of developing thermostable vaccines. *Expert Review of Vaccines* 8(5), 547–557 (2009).

76. *A Study of AeroVanc for the Treatment of MRSA Infection in CF Patients*, (2017, ClinicalTrials.gov: U.S. National Library of Medicine.
77. Sou, T., Orlando, L., McIntosh, M.P., Kaminskas, L.M. & Morton, D.A. Investigating the interactions of amino acid components on a mannitol-based spray-dried powder formulation for pulmonary delivery: A design of experiment approach. *International Journal of Pharmacy* 421(2), 220–229 (2011).
78. Alhajj, N., O'Reilly, N.J. & Cathcart, H. Leucine as an excipient in spray dried powder for inhalation. *Drug Discovery Today* 26(10), 2384–2396 (2021).
79. Yurtsever, Z., Erman, B. & Yurtsever, E. Competitive hydrogen bonding in aspirin-aspirin and aspirin-leucine interactions. *Turkish Journal of Chemistry* 36, 383–398 (2012).
80. Mangal, S. *et al.* Physico-chemical properties, aerosolization and dissolution of co-spray dried azithromycin particles with L-leucine for inhalation. *Pharmaceutical Research* 35(2), 28 (2018).
81. FDA Label, TOBI Podhaler (tobramycin inhalation powder), for oral inhalation use. FDA: Novartis, 2020.
82. Thompson, J.W., Kaiser, T.J. & Jorgenson, J.W. Viscosity measurements of methanol-water and acetonitrile-water mixtures at pressures up to 3500 bar using a novel capillary time-of-flight viscometer. *Journal of Chromatography: Part A* 1134(1–2), 201–209 (2006).
83. Gu, T., Gu, Y. & Zheng, Y. Phase separation of acetonitrile-water mixture in protein purification. *Separations Technology* 4(4), 258–261 (1994).
84. Parumasivam, T. *et al.* The delivery of high-dose dry powder antibiotics by a low-cost generic inhaler. *The AAPS Journal* 19(1), 191–202 (2017).

Nanoparticles as Specific Drug Carriers

10

Thaís Larissa do Amaral Montanheiro,
Karla Faquine Rodrigues,
Renata Guimarães Ribas,
Vanessa Modelski Schatkoski,
Raissa Monteiro Pereira, and
Gilmar Patrocínio Thim

Contents

DOI: 10.1201/9781003182566-13

10.1 INTRODUCTION

One of the leading causes of death and disability worldwide involves respiratory tract diseases. About nine million deaths were related to respiratory disease in 2016, which corresponds to 15% of the death causes around the world, according to the World Health Organization. Lung cancer, tuberculosis, chronic obstructive pulmonary diseases, lower respiratory infections, asthma, idiopathic pulmonary fibrosis, and pulmonary hypertension are respiratory diseases listed in the top ten causes of death in the world[1,2] and will become one of the leading causes of death worldwide in the near future.[3]

Inhalation therapy is one of the oldest approaches to treat respiratory disease. Currently, it is accepted as the most effective and safest treatment to deliver drugs directly to the airways because the drug goes directly through the respiratory system to the lungs, avoiding contact with other tissues and acting *in situ*. However, particle size limits the application, especially when the drug is administrated through airways.[4] In cancer treatment, like lung cancer, small molecules used as agents of chemotherapeutics have some restrictions in clinical applications: low water solubility, nonspecific biodistribution, and lack of targeting as well as low therapeutic indices are some of them.[5] Thus, there is great interest in tailoring particle size to deliver drugs in specific areas of the respiratory tract. The synthesis development of nanoparticles (NPs) can be an option to improve drug delivery systems (DDS).

Nanotechnology is a multidisciplinary area capable of engineering NPs ranging from 1–500 nm.[6] These NPs can be used to study and understand lethal biological problems and to diagnose and cure diseases.[7] Human living cells have a complex behavior that includes biological activity, cell signaling, metabolism, energy production, and nutrient transport. Each element of the cell is fundamental for its health function and plays an important role in biochemical chain reactions.[8] The advantage of NPs' use is that it consists of an easy cell interaction that can modify specific cell components, enabling less toxic and more efficient therapeutic performance. By this, the NPs are highly recommended for drug delivery due to their large surface area that enhances bioactivity, facilitates targeting, and can regulate solubility and stability. Therefore, the use of NPs with therapeutics purposes is expected to solve many severe diseases in the least invasive way possible.[9]

NPs can infiltrate almost any tissue site, and for this reason, they are the current promise for delivering drugs to treat lung diseases. The pulmonary drug delivery route presents many characteristics that makes the use of NPs suitable. The lung presents a large alveolar surface area available for drug absorption, with a highly permeable epithelial layer. Also, it has an extensive vascularized tissue combined with a relatively low level of endogenous enzymatic/proteolytic that facilitates the medicine interaction. Another relevant aspect is the possibility to deliver drugs directly to the site of lung disease, avoiding the first-pass metabolism by the hepatic portal system with pH variations.[10] This way, many types of NPs can be synthesized from various organic or inorganic materials to be used in drug delivery.[11]

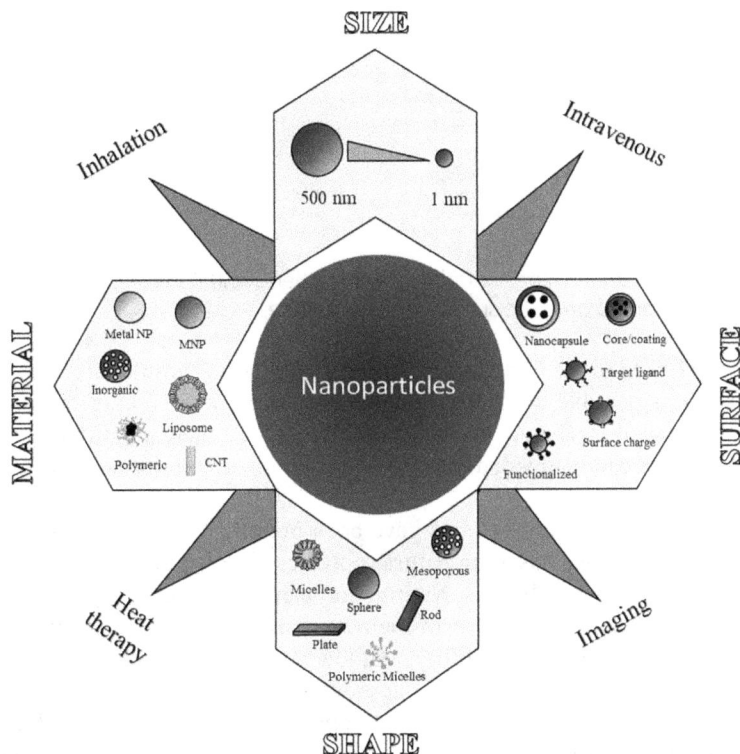

FIGURE 10.1 Different types of nanoparticles, shapes, and applications.

The development of nanocarriers for drug delivery and targeting to the lung has been widely studied by the scientific community in recent decades and more recently due to the global spreading disease SARS-CoV-2, which was first recognized in December 2019.[2,12] In general, the use of carrier systems composed of NPs is conceptually attractive for the use of drugs that act on the respiratory system. This system of delivering drugs can cause retention of the particles in the lungs accompanied by a prolonged drug release if large porous nanoparticle matrices are used.[13]

Different NPs can be synthesized according to the application, and existing NPs can be modified to obtain the desired features (Figure 10.1). In this chapter, the most common NPs used for pulmonary diseases treatments have been cited, with their main advantages as drug carriers to the lungs.

10.2 POLYMERIC NANOPARTICLES

Polymeric nanoparticles applied to controlled drug release refer to two different types of structures: nanospheres and nanocapsules. Nanospheres are systems in which an active ingredient is homogeneously dispersed or dissolved within the polymer matrix

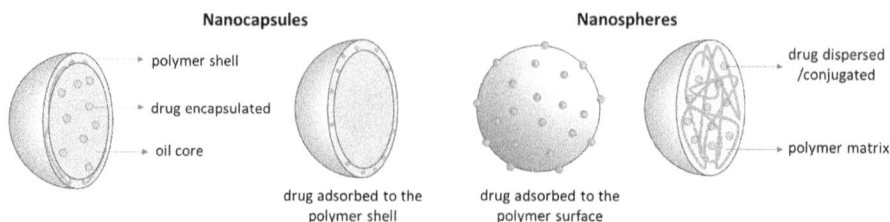

FIGURE 10.2 Schematic representation of nanospheres and nanocapsules with the drug entrapped or adsorbed onto the surface of nanoparticles.

or covalently linked to the particle. On the other hand, nanocapsules are vesicular systems, where it is possible to identify a core that generally consists of oil surrounded by a polymeric shell[14,15] (Figure 10.2). For this type of NP, there are different synthesis techniques, which can be divided into methods that involve preformed polymers or *in situ* polymerization.[16]

The polymeric delivery systems have been broadly categorized into two main groups: (i) nanoparticles based on natural polymers and (ii) nanoparticles based on synthetic biodegradable polymers. Natural polymers have been widely used in pharmaceutical and medical areas due to their favorable biological properties, including biodegradability, biocompatibility, and low toxicity. Coupled with low cost and Food and Drug Administration (FDA) approval, chitosan and alginate are the most popular polymeric materials used in pulmonary DDS.[14] Chitosan is obtained by alkaline deacetylation of chitin, derived from the exoskeleton of crustaceans. The safety and tolerability of chitosan are synergistic characteristics towards its application in drug delivery via pulmonary route. Despite the natural properties, chitosan has some disadvantages, such as poor solubility at physiological pH and passive effect on drug targeting. Thus, combined with the presence of reactive amine groups in the chemical structure of chitosan, chemical modifications through the conjugation of various functional groups allow the control of hydrophilicity and solubility at neutral and basic pH, opening new opportunities to expand the application of this natural polymer as a drug carrier.[17]

10.2.1 Natural Polymers

Chitosan nanoparticles have good mucoadhesive and membrane permeability-enhancing properties improving the uptake of hydrophilic drugs in the lungs.[15,18] On the other hand, mucoadhesive properties of chitosan and derivatives may also be adverse once adhesion of delivery systems at the upper respiratory tract and airways can also occur, thus limiting the amount of carrier that effectively reaches the deep lung.[17] In addition, in the area of inhalation therapy, nanoparticles can be rapidly eliminated by macrophages of the alveolar region which results in rapid phagocytosis of carrier particles and loss of the therapeutic molecules.[19] However, it is possible to improve the drug circulation time and biodistribution by modulating some of the physical-chemical properties of nanoparticles such as size, shape, density, composition, and surface charge.[15]

Grafting of hydrophilic polymers such as polyethylene glycol (PEG) onto the chitosan backbone has been carried out to improve chitosan physicochemical properties by forming a swelling/viscous crown around the drug-loaded microparticles to temporarily repulse macrophages.[17,19] Poly(lactic-*co*-glycolic acid) (PLGA) nanoparticles were attached to chitosan-*g*-PEG for sustained pulmonary delivery of curcumin using dry powder inhalers for the treatment of various pulmonary diseases. The developed carriers (average size 3.1–3.9 μm) attained high swelling within a few minutes and showed low moisture content as dry powders (0.9–1.8%). The low moisture content decreased the particle density and accordingly enhanced the aerodynamic performance of the particles through the inhalation process. The chitosan-*g*-PEG attached to PLGA nanoparticles provides desirable biodegradation rates, high drug loading (up to 97%), and good sustained release.[19]

Additionally, antimicrobial activity for different types of chitosan and derivatives has been reported.[18,20,21] The electrostatic interaction between the protonated amino groups of chitosan and the phosphoryl groups and lipopolysaccharides of bacterial cell membranes destroys the membrane and releases the cellular contents resulting in the chitosan antibacterial effects.[22] Thus, because of their unique membrane interruption ability in addition to antimicrobial effects, chitosan and its derivatives are good candidates to effectively sensitize multidrug-resistant bacteria to classical antibiotics.[21] The antimicrobial synergy between chitosan and relevant antibiotics (amikacin, tazobactam, tobramycin, rifampicin, and novobiocin) performed in *in vivo* lung infection models proves to be effective against drug-resistant pathogens such as *A. baumannii* and methicillin-resistant *Staphylococcus aureus*.[21]

Chitosan has also been investigated for non-viral gene delivery in the form of deoxyribonucleic acid (DNA)-chitosan complexes or as nanoparticles due to its cationic nature.[23,24] Ionic interactions between primary amine of chitosan and the negatively charged phosphate backbone of DNA protect it from nuclease degradation and are hence found effective in DNA-based vaccine delivery.[25] Chitosan nanoparticles have been employed in pulmonary delivery of DNA vaccines against tuberculosis increasing immune responses at mucosal sites.[23] A chitosan–DNA nanoparticle encoding human HLA-A*0201-restricted T cell-epitopes of six M. tuberculosis proteins was evaluated in transgenic mice. Two immunization strategies (non-invasive endotracheal and intramuscular injection) using the polyepitope DNA vaccine were investigated. The nanoparticle-based DNA created induced the maturation of dendritic cells and increased the IFN-γ secretion from T-cells after pulmonary mucosal immunization.[23]

10.2.2 Synthetic Polymers

Despite being promising materials in the drug loading area, natural polymers faced many problems such as stability, reproducibility, changes in storage aesthetics, and uncontrollable formulation characteristics. On the other hand, synthetic polymers can be custom designed to meet specific needs.[26] Among emerging synthetic biodegradable polymers proposed for pulmonary delivery, the most commonly used polymers are poly(lactic acid), PLGA, and poly(ε-caprolactone) (PCL).[14,27,28] Synthetic polymers have the advantage of allowing the sustained release of the drug, as they generally have slower degradation than natural polymers. PCL, for example, undergoes total degradation in two to four years,[29] while chitosan is degraded in a few days or months, depending on its degree of deacetylation.[30]

PLGA nanoparticles are one of the most explored biodegradable polymeric drug carriers to promote either fast or prolonged drug release with applications in cancer treatment,[31] cystic fibrosis,[32] and in the treatment of pulmonary tuberculosis.[33] PLGA degrades slowly *in vivo,* and the by-products like lactic and glycolic acid are easily metabolized and excreted.[32] Therefore, PLGA nanoparticles can entrap both water-soluble and water-insoluble molecules becoming continuously evaluated for the delivery of drugs, genetic materials, and proteins to *in vitro* and *in vivo* studies. These nanoparticulate systems are rapidly endocytosed by cells followed by the release of their therapeutic payload.[32] However, the slow degradation rate of PLGA is a disadvantage for pulmonary drug delivery, especially when repeated administrations are required.[34]

The drug resistance that develops in time by cancer cells remains the main challenge in chemotherapy. To overcome the mechanisms of multidrug resistance in lung cancer cells, a system of PLGA nanoparticles loaded with docetaxel (DOC) and vitamin E TPGS (D-tocopheryl polyethylene glycol succinate) has been proposed. DOC is a common antineoplastic agent used to treat many types of cancer that interfere with microtubule function leading to altered mitosis and cellular death, whereas vitamin E TPGS inhibits multidrug resistance-related proteins, thereby improving the anticancer efficiency of DOC.[31,35] In *in vitro* tests, the use of 20% vitamin E TPGS in a vitamin E TPGS/PLGA mixture showed an increased death rate in HeLa cells after 48 h. The IC_{50} values of 20% vitamin E TPGS/PLGA formulation (0.009 μg/mL) were 52.7-fold more effective than the free vitamin E TPGS nanoparticles (2.619 μg/mL). In addition, a xenograft tumor model showed that the vitamin E TPGS-loaded PLGA nanoparticles have a significantly better anti-tumor effect compared with the use of DOC alone.[31]

The primary modality to treat lung cancer patients has been systemic chemotherapy. However, its effectiveness is limited once the chemotherapeutic drug is targeted to lung tumor sites consequently resulting in normal cells' damage, causing significant toxicities and undesirable side effects.[36] So, aerosol delivery of chemotherapeutic agents is a direct local delivery method that offers a novel therapeutic approach for lung cancer therapy. Polymeric micelles have been developed to entrap anticancer drugs due to their ability to solubilize hydrophobic drugs, good biocompatibility, long circulation, and selective tumor targeting. Polymeric micelles are nano-sized core/shell structures formed by amphiphilic block copolymers. The hydrophobic cores usually serve as reservoirs for a hydrophobic drug, whereas the hydrophilic shell can provide the necessary steric protection to stabilize the cores. The hydrophilic shell has the function to maintain the dispersion and stability of the micelles and prevent rapid phagocytosis by macrophages *in vivo.* As a typical polymeric micelle, PLGA-*co*-PEG (PLGA-PEG) has been broadly used for drug delivery. However, PLGA-polyspermine (PSPE) polymeric micelles have been developed to overcome some drawbacks associated with PEG such as enhanced serum protein binding, reduced uptake by target cells, and the elicitation of an immune response which facilitates clearance *in vivo.*[36] *In vitro* and *in vivo* tests have shown that dihydroergotamine tartrate encapsulated into PLGA-PSPE polymeric micelles can significantly suppress lung cancer cell survival and improve anticancer effect administration with no potential systemic toxicity after being delivered to the lung via an aerosol.

PCL is a viable material for use as nano-drug delivery vesicles especially when long-term drug delivery is desired due to its slow degradation rate. The biodegradability of PCL is adjustable through forming of blends, composites, and copolymers. For example, the biodegradability of PCL can be enhanced by copolymerization with PEG.[37,38] PEG is suitable to construct caprolactone block copolymers (two or three block copolymers) because of its hydrophilicity, nontoxicity, and absence of antigenicity and immunogenicity.[37] In recent years, the PCL-PEG triblock copolymer nanoparticles have attracted wide attention due to their core-shell structure that allows hydrophobic anticancer drugs to enter the inner core. A study performed using nanoparticles prepared from a PCL-PEG triblock copolymer loaded with an antineoplastic agent (paclitaxel) showed the significant anti-tumor efficacy of nanoparticles in combination with chronomodulated chemotherapy in lung cancer.[38] Besides this, it releases drugs in a slow and sustained manner at a later stage. Their hydrophilic outer shell prevents the rapid elimination of the drugs from blood circulation and they avoid being captured by the reticuloendothelial system.[38]

The behavior of different NPs, including natural and synthetic polymer-based nanoparticles (gelatin, chitosan, alginate, PLGA, PLGA–chitosan, and PLGA–PEG), was screened for pulmonary protein/DNA delivery both *in vitro* and *in vivo*. PLGA-based NPs had the highest cytocompatibility, and natural polymer NPs showed the highest *in vitro* uptake at specified concentrations by type 1 alveolar epithelial cells. Upon nebulization and inhalational delivery into rat lungs, PLGA NPs yielded more uniform and sustained tissue distributions of the payload compound than gelatin NPs. Overall, the study favored PLGA and gelatin NPs as promising carriers for pulmonary protein/DNA delivery.[39] The properties observed *in vitro* conditions such as cellular uptake and cytotoxicity may not completely reflect their behavior *in vivo*. Therefore, it is important to validate the *in vitro* with *in vivo* results to choose the most favorable nanocarrier for the desired application.[39]

Synthetic biodegradable copolymers NPs such as poly(glycerol adipate-*co*-ω-pentadecalactone) (PGA-co-PDL) have the potential to be used for gene delivery and specific cell targeting. However, the hydrophobic nature of NPs makes it difficult to load microRNA (miRNA) into NPs due to the absence of electrostatic interaction. However, cationic additives such as chitosan or cationic lipids such as 1,2-dioleoyl-3-trimethylammonium-propane (DOTAP) can be added to the surface pre or post-formation of NPs promoting the efficiency of miRNA transfection.[40,41] In a preliminary *in vitro* study, PGA-co-PDL was covered with DOTAP aiming to improve the miR-146a adsorption to reduce target gene IRAK1 expression in chronic obstructive pulmonary disease (COPD). The results showed that 15% (w/w) of DOTAP on PGA-co-PDL NPs can effectively adsorb 32.25 ± 2.0 µg miR-146a per 10 mg NPs after 2 h. As a result, the high miR-146a-NPs concentration reduced target gene IRAK1 expression to 40% claiming the potential of cationic NPs for delivery of miR-146a in the treatment and management of COPD.[41] Additionally, a study comparing poly(β-amino ester) formulated with PEG-lipid to deliver both messenger RNA (mRNA) or DNA *in vivo* indicates that different nucleic acids require tailored delivery vectors. *In vitro* assays showed that there was little difference between the two nucleic acids in their ability to produce the luciferase protein in HeLa cells. However, *in vivo* assays showed that mRNA was two orders of magnitude greater than plasmin DNA (pDNA) to induce protein production in the lungs of mice following systemic delivery.[42]

10.3 LIPID NANOPARTICLES

Lipid nanoparticles (LNPs), including solid lipid nanoparticles (SLNP), nanostructured lipid carriers (NLC), cationic lipid–nucleic acid complexes (lipoplexes), and liposomes (an early version of LNPs), are a versatile nanocarrier platform because they can transport hydrophobic or hydrophilic molecules, including small molecules, proteins, and nucleic acids.[43] Lipid-based nanocarriers were developed to improve the performance of nanoemulsions, in which the liquid phase is substituted with solid one (SLNP) or a blend of solid and liquid lipids.[44] Lipoplexes are a complex formed by a combination of cationic liposomes with negatively charged DNA that can be used as gene vectors.[45]

LNPs have been synthesized and used for delivering conventional drugs or genetic drugs including plasmid DNA-containing therapeutic genes, antisense oligonucleotides (ASO), and small interfering RNA (siRNA) both *in vitro* and *in vivo*. However, their application in gene delivery is limited due to low efficiency.[46] To overcome this problem, new lipids are being synthesized and new approaches for complex formation are being developed continuously.[47]

There are various potential therapeutic applications of siRNA in the lung, including treatment cystic fibrosis, tumor metastasis, and asthma. In this way, systemic administration of siRNA via the intravascular route with cationic liposomes has shown success for siRNA delivery into the lungs.[48] A study tested six cationic cholesterol derivatives, 11 cationic glycerol-based derivatives, and 17 cationic liposomes composed of cationic lipid and 1,2 dioleoyl phosphatidylethanolamine to compare the efficiency of Tie2 siRNA delivery to lung tissue when injected intravenously in mice. The cationic cholesterol derivative-based lipoplexes demonstrated very efficient gene silencing, while glycerol-derivatives with short-length alkyl chains and long linker arms decreased the efficiency of gene silencing. However, some formulations showed a high accumulation of siRNA in the lung. Furthermore, injections with 3 glycerol-based derivatives with protein kinase N3 (PKN3) siRNA could suppress the increased tumor growth in mice Lewis lung carcinoma. Therefore, the siRNA biodistribution and *in vivo* knockdown efficiency are strongly affected by the type of cationic lipid of cationic liposomes.[48] Each lipid carrier has a distinctive structure and function to fit its application. Therefore, proper selection of lipid vehicles combined with formulation techniques and coherent design of the delivery system are indispensable elements to engineer lipid-based delivery systems.[49]

Cationic lipids have a short residence time in blood circulation resulting in their elimination from the bloodstream by the reticuloendothelial system after systemic administration. This problem was partially solved by covering their surface with other functional groups such as PEG. However, the delivery of different types of payloads requires different properties of carriers, including their surface charge.[46] For example, modified uncharged nucleotides can be delivered by neutral or slightly charged liposomes whereases native negatively charged such as siRNA or DNA molecules required cationic liposomes.

PEGylated LNPs were investigated to deliver doxorubicin (DOX) and ASO while DOTAP was used to deliver negatively charged siRNA. Liposomal drug formulations provided more efficient intracellular delivery of DOX, ASO, and siRNA *in vitro* when compared with free drugs. PEGylated and cationic liposomes with respective payload were used to compare two distinct routes of administration, systemic intravenous and local intratracheal, on mice. The study showed that intratracheal delivery of both types of liposomes *in vivo* led to higher peak concentrations and much longer retention of liposomes, DOX, ASO, and siRNA in the lungs when compared with systemic administration.[46] Another study showed that nanostructured lipid carriers (NLCs) used for inhalation delivery of anticancer drugs and siRNA effectively delivered their payload into lung cancer cells leaving healthy lung tissues intact and significantly decreasing the exposure of healthy organs when compared with intravenous injection. In addition, the NLCs showed enhanced antitumor activity when compared with intravenous treatment. Drug inhalation enables rapid deposition in the lungs and induces fewer side effects than administration by other routes.[50]

Lipid–polymer hybrid nanoparticles are a new structure of the delivery system that utilize the unique attributes of liposomes and polymeric NPs that led to their initial clinical success. This configuration overcomes limitations like structural disintegration, limited circulation time, and content leakage. The polymeric core facilitates encapsulation of hydrophobic drugs whereases a lipid monolayer surrounding the polymer mitigates the loss of entrapped drugs and protects the core from degradation by preventing the diffusion of water into the inner core.[51]

Pulmonary drug delivery offers opportunities to improve drug therapies systemically and locally using advanced DDS such as polymeric and lipid-based nanoparticles. However, the prolonged use of the drug often leads to nephrotoxicity, neurotoxicity, and irreversible ototoxicity.[52] In this way, the entrapment and controlled release of the drug into polymeric or lipid-based nanoparticles could reduce the required dose remarkably and hence reduce the associated toxicity.

Among clinically approved nanoparticle formulations whether in the United States by the FDA or in the European Union by the European Medicines Agency (EMA), 35% include polymeric-based nanoparticles and 29% include lipid-based nanoparticles.[53] Many clinically approved nanoparticle formulations are used for the treatment of different cancers. For example, Doxil is a PEGylated liposome type of nanocarrier used for treating multiple cancers, and it was the first approved cancer nanomedicine (FDA 1995).[53] Most recently, an albumin-bound paclitaxel nanoparticle (Abraxane®) was approved in 2012 by the FDA for cancer treatment.[53,54] It has been used for the treatment of a large list of cancer including non-small cell lung carcinoma, and pancreatic and prostate cancer. In addition to approved nanoparticle therapies, updates on reported nanoparticle clinical trials that have not been clinically approved and are currently undergoing clinical trials are presented in Table 10.1.

10.4 CELLULOSE NANOCRYSTALS

Nanocellulose is a natural material extracted from native cellulose, with remarkable properties such as having no cytotoxicity, high elastic modulus and tensile strength,

TABLE 10.1   FDA Approved drug-loaded polymer and lipid-based nanoparticles and updates on nanoparticles that have not been clinically approved yet

NAME	MATERIAL DESCRIPTION	INDICATIONS	YEAR APPROVED	REF.
Doxil Caelyx (Janssen)	Liposomal nanoparticle	Various cancers including: solid malignancies, ovarian, breast, leukemia, lymphomas, prostate, metastatic, or liver	1995	54
Pfizer-BioNTech	Liposomal nanoparticle	COVID-19	2020	53
Moderna	Liposomal nanoparticle	COVID-19	2020	53
Poractant Alfa	Liposome-proteins SP-band SP-C	Pulmonary surfactant for respiratory distress syndrome	1999	53,55
Abraxane	Albumin-particle bound paclitaxel	Lung cancer, metastatic breast cancer, metastatic pancreatic cancer	2005	54
Oncoprex (Genprex)	Liposomal nanoparticle	Lung cancer	Phase I e II Active (2016)	54
BIND-014 (BIND Therapeutics)	PSMA targeted (via ACUPA) docetaxel PEG-PLGA or PLA–PEG particle	Prostate, metastatic, non-small cell lung, cervical, head and neck, or KRAS positive lung cancers	Phase II completed (2016)	54
ND-L02-s0201 (Nitto Denko)	siRNA lipid nanoparticle conjugated to vitamin A	Hepatic fibrosis and pulmonary fibrosis	Phase I completed (2016) Phase II recruiting (2019)	54

hydrophilicity, good colloidal stability, high surface area, and the possibility of surface modification.[56,57] There are three main types of nanocellulose: cellulose nanocrystals (CNC) or nanowhiskers (CNW), cellulose nanofibers (CNF), and bacterial cellulose (BC).[56,58] CNCs are usually obtained by acid or enzymatic hydrolysis of cellulose and CNFs are usually mechanically processed.[56,57,59] BC are synthesized by bacteria such as *Acetobacter xylinum*, with no need for further purification.[58]

Several studies have shown the non-toxicity of CNCs, and the potential for use as biomaterials[56,59,60]; however, when CNCs are inhaled under a high concentration, there may be some cytotoxicity and inflammation occurrence.[61] CNCs sizes and surface energy directly affect the interactions with respiratory mucus and cells, affecting the

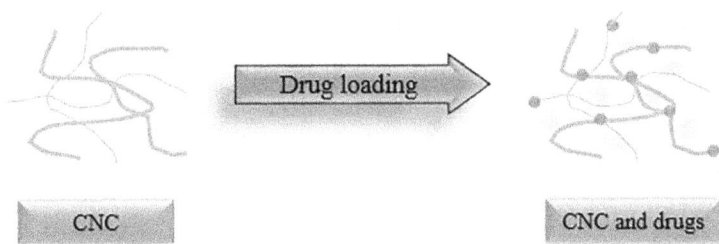

FIGURE 10.3   CNC NPs before and after drug loading.

respiratory tract,[62] still, studies relating to these properties are very limited. Apparently, longer CNCs may lead to long-term consequences because they can sit longer on the lung epithelial cells.[63] Modified CNCs have been shown to increase the up-regulation of inflammatory cytokines in mice's lungs.[64]

Cellulosic materials are often used in the preparation of pharmaceutical dosage forms. CNCs can be used as DDS, for encapsulation and delivery of biomolecules, due to their good colloidal stability. To achieve the desired properties, usually, CNCs are grafted or coated with other materials, such as chitosan and sodium alginate to form films or microcapsules. The presence of CNC may induce a slower drug release, resulting in a steric effect. Besides that, the vast possibilities of converting the hydroxyl group on CNC's surface allow providing programmed drug releases.[65,66] CNCs can also be used as dispensers for cancer theranostic agents, once several anti-cancer agents have presented many side effects, such as toxicity, neuropathy, anorexia, and cognitive and motivational deficits fatigue, among others.[67] Figure 10.3 presents a schematic of the structure of CNC NPs being loaded with some type of drug.

Core-shell structures with CNC as the core can be obtained using the layer-by-layer technique, for example.[66] Chemotherapeutic drugs such as DOX and hyaluronic acid can be used to form the layers, based on electrostatic interactions between positive and negative charges, through an eco-friendly approach. Hyaluronic acid is employed to enclose the CNC-DOX structure and to provide selective drug delivery to CD44 receptor-positive lung adenocarcinoma (A549) cells. The prepared material was tested *in vitro* to evaluate cell accumulation, anticancer activity, tumor infiltration, and the *in vivo* tests were for biodistribution and systemic toxicity of the engineered nanosystems after intravenous administration in normal mice. This core-shell structure presented improved tumor penetration potential, reactive oxygen species (ROS) production, and cancer-killing capacity, along with promising *in vivo* results if compared to pure DOX or DOX-CNC structure.

The dissemination of melanoma cells from the initial tumor location to other parts of the body, such as the lungs, occurs via the circulatory and lymphatic systems. CNCs have the potential to embolize into neovascularization of metastatic tumors once they accumulate in the lung vasculature. Using this concept, CNCs could be used to deliver drugs to metastatic melanoma in the lung; moreover, CNCs could be radiolabeled with radioisotopes to obtain a theranostic system. Lutetium-labeled CNC loaded with vemurafenib was developed to investigate the synergistic effects of radio and chemotherapy. CNC were evaluated through *in vitro* tests of cell cytotoxicity, cell uptake, cell survival,

TABLE 10.2   Use of CNC in the treatment of lung cancer

NANOPARTICLE	DISEASE	TREATMENT/DRUG	REF.
CNC	Lung cancer	DOX/Hyaluronic acid	71
		Radiolabeled/Vemurafenib	72
		Fluorescent labeling/CAD	73

and *in vivo* biodistribution. In addition, therapeutic studies of NPs were conducted in mice. CNC proved to be a potential renewable and natural platform for the development of theranostic systems to treat metastatic melanoma in the lung using radiotherapy and sustained release of vemurafenib.[68]

Rod-like CNC is beneficial for enhanced permeability and retention effect in tumor tissues and is a convenient drug delivery platform, which can be transformed into fluorescence-visible nanoparticles through fluorescent labeling. This fluorescent CNC can be labeled with cis-aconityl-doxorubicin (CAD) and be used in lung cancer therapies. The obtained fluorescent CNC-CAD is simply fabricated and has improved cellular uptake and intracellular controlled release. When tested, *in vitro*, against human large cell lung cancer cell line (NCI-H460), CNC-CAD showed considerable ability as a fluorescence-visible DDS.[69]

Nanocrystals, in general, have suitable morphology for pulmonary drug delivery. Drug-loaded nanocrystals are expected to present selective cellular internalization. The possibility of surface functionalization increases the possibility of having a more prolonged and specific delivery of drugs into lung cells.[70] CNCs are promising nanocrystals because of their intrinsic properties and vast possibilities of surface modification. However, besides having auspicious results, few studies are available, and there is the need for further investigation combined with *in vivo* assays. Table 10.2 summarizes the use of CNC in the treatment of lung cancer, showing its association with different drugs.

10.5 CARBON NANOPARTICLES

The search for highly efficient materials has intensified in recent years, especially for nanomedicine applications. In this sense, carbonaceous nanostructures have been presented as a very promising materials class to meet the needs of medical and biological science. This is, due to their ability to directly interact with biomolecules, including peptides, lipids, nucleic acids, and proteins, for the delivery of specific drugs.[74] Studies show that carbon nanostructures are ideal for the production of drug nanocarriers because they are capable of encapsulating substances.[75] As well as this, carbon-based nanocarriers can be easily adapted for targeted delivery, resulting in a higher drug concentration at the site for designated drug action.[76] In addition, carbon nanostructures also have other characteristics suitable for drug carriers, such as high surface area, easy functionalization, improved cell uptake, biocompatibility, and antiviral properties.[77,78]

Carbonaceous nanomaterials can be synthesized in different structures and geometries, such as nanoparticles, nanotubes, nanodisks, nanoshells, nanobuds, nanowires, and nanocages, among others.[75,78] Some of the carbonaceous nanomaterials that can be

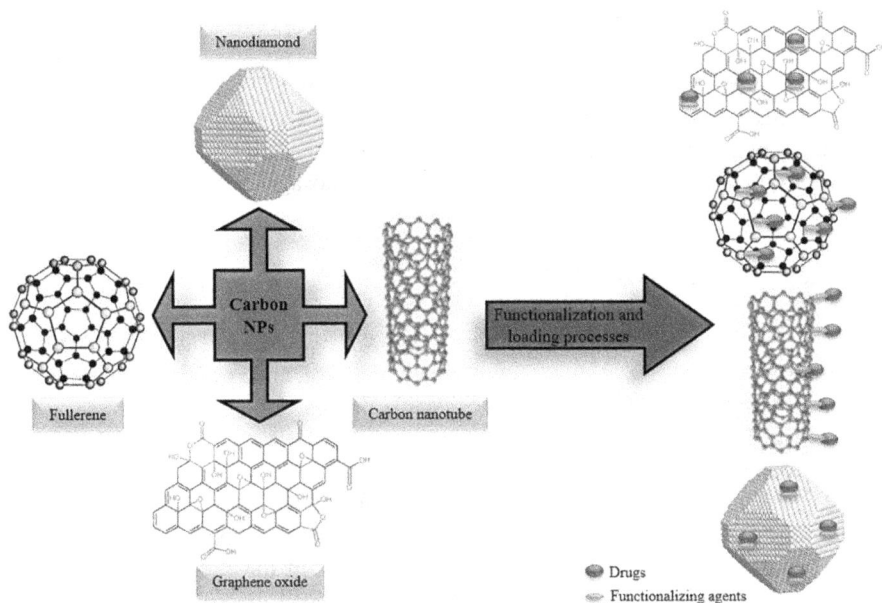

FIGURE 10.4   Structure of carbon NPs.

described as carbon allotropes are fullerene (C60), carbon nanotube (CNT), graphene (GR), and nanodiamond (ND). Allotropic forms of carbon-based materials can have zero, one, two, or three dimensions.[78]

The carbon nanostructures mentioned (Figure 10.4), C60, GO, CNT, and ND, are ideal drug carriers for lung diseases, whether viral, antimicrobial, or carcinogenic.[79] It is known that lung cancer is extremely lethal since this disease is the type of cancer that causes the most deaths in the world,[80] and the harmful effects of SARS-CoV-19, among other viral diseases, were responsible for millions of deaths in the last two years. In this way, carbonaceous nanostructures help to obtain increasingly efficient materials for the treatment of these pathologies.

10.5.1 Fullerene

C60 consists of 60 carbon atoms with sp^2 hybridization, arranged in hexagons and pentagons to form a spherical and hollow structure, of zero dimension.[81] The C60 has excellent symmetry and therefore has high structural and chemical stability. Furthermore, it has properties such as low toxicity, scavenging of free radicals, and it is easy to insert functional groups on its surface. These features make the C60 attractive to transport drugs in the human body in a targeted way.[76,78]

Tris-aminocaproic acid chemically bound to the surface of C60 hydrates (FTACAH) was prepared and tested (*in vitro*) for antiviral activity against the respiratory syncytial virus (RSV). RSV is responsible for infectious pathologies of the respiratory system and affects mainly newborns and children. A comparative study of the cytotoxicity of

FTACAH and the drug ribavirin, which can be used to fight the RSV virus, was also conducted. Cytotoxicity results indicated that FTACAH was more effective than the standard drug since that it was used up to a concentration of 100 g/mL. In addition, the antiviral activity study showed that FTACAH exhibited antiviral activity against RSV, if administrated within two hours of infection or simultaneously with the virus. Besides that, the efficiency of FTACAH was dependent on its dosage in the medium.[82]

10.5.2 Nanodiamond

ND is a zero-dimensional material, composed of sp^3 type hybridization in its interior, and the surface can be stabilized by converting sp^3 hybridization to sp^2 hybridization.[81,83] The properties of ND such as low toxicity, stable fluorescence, easy functionalization, and intrinsic biocompatibility indicate ND as an appropriate material for drug loading by the human body.[84]

ND covalently bonded to PTX was prepared for therapy against human lung carcinoma. For this, *in vivo* tests were conducted, so that the proposed biomaterial was injected subcutaneously in the area of the right flank in mice. The covalent conjugation between ND and PTX was confirmed and the cell viability tests proved that ND-paclitaxel blocked both tumor advancement and the formation of cancer cells, suggesting that the proposed material is indicated for the treatment of human lung carcinoma.[80] In contrast, ND particles were shown not to provoke mitotic blockade and apoptosis in lung cancer cells. Thus, it was found that ND is a benign nanomaterial for drug delivery based on its non-cytotoxicity and biocompatibility.[80]

10.5.3 Graphene

GR is a two-dimensional material composed of sp^2 type hybridization compacted forming hexagonal structures similar to a honeycomb; the hexagon tips are composed of sp^3 type hybridization.[76] GR can also be frequently found in other derivative forms, such as graphene oxide (GO) and reduced graphene oxide. GR and its derivatives have excellent physicochemical properties such as biocompatibility, high surface area, easy surface modification, and good mechanical strength, thus becoming promising materials for drug loading.[76]

β-cyclodextrin-functionalized GO was prepared to load curcumin in the treatment against RSV. Curcumin is a natural polyphenol used as an antioxidant, antifungal, antibacterial, anti-inflammatory, and antiviral agent. Due to its properties, curcumin can be used against the RSV virus. The main *in vitro* tests results indicated highly efficient inhibition of RSV infection and biocompatibility with host cells. The efficiency against RSV infection was dependent on the administered antiviral dose.[85]

10.5.4 Carbon Nanotube

Since the publication of the Japanese physicist Sumio Iijima in 1991,[86] CNTs have been widely studied and used in several fields of chemistry, physics, and engineering. CNT is a one-dimensional material, composed of carbon atoms linked by sp² type hybridizations, forming hexagons rolled like cylinders.[81,87] CNT has unique properties, such as high aspect ratio, very low density, cell penetration capacity, high surface area, and appropriate mechanical resistance. Thus, it is often used as a carrier for a wide variety of therapeutic agents.[76]

CNT can be used as a chemotherapeutic agent when functionalized with hyperbranched polycitric acid (PCA) and loaded with paclitaxel (PTX). The functionalizing agent PCA improves the hydrophilicity and functionality of the CNTs. PTX is a potent anticancer agent often used in chemotherapy. *In vitro* results indicated that the proposed material had a more cytotoxic effect than the free drug in a shorter incubation time, suggesting that the material has better cell penetration capacity. Thus, the drug carrier based on the CNT/PCA/PTX conjugate holds promise for lung cancer therapy.[88]

To assess the best composition for combating cancer cells, CNT had its surface investigated after functionalization with different chemical groups and subsequent loading with different anti-cancer agents. The functionalizing agents used were antifouling polymer PEG and tumor recognition modules (folic acid (FA)/hyaluronic acid /estradiol (ES)). Three different anticancer agents, methotrexate (MTX), DOX, and PTX, were loaded into each functionalized CNT preparation. *In vitro* cytotoxicity assays indicated that for the A549 cell line, samples CNT/ES/MTX and CNT/ES/DOX showed the greatest cytotoxic effect.[89]

Since the beginning of the COVID-19 pandemic, there has been a relentless search for drugs that would effectively combat the virus. Several studies address the issue in the nanobiomedicine field, to implement nanomaterials to treat COVID-19. In this sense, CNT was studied by computer simulations to assess its efficiency as carriers of the drug Remdesivir, to act in the control of the COVID-19 virus. For this, the drug interaction was tested with pure CNT and CNT functionalized with carboxylic groups and CNT doped with sulfur (S), aluminum (Al), and silicon (Si). The computational study relied on density functional theory and time-dependent density functional theory calculations. Computational calculations attributed Si-doped CNT as the best interaction with Remdesivir, making it the most promising material for drug loading to the lungs.[74]

Single-wall carbon nanotubes (SWCNT) and GO have been combined to load and potentiate the bioactive drug PTX, to fight lung cancer. To assess the efficacy of the drug carrier prepared, *in vitro* tests were conducted on two lung cancer cell lines, A549 and NCI-H460. The results obtained showed that there was an increase in cell death after the combined treatment of SWNT/GO/PTX, indicating a synergistic effect of the proposed material. However, it was found that the positive effect of SWNT/GO/PTX depends on the presence of ROS in the medium, as these species can increase the susceptibility of cancer cells. Thus, the ability of SWCNT and GO to generate ROS is crucial for the successful use of SWCNT/GO/PTX as a drug carrier. In addition, the study also showed that the two cell lines used were more vulnerable to GO than to SWCNT, which can be attributed to variations in different carbon nanostructures. The positive results regarding the use of SWCNT/GO/PTX proved the synergy between the components, thus, it was a promising material for the treatment of lung cancer.[90]

TABLE 10.3   Use of carbon nanoparticles to treat lung disease

NANOPARTICLE	DISEASE	TREATMENT/DRUG	REF.
C60	Respiratory syncytial virus	Tris-aminocaproic acid	91
ND	Lung cancer	PTX	71
GO	Respiratory syncytial virus	Curcumin	85
CNT	Lung cancer	Chemotherapy/PTX	92
	COVID-19	MTX, DOX, and PTX	93,94
		Remdesivir	95
CNT/GO	Lung cancer	PTX	90

10.5.5 Final Considerations on the Use of Carbon Nanoparticles

Carbon nanostructures for application as a drug carrier in the treatment of lung diseases exhibited positive results regarding the treatment of lung cancer and viral diseases that affect the lungs. But there was still a lot to explore and unravel. In this sense, the future requires the development of new treatments based on carbonaceous structures nanocarriers to fight cancer and other deadly respiratory diseases. The aid of computer simulations to study the interaction between the proposed nanoparticles and the virus or cancer cell under study is of paramount important. In addition, *in vitro* and *in vivo* assays are essential to obtain an effective material for clinical study. Table 10.3 summarizes the use of carbon nanoparticles to treat lung disease.

10.6 INORGANIC NANOPARTICLES

Inorganic NPs can be derived from their macromolecule counterparts such as silica or calcium phosphate.[11] Nonmetallic NPs can be surface modified using functionalization to improve controlled release, environmental response, targeting, and imaging,[93] as illustrated by Figure 10.5. Due to their tunable surface modification and adjustable size strategies they can be used as drug carrier systems.[96] NPs are characterized by their easy modification and detection, high drug loading capacity, chemical stability, and optical and magnetic properties. However, inorganic NPs are difficult to degrade *in vivo*, which limits their usage in pharmacology. But their broad application prospects in the pharmaceutical field and drug loading treatments should still be recognized.[96]

10.6.1 Silica Nanoparticles

Silica is an inorganic nanoparticle that presents highly porous amorphous structures and a large surface area. Mesoporous silica nanoparticles (MSNs) are a sub-classification of silica and present attractive properties of biocompatibility, ease functionalization, and

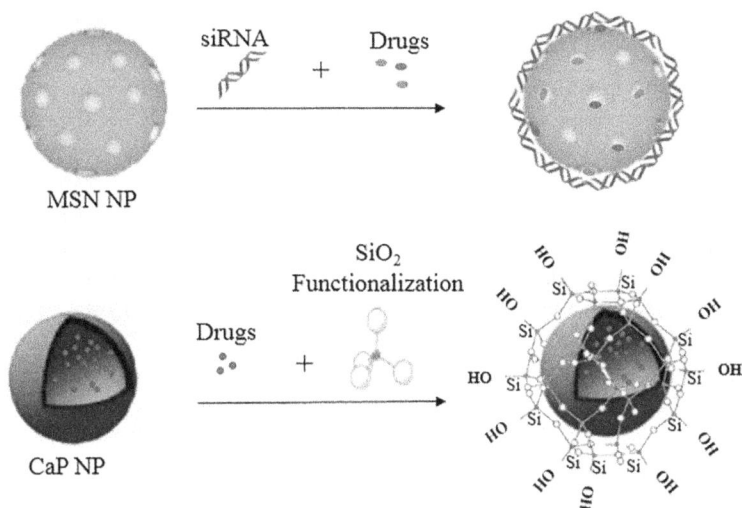

FIGURE 10.5 Structure of inorganic NPs.

highly porous framework. Because of this, they are vastly used as important carrier tools in controlled DDS. The pores of the MSNs permit the loading of different types of drugs, which facilitates a dual therapy for cancer treatment[97] (Figure 10.5).

Aiming to treat lung cancer, it was proposed to synthesize a MSNs conjugated with the drug cetuximab targeting epidermal growth factor receptor and delivering siRNA against polo-like kinase 1 (PLK1). PLK1 inhibition can lead to the death of cancer cells by interfering with multiple stages of mitosis.[98] The MSNs helped with the tumor growth reduction and prolonged survival of the healthy cells.[99] Another study demonstrated that MSNs coated with albumin were used to targeted-controlled release of paclitaxel. It was used A549 cells to perform *in vitro* cytotoxicity study. The results showed significant anti-proliferative activity of albumin-coated MSNs in lung cancer treatment.[100]

Another approach to treat lung cancer using MSNs was using siRNA. The RNA interference mechanism has been developed for endogenous post-transcriptional gene silencing inside cells. In this line of research, MSNs are viewed as promising candidates for siRNA because they are a non-viral vectors-based gene delivery and provide space and binding sites to accommodate siRNA. For this purpose, the MSNs are modified with positively charged polymers such as poly L-lysine or polyethylenimine for binding of negatively charged nucleic acids via electrostatic interactions. In the study, MSNs loaded with carfilzomib (CAR) – a proteasome inhibitor – and anticancer drugs etoposide (ETO) or DOC were compared for a co-delivery therapy with MSNs prepared with a survivin siRNA. The principles of proteasome agents are to induce apoptosis and tumor regression either individually or in combination through synergism effect. On the other side, siRNA acts inducing specific silencing of genetic targets, in this case it was the agent surviving, whose expression has been associated with lung cancers. Using tetraethyl orthosilicate as silica precursor, it was obtained MSNs, by sol-gel method with combined drug formulations of MSNs (DOC+CAR), MSNs (ETO+CAR), MSNs (DOC+CAR)-si, and MSNs (ETO+CAR)-si (-si samples: siRNA conjugated). After analysis of intracellular uptake of fluorescein amidite with A549 lung cells, mitochondrial membrane potential loss, and *in vitro* cytotoxicity, it was reported that these drug-loaded MSNs formulations illustrated good dispersibility, sustained drug release activity, biocompatibility, and low toxicity. Because of better cellular uptake along with suppression of surviving expression, both formulated combined drug-loaded NPs exhibited superior *in vitro* cytotoxicity. Adding to this, the study of apoptotic events executed by combined drug-loaded MSNs and siRNA complexed combined drug-loaded MSNs in A549 cells by flow cytometry revealed that siRNA conjugated combined drug-loaded MSNs has resulted in higher apoptotic cell death as compared to combined drug-loaded MSNs. In this regard, MSNs mediated RNAi-based therapeutic strategy may emerge as a better approach for lung cancer therapy.[101]

10.6.2 Calcium Phosphate Nanoparticles

In contrast to many other kinds of inorganic nanoparticles, calcium phosphate nanoparticles (CaP NPs) are considered biodegradable in a biological environment when compared to bio-persistent materials like gold, ND, magnetite, or carbon nanotubes. Adding to this, CaP NPs present an efficient delivery system, that is, the ability to incorporate drugs or biomolecules both inside and on the surface of the particles (Figure 10.5). This can be accomplished either by being physically or covalently bound. This ability turns the material able to retain the biomolecules until the particle has reached the target site. After that, the NPs are dissolved generating harmless compounds, which are calcium and phosphate ions.[102] CaP NPs exhibit many advantages as a carrier system for biomedical applications. Their main characteristics are non-toxicity, ability to be multi-functionalized, theranostic properties, high affinity to nucleic acids, good biodegradability, and high biocompatibility. These NPs can be synthesized following different routes such as wet-chemical precipitation, sol-gel chemistry, flame spray pyrolysis, and solid-state reactions. In parallel, the efficient action of CaP NPs in biological systems depends on the combination of the core composition as well as on the surface properties. Because CaP NPs are ionic compounds that cannot be covalently functionalized, the strategies used to modify the surface are the electrostatic approach or the covalent approach by using an outer silica shell.[102]

The surface modification can be used for applying siRNA, which is a gene silencer, and was widely investigated.[103-105] In this context, CaP NPs were designed with a lipid bilayer coating for targeted delivery of siRNA by water-in-oil micro-emulsion method. It was employed an anionic type of lipid called dioleoylphosphatydic acid in order to protect the CaP NPs and make them soluble in organic solvent. The siRNA was entrapped in the core of the NPs and the materials were tested against human H460 lung cancer cells to verify the delivery activity. Although the study did not verify the therapeutic activity of these NPs, it demonstrated that CaP NPs can effectively deliver siRNA to the solid tumor in a xenograft model.[105]

With the increase of nanoparticle types and applications, it is also clear that the potential toxicities of these novel materials and the properties driving such toxic responses must also be understood. The excess production of ROS has been reported as one of the main mechanisms of MSNs toxicity. The production of ROS induced by NPs has been proposed to occur via mitochondrial membrane depolarization, electron transport chain impairment, and activation of nicotinamide adenine dinucleotide

TABLE 10.4 Advantages and disadvantages of inorganic nanoparticles.

MATERIAL	ADVANTAGE	DISADVANTAGE	REFERENCE
MSNs	High loading capacity, controllable release rate, flexible platforms for triggered release	Toxicity from surface-exposed silanol groups, increased ROS production	94
CaP	Load cargo molecules into the particles	pH dependent degradation may fail to meet the requirements for prolonged drug release	102,107

phosphate oxidases. Although many *in vitro* studies showed non-toxic effects of MSNs at doses of up to 100 µg/ml, high doses have induced cytotoxicity.[106] By the other side, CaP NPs has been considered very biocompatible when used as DDS. The degradation products of CaP NPs, Ca^{2+}, and PO_4^{3-} are intrinsic to the body and would not lead to an immunogenic response or pose a threat to the system.[107] However, there exist some concerns about biological effect of nanoparticles treatment, the literature shows that CaP NPs have inherent toxicity. What was observed is that CaP can lead to an increase of the intracellular calcium concentration after endosomal uptake and lysosomal degradation. However, cells are able to clear the calcium from the cytoplasm within a few hours, unless very high doses of calcium phosphate are applied.[108] The advantages and disadvantages of inorganic nanoparticles are listed in Table 10.4.

10.7 METALLIC AND MAGNETIC NANOPARTICLES

Different NPs have been studied in the biomedical field as DDS or as stand-alone therapeutic agents. Metallic nanoparticles can be applied in simultaneous diagnosis and therapy for many diseases (Table 10.5), including cancer therapies due to their distinct properties, for instance, easy modification and detection, high drug loading capacity, chemical stability, and magnetic properties.[6,9,11,71,72,96,109–116] These nanoparticles have great potential as anticancer therapeutic agents, and one of the reasons is their reduced size (< 50 nm), compared to other nanoparticles, that provides a large surface area to carry large medicaments doses[117] and easily penetrate the cell membranes and biological barriers.[118] Among all the metallic NPs that are used in biomedical applications, gold NPs (AuNPs), silver NPs (AgNPs), zinc and iron oxides, such as maghemite and magnetite, are the most popular.

10.7.1 Gold Nanoparticles

AuNPs have singular properties such as chemical stability, inert character, high electron density, high surface-to-volume ratio, good biocompatibility, and affinity to

TABLE 10.5 Metallic nanoparticles applications for different diseases

NANOPARTICLE	DISEASE	TREATMENT/DRUG	REFERENCE
Au	Lung cancer	DOC, FA	71
		Asparaginase	72
		Oxaliplatin	73
		Photodynamic therapy (AlPcS4Cl)	119
Ag	Lung cancer	Photodynamic therapy (Hypocrellin B)	91
	Influenza	Methotrexate	120
		Virus-inactivated flu vaccine	113
Zn NP	Lung cancer	Camptothecin	114
MNP	Lung cancer	Magnetic resonance imaging/diagnostics	92–94
	Tuberculosis	DOX or cisplatin	95
		Metallic iron (Fe) core and a shell of	2
		Fe3O4 (coated with PEG)	109,110
		PEM	
		MTX/DOX	
		Q203/bedaquiline	

biomolecules which allow them to be functionalized with several molecules, making them potential particles for drug carriers and a tool for diagnosis.[6,121] Nevertheless, some aspects must be considered when these particles are used *in vivo*. It is important, for instance, to avoid particles agglomeration, which can cause minor pulmonary inflammation.[121,122] A previous study *in vivo* showed that changes in lung histopathology and function in high-dose of Ag administration (20 µg/m³) resulted in lowest observed adverse effect level (LOAEL), and in the middle concentration (0.38 µg/m³), there was no observed adverse effect level (NOAEL).[123]

One of the serious and deadliest respiratory tract diseases is lung cancer and it is one of the biggest concerns among scientists and researchers nowadays. Lung cancer is one of the most common cancer types worldwide, responsible for 13% of all new cancer cases and higher cancer mortality, with over 1.8 million deaths annually[124] and about 20% of cancer-related deaths worldwide.[119,125] Drug-resistant development, shortly after initial treatment, reduces the efficacy of conventional chemotherapeutics and newer targeted therapeutic agents. However, using NPs to deliver small molecules with therapeutic properties can be an alternative to overcome these limitations. AuNPs play a notable role in pharmacology, being an excellent candidate for target drug delivery, especially against lung cancerous cells.

The cytotoxic activity of AuNPs against different cancerous cell lines such as A549, H460, and H520, have been proven, showing potential against lung cancer.[71,72,126] Commonly, these particles are loaded with drugs for chemotherapy, including DOC, asparaginase, DOX, gemcitabine hydrochloride, 5-fluorouracil, PTX, daunorubicin,[5,73,126,127] and are used as target drug delivery.

In a recent study, the cytotoxic activity of AuNPs loaded with DOC and FA to treat cancer was evaluated.[71] Different concentrations and times intervals were used *in vitro* tests to evaluate the cytotoxicity of AuNPs/DOC/FA nanoconjugates. The results showed that the combination of AuNPs, DOC, and FA components simultaneously triggered a formidable decrease in cell cancer line H520, especially with the concentration of 25 µM, representing almost 50% of the control (free DOC). This is one example that shows that AuNPs have excellent responses in biomedical and pharmacological applications *in vitro,* particularly in targeted certain drug deliveries and therapies for cancer treatment.

Certain drugs used in chemotherapy present restrictions on their use against cancer: side effects, lack of specificity, quantity limitations, and resistance of some cancerous cells. Platinum-based anticancer drugs such as cisplatin, carboplatin, and oxaliplatin are other examples of essential components of chemotherapy but are restricted by severe dose-limiting side effects (neurotoxicity, nausea, and vomiting) and the ability of certain tumors to develop resistance in a short time.[73] Due to the possibility for surface modification, functionalized AuNPs are a promising approach for drug delivery, owing to their unique dimensions, tunable surface functionalities, and controllable drug release.[128,129]

In previous study,[72] AuNPs were used to mediate the delivery of asparaginase, an antineoplastic chemotherapy drug that is obtained from the fungal strain *Aspergillus terreus* and is used in cancer treatment. The AuNPs were synthesized using auric chloride and then functionalized with asparaginase using glutaraldehyde as a binder. MTT assay was carried out to examine the cytotoxicity of this nanomaterial against lung cancer cell line A549 and the data showed that the increase of asparaginase concentration in the nanocomposite entails a decrease in the cell viability. Thus, the AuNPs/asparaginase combination is another system that has a high potential to be an effective and novel drug against lung cancer.

A significant number of investigations on nanoparticles use different polymers as functionalization agents to develop new biomaterials for cancer treatment. In one of these studies,[73] naked AuNPs were functionalized with a thiolated PEG monolayer circumscribed with the carboxylate group. After the functionalization, the active component of oxaliplatin was added to the surface. One interesting point to highlight is that the thiol-gold bond is susceptible to displacement by strong nucleophiles commonly found *in vivo.* To overcome this, the researchers used a cyclic disulfide to bind the linker to the nanoparticles. Additionally, the monolayer also contains a stabilizing linkage that is hydrophobic on the inner core of the nanoparticle and hydrophilic on the outer part of the sphere to make it compatible with a biological environment. The platinum-tethered nanoparticles demonstrated an unusual ability to penetrate the nucleus in the lung cancer cells and a better, or at least similar, cytotoxicity than oxaliplatin alone in all the cell lines.

Cancer stem cells are responsible for tumor growth and recurrence after drug-induced cell death, diminishing the effect of traditional cancer therapy and contributing to lung cancer mortality rates. Unfortunately, recent tests have shown that conventional cancer treatments can be resisted.[130] Traditional therapies, such as chemotherapy, radiation, and surgery, being tough but effective, cause side effects, including nausea, vomiting and diarrhea, hair loss and alopecia, hospitalization for several days/weeks, mucositis, skin toxicity, and xerostomia.[131–133] Current research is focused on improving alternative treatment modalities, such as photodynamic therapy. Photosensitizer drugs, light, and oxygen are the three fundamental factors in photodynamic therapy. First, the photosensitizer drug is administrated to a patient, and it accumulates within a tumor site. Once this drug is exposed to a specific wavelength of light, it is stimulated to produce ROS, which causes tumor destruction. However, the efficacy of the therapy is highly dependent on the accumulation of the photosensitizer in tumor cells.[134] Therefore, many studies have been carried out to develop specific receptors-based photosynthetic nanocarrier drugs, to promote the active uptake and absorption of photosynthetic drugs in tumor sites only, avoiding undesirable side effects.[91,134,135]

Photodynamic therapy can be improved using AuNPs along with target antibody-mediated selection of cancer stem cells, to successfully treat lung cancer.[119] In this study, AuNPs were functionalized with PEG and then a nanobioconjugate was prepared to combine the functionalized nanoparticles with the targeted antibody and the photosensitizer (AlPcS$_4$Cl). Conjugation of the nanocomposite was well succeeded, and all the nanobioconjugates were located into the organelles involved in cell homeostasis. Moreover, the combination of AuNPs with the photosensitizer and the antibody showed significant cell toxicity and cell death compared to free AlPcS4Cl. The effectiveness of photodynamic therapy on lung cancer stem cells destruction was intensified to the point of eradication.

10.7.2 Silver Nanoparticles

Another metallic nanoparticle widely used in the biomedical field is AgNPs because of their high conductivity, lower toxicity in small doses, and therapeutic effects.[136] AgNPs' toxicity in inhalation route was studied, and results demonstrated a dose- and time-dependency with NPs concentration increase in blood, causing increases in alveolar inflammation and small granulomatous lesions in lung tissue.[137,138] Besides these toxicity limitations, AgNPs can also be used for the enhancement of photodynamic therapy.[91,134,135] Hypocrellin B loaded poly lactide-co-glycolide nanoparticle formulations were incorporated with AgNPs in a former investigation.[91] DDS reported enhanced singlet oxygen production with light exposure at a cellular level and significantly induced 82.2% on A549 cells death with limited recovery. Moreover, another study[135] showed that AgNPs can also be used in photodynamic therapy without any photosensitizer. Laser irradiated silver NPs exhibited photodynamic activity in lung cancer cells (A549) by promoting a decrease in viability and proliferation, with increased cytotoxicity and a significant 80% increase of induced apoptotic programmed cell death.

Along with AuNPs, AgNPs have been successfully used both *in vitro* and *in vivo* anticancer therapies because they are stable and easy to make.[139] Conjugates of AgNPs and methotrexate were obtained with a narrow size distribution to improve the treatment efficacy in cancer therapy.[120] In this study, different concentrations of methotrexate were used to load AgNPs: 28, 31, and 40%. *In vitro* drug release tests showed equivalent release profiles, liberating between 77 and 85% of the initial methotrexate loaded. The addition of the nanocarrier delayed the methotrexate release and changed its pharmacokinetics. Although the free methotrexate releases following first-order kinetic modes, the presence of AgNPs fitted a Higuchi model, where the solubilization is controlled by the diffusion process. The nanoconjugate decreased the percentage of living cells in a colon and lung cancer cell line, HTC116 and A549, respectively. The last test performed was a zebrafish assay, which did not show any significant cytotoxic effect, confirming the reduction of systemic drug toxicity achieved by combining methotrexate with AgNPs. This reduction in toxicity suggests an improvement of the usage of this nanocarrier in chemotherapy against human cancers since its activity appears to be selective: killing cancerous cells but not affecting healthy systems.

The mechanism of cancer cells death caused by AgNPs is still under investigation. However, in terms of nanoscale, much research indicates that size is considered as one of the important parameters that determine the physicochemical properties of nanoparticles and ultimately their biological behavior. In this regard, the molecular mechanism of cancer cell death caused by AgNPs of different sizes was investigated.[118] The influence of different AgNPs sizes (13, 45, and 92 nm) against A549 lung adenocarcinoma cells was evaluated, and the results exhibited that the smaller nanoparticles were more toxic and the migratory and invasive abilities of A549 cells were significantly suppressed. By inducing apoptosis, AgNPs with 13 nm inhibited the growth and invasion of lung cancer cells *in vitro*. The same effect starts decreasing with the size of 45 nm and completely vanishes for 92 nm AgNPs. This suggests that the size of AgNPs plays a significant role in nanoparticles effectiveness against lung adenocarcinoma, and further experiments need to be performed to optimize other nanoparticles' sizes for applications in cancer therapies.

Although being used as an anticancer agent, the main use of AgNPs is as an antibacterial agent,[6] which is very interesting since it is beneficial for maintaining formulation sterility for extended periods.[140] Thereby, AgNPs were included in the virus-inactivated flu vaccine to evaluate his influence in the reduction of viral loads and prevention of excessive lung inflammation followed by influenza infection.[113] Mice were used to investigate the effects of the vaccine containing AgNPs. The data demonstrated that AgNPs are capable of increasing cytokines (CCL-5, CCL-2, IL-12, and IL-6) levels in the bronchoalveolar lavages. Additionally, when administered intra-pulmonary, the metallic nanoparticles increased antigen availability, the retention of the antigen in the lung compartment, and the local immune stimulation. AgNPs stimulated stronger antigen-specific immunoglobulins production with lower toxicity by promoting bronchus-associated lymphoid tissue neogenesis and acted as a genuine mucosal adjuvant. Thus, the study proved that the vaccine combined with AgNPs protected mice from lethal flu, decreasing mortality rates.

10.7.3 Zinc Oxide Nanoparticles

Besides metallic nanoparticles, a variety of metal oxide nanoparticles have shown success for use as vehicles for drug delivery, targeted gene delivery, and tumor imaging, especially against cell lung cancer and other cancer cell lines.[141,142] Considering a strong safety record, zinc oxide nanoparticles (ZnO NPs) are often used in the biomedical field due to their singular properties, namely favorable bandgap, electrostatic charge, surface chemistry, and potentiation of redox-cycling cascades, among others. Strikingly, ZnO NPs appear to have inherent anticancer cytotoxicity. Zinc oxide is an inorganic semiconductor compound that is practically insoluble in water, can absorb ultraviolet light at waves of 350 to 380 nm,[143,144] beyond being non-toxic and biocompatible.[145] Nevertheless, ZnO has some toxicity limitations and appeared to be, in metal form, more toxic in relative low concentrations if compared to other metal such as tungsten.[146] Previous studies reported that particles with less than 100 nm in hydrodynamic diameter influence different cancerous cells *in vitro*,[147] probably due to Zn^{2+} that triggers ROS production.[148,149] A research group reported that ZnO protects macrophages from the cytotoxic effects of an anticancer drug. Conversely, another group mentioned that intravenously administered ZnO NPs accumulate in multiple tissues, especially lung tissues, and elicit ROS production.[150–152] Ultimately, these results imply that ZnO NPs may target small-cell lung cancer cells via a pathway distinct from that of traditional chemotherapies, which makes this nanomaterial an alternative approach against lung cancer.

ZnO NPs were tested against diverse cancer cell lines, such as NCI-N417 (N417), H82, and H187, to investigate anticancer effects *in vitro* by generating ROS.[153] ZnO NPs were proved to be effectively cytotoxic against cancer cells, with only N417 cells having acquired resistance, but less active against normal lung cells. When administered intravenously, ZnO NPs are also genotoxic *in vivo* against lung cancer cells, without any undesirable side effects through the end of the experiment. It is important to highlight that particles less than 100 nm not only minimize the risk of venous thrombosis but also maximize delivery efficiency.[142] The authors also noticed that because of high nanoparticles stability, it is advantageous to use this nanomaterial prepared once for many subsequent experiments, enhancing reproducibility and convenience. This stability is also desirable in materials to produce drugs because extends the shelf life of the final product. Therefore, they first collected empirical evidence that ZnO NPs have genotoxic anticancer effects in an orthotopic mouse model of human small-cell lung cancer and could be used for novel small-cell lung cancer treatments.[153]

ZnO NPs as a DDS have been the focus of several studies.[114,154] ZnO NPs were synthesized by co-precipitation method, functionalized with N-acetyl-L-cysteine, and combined with antitumor camptothecin to use as a new drug system to treat cancer.[114] The incorporation of camptothecin increased the NPs size going from a mean size of 62 to 78 nm. Although the size expansion, the particles were maintained in the optimized range for long-circulating and accumulation in tumors.[147] In the MTT assay, the conjugated nanomaterial killed 85.96% of A549 cancer cells, showing the potential of ZnO NPs conjugated with camptothecin for new therapeutic endeavors.

10.7.4 Magnetic Nanoparticles

Another oxide extendedly used in the biomedical field is iron oxides, normally maghemite and magnetite. These nanomaterials have been used due to properties such as biocompatibility and biodegradability, and especially because of their magnetic and heat-mediated characteristics coupled with tunable size and functionality.[93,155] Because of these characteristics, these magnetic nanoparticles (MNPs) can be used in different applications including targeted drug delivery and hyperthermia-based therapy.[110,111,116,155] However, toxicity limitations are observed in literature. Previous results showed that iron NPs inhalation exposure may induce cytotoxicity via oxidative stress and lead to biphasic inflammatory responses in the Wistar rat.[156] Thus, it is very important that for all MNPs, preliminary studies define exactly their toxicity limits to avoid side effects in clinical applications. Lung cancer and tuberculosis are some of the diseases that can be treated with MNPs.[92,109,111,157] Lung cancer is one of the most common diseases of this type and can be divided into small-cell lung cancers (SCLCs) and non-small-cell lung cancers (NSCLCs). Because more than 85% of the total cases are NSCLCs, the focus of the treatments is mitigating this type of cancer. For a majority of patients with NSCLC, the first-line treatments are systematic chemotherapy, immunotherapy, or oncogene targeted therapy. This way, early surgery is avoided due to the deficiency in early-stage diagnostics and local invasion.[93]

Moreover, MNPs can be applied as contrast agents for magnetic resonance imaging, contributing to identifying tumors and helping in earlier diagnostics.[92] Size, composition, and particle shape have a direct influence on magnetic properties.[155] Although MNPs have the approval of the FDA, variables could affect their toxicity, for example, route of administration, the location of the particles about the cells, and dosage. The free iron release can be associated with free radicals, which could induce harmful side effects such as atherosclerosis, Alzheimer's disease, and age-related macular degeneration. Thus, for *in vivo* applications, MNPs are used together with a coating material once it is proven that they have a positive impact on cytotoxicity. Commonly, these coatings are hydrophilic and electrically neutral, for instance, liposomes, surfactants, polymers, and inorganic salts.[95,110–112]

Maghemite (γ-Fe_2O_3) is a predominant form of iron oxide NPs used for biomedical applications. This structure presents ferromagnetic properties exhibiting all iron atoms in Fe (III) oxidation state. Ions of Fe (III) are commonly found in the human body and are less toxic than Fe (II), which makes them favorable as core material. Fe_2O_3 NPs for drug delivery generally consist of a magnetic core composed of an outer coating obtained by functionalization. The charge can be encapsulated either inside the particle shell or within the co-embedded mesoporous particles. Alternatively, the charges can also be bound to surface moieties. By this, a synergistic combination with hyperthermic properties of the Fe_2O_3 and stimuli-responsive elements can promote triggered charge release.[94] As an example, it was designed a Fe_2O_3 nanostructure featured with a multidomain magnetite core and cross-linked starch matrix terminal cations that can be loaded with the drug DOX or cisplatin. This combination is applied as a therapeutic agent with high capacity of penetrative delivery and retention in the deep tumor. When combined with magnetic resonance imaging and inductive heating, Fe_2O_3 NPs can provide multimodal cancer treatment.[93,94]

One of the biggest goals in cancer treatment is that the drug kills only cancerous cells and does not affect negatively normal ones. In this regard, PEG-coated Fe/Fe_3O_4 core-shell nanoparticles were produced to investigate the effect of these MNPs on A549 cells and mouse fibroblast NIH3T3 cells (non-cancerous cells).[95] The particle was formed by a metallic iron (Fe) core and a shell of Fe_3O_4 and coated with PEG. The results demonstrated that these nanoparticles presented ten times more toxicity against A549 cells than Paclitaxel, an anti-cancer drug. The degradation of Fe_3O_4 exposes Fe core, which accelerates the release of iron ions leading to cell death. Conversely, according to scratch tests, the MNPs did not have any inhibitory effect on the motility of NIH3T3 cells, only for the cancerous cells, which indicates that these nanoparticles are toxic only against cancer, not to healthy cells.

Due to their magnetic properties, MNPs are widely used in DDS since they effectively deliver drug molecules to the desired location by applying an external magnetic field.[2] The accumulation of higher doses in the tumor microenvironment reduces the systemic distribution in the organism and decreases potential side effects. Thus, many studies using MNPs loaded with different anti-cancer drugs have been developed. In one of them, the authors loaded pemetrexed (PEM) drug into magnetic O-carboxymethyl chitosan nanoparticle (PMCMC) by absorption method. The magnetic characteristics of PMCMC are provided by Fe_3O_4 NPs that were encapsulated into the PEM-loaded modified chitosan. They used A549 and CRL5807 (bronchioalveolar carcinoma) cells to evaluate the cytotoxicity of these PMCMC and the pure PEM. *In vivo* tests showed that after the 18th day of treatment, there was no tumor present in mice using PMCMC with exposure to a magnetic field, while the mice treated with only PEM died or still had tumors. Additionally, PMCMC has target antitumor activity without toxicity in healthy tissues and anemia potential, unlike PEM treatment.

As a strategy to achieve better results, researchers have been using combined therapy by integrating two or more therapeutic agents in only one nanoparticle platform. One of these studies[116] developed a DDS combining Fe_3O_4 MNPs with the combined drugs cetuximab and DOX.[158,159] The MNPs presented significant cytotoxicity against A549 cells and permitted a considerable surface for drug loading, which could improve drugs pharmacokinetics and biological distribution. In a different study,[110] the authors prepared another DDS with MTX, DOX, and PEG-coated magnetic hollow-nanosphere (Fe_3O_4). Because of the hollow structure, it was possible to load both hydrophilic and hydrophobic drugs for co-delivery. The MNPs loaded with MTX and DOX presented higher cytotoxicity *in vitro* against A549 cells than the same combination of drugs without the nanospheres. Moreover, this system was developed to be used as local delivery through inhalation, which could be an alternative route to deliver higher drug concentration in contrast with the traditionally intravenous applications.

Besides many cancer studies, MNPs also are being used to treat other diseases, tuberculosis for instance. Tuberculosis (TB) is an acute respiratory infection, poverty-related disease and is responsible for the death of more persons than any other microbial pathogen, with about 1.5 million deaths in 2018.[160-163] TB is caused by the inhalation of *Mycobacterium tuberculosis* bacilli, which further colonize in alveolar macrophages.[164] The treatment of TB is performed using various anti-TB drugs with long treatment schedules. As a result, poor patient compliance is observed, increasing the risk of treatment failure.[165,166] To overcome this drawback, a spherical poly(D, L-lactide-co-glycolide) drug carrier loaded with superparamagnetic iron oxides (Fe_3O_4/FeO), Q203, and bedaquiline was developed.[109] The particles were not prejudicial to normal tissue, and *in vitro* results demonstrated better dispersion and deposition into the lungs through an external magnetic field, with minimal losses. The combination Q203 and bedaquiline had good synergic antibacterial properties, better than other existing pulmonary systems. Additionally, it presented better efficiency in deposition, targeting, and dispersion into the alveolar tissue, which makes these MNPs a potential drug carrier for TB treatment. Nevertheless, more studies, especially *in vivo*, need to be carried out before any clinical applications.

Research in nanotechnology for medical diagnosis, anticancer treatment, drug delivery, and thermotherapy has significantly risen in the last years. Among all the nanomaterials available, metallic NPs, and their oxides have become potential

TABLE 10.6 Advantages and limitations of metallic and magnetic nanoparticles in respiratory treatments

NANOPARTICLE	ADVANTAGES	LIMITATIONS	REF.
Au	Chemical stability, inert character, high electron density, high surface-to-volume ratio, good biocompatibility, affinity to biomolecules, permits functionalization	Agglomerations Solubility limit Toxicity limitations	6,121, 121,122,171
Ag	High conductivity, lower toxicity in small doses, therapeutic effects, antibacterial agent used for the enhancement of photodynamic therapy	Agglomerations Toxicity limitations	136. 91,134,135
Zn NP	Favorable bandgap, electrostatic charge, surface chemistry, and potentiation of redox-cycling cascades non-toxic and biocompatible	Insoluble in water	145,141,142
MNP	Unique electrical and magnetic characteristics, biocompatibility and biodegradability, tunable size and functionality	Toxicity limitations Behavior in long-term treatment unknown	93,155

candidates in respiratory disorders therapy, alongside some disadvantages (Table 10.6). AuNPs, AgNPs, MNPs, and zinc oxide nanoparticles have shown great potential for biomedical and pharmacological applications *in vitro*, especially in targeted drug deliveries and therapies. MNPs have been showing good results in clinical trials and in commercial products. Metal and magnetic nanoparticles have been widely studied, and many new nanoparticle products are currently being clinically tested.[138,167–170] Iron NPs, for instance, have been already approved for being used in anemia and iron deficiency, along with ultrasound contrast agent and imaging node metastases. Besides, their use in thermal ablation for cancer are already in clinical tests (first trial complete).[54] Moreover, AuNPs have been also showing good results as drug delivery applications, and many clinical trials have been carried out in advanced phases for this nanoparticle in intravenous route, including therapies against primary and/or metastatic lung tumors and NSLC (non-small lung cancer) (NCT00356980; NCT01679470).[169] Recent studies have been proven that MNPs, assisted with a magnetic field, could be used as drug carriers, making treatment fastest, more efficient, and with less harm to normal cells. Nevertheless, limited studies with *in vivo* assays have been published, and more studies are still required to better understand their behavior in long-term treatment and optimize targeted delivery of metallic nanoparticles. Thus, this leaves an opportunity for thorough research to guarantee that the treatment is safe and efficient for patients.

10.8 CONCLUSIONS AND FUTURE PERSPECTIVES

Nanotechnology progress led to new applications in therapeutic drug delivery and the development of treatments for a variety of diseases and disorders. Nanoparticles allow obtaining exclusive properties resulting from their small size. Besides this, the opportunity of controlling the size and shape of the nanoparticle core provides yet another dimension of physical control that can be used to tailoring specific functions.

The complexity and lethality of respiratory diseases have caused industry and academia around the world to work incessantly to find plausible solutions to cure or prevent the advancement of these diseases. In support of this, nanotechnology proposes innovative perspectives to solve many problems, specifically in the medical and biological fields. Thus, the application of nanocarriers for the treatment of pulmonary pathologies is a viable strategy. The kind of nanoparticle to be used depends on the administration route, the therapeutic indication, the drug's property, and many other aspects. In this way, several strategies can be developed for a successful release. Efficacy and safety are the main aspects of any therapy. So, the drug concentration must be high enough at the site of action to have the therapeutic effect but at the same time not too high to cause the toxic side effects. Therefore, the drug concentration must be essentially constant within the therapeutic window.

Research efforts have focused on enhancing the target drugs to the lung through different delivery systems as well as maximizing the efficacy and control of the side effects. However, understanding the interactions of particles with biological systems remains a challenge for nanoparticulate drug delivery to the lungs. Computer simulations could be employed to study the interaction between the proposed nanoparticles and the virus or cancer cell under study.

Lately, several nanomedicines have been widely used, and some are already in clinical trials. Although some successes have been achieved, many challenges must be conquered to accelerate the clinical transformation of nanomedicines. First, the biological effects of these drug carriers' nanostructures are not well established. For this, it is necessary for further detailed investigations to develop standardized methods for the evaluation of the biological impacts of nanostructures before they can be used in clinical trials. Second, considering that the biosafety of the nanostructures is the foundation for their biomedical application, the nanotoxicology aspect must be strictly defined. This means that until now, many studies have accomplished *in vitro* analyses. However, further *in vivo* investigations of pharmacokinetics, pharmacodynamics, and metabolism in animal models must be conducted before these nanostructures can be used in humans.

BIBLIOGRAPHY

1. WHO. *The top 10 causes of death*. World Health Organization. (2019). https://www.who.int/news-room/fact-sheets/detail/the-top-10-causes-of-death.

2. Menezes, B. R. C. de *et al.* Current advances in drug delivery of nanoparticles for respiratory disease treatment. *J. Mater. Chem. B* 9(7), 1745–1761 (2021).

3. Patel, K. & Patel, K. Challenges and recent progress of nano sized drug delivery systems for lung cancer therapy : A review. *Himal. J. Heal. Sci.* 5, 58–62 (2020).

4. Lavorini, F., Buttini, F. & Usmani, O. S. 100 years of drug delivery to the lungs. *Handb. Exp. Pharmacol.* 260, 143–159 (2019).

5. Jahangirian, H. *et al.* A review of small molecules and drug delivery applications using gold and iron nanoparticles. *Int. J. Nanomedicine* 14, 1633–1657 (2019).

6. Vaghasiya, K., Sharma, A., Ray, E., Adlakha, S. & Verma, R. K. Methods to characterize nanoparticles for mucosal drug delivery. (2020). https://doi.org/10.1007/978-3-030-35910-2_2.

7. Sahu, T. *et al.* Nanotechnology based drug delivery system: Current strategies and emerging therapeutic potential for medical science. *J. Drug Deliv. Sci. Technol.* 63, 102487 (2021).

8. Xie, M. & Fussenegger, M. Designing cell function: Assembly of synthetic gene circuits for cell biology applications. *Nat. Rev. Mol. Cell Biol.* 19(8), 507–525 (2018).

9. Abdelaziz, H. M. *et al.* Inhalable particulate drug delivery systems for lung cancer therapy: Nanoparticles, microparticles, nanocomposites and nanoaggregates. *J. Control. Release* 269, 374–392 (2018).

10. Mohamud, R. *et al.* The effects of engineered nanoparticles on pulmonary immune homeostasis. *Drug Metab. Rev.* 46(2), 176–190 (2014).

11. Chenthamara, D. *et al.* Therapeutic efficacy of nanoparticles and routes of administration. *Biomater. Res.* 23, 1–29 (2019).

12. Chowdhuryz, N. K. *et al.* Nanoparticles as an effective drug delivery system in Covid-19. *Biomed. Pharmacother.* 112162 (2021). https://doi.org/10.1016/j.biopha.2021.112162.

13. Azarmi, S., Roa, W. H. & Löbenberg, R. Targeted delivery of nanoparticles for the treatment of lung diseases. *Adv. Drug Deliv. Rev.* 60(8), 863–875 (2008).

14. d'Angelo, I., Conte, C., Miro, A., Quaglia, F. & Ungaro, F. Pulmonary drug delivery: A role for polymeric nanoparticles? *Curr. Top. Med. Chem.* 15(4), 386–400 (2015).

15. Castro, A. *et al.* Docetaxel in chitosan-based nanocapsules conjugated with an anti-Tn antigen mouse/human chimeric antibody as a promising targeting strategy of lung tumors. *Int. J. Biol. Macromol.* 182, 806–814 (2021).

16. Vauthier, C. & Bouchemal, K. Methods for the preparation and manufacture of polymeric nanoparticles. *Pharm. Res.* 26(5), 1025–1058 (2009).

17. Andrade, F. *et al.* Chitosan-grafted copolymers and chitosan-ligand conjugates as matrices for pulmonary drug delivery. *Int. J. Carbohydr. Chem.* 2011, 1–14 (2011).

18. Garg, T., Rath, G. & Goyal, A. K. Inhalable chitosan nanoparticles as antitubercular drug carriers for an effective treatment of tuberculosis. *Artif. Cells Nanomed. Biotechnol.* 44(3), 997–1001 (2016).

19. El-Sherbiny, I. M. & Smyth, H. D. C. Controlled release pulmonary administration of curcumin using swellable biocompatible microparticles. *Mol. Pharm.* 9(2), 269–280 (2012).

20. Hosseinnejad, M. & Jafari, S. M. Evaluation of different factors affecting antimicrobial properties of chitosan. *Int. J. Biol. Macromol.* 85, 467–475 (2016).

21. Si, Z. *et al.* Antimicrobial effect of a novel chitosan derivative and its synergistic effect with antibiotics. *ACS Appl. Mater. Interfaces* 13(2), 3237–3245 (2021).

22. Islam, N. & Ferro, V. Recent advances in chitosan-based nanoparticulate pulmonary drug delivery. *Nanoscale* 8(30), 14341–14358 (2016).

23. Bivas-Benita, M. *et al.* Pulmonary delivery of chitosan-DNA nanoparticles enhances the immunogenicity of a DNA vaccine encoding HLA-a*0201-restricted T-cell epitopes of Mycobacterium tuberculosis. *Vaccine* 22(13–14), 1609–1615 (2004).

24. Köping-Höggård, M. *et al.* Chitosan as a nonviral gene delivery system: Structure-property relationships and characteristics compared with polyethylenimine in vitro and after lung administration in vivo. *Gene Ther.* 8(14), 1108–1121 (2001).

25. Khademi, F. *et al.* Are chitosan natural polymers suitable as adjuvant/delivery system for anti-tuberculosis vaccines? *Microb. Pathog.* 121, 218–223 (2018).

26. Bhatia, S. Natural polymers vs synthetic polymer. In *Natural polymer drug delivery systems* 95–118 (Springer International Publishing, 2016). https://doi.org/10.1007/978-3-319-41129-3_3.

27. Paranjpe, M. & Müller-Goymann, C. C. Nanoparticle-mediated pulmonary drug delivery: A review. *Int. J. Mol. Sci.* 15(4), 5852–5873 (2014).

28. Sung, J. C., Pulliam, B. L. & Edwards, D. A. Nanoparticles for drug delivery to the lungs. *Trends Biotechnol.* 25(12), 563–570 (2007).

29. Woodruff, M. A. & Hutmacher, D. W. The return of a forgotten polymer—Polycaprolactone in the 21st century. *Prog. Polym. Sci.* 35(10), 1217–1256 (2010).

30. Kean, T. & Thanou, M. Biodegradation, biodistribution and toxicity of chitosan. *Adv. Drug Deliv. Rev.* 62(1), 3–11 (2010).

31. Zhu, H. *et al.* Co-delivery of chemotherapeutic drugs with vitamin E TPGS by porous PLGA nanoparticles for enhanced chemotherapy against multi-drug resistance. *Biomaterials* 35(7), 2391–2400 (2014).

32. Vij, N. *et al.* Development of pegylated PLGA nanoparticle for controlled and sustained drug delivery in cystic fibrosis. *J. Nanobiotechnology* 8, 1–18 (2010).

33. Haque, S. *et al.* The impact of size and charge on the pulmonary pharmacokinetics and immunological response of the lungs to PLGA nanoparticles after intratracheal administration to rats. *Nanomed. Nanotechnol. Biol. Med.* 30, 102291 (2020).

34. Beck-Broichsitter, M., Merkel, O. M. & Kissel, T. Controlled pulmonary drug and gene delivery using polymeric nano-carriers. *J. Control. Release* 161(2), 214–224 (2012).

35. Tkaczuk, K. & Yared, J. Update on taxane development: New analogs and new formulations. *Drug Des. Devel. Ther.* 371 (2012). https://doi.org/10.2147/DDDT.S28997.

36. Qiao, J.-B. *et al.* Aerosol delivery of biocompatible dihydroergotamine-loaded PLGA-PSPE polymeric micelles for efficient lung cancer therapy. *Polym. Chem.* 8(9), 1540–1554 (2017).

37. Barghi, L., Asgari, D., Barar, J. & Valizadeh, H. Synthesis of PCEC copolymers with controlled molecular weight using full factorial methodology. *Adv. Pharm. Bull.* 5(1), 51–56 (2015).

38. Hu, J. *et al.* Paclitaxel-loaded polymeric nanoparticles combined with chronomodulated chemotherapy on lung cancer: In vitro and in vivo evaluation. *Int. J. Pharm.* 516(1–2), 313–322 (2017).

39. Menon, J. U. *et al.* Polymeric nanoparticles for pulmonary protein and DNA delivery. *Acta Biomater.* 10(6), 2643–2652 (2014).

40. Cosco, D. *et al.* Delivery of miR-34a by chitosan/PLGA nanoplexes for the anticancer treatment of multiple myeloma. *Sci. Rep.* 5, 17579 (2015).

41. Mohamed, A., Kunda, N. K., Ross, K., Hutcheon, G. A. & Saleem, I. Y. Polymeric nanoparticles for the delivery of miRNA to treat chronic obstructive pulmonary disease (COPD). *Eur. J. Pharm. Biopharm.* 136, 1–8 (2019).

42. Kaczmarek, J. C. *et al.* Systemic delivery of mRNA and DNA to the lung using polymer-lipid nanoparticles. *Biomaterials* 275, (2021).

43. Tenchov, R., Bird, R., Curtze, A. E. & Zhou, Q. Lipid nanoparticles—From liposomes to mRNA vaccine delivery, a landscape of research diversity and advancement. *ACS Nano* (2021). https://doi.org/10.1021/acsnano.1c04996.

44. Puri, A. *et al.* Lipid-based nanoparticles as pharmaceutical drug carriers: From concepts to clinic. *Crit. Rev. Ther. Drug Carr Syst.* 26(6), 523–580 (2009).

45. Hattori, Y. *et al.* Effect of cationic lipid in cationic liposomes on siRNA delivery into the lung by intravenous injection of cationic lipoplex. *J. Drug Target.* 27(2), 217–227 (2019).

46. Garbuzenko, O. B. *et al.* Intratracheal versus intravenous liposomal delivery of siRNA, antisense oligonucleotides and anticancer drug. *Pharm. Res.* 26(2), 382–394 (2009).

47. Thapa, B. & Narain, R. *Mechanism, current challenges and new approaches for non viral gene delivery. Polymers and nanomaterials for gene therapy* (Elsevier Ltd., 2016). https://doi.org/10.1016/B978-0-08-100520-0.00001-1.

48. Hattori, Y. *et al.* siRNA delivery to lung-metastasized tumor by systemic injection with cationic liposomes. *J. Liposome Res.* 25(4), 279–286 (2015).

49. Ngan, C. L. & Asmawi, A. A. Lipid-based pulmonary delivery system: A review and future considerations of formulation strategies and limitations. *Drug Deliv. Transl. Res.* 8(5), 1527–1544 (2018).

50. Taratula, O., Kuzmov, A., Shah, M., Garbuzenko, O. B. & Minko, T. Nanostructured lipid carriers as multifunctional nanomedicine platform for pulmonary co-delivery of anticancer drugs and siRNA. *J. Control. Release* 171(3), 349–357 (2013).

51. Mukherjee, A. *et al.* Lipid–polymer hybrid nanoparticles as a next-generation drug delivery platform: State of the art, emerging technologies, and perspectives. *Int. J. Nanomedicine* 14, 1937–1952 (2019).

52. Mangal, S., Gao, W., Li, T. & Zhou, Q. T. Pulmonary delivery of nanoparticle chemotherapy for the treatment of lung cancers: Challenges and opportunities. *Acta Pharmacol. Sin.* 38(6), 782–797 (2017).

53. Abdellatif, A. A. H. & Alsowinea, A. F. Approved and marketed nanoparticles for disease targeting and applications in COVID-19. *Nanotechnol. Rev.* 10(1), 1941–1977 (2021).

54. Anselmo, A. C. & Mitragotri, S. Nanoparticles in the clinic: An update. *Bioeng. Transl. Med.* 4(3), 1–16 (2019).

55. Patra, J. K. *et al.* Nano based drug delivery systems: Recent developments and future prospects. *J. Nanobiotechnology* 16(1), 71 (2018).

56. Montanheiro, T. L. do A. *et al.* A brief review concerning the latest advances in the influence of nanoparticle reinforcement into polymeric-matrix biomaterials. *J. Biomater. Sci. Polym. Ed.* 1–25 (2020). https://doi.org/10.1080/09205063.2020.1781527.

57. Ferreira, S. D. O., Montanheiro, T. L. do A., Ontagna, L. S. & Lemes, A. P. Study of cellulose nanocrystals and zinc nitrate hexahydrate addition in chitosan. *Mater. Res.* 22, 1–10 (2019).

58. Lin, N. & Dufresne, A. Nanocellulose in biomedicine: Current status and future prospect. *Eur. Polym. J.* 59, 302–325 (2014).

59. Montanheiro, T. L. do A. *et al.* Evaluation of cellulose nanocrystal addition on morphology, compression modulus and cytotoxicity of poly (3-hydroxybutyrate- co –3-hydroxyvalerate) scaffolds. *J. Mater. Sci. Mater. Life Sci.* 54(9), 7198–7210 (2019).

60. Montanheiro, T. L. A. *et al.* Cytotoxicity and physico-chemical evaluation of acetylated and pegylated cellulose nanocrystals. *J. Nanopart. Res.* 20(8), 206 (2018).

61. Seabra, A. B., Bernardes, J. S., Fávaro, W. J., Paula, A. J. & Durán, N. Cellulose nanocrystals as carriers in medicine and their toxicities: A review. *Carbohydr. Polym.* 181, 514–527 (2018).

62. Roman, M. Toxicity of cellulose nanocrystals: A review. *Ind. Biotechnol.* 11(1), 25–33 (2015).

63. Sunasee, R., Hemraz, U. D. & Ckless, K. Cellulose nanocrystals: A versatile nanoplatform for emerging biomedical applications. *Expert Opin. Drug Deliv.* 13(9), 1243–1256 (2016).

64. Yanamala, N. *et al.* In vivo evaluation of the pulmonary toxicity of cellulose nanocrystals: A renewable and sustainable nanomaterial of the future. *ACS Sustain. Chem. Eng.* 2(7), 1691–1698 (2014).

65. Grishkewich, N., Mohammed, N., Tang, J. & Tam, K. C. Recent advances in the application of cellulose nanocrystals. *Curr. Opin. Colloid Interface Sci.* 29, 32–45 (2017).

66. Seo, J. H. *et al.* Multi-layered cellulose nanocrystal system for CD44 receptor-positive tumor-targeted anticancer drug delivery. *Int. J. Biol. Macromol.* 162, 798–809 (2020).

67. Lugoloobi, I. *et al.* Cellulose nanocrystals in cancer diagnostics and treatment. *J. Control. Release* 336, 207–232 (2021).

68. Imlimthan, S. *et al.* A theranostic cellulose nanocrystal-based drug delivery system with enhanced retention in pulmonary metastasis of melanoma. *Small* 17(18), 2007705 (2021).

69. Li, N. *et al.* Rod-like cellulose nanocrystal/cis-aconityl-doxorubicin prodrug: A fluorescence-visible drug delivery system with enhanced cellular uptake and intracellular drug controlled release. *Mater. Sci. Eng. C Mater. Biol. Appl.* 91, 179–189 (2018).

70. Kumar, M., Jha, A., Dr, M. & Mishra, B. Targeted drug nanocrystals for pulmonary delivery: A potential strategy for lung cancer therapy. *Expert Opin. Drug Deliv.* 17(10), 1459–1472 (2020).

71. Thambiraj, S., Shruthi, S., Vijayalakshmi, R. & Ravi Shankaran, D. Evaluation of cytotoxic activity of docetaxel loaded gold nanoparticles for lung cancer drug delivery. *Cancer Treat. Res. Commun.* 21, 100157 (2019).

72. Baskar, G., Garrick, B. G., Lalitha, K. & Chamundeeswari, M. Gold nanoparticle mediated delivery of fungal asparaginase against cancer cells. *J. Drug Deliv. Sci. Technol.* 44, 498–504 (2018).

73. Brown, S. D. *et al.* Gold nanoparticles for the improved anticancer drug delivery of the active component of oxaliplatin. *J. Am. Chem. Soc.* 132(13), 4678–4684 (2010).

74. Jomhori, M., Mosaddeghi, H. & Farzin, H. Tracking the interaction between single-wall carbon nanotube and SARS-Cov-2 spike glycoprotein: A molecular dynamics simulations study. *Comput. Biol. Med.* 136, 104692 (2021).

75. Jha, R., Singh, A., Sharma, P. K. & Fuloria, N. K. Smart carbon nanotubes for drug delivery system: A comprehensive study. *J. Drug Deliv. Sci. Technol.* 58, 101811 (2020).

76. Dawre, S. & Maru, S. Human respiratory viral infections: Current status and future prospects of nanotechnology-based approaches for prophylaxis and treatment. *Life Sci.* 278, 119561 (2021).

77. Wong, B. S. *et al.* Carbon nanotubes for delivery of small molecule drugs. *Adv. Drug Deliv. Rev.* 65(15), 1964–2015 (2013).

78. Riley, P. R. & Narayan, R. J. Recent advances in carbon nanomaterials for biomedical applications: A review. *Curr. Opin. Biomed. Eng.* 17, 100262 (2021).

79. Ghaemi, F., Amiri, A., Bajuri, M. Y., Yuhana, N. Y. & Ferrara, M. Role of different types of nanomaterials against diagnosis, prevention and therapy of COVID-19. *Sustain. Cities Soc.* 72, 103046 (2021).

80. Liu, K.-K. *et al.* Covalent linkage of nanodiamond-paclitaxel for drug delivery and cancer therapy. *Nanotechnology* 21(31), 315106 (2010).

81. Karfa, P., De, S., Majhi, K. C., Madhuri, R. & Sharma, P. K. Functionalization of carbon nanostructures. In *Comprehensive nanoscience and nanotechnology* vols 1–5 123–144 (Elsevier, 2019).

82. Falynskova, I. N. *et al.* Antiviral activity of fullerene-(tris-aminocaproic acid) hydrate against respiratory syncytial virus in HEp-2 cell culture. *Pharm. Chem. J.* 48(2), 85–88 (2014).

83. Wen, B. & Tian, Y. Synthesis, thermal properties and application of nanodiamond. In *Thermal transport in carbon-based nanomaterials* 85–112 (Elsevier, 2017), https://doi.org/10.1016/B978-0-32-346240-2.00004-2.

84. Qin, J.-X. *et al.* Nanodiamonds: Synthesis, properties, and applications in nanomedicine. *Mater. Des.* 210, 110091 (2021).

85. Yang, X. X., Li, C. M., Li, Y. F., Wang, J. & Huang, C. Z. Synergistic antiviral effect of curcumin functionalized graphene oxide against respiratory syncytial virus infection. *Nanoscale* 9(41), 16086–16092 (2017).

86. Iijima, S. Helical microtubules of graphitic carbon. *Nature* 354(6348), 56–58 (1991).

87. Selvaraj, M., Hai, A., Banat, F. & Haija, M. A. Application and prospects of carbon nanostructured materials in water treatment: A review. *J. Water Process Eng.* 33, 100996 (2020).

88. Sobhani, Z., Dinarvand, R., Atyabi, F., Ghahremani, M., & Adeli, M. Increased paclitaxel cytotoxicity against cancer cell lines using a novel functionalized carbon nanotube. *Int. J. Nanomedicine* 705, (2011). https://doi.org/10.2147/IJN.S17336.

89. Das, M., Singh, R. P., Datir, S. R. & Jain, S. Surface chemistry dependent "switch" regulates the trafficking and therapeutic performance of drug-loaded carbon nanotubes. *Bioconjug. Chem.* 24(4), 626–639 (2013).

90. Arya, N., Arora, A., Vasu, K. S., Sood, A. K. & Katti, D. S. Combination of single walled carbon nanotubes/graphene oxide with paclitaxel: A reactive oxygen species mediated synergism for treatment of lung cancer. *Nanoscale* 5(7), 2818 (2013).

91. Natesan, S. *et al.* Hypocrellin B and nano silver loaded polymeric nanoparticles: Enhanced generation of singlet oxygen for improved photodynamic therapy. *Mater. Sci. Eng. C Mater. Biol. Appl.* 77, 935–946 (2017).

92. Sadhasivam, J. & Sugumaran, A. Magnetic nanocarriers: Emerging tool for the effective targeted treatment of lung cancer. *J. Drug Deliv. Sci. Technol.* 55, 101493 (2020).

93. Wang, W. *et al.* Nanomedicine in lung cancer: Current states of overcoming drug resistance and improving cancer immunotherapy. *Wiley Interdiscip. Rev. Nanomed. Nanobiotechnology* 13(1), 1–22 (2021).

94. Luther, D. C. *et al.* Delivery of drugs, proteins, and nucleic acids using inorganic nanoparticles. *Adv. Drug Deliv. Rev.* 156, 188–213 (2020).

95. Domac, B. H. *et al.* Effects of pegylated Fe–Fe_3O_4 core-shell nanoparticles on NIH_3T_3 and A_{549} cell lines. *Heliyon* 6(1), 4–9 (2020).

96. Li, W. *et al.* AuNPs as an important inorganic nanoparticle applied in drug carrier systems. *Artif. Cells Nanomed. Biotechnol.* 47(1), 4222–4233 (2019).

97. Thakuria, A., Kataria, B. & Gupta, D. Nanoparticle-based methodologies for targeted drug delivery—An insight. *J. Nanopart. Res.* 23(4), 87 (2021).

98. Liu, Z., Sun, Q. & Wang, X. PLK1, A potential target for cancer therapy. *Transl. Oncol.* 10(1), 22–32 (2017).

99. Reda, M. *et al.* PLK1 and EGFR targeted nanoparticle as a radiation sensitizer for non-small cell lung cancer. *Cancer Lett.* 467, 9–18 (2019).

100. Tasciotti, E. *et al.* Mesoporous silicon particles as a multistage delivery system for imaging and therapeutic applications. *Nat. Nanotechnol.* 3(3), 151–157 (2008).

101. Dilnawaz, F. & Sahoo, S. K. Augmented anticancer efficacy by si-RNA complexed drug-loaded mesoporous silica nanoparticles in lung cancer therapy. *ACS Appl. Nano Mater.* 1(2), 730–740 (2018).

102. Sokolova, V. & Epple, M. Biological and medical applications of calcium phosphate nanoparticles. *Chem. Eur. J.* 27(27), 7471–7488 (2021).

103. Lee, M. S. *et al.* Target-specific delivery of siRNA by stabilized calcium phosphate nanoparticles using dopa–hyaluronic acid conjugate. *J. Control. Release* 192, 122–130 (2014).

104. Xu, X., Li, Z., Zhao, X., Keen, L. & Kong, X. Calcium phosphate nanoparticles-based systems for siRNA delivery. *Regen. Biomater.* 3(3), 187–195 (2016).

105. Li, J., Yang, Y. & Huang, L. Calcium phosphate nanoparticles with an asymmetric lipid bilayer coating for siRNA delivery to the tumor. *J. Control. Release* 158(1), 108–114 (2012).

106. Hozayen, W. G. *et al.* Cardiac and pulmonary toxicity of mesoporous silica nanoparticles is associated with excessive ROS production and redox imbalance in Wistar rats. *Biomed. Pharmacother.* 109, 2527–2538 (2019).

107. Piao, Y. *et al.* Calcium phosphate nanoparticle-based systems for therapeutic delivery. In *Theranostic bionanomaterials* 147–164 (Elsevier, 2019). https://doi.org/10.1016/B978-0-12-815341-3.00006-7.

108. Epple, M. Review of potential health risks associated with nanoscopic calcium phosphate. *Acta Biomater.* 77, 1–14 (2018).

109. Poh, W. *et al.* Active pulmonary targeting against tuberculosis (TB) via triple-encapsulation of Q_{203}, bedaquiline and superparamagnetic iron oxides (SPIOs) in nanoparticle aggregates. *Drug Deliv.* 26(1), 1039–1048 (2019).

110. Nozohouri, S., Salehi, R., Ghanbarzadeh, S., Adibkia, K. & Hamishehkar, H. A multilayer hollow nanocarrier for pulmonary co-drug delivery of methotrexate and doxorubicin in the form of dry powder inhalation formulation. *Mater. Sci. Eng. C Mater. Biol. Appl.* 99, 752–761 (2019).

111. Ak, G. *et al.* Delivery of pemetrexed by magnetic nanoparticles: Design, characterization, in vitro and in vivo assessment. *Prep. Biochem. Biotechnol.* 50(3), 215–225 (2020).

112. Liu, D. *et al.* Targeted destruction of cancer stem cells using multifunctional magnetic nanoparticles that enable combined hyperthermia and chemotherapy. *Theranostics* 10(3), 1181–1196 (2020).

113. Sanchez-Guzman, D. *et al.* Silver nanoparticle-adjuvanted vaccine protects against lethal influenza infection through inducing BALT and IgA-mediated mucosal immunity. *Biomaterials* 217, 119308 (2019).

114. Li, C., Zhang, H., Gong, X., Li, Q. & Zhao, X. Synthesis, characterization, and cytotoxicity assessment of N-acetyl-l-cysteine capped ZnO nanoparticles as camptothecin delivery system. *Colloids Surf. B: Biointerfaces* 174, 476–482 (2019).

115. Mohiyuddin, S., Naqvi, S. & Packirisamy, G. Enhanced antineoplastic/therapeutic efficacy using 5-fluorouracil-loaded calcium phosphate nanoparticles. *Beilstein J. Nanotechnol.* 9, 2499–2515 (2018).

116. Zhang, Q. *et al.* Cetuximab and doxorubicin loaded dextran-coated Fe_3O_4 magnetic nanoparticles as novel targeted nanocarriers for non-small cell lung cancer. *J. Magn. Magn. Mater.* 481, 122–128 (2019).

117. Yih, T. C. & Al-Fandi, M. Engineered nanoparticles as precise drug delivery systems. *J. Cell. Biochem.* 97(6), 1184–1190 (2006).

118. Que, Y. M. *et al.* Size dependent anti-invasiveness of silver nanoparticles in lung cancer cells. *RSC Adv.* 9(37), 21134–21138 (2019).

119. Crous, A. & Abrahamse, H. Effective gold nanoparticle-antibody-mediated drug delivery for photodynamic therapy of lung cancer stem cells. *Int. J. Mol. Sci.* 21(11), 3742 (2020).

120. Rozalen, M., Sánchez-Polo, M., Fernández-Perales, M., Widmann, T. J. & Rivera-Utrilla, J. Synthesis of controlled-size silver nanoparticles for the administration of methotrexate drug and its activity in colon and lung cancer cells. *RSC Adv.* 10(18), 10646–10660 (2020).

121. Kaur, G., Narang, R. K., Rath, G. & Goyal, A. K. Advances in pulmonary delivery of nanoparticles. *Artif. Cells Blood Substit. Biotechnol.* 40(1–2), 75–96 (2012).

122. Gosens, I. *et al.* Impact of agglomeration state of nano- and submicron sized gold particles on pulmonary inflammation. *Part. Fibre Toxicol.* 7(1), 37 (2010).

123. Sung, J. H. *et al.* Subchronic inhalation toxicity of gold nanoparticles. *Part. Fibre Toxicol.* 8, 1–18 (2011).

124. Araujo, L. H. *et al.* Lung cancer in Brazil. *J. Bras. Pneumol.* 44(1), 55–64 (2018).

125. Maiuthed, A., Chantarawong, W. & Chanvorachote, P. Lung cancer stem cells and cancer stem cell-targeting natural compounds. *Anticancer Res.* 38(7), 3797–3809 (2018).

126. Ramalingam, V., Varunkumar, K., Ravikumar, V. & Rajaram, R. Target delivery of doxorubicin tethered with PVP stabilized gold nanoparticles for effective treatment of lung cancer. *Sci. Rep.* 8(1), 3815 (2018).

127. Pooja, D. *et al.* Natural polysaccharide functionalized gold nanoparticles as biocompatible drug delivery carrier. *Int. J. Biol. Macromol.* 80, 48–56 (2015).

128. Alkilany, A. M. & Murphy, C. J. Toxicity and cellular uptake of gold nanoparticles: What we have learned so far? *J. Nanopart. Res.* 12(7), 2313–2333 (2010).

129. Shukla, R. *et al.* Biocompatibility of gold nanoparticles and their endocytotic fate Inside the cellular compartment: A microscopic overview. *Langmuir* 21(23), 10644–10654 (2005).

130. Phi, L. T. H. *et al.* Cancer stem cells (CSCs) in drug resistance and their therapeutic implications in cancer treatment. *Stem Cells Int.* 2018, 1–16 (2018).

131. Stubbe, C. E. & Valero, M. Complementary strategies for the management of radiation therapy side effects. *J. Adv. Pract. Oncol.* 4, 219–231 (2013).

132. Sasaki, H. *et al.* Patient perceptions of symptoms and concerns during cancer chemotherapy: 'Affects my family' is the most important. *Int. J. Clin. Oncol.* 22(4), 793–800 (2017).

133. Shiono, S., Abiko, M. & Sato, T. Postoperative complications in elderly patients after lung cancer surgery. *Interact. Cardiovasc. Thorac. Surg.* 16(6), 819–823 (2013).

134. Mokwena, M. G., Kruger, C. A., Ivan, M. T. & Heidi, A. A review of nanoparticle photosensitizer drug delivery uptake systems for photodynamic treatment of lung cancer. *Photodiagn. Photodyn. Ther.* 22, 147–154 (2018).

135. Abrahamse, H., Abdel Harith, M., Hussein, A. & Tynga, I. Photodynamic ability of silver nanoparticles in inducing cytotoxic effects in breast and lung cancer cell lines. *Int. J. Nanomedicine* 9, 3771 (2014).

136. Wadhwa, R. *et al. Nanoparticle-based drug delivery for chronic obstructive pulmonary disorder and asthma. Nanotechnology in modern animal biotechnology* (Elsevier Inc., 2019). https://doi.org/10.1016/b978-0-12-818823-1.00005-3.

137. Sung, J. H. *et al.* Lung function changes in Sprague-Dawley rats after prolonged inhalation exposure to silver nanoparticles. *Inhal. Toxicol.* 20(6), 567–574 (2008).

138. Ajdary, M. *et al.* Health concerns of various nanoparticles: A review of their in vitro and in vivo toxicity. *Nanomaterials* 8(9), 634 (2018).

139. Zhao, X. *et al.* Fungal silver nanoparticles: Synthesis, application and challenges. *Crit. Rev. Biotechnol.* 38(6), 817–835 (2018).

140. Rai, M., Yadav, A. & Gade, A. Silver nanoparticles as a new generation of antimicrobials. *Biotechnol. Adv.* 27(1), 76–83 (2009).

141. Rasmussen, J. W., Martinez, E., Louka, P. & Wingett, D. G. Zinc oxide nanoparticles for selective destruction of tumor cells and potential for drug delivery applications. *Expert Opin. Drug Deliv.* 7(9), 1063–1077 (2010).

142. Wilhelm, S. *et al.* Analysis of nanoparticle delivery to tumours. *Nat. Rev. Mater.* 1(5), 16014 (2016).

143. Serpone, N., Dondi, D. & Albini, A. Inorganic and organic UV filters: Their role and efficacy in sunscreens and suncare products. *Inorg. Chim. Acta* 360(3), 794–802 (2007).

144. Sato, M. *et al.* Preparation, characterization and properties of novel covalently surface-functionalized zinc oxide nanoparticles. *Appl. Surf. Sci.* 256(14), 4497–4501 (2010).

145. Pugazhendhi, A., Edison, T. N. J. I., Karuppusamy, I. & Kathirvel, B. Inorganic nanoparticles: A potential cancer therapy for human welfare. *Int. J. Pharm.* 539(1–2), 104–111 (2018).

146. Dankers, A. C. A. *et al.* A practical approach to assess inhalation toxicity of metal oxide nanoparticles in vitro. *J. Appl. Toxicol.* 38(2), 160–171 (2018).

147. Wang, J., Gao, S., Wang, S., Xu, Z. & Wei, L. Zinc oxide nanoparticles induce toxicity in CAL_{27} oral cancer cell lines by activating $PINK_1$/Parkin-mediated mitophagy. *Int. J. Nanomedicine* 13, 3441–3450 (2018).

148. De Berardis, B. *et al.* Exposure to ZnO nanoparticles induces oxidative stress and cytotoxicity in human colon carcinoma cells. *Toxicol. Appl. Pharmacol.* 246(3), 116–127 (2010).

149. Song, W. *et al.* Role of the dissolved zinc ion and reactive oxygen species in cytotoxicity of ZnO nanoparticles. *Toxicol. Lett.* 199(3), 389–397 (2010).

150. Wang, J., Lee, J. S., Kim, D. & Zhu, L. Exploration of zinc oxide nanoparticles as a multitarget and multifunctional anticancer nanomedicine. *ACS Appl. Mater. Interfaces* 9(46), 39971–39984 (2017).

151. Fujihara, J. *et al.* Pro-inflammatory responses and oxidative stress induced by ZnO nanoparticles in vivo following intravenous injection. *Eur. Rev. Med. Pharmacol. Sci.* 19(24), 4920–4926 (2015).

152. Fujihara, J. *et al.* Distribution and toxicity evaluation of ZnO dispersion nanoparticles in single intravenously exposed mice. *J. Med. Investig.* 62(1–2), 45–50 (2015).

153. Tanino, R. *et al.* Anticancer activity of ZnO nanoparticles against human small-cell lung cancer in an orthotopic mouse model. *Mol. Cancer Ther.* 19(2), 502–512 (2020).

154. Palanikumar, L., Ramasamy, S., Hariharan, G. & Balachandran, C. Influence of particle size of nano zinc oxide on the controlled delivery of amoxicillin. *Appl. Nanosci.* 3(5), 441–451 (2013).

155. El-Sherbiny, I. M., Elbaz, N. M., Sedki, M., Elgammal, A. & Yacoub, M. H. Magnetic nanoparticles-based drug and gene delivery systems for the treatment of pulmonary diseases. *Nanomedicine* 12(4), 387–402 (2017).

156. Srinivas, A. *et al.* Oxidative stress and inflammatory responses of rat following acute inhalation exposure to iron oxide nanoparticles. *Hum. Exp. Toxicol.* 31(11), 1113–1131 (2012).

157. Wu, C. Y. & Chen, Y. C. Riboflavin immobilized Fe_3O_4 magnetic nanoparticles carried with n-butylidenephthalide as targeting-based anticancer agents. *Artif. Cells Nanomed. Biotechnol.* 47(1), 210–220 (2019).

158. Roskoski, R. The ErbB/HER family of protein-tyrosine kinases and cancer. *Pharmacol. Res.* 79, 34–74 (2014).

159. Numico, G. *et al.* Single-agent pegylated liposomal doxorubicin (Caelix®) in chemotherapy pretreated non-small cell lung cancer patients: A pilot trial. *Lung Cancer* 35(1), 59–64 (2002).

160. Daniel, T. M. The history of tuberculosis. *Respir. Med.* 100(11), 1862–1870 (2006).

161. Merker, M. *et al.* Evolutionary history and global spread of the Mycobacterium tuberculosis Beijing lineage. *Nat. Genet.* 47(3), 242 (2015).

162. *Global tuberculosis report 2021.* World Health Organization. (2021). Licence: CC BY-NC-SA 3.0 IGO.

163. Sulis, G., Roggi, A., Matteelli, A. & Raviglione, M. C. Tuberculosis: Epidemiology and control. *Mediterr. J. Hematol. Infect. Dis.* 6(1), e2014070 (2014).

164. Vieira, A. C. C. *et al.* Mucoadhesive chitosan-coated solid lipid nanoparticles for better management of tuberculosis. *Int. J. Pharm.* 536(1), 478–485 (2018).

165. Zumla, A., Nahid, P. & Cole, S. T. Advances in the development of new tuberculosis drugs and treatment regimens. *Nat. Rev. Drug Discov.* 12(5), 388–404 (2013).

166. Costa, A. *et al.* The formulation of nanomedicines for treating tuberculosis. *Adv. Drug Deliv. Rev.* 102, 102–115 (2016).

167. El-Boubbou, K. Magnetic iron oxide nanoparticles as drug carriers: Clinical relevance. *Nanomedicine* 13(8), 953–971 (2018).

168. Jiang, X., He, C. & Lin, W. Supramolecular metal-based nanoparticles for drug delivery and cancer therapy. *Curr. Opin. Chem. Biol.* 61, 143–153 (2021).

169. Bayda, S. *et al.* Inorganic nanoparticles for cancer therapy: A transition from lab to clinic. *Curr. Med. Chem.* 25(34), 4269–4303 (2017).

170. Huang, H., Feng, W., Chen, Y. & Shi, J. Inorganic nanoparticles in clinical trials and translations. *Nano Today* 35, 100972 (2020).

171. Mitchell, M. J. *et al.* Engineering precision nanoparticles for drug delivery. *Nat. Rev. Drug Discov.* 20(2), 101–124 (2021).

SECTION IV

Advancing Established Technologies

Surface Modification of Micronized Drug Particles for Aerosolization

11

Tania Bajaj, Vishav Prabhjot Kaur, Urvashi Anwekar, Deepak Chitkara, and Charan Singh

Contents

DOI: 10.1201/9781003182566-15

11.1 INTRODUCTION

Lung diseases include any disorder that hampers the normal working of the lungs and impacts the functioning of the respiratory system or the breathing potential. These diseases could be due to bacteria, viruses, fungi, and environmental factors such as asthma or lung cancer.[1,2] Many people all over the world are affected by diseases of the lungs.[3] In the last two decades, the death rate because of or linked to chronic obstructive pulmonary disease (COPD) has been continuously augmenting in the United States.[4] In the United States for the year 2018, the numbers for a chronic lung disorder like lung cancer were calculated at 121,680 for men and 112,350 for women, which means 641 new lung cancer cases are detected daily.[5] In the United States, especially lower respiratory tract diseases including COPD, emphysema, and chronic bronchitis are prime causes of death.[3] In asthma and COPD, the flow of air is reduced because of the tapering of airways, while in pulmonary fibrosis, a tissue of the lungs gets disfigured, and in pneumonia, an infection (either bacterial or viral) occurs which loads the air sacs with fluid. Apart from these airway diseases, lung cancer is a disorder wherein the cells do not develop normally.

Globally, lung cancer has become the cause of death for over one million citizens over the period from 2001 to 2020. In a study, it is reported that the use of tobacco is responsible for raising the incidence rate of lung cancer.[6,7] Lung cancer begins in the bronchi (in the lining of cells) and extends over to other regions of the lungs, such as bronchioles and alveoli. Broadly, lung cancer is classified into two categories which are handled dissimilarly: non-small cell lung cancer (NSCLC) and small cell lung cancer (SCLC).[8] Lung cancer is the most common cancer in terms of total cases (11.6%) and an major cause of cancer death (18.4%) in males and females. The next most common cancers for incidence are breast cancer, prostate cancer, colorectal cancer, stomach cancer, and liver cancer.[9] Lungs are an appealing choice for the delivery of drugs for local action, as the lungs are the only organ that is exposed to the external environment directly, therefore, inhalation drug delivery to treat pulmonary disorders is highly recommended.[10] Inhalation or pulmonary delivery could be a better strategy to treat a variety of lung diseases, such as allergy, asthma, idiopathic pulmonary fibrosis (IPF), cystic fibrosis (CF), acute lung injury (ALI), COPD, lung cancer, and tuberculosis.[1,11] Delivering the drugs by inhalation route possesses a few limitations; the first limitation is that the safeguarding operations of the respiratory tract do not allow the inhaled particles to enter the lungs – additionally, they inactivate them if they are deposited. The second limitation is that the patient requires an inhaler device and the proper understanding of the working of the device to target the drugs into the lungs. But sometimes patients are not able to meet these requirements, which serves as a huge snag.[12] Further, if the drug is delivered at its targeted site of pharmacological effect, it could lower the dose or frequency of dosing, ultimately leading to reduced systemic side effects.

Apart from localized delivery, when the drug is targeted to the deep lung region, absorption through the epithelial cells results in the accumulation of higher concentrations of the drug in the blood, promoting the quick onset of action as well as the bypassing first-pass metabolism.[12] The inhalation or lung targeted delivery is advantageous over the other routes of drug administration (for instance, oral or parenteral) for the treatment of any kind of lung disease.[11] The solute permeability of lungs is huge, possesses enormous absorption area for drug absorption, finite enzymatic activity, and the inhalation drug delivery is painless.

An inter-disciplinary process that delivers nanotechnology-enabled drug delivery systems with intended properties such as particle size, particles density, surface topography, and morphology is termed particle engineering. The nanoparticles can be formulated using various processes, such as top-down approach, bottom-up approach, lyophilization, supercritical fluid technology, and nano spray drying.[13] For synthesizing microparticles of drugs for inhalation therapy, the spray drying technique has been very commonly used. Recently, Jun et al. developed and evaluated sodium cromoglycate-loaded porous particles to enhance their powder flow properties via dry powder inhalers. In the study, the authors employed an anti-solvent precipitation method followed by a spray drying technique to obtain the micron-sized spherical microparticles. In vitro aerosol deposition studies revealed remarkable improvement in the aerosolization efficiency from the sodium cromoglycate containing agglomerates vis-à-vis its free form. Further, the supercritical-assisted atomization (SAA) process resulted in a good particle size pattern owing to its mild operating experimental conditions.[14] Moreover, Roa et al. assessed the therapeutic efficacy of doxorubicin (DOX)-loaded nanoparticles (NPs) in the orthotropic cancer mice model. In this study, they used the spray and freeze-drying technology to mix the DOX-loaded NPs with the suitable inhalation carriers' particles. Cytotoxicity studies were performed on the human non-small cell lung carcinoma cell line NCL-H460. Finally, the authors concluded that DOX-loaded NPs reduced the cardiotoxicity and enhanced the survival time of the tumor-bearing mice via inhalation delivery in comparison to intravenous dosing of the drug at an equivalent dose.[15] Similarly, Kalantarian et al. designed 5-fluorouracil (5-FU) NPs intended for lung delivery by using a supercritical anti-solvent process.[16] The authors optimized various experimental conditions such as type of solvents, temperature, flow rate, and pressure. In vitro lung aerodynamic studies using twin-stage liquid impinger revealed improved powder flow characterization properties. In inhalation therapies, the mechanism of particles deposition in the respiratory airways is of great importance as this could impact the uptake and efficiency of the drug delivery.[17]

11.2 MECHANISM OF PARTICLE DEPOSITION IN THE LUNGS

An airway tree is the constituent of the lungs, which begins from the trachea and ends at the alveoli. These airways are further cleaved into two segments: the tracheobronchial part and the pulmonary part.[18] As already discussed, the lungs possess enormous surface area; thereby, they could be used as the paramount spot for particle deposition, for action at the localized site, or entering the blood circulation for systemic effects.[19,20]

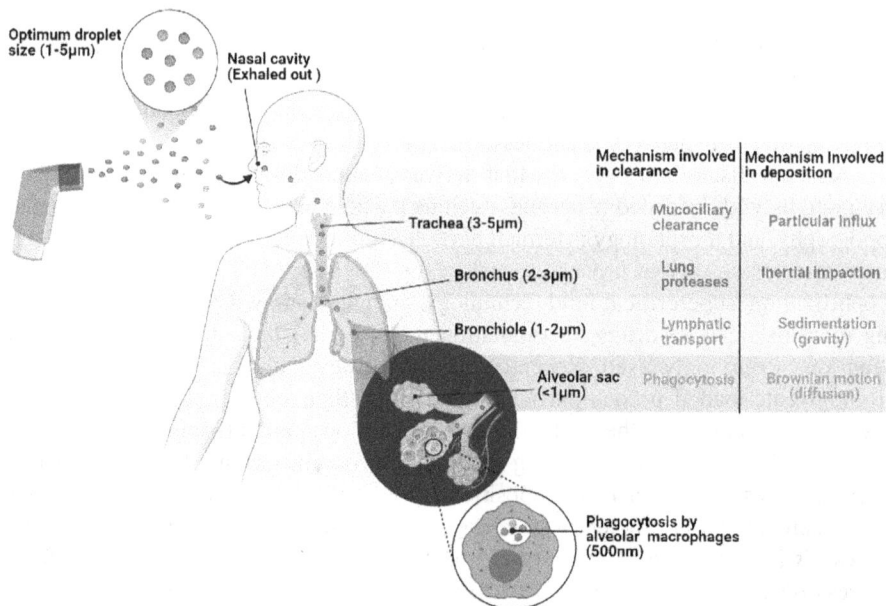

FIGURE 11.1　Various mechanisms of particle deposition in and clearance from the lungs.

Generally, the volume of the lungs enlarges during inhalation, and it contracts during exhalation, which modifies the geometry of airways. Deposition refers to an episode of particle adherence to the surface[21] and is regulated with three operations: inertial impaction, gravitational sedimentation, and Brownian diffusion. Apart from these, the mechanisms such as mixing induced by turbulent flows, electrostatic precipitation, and interception (for the particles of large size) could also lead to aerosol deposition in certain cases. Each mechanism's contribution to deposition is influenced by lung structure and size, the degree of airway obstruction, the breathing pattern, and the particle size distribution.[19]

To conclude, a variety of forces are prone to be linked with the foreign airborne particles in the complete length of the respiratory tract, and those forces can be called gravitational force, the resistant force of the air which is inhaled, and the inertial force. The mechanism of the settling of particles in the lungs is governed through the balance between these forces and the properties of the aerosol as depicted in Figure 11.1.

11.2.1　Primary Mechanisms of Particle Deposition

11.2.1.1　Inertial impaction

Inertial impaction is found to be the chief mechanism of settling of the particles in the airway tract for particles > 5μm in size and for particles of size < 2 μm, depending on the flow rate. Inertial impaction occurs in the case when the direction of the flow swaps instantly, leading to the deflection of the particles from the air streamlines;

particles collide with the airway walls. Strokes' number (Stk) could be used as a means to describe the particles that deviate from the aerodynamics of air as

$$\text{Stk} = \frac{\rho p d 2 p u}{18 \mu d}$$

where dp and ρp refer to the particle diameter and density; u and μ denote the mean velocity and dynamic viscosity of the carrier gas; and d refers to the airway diameter. The dimensionless Strokes' number, Stk, as already described, denotes the possibility of settling particles in the respiratory tract through the process of impaction. It could therefore be predicted that the greater the Strokes' number, the more efficiently the particles are supposed to settle. Thereby, looking at the bifurcated architecture of the lungs, the large size particles that mediate through the respiratory tract with inflated momentum are supposed to deposit in the upper airway tract.[17] Inertial impaction prevails when these airborne particles have sufficient impulse to stay in the particular orientation so that they can strike the lining of the respiratory tract. Particles having a size range > 1 μm and whose higher doses are to be delivered to the body can be easily delivered via this method.

With the process of inertial impaction, even the gigantic lump of aerosol particles could also settle on the lungs' surface instantly. As reported in the literature, this mechanism could be used to incorporate the aerosols on the cell's surface in commercially available particle sizing devices and modified commercial devices. The commercial sizing devices possess a few limitations, as only a finite number of particles only get delivered to the target zone owing to their complex design and therefore, a self-designed delivery device or a custom-designed device could serve the purpose, by which the size range, as well as the deposition pattern of settled particles, could be controlled. In a study, a device has been manufactured which tends to deliver the particles present in aerosol to a predictable region, i.e., to the surface of cells grown at the ALI using inertial impaction, and it can be propagated. To formulate a device with sub-micron d50, it should be constructed in such a way that it possesses tiny slits with giant air momentum, as the small slits lead to irregular settling of particles, and huge-sized slits do not permit the settling of particles.[22] When the pressurized metered-dose inhalers (pMDIs) are actuated, they produce a freaked-out response which leads to the settling of molecules through inertial impaction. Contrary to this, the aerosols that are produced by nebulizers are predicted to be revolving around the respiratory fashion of the individual. Sangwan et al., in their study, have assessed the settling behaviors of the particles from aerosols produced by Misty-Neb® (Median Mass Aerodynamic Diameter, MMAD=3.1 m) and AeroEclipse® (MMAD=2.2 m) for better lung delivery.[17] Several studies have explored the effects of means of the settling of particles in the respiratory tract. For instance, research showed that the settling of particles by the process of gravitation is predicted to arouse in the peripheral passageway, where neither impaction nor diffusion can occur.[23] Additionally, another research group hypothesized that inertial impaction is an important mechanism of particle deposition for particles that are in the range of micron size.[24] If inertial impaction is thought to be a deposition mechanism for the in vitro studies, there could be many hurdles in the pathway; the first hurdle being the requirement of a concentrated aerosol. Secondly, when the particles settle through this mechanism, they settle irregularly throughout the surface of the cell. By modifying the configuration and sizes of the jets used for performing inertial impaction, the regularity or the alignment of the deposited particles could be maintained.[22]

11.2.1.2 Gravitational sedimentation

In the respiratory tract, deposition by gravitational sedimentation is the only precise method for the molecules falling in the size range of 1–8 μm, as the bigger molecules settle by the principle of inertial impaction and the minute molecules settle by the principle of Brownian diffusion. The particles falling under this category cannot either be a constituent of Brownian diffusion or inertia. The mechanism of gravitational sedimentation is generally governed by the balance between streamlined and planetary motion.[25] Gravitational sedimentation means the molecules' deposition by the force of gravity. The molecules attain the terminal settling velocity when the downward pull (termed as gravity) matches the antagonizing viscous resistive forces of the air, which could be expressed using the following equation:

$$vs = \frac{\rho p d2 p}{18\mu} g$$

Where g is the gravitational acceleration.

Overall, the morphology of the human lung remains the same in all individuals, but there could occur some regional differences in the oxygenation process by the downward pull (i.e., gravity effect). These changes might also influence the settling and dispersal of the molecules inhaled.[26] In reference to this, Tsuda et al. discussed in their research on the 2D alveolated duct, which possesses vital significance for particles settling through the mechanism of gravitational sedimentation. More recently, Haber et al. discussed in their research about the critical importance of alveolar wall motion.[25]

Computational fluid-particle dynamics (CFPD) simulations for the particles settling through the process of gravitational force began in the late 90s, which focused on small bronchial airways and alveolar ducts or sacs. In reference to that, Hofmann et al. imitated the gravitational deposition of particles in a non-uniform, uni-directional airway model and concluded that the angle of gravity played a vital role in identifying the localized doses.[27] Haber et al. infused the process of deposition through gravitational force with wall movements, using a 3D hemispherical alveolus model.[28]

11.2.1.2.1 Brownian diffusion

The Brownian diffusion arises because of the erratic movement of the particles caused by their crashing with the gas molecules. The diffusion rate is equivalent to the Brownian diffusion coefficient as given in the following equation:

$$DB = \frac{ckT}{3\pi\mu dp}$$

Where k represents the Boltzmann's constant, T is the absolute temperature, and c is the Cunningham correction factor. For the molecules possessing density as one (molecules of diameters less than 0.5μm), Brownian motion is significant, and for larger particles, sedimentation is a significant mechanism of deposition.[29] Similar to impaction and sedimentation, it is predicted that the settling that occurs by the process of Brownian diffusion enhances with the dropping particle size, and it is the only mechanism responsible for settling of particles $< 0.5\mu m$ in diameter. The mechanism of Brownian diffusion transpires basically in the pulmonary acinus, although it should be noted that for very small particles (possessing particle diameter < 0.01 μm), the settling of particles by this process is also significant in the nose, mouth, and pharyngeal airways. As already known, the flow of air into the nose and larynx is disorderly; the Brownian diffusion process, however, regulates the formation of the boundary layers in the airways.[30] The settling of particles by Brownian diffusion declines with an increase in the size of particles and is not based upon the flow rate.[31]

11.2.1.3 Other deposition mechanisms

11.2.1.3.1 Turbulent flows
A cascade of flow is governed by the Reynolds number (Re). In an infinitely long cylindrical respiratory tract, the flow is said to be laminar if the Re value falls below 2100, and it is said to be turbulent if it goes above 2100. The flow in the airways could be mentioned by its mean value over which the oscillations by the disruption of the flow are superimposed. These flow disruptions lead to the occurrence of turbulent flows, which lead to alterations in both the magnitude and direction of the pathway of the particles. A study by Matida *et al.* describes that the mixing caused by the turbulent flow is as significant as the inertial impaction is for particle deposition.[32]

11.2.1.3.2 Electrostatic precipitation
Deposition by the process of electrostatic precipitation is usually considered unimportant compared with the mechanisms of impaction, sedimentation, and diffusion, and thus the literature on the effect of electrostatic charges on aerosol deposition in the lung is rather scant.

11.2.1.3.3 Interception
Deposition by interception occurs when a particle comes close enough to an airway wall that an edge touches its surface. It is an important mechanism for elongated particles such as fibers for which the ratio between length and diameter is large.

11.3 PARTICLE ENGINEERING FOR LUNG DELIVERY

Of late, the role of nanotechnology in the area of management and treatment of lung diseases has evolved tremendously. In this regard, nanotechnology-enabled drug delivery systems, including nano- and micro-sized particles, have shown great outcomes and are expected to provide new and advanced avenues in the delivery of drugs and biologics.[33] It is well reported in the literature that after the administration of drugs and biotherapeutics, the absorbed particles would be interacting with the blood cells and plasma. This interaction will depend on the particles' surface properties such as charge, morphology, hydrophilicity, and surface decoration with some ligands.[34] For the treatment of lung disorders, the carrier systems that could be used are organic (lipid, polymer, lipid-polymer hybrid) and inorganic nanoparticles (metal-organic frameworks, silica nanoparticles), and some other newer systems (carbon nanotubes, quantum dots). In addition, a summary and illustration of the methods for surface engineering for better aerosolization are presented in Table 11.1 and Figure 11.2, respectively. In this section,

TABLE 11.1   Summary of the methods for surface engineering for better aerosolization

NO.	METHOD	ADVANTAGES	LIMITATIONS	REFERENCES
1.	Spray drying	Versatile and prompt process Free-flowing particles with mono-dispersed size A simple method for converting moist substances into desiccated forms	The tedious process to generate nano-sized particles	35–37
2.	Nano-in-micro	Improved therapeutic properties of the drug Stable product Potent technique to shield the synthetic substances	Harsh processing conditions can negatively impact the integrity of the micro-capsules A very limited number of matrix/coating/excipients materials have been approved for use Liquid flowing inwards can either carry polar or non-polar molecule(s) The process of freezing is a mandate	38–40
3.	Dialysis method	Convenient method The use of potentially toxic solvents can be avoided Greater release of drug Economic	Not suitable when the drug binds to the polymer or membrane Cumbersome setup procedure Slow and sustaining process Drug loading in micellar particles is a complex process	41–44
4.	Solvent evaporation method	Operate at low temperatures Nano/micro-sized particles can be effectively achieved	Scale-up of the formulation is difficult Impaired drug loading capacity	45–47

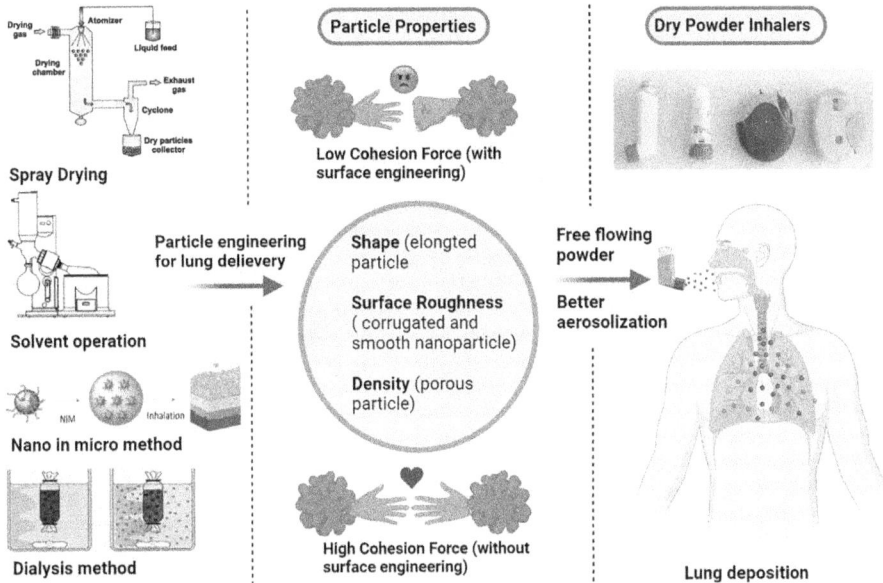

FIGURE 11.2 Various methods for surface engineering of the particles for lung delivery.

we briefly discuss various nano-carriers explored in the area of inhalation delivery by surface engineering of particles for better delivery of therapeutics using sugars, amino acids, cyclodextrins as shown in Figure 11.3.

Among various carrier systems, lipid-based carriers such as liposomes and solid lipid nanoparticles have been explored. Liposomes consist of nano-sized spherical vesicles that allow them to encapsulate both hydrophilic drugs and hydrophobic in an aqueous center and lipid bilayers, respectively. Liposomes offer diverse advantages such as being biocompatible, easy surface modification, stable, and longer duration of retention at the local site of action. Liposomes consist of cholesterol and phospholipids (phosphatidylethanolamine and phosphatidylcholine) in their structure in the 0.05–5 µm size range. There are multiple mechanisms through which the liposomes deliver the drugs to the local target, such as active (surface anchoring of some ligands) targeting, passive targeting (PEGylated), and responsive (magnetic, temperature, pH).[33] These surface modifications result in improved biopharmaceutical attributes as well as control the drug release from the nanoformulations. This may further improve the toxicity profile of the delivered drug at the targeted site. Apart from liposomes, another lipidic system, which is solid lipid nanoparticles (SLNs), are made up of solid lipid (0.1–30%) and surfactants (0.5–5%). These carrier systems provide numerous advantages such as the use of biodegradable and biocompatible lipids, enhanced stability with improved toxicity profile of the drugs as well as avoidance of first-pass metabolism compared to other colloidal carriers.[33] Although, there are some drawbacks of these carriers, including low drug loading and formation of crystalline structure in the lipid matrix. Owing to the limitations associated with SLNs, research led to the development of second-generation SLNs, termed nanostructured lipid carriers.[25] These NLCs contain a mixture of solid and liquid lipid, which are responsible for higher drug loading and the reduction of drug

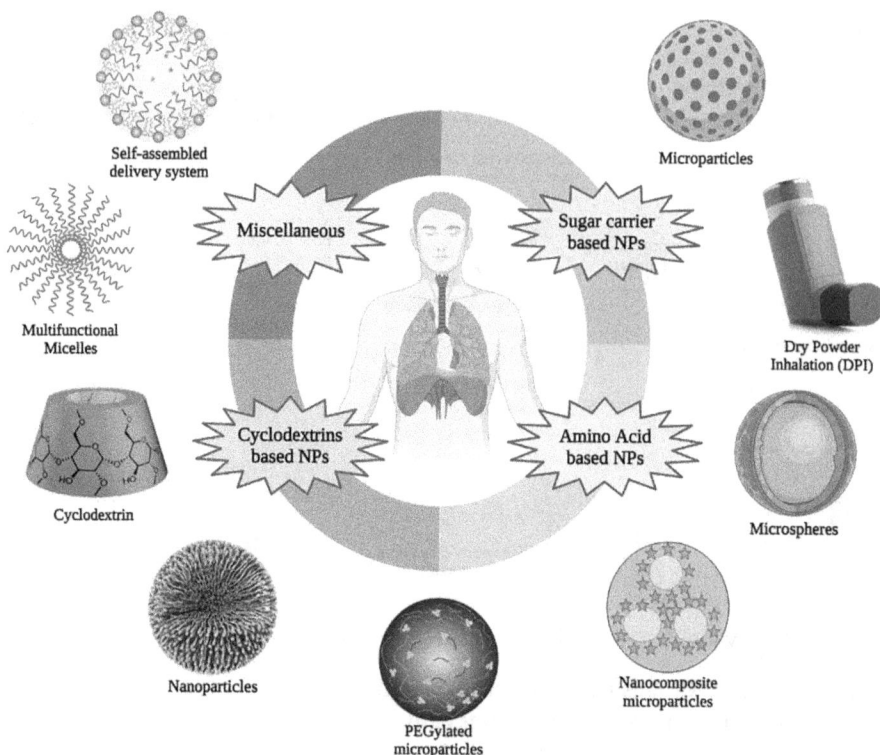

FIGURE 11.3   Strategies of particle engineering for pulmonary drug delivery.

expulsion. Apart from the lipidic systems, there are diverse polymeric carriers wherein both hydrophilic (chitosan, dextran, gelatin, alginate, etc.) and hydrophobic polymers (polyesters, polycarbonates, poly anhydrides, etc.) for biomedical applications. These carriers are gaining huge attention to treat various ailments as per the need in the area of nanotechnology. In a study, docetaxel-loaded hyaluronan/polyethyleneimine-coated polymeric nanoparticles to target the cancer cells via a cluster of differentiation 4 i.e., CD44 receptors were reported.[48] For targeted delivery, polymeric micelles (PMs) have also been explored, which are made up of hydrophobic core and hydrophilic shell to deliver the therapeutics.[49] For example, α-Conotoxin ImI coated PMs have been used to target the alpha 7 nicotinic acetylcholine receptor (α7-nAChR) gene to treat lung cancer.[50] Dendrimers (DMs) which are radially branched bifurcated nano-sized structures ranging from 10 to 100 nm have been reported. These are excellent drug delivery systems due to the presence of functional groups on their surface.[33] Aerosol delivery of polyethylene glycol-coated dendrimers (PEG-coated DMs) is also reported in the literature to target the lungs.[51] Further, superparamagnetic material of a size greater than 25 nm, known as magnetic nanoparticles (MNPs), has been explored in the field of drug delivery. MNPs could be biodegradable or non-biodegradable. The non-biodegradable MNPs are coated with some special material to facilitate the excretion through the kidney.[33] In a study, cisplatin encapsulated functionalized iron oxide (Fe_3O_4) nanoparticles have been studied to improve their anti-cancer activity. The results of the studies revealed improved antitumor activity of the drug against lung cancer.[50] Carbon nanotubes (CNTs) are another carrier system that is explored to deliver the drugs to the local site of action. These contain carbon atoms from 4 nm to 100 nm diameter; however, the diameter depends on the arrangement of the graphene molecules.[33] These have issues of solubility in the organic and aqueous solvents, along with their intrinsic toxicity in the biological fluids.[53] In a study, doxorubicin–pluronic complexes and plain doxorubicin showed cytotoxicity against human breast cancer cell lines (MCF-7) containing estrogen, progesterone, and glucocorticoid receptors.[54] Of late, nano-sized colloidal particles containing a core and a 'cap' or 'shell' quantum dots (QDs) have been explored for various biomedical applications. QDs possess large photobleaching and absorption spectra along with stability.[55,56] There are multiple applications of QDs from imaging (biological, cellular, and molecular), labeling, and detection to estimate toxicity.[57] Various strategies explored for the surface engineering of the nano-carriers for enhanced lung delivery are shown in Table 11.2 and Figure 11.3.

11.3.1 Sugar Carrier-Based Surface Engineering

Nowadays, various polysaccharides and sugar molecules are gaining tremendous attention in the area of drug delivery and tissue engineering. These are the most widely used carriers due to their biocompatible nature, easy availability, and validated surface engineering protocols. A few sugar molecules such as dextran and heparin have the capability to prevent opsonization and complement activation. In addition to this, some polysaccharides, for instance, chitosan, hyaluronic acid, and chondroitin sulfate have been used as ligands. These could be used to coat via electrostatic interactions and/or be conjugated by some chemical bonds onto the NPs surface.[58] So far, US Food and Drug Administration (FDA)-approved sugars are concerned; lactose monohydrate is the only sugar. It is available in the crystalline (α- and anhydrous lactose monohydrate) and amorphous (lactose) forms.[59] The convenience of using lactose as the continually used carrier in DPIs is because of its thoroughly researched toxicity profile, physic-chemical steadiness, and its harmony with a wide range of drugs, its availability, and cost. The majority of the DPI formulations available in the market possess α-lactose monohydrate as the carrier system incorporated into them.[60,61] In a study, lactose-containing spray-dried nanoparticles with or without gelatin or poly(butylcyanoacrylate) were explored via inhalation delivery.[62] Singh *et al.* evaluated fluticasone propionate loaded surface-modified lactose (SML) particles for inhalation delivery. Physicochemical characterization studies revealed the crystalline nature of the particles. The *in vitro* powder flow characterization studies showed improved flow properties and surface roughness. *In vitro* aerosolization studies showed a good fine particle fraction (FPF) upon lactose modification. Stability studies at 40 °C/75% Relative Humidity (RH) demonstrated no significant change in the fine particle fraction. Thus, the authors concluded that SML microparticles possessed excellent inhalational properties.[63] In another study, Grenha *et al.* developed and evaluated mannitol and lactose modified protein-loaded chitosan nanoparticles for lung delivery. The authors reported the effect of chitosan concentration on the surface morphology of the microspheres. They also reported high protein

TABLE 11.2 Surface engineering of the nano-carriers for enhanced lung delivery

CARRIER SYSTEM	METHOD USED	MAJOR OUTCOME	REFERENCES
Sugar-based carrier systems			
Dry powder inhalation (DPI) formulation	Lactose modified particles	Improved flow properties and reduced surface roughness Enhanced fine particle fraction (FPF) value and inhalation properties	63
Chitosan nanoparticles	Micro-encapsulation	Increased loading capacity and faster release	64
Microspheres	Spray drying	Enhanced FPF Good deposition of microspheres in the lungs	62
DPI	DoE	Optimized L-leucine concentration	65
DPI	Spray drying	Optimized amount of amino acids (trehalose/leucine) to serve as inhalable systems	67
DPI	Spray drying	High-performing aerosols were obtained with uniform dispersal of the particles	68
Nanocomposites	Spray drying	Feed concentration affected the formulation	69
Self-assembled delivery system		Stable formulation with respirable size	70
Amino acid-based carrier systems			
Hybrid core-shell nanoparticles	Solvent evaporation	Inhalable nanocomposites showed better performance	73
DPI	Spray drying, Co-Jet milling, mechanofusion	Coated formulation with good inhalation potential	71
DPI	Spray drying	MMAD suitable for pulmonary deliver	75
DPI	Spray drying	Histidine (HIS-) and Leucine (LEU-) modified powders with high FPF values	72
Nanoparticle aggregate powders	Spray drying	High IgG titers value	73
Microparticles	Mechanistic models	Rapid synthesis of microspheres	78
Powder	Co-spray drying on aerosolization	Increased FPF value for deep lung delivery	79
Lactose solutions	Spray drying	Significantly enhanced aerosol efficiency	80

(Continued)

TABLE 11.2 (CONTINUED) Surface engineering of the nano-carriers for enhanced lung delivery

CARRIER SYSTEM	METHOD USED	MAJOR OUTCOME	REFERENCES
PEGylated polystyrene microparticles		Large accumulation in the lung cancer domain	81
Nanoscale complex	pH-dependent	The higher therapeutic effect boosted the cancerous cell death	82
(methoxy poly(ethylene glycol)-b-poly(L-glutamic acid-co-L-phenylalanine) (mPEG-b-P(Glu-co-Phe))-based nanoparticles		High drug loading content and pH-dependent release with high antiproliferative activity	83
Cyclodextrin based carrier systems			
Nanoporous/ nanoparticulate microparticles (NPMPs)	Spray drying	Suitable FPF with remarkable MMAD for targeted delivery	85
DPI	Spray drying	Marked shape and desired particles size required for inhalation delivery	74
Miscellaneous			
Micronized powders	Mechanofusion	Free-flowing powder with high aerosolization	86
Magnesium stearate coated particles	Mechanofusion	Improved aerosol performance	87
Nano complex	Spray drying	Increased drug release and cytotoxicity potential	88

loading (65–80%) and burst release (75–80% in 15 min) after sugars coating. There was no significant change in the particle size and potential of the microparticles in the aqueous media.[64] In another research work, spray-dried Isoniazid (INH) loaded chitosan microspheres using lactose and l-leucine as bulking and dispersing agents, respectively, were evaluated. The particle size analysis data showed 4–6 μm, which indicated a good size range for lung delivery. Additionally, there was high drug loading (88–108%) of INH and good FPF (55–67%) of the microparticles.[65] A demerit of using lactose, basically α-lactose monohydrate as the carrier molecule in DPI formulations, is its contribution in the Maillard decomposition reactions when it is used with low molecular weight drugs.[58] Thereby, Focaroli *et al.* studied the effect of l-leucine concentration and experimental conditions on the properties of spray-dried trehalose-based dry powder formulation by employing the Design of Experiment (DoE) approach. Various experimental parameters such as inlet and outlet temperature, gas flow, feed solution, and flow rate were optimized. There was an impact of gas flow rate on the particle size and drying chamber temperature and feed rate on the yield and residual moisture, respectively. Finally, they concluded that high leucine concentration prevented the crystallization of amorphous trehalose.[66] In a study, a combination of sugars (mannitol, trehalose) and amino acids (glycine, alanine) were studied to form a stable amorphous glassy matrix. In this study, leucine was used as a particle formation and powder flow enhancing agent. *In vitro* aerosolization studies showed high FPFs from various formulations. The authors of the study concluded that a good combination of trehalose and leucine could result in better lung delivery.[67] In another approach, mannitol containing spray-dried antibiotics (tobramycin and azithromycin) loaded dry powders were formulated. The results of the studies demonstrated narrow particle size with smooth surface and low residual moisture content. *In vitro* aerosolization studies showed good FPF, a respirable fraction (RF), and MMAD of drug-loaded particles.[68] Wang et al. examined spray-dried curcumin-loaded acetylated dextran–based nanocomposites using the DoE approach for deep lung delivery. The authors found that feed concentration affects the final formulation in terms of aerosol properties. The optimized experimental parameters were drug loading (80%), feed concentration (0.5%), and inlet temperature (below 130 °C).[69] In another study, Muddineti *et al.* developed cholesterol-modified low molecular weight chitosan co-encapsulated small interfering RNA (siRNA) and curcumin self-assembled delivery system (C-CCM/siRNA) for lung delivery. In this, the condensation studies showed minimum nitrogen to phosphorous (N/P) ratio equivalent to 40. *In vitro* cell uptake studies showed higher uptake of C-CCM/siRNA in the lung cancer cells in a time-dependent manner. Finally, stability studies demonstrated the stable formulation of siRNA and curcumin at 4 °C. Thus, the feasibility of the siRNA and curcumin has great potential to treat lung cancer.[70]

11.3.2 Amino Acid-Based Surface Engineering

Protein-based nano-carriers play a vital role in the process of surface modification to change the surface properties and increase the ability to target the cells. Albumin possesses a number of binding sites and functional groups, which provide the ability for surface modification of albumin-based nano-carriers.[71] Albumin is such a protein that is present in a plentiful amount in the body. Also, it is widely used owing to its advantages as it is compatible with the biological environment as well as with many drugs, thereby, the drugs can adhere to albumin through covalent or non-covalent bonds and it works on the principle of endocytosis. It is biodegradable and to date, no reports have depicted its toxicity profile. The albumins generally used for synthesizing nano-formulations are of two types, namely, bovine serum albumin (BSA) and human serum albumin (HSA). Although HSA is costly, the market formulations containing nanoformulations of albumin generally contain HSA in them, as BSA has a limitation of inducing immunogenicity. Sie Huey Lee *et al.* formulated nanoparticles of BSA with the help of a nanospray drier.[72] New materials comprising phospholipids, notably lecithin and amino acids (lysine, polylysine) are the molecules extensively used in research for the synthesis of pulmonary targeted delivery systems.[62] In a recent research, Kamel *et al.* studied hybrid lipid nanocore-protein shell nanoparticles (HLPNPs) co-encapsulated all-trans retinoic acid (ATRA) and genistein (GNS) nanocomposites by employing the solvent evaporation method. In this study, the authors found remarkable powder flow properties using a mixture of mannitol/hydroxypropyl-β-cyclodextrin (HPβCD)/leucine. *In vivo* animal studies results displayed better performance of inhalable nanocomposites than the intravenous nanoparticle suspension at an equivalent dose of the drug against lung cancer-bearing mice.[73] Lakio *et al.* formulated L-arginine (ARG) loaded dry powder inhalation (DPI) formulation without the carrier. *In vitro* lung deposition studies showed excellent inhalable properties. The authors suggested the impact of magnesium stearate and l-leucine on the L-arginine particles as additives in the DPIs.[74] In another research, Rattanupatam *et al.* formulated budesonide loaded l-leucine, and l-leucine sieved mannitol dry powders for inhalation delivery. The solid-state characterization confirmed no relationship was observed between budesonide and L-leucine after the particles were co-sprayed. *In vitro*, the aerosol performance of co-spray dried budesonide-L-leucine showed appropriate MMAD and high FPF for deep lung delivery.[75] Similarly, Yang *et al.* evaluated spray-dried powder Aztreonam (AZT) loaded amino acids modified (glycine (GLY)), HIS, and LEU particles for inhalation delivery. The characterization results revealed that the GLY-AZT modified powders generated lumps (144.51 μm), which hindered it from getting targeted to the pulmonary area. However, HIS-modified spray-dried powders possessed enhanced powder flow properties, while the LEU-containing particles showed indented morphology with remarkably lowered densities. Nonetheless, the FPF value for HIS- (51.4% w/w) and LEU-modified powders (61.7% w/w) was enhanced remarkably as compared to AZT spray-dried powders (45.4% w/w).[76] In a study, Muttil *et al.* studied leucine modified spray-dried recombinant hepatitis B surface antigen (rHBsAg) with polylactic-co-glycolic acid/polyethylene glycol (PLGA/PEG) nanoparticles: the physical mixture of PLGA/PEG and PLGA/PEG nanoparticles plus free antigen. These formulations were dosed to guinea pigs *via* inhalation route to examine the production of IgA and IgG titers. *In vivo* animal studies revealed the presence of IgG titer values higher than 1,000mIU/ml in AgNASD vaccinated or inoculated guinea pigs.[77] In another work, Feng *et al.* demonstrated spray-dried l-leucine and trehalose microparticles for effective lung delivery. From the studies, they concluded that the combinations of these two excipients could be useful for targeted action via inhalation delivery.[78] Recently, Adhikari *et al.* studied the effect of multiple amino acids (valine, methionine, phenylalanine, and tryptophan) on the aerosolization efficiency of co-sprayed kanamycin. *In vitro* aerosolization studies revealed that methionine-containing kanamycin formulation showed the highest FPF in comparison to other amino acids. Moreover, methionine-containing kanamycin formulation exhibited better aerosol stability among other amino acid-based powders.[79] In another study, different amino acids were employed to hike the lung deposition potential of inhalable spray-dried powders for gene targeting. In this work, lipid/polycation/plasmid DNA i.e., pDNA (LPD) vectors were dissolved in lactose with or without amino acids for spray drying purposes. *In vitro* cells transfection studies revealed aspartic acid and threonine-based formulations showed damage to the A549 cells and might lower the performance of the LPD formulation. The authors finally suggested that all the used amino acids result in the lung deposition potential of the spray-dried powder.[80] In a different study, Chao and colleagues synthesized norvaline (Nva) α-amino acid prodrug of camptothecin (CPT) PEGylated polystyrene microparticles (MPs). The *in vivo* studies revealed that the CPT plasma concentrations were low and stagnant for a period of four days after one *i.v.* dosing of microparticles in contrast to that of free CPT. Additionally, anticancer efficacy was assessed in a xenograft murine model, and it was collated to a bolus injection of CPT. The results indicated that the animals that were administered with free CPT or CPT-Nva-MPs possessed notably minute lung cancer domain.[81] Similarly, a pH-dependent nanoscale complex of polyglycolic acid/Doxorubicin (PGA/DOX-amphiphile) as a carrier system was proposed for the management of non-small cell lung cancer. Extemporaneously, the formulated complex was converted into NPs in the aqueous solutions. The *in vitro* analysis data depicted that the block co-polypeptide was neither harmful to the cell nor to the components of blood, and the residence of co-polypeptide carrier could remarkably decrease the hemolysis ratio of doxorubicin. The drug-loaded micellar nanoparticles possessed enhanced pharmacological effect, enhanced cancerous tissues death, and lessened hematological toxicity in the xenograft murine model in contrast to the unformulated doxorubicin. Moreover, the *in vivo* pharmacokinetic studies demonstrated that micellar nanoparticles remarkably enhanced the mean residence time of the drug in the blood.[82] In a similar study, doxorubicin-loaded amphiphilic polypeptide (methoxy poly(ethylene glycol)-b-poly(L-glutamic acid-co-L-phenylalanine) (mPEG-b-P(Glu-co-Phe))-based nanoparticles (DOX-NP) were fabricated for lung cancer treatment. The formulated NPs showed inflated loading of drug and pH-dependent drug release. The *in vitro* studies depicted that DOX-NP possessed a greater tendency to retard the growth of cells, and enhanced cell uptake was observed in A549 cell lines in contrast to that of free doxorubicin. Finally, *in vivo* studies on the lung cancer xenograft nude mice model depicted that the DOX-NPs possessed remarkable anti-cancer activity and increased the deposition of the tumor, indicating the enhanced circulation in blood. The authors concluded that the permeation and retention effects were enhanced as compared with unformulated DOX.[83]

11.3.3 Cyclodextrin-Based Surface Engineering

Cyclodextrin belongs to the category of oligosaccharides which possess hydrophilic outer surface and lipophilic center. Cyclodextrins are basically used in pulmonary delivery to enhance the stability, solubility, and dissolution profile of water-insoluble drugs, ultimately causing an increase in the absorption of the drug and a reduction in its clearance. They do not cause a reduction in the pulmonary deposition of the drugs when used in the inhalation devices.[84] Amaro *et al.* synthesized carbohydrate-grounded salmon calcitonin (sCT) loaded nanoporous/nanoparticulate microparticles (NPMPs) and spray-dried using raffinose or trehalose with or without HP-β-CD. *In vitro* lung deposition studies showed a remarkable FPF with better MMAD for lung delivery. Spray-dried sCT powders with raffinose and trehalose showed 100% and 70–90% bioactivity, respectively, *vis-à-vis* unformulated sCT. Hence, based on the *in vitro* and *in vivo* analysis author concluded the potential of spray-dried sCT powders for inhalation delivery.[85] In another research work, Singh *et al.* investigated the effect of Vit C, cyclodextrin and their combination on the aerosolization efficiency of the rifampicin loaded spray dried liposheres. Upon addition of these excipients, the liposheres showed better powder flow properties, and optimum

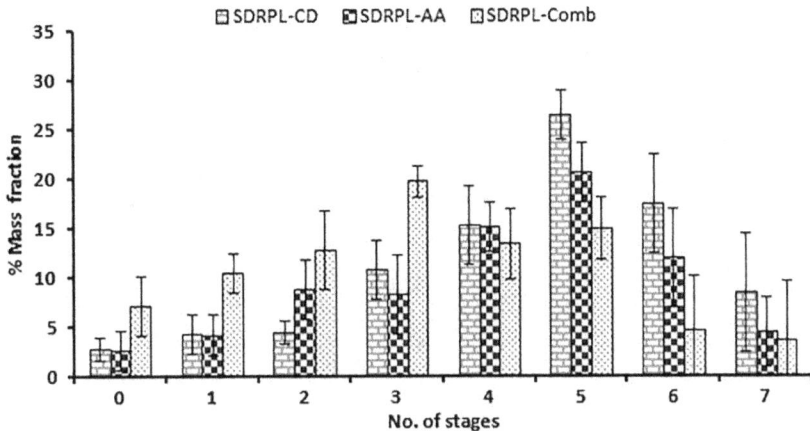

FIGURE 11.4 *In vitro* aerosol performance of lipospheres by using ACI. Reprinted from Ref (10), licensed under CC BY NC ND 4.0 (https://creativecommons.org/licenses/by-nc -nd/4.0/). Copyright 2015 Singh C, Seshu Kumar LV, Singh A, and Suresh S. Published by Shenyang Pharmaceutical University.

MMAD and FPF. Additionally, lipospheres exhibited improved *in vitro* antimycobacterial activity on $H_{37}Rv$ strain due to probable cyclodextrin–cholesterol complex formation in the bacteria cell wall.[10] Figure 11.4 shows the *in vitro* aerosol performance pattern of the various formulations containing Vit C and cyclodextrin by using eight-stage Anderson Cascade Impactor (ACI). Finally, the authors concluded that cyclodextrin loaded lipospheres showed better outcomes in terms of aerosolization efficiency and *in vitro* efficacy studies compared to Vit C and combination formulations. The advantages and limitations of different approaches has been outlined in the Table 11.3.

11.3.4 Miscellaneous

In an investigation, magnesium stearate coated pulverized salbutamol sulfate and salmeterol xinaofoate powders were prepared for inhalation delivery. The prepared powders were further characterized using Spraytec and twin stage impinger for *in vitro* aerosol efficiency. The Spraytec results demonstrated better de-agglomeration efficiency of the pulverized powder. On the other hand, twin stage impinger cascade impactor studies revealed remarkable FPF, which is suitable for deep lung delivery. Finally, based on optimum cohesive forces, the authors concluded that pulverized formulation has potential for lung delivery.[86] On similar lines, magnesium stearate-coated salbutamol sulfate particles were synthesized upon principle mechanofusion. The X-ray photoelectron spectroscopy confirmed the mechanofusion caused coating onto the surface of drug particles. Coating of the particles results in negligible changes and improved aerosolization of the coated formulations *vis-à-vis* uncoated formulation.[87] Abd *et al.* formulated lactoferrin–chondroitin sulfate modified doxorubicin and ellagic acid-loaded nanocrystals for lung delivery. Following the spray drying process, these nanoformulations were transformed into respirable nanocomposites. *In vitro* cell line studies on A549 lung cancer cells revealed

TABLE 11.3 Merits and demerits of these carriers for improved delivery of drugs via an aerosol route of administration

S. NO.	CARRIER SYSTEMS	MERITS	DEMERITS
1.	Sugar-based	• Physico-chemical steadiness (stability) • Harmony with a wide range of drugs • Easy availability • Cost-effective • Potential to prevent opsonization	• α-lactose monohydrate participates in Maillard decomposition reactions
2.	Amino acid- based	• Bio-degradable • Non-toxic • Have plenty of binding regions and functional groups • Component of human body	• Costly • Can induce immunogenicity
3.	Cyclodextrin- based	• Enhance the solubility and absorption of water-insoluble drugs	• Limited routes of administration

higher toxicity potential and better internalization. This could be attributed to the transferrin (Tf) and CD44 receptors mediated endocytosis. Further, *in vitro* cascade impactor studies demonstrated remarkable FPF for potential lung delivery.[88]

11.4 CONCLUSIONS AND FUTURE PERSPECTIVES

Lungs constitute an airway tree, which begins from the bottom of the trachea and finishes at alveoli. This pulmonary organ is the nucleus of the respiratory system. This system is divided into the upper and lower respiratory tract. Lungs are a self-cleaning organ, but at times, there may occur a respiratory disorder, which sometimes may be acute and other times could be chronic. Some types of respiratory disorders might cause or might be a sign of lung disease. The typical ailments that could occur in the lungs are asthma, bronchitis, COPD, pneumonia, tuberculosis, pulmonary fibrosis, lung cancer, etc. The general causes of these diseases result from exposure to bacteria, viruses, molds, chemicals, indoor air, or cigarette or tobacco smoking. The treatment strategies for lung disorders depend upon the cause of the lung disorders. It is reported that inhalation delivery has the potential to treat multiple lung disorders. Currently, several treatment strategies and analysis methods are in practice that could be used to treat lung diseases. The inhalation drug delivery offers numerous favorable characteristics *vis-à-vis* the conventional route of administrations, such as low dosing frequency, quick onset of action, and by-passing first-pass metabolism. The size of the lungs inflates during inhalation, and particle deposition to lungs is governed by a few mechanisms (primary and secondary); the primary mechanisms are inertial impaction (particle size greater than 5μm and less than 2 μm), gravitational sedimentation (size of the particles 1–8 μm), and Brownian diffusion (for the random motion particles) and the secondary mechanisms are electrostatic precipitation, mixing induced by turbulent flows (occurs during flow fluctuations), and an interception (in the case of elongated particles). Each mechanism's input is impacted by the lungs' structure and size. Particle engineering (in terms of nanotechnology) is needed to improve the physical stability and the physicochemical characteristics of the formulation. The novel drug delivery systems are stemming out as a propitious road, which could be relied on in the near future for delivering and targeting the drugs to obtain the intended pharmacological action. To enrich with the nanotechnology-enabled carrier systems that could be prepared for delivering the drug particles into the lungs, we have surveyed multiple carrier systems, and among the gathered delivery systems, it was observed that researchers have performed sugar-, amino acid-, and cyclodextrin-based particle engineering to date. The use of nanotechnology *in vivo* is a rapidly expanding field. The emerging nanotechnology serves as a tool for the analysis and treatment regimen for lung diseases. Furthermore, to enhance the therapeutic effect of target delivery to lungs, the appropriate receptor(s) could be determined, which would be specific for the lungs, and the identification of that particular receptor would lead to the enhancement of therapeutic effect in bronchioles and alveoli. Additionally, to eliminate the toxicity to the cells, the nanoparticles could be optimized for controlled release. One should consider the costs of nanomedicines and large-scale manufacturing issues as the important aspects to be considered while performing clinical trials. Moreover, among the nano-formulations, metal-organic frameworks could be designed for the effective loading of poorly soluble or poorly permeable drugs.

CONFLICT OF INTEREST

The authors declare no conflict of interest.

ACKNOWLEDGEMENT

Authors are thankful to Biorender.com for providing an online platform for making illustrations.

REFERENCES

1. Ding, L., Tang, S., Wyatt, T.A., Knoell, D.L., Oupický, D. Pulmonary siRNA delivery for lung disease: Review of recent progress and challenges. *J. Control. Release* 330, 977–91 (2020).

2. Kaur, R., Kaur, R., Singh, C., Kaur, S., Goyal, A.K., Singh, K.K., Singh, B. Inhalational drug delivery in pulmonary aspergillosis. *Crit. Rev. Ther. Drug Carrier Syst.* 36(3), 183–217 (2019).

3. https://www.niehs.nih.gov/health/topics/conditions/lung-disease/index.cfm.

4. Mannino, D.M. COPD: Epidemiology, prevalence, morbidity and mortality, and disease heterogeneity. *Chest* 121, 121S–6S (2002).

5. Hofmann, W., Balásházy, I., Koblinger, L. The effect of gravity on particle deposition patterns in bronchial airway bifurcations. *J. Aerosol Sci.* 26(7), 1161–8 (1995).

6. Spiro, S.G., Silvestri, G.A. One hundred years of lung cancer. *Am. J. Respir. Crit. Care Med.* 172(5), 523–9 (2005).

7. Witschi, H. A short history of lung cancer. *Toxicol. Sci.* 64(1), 4–6 (2001).

8. Goldstraw, P., Ball, D., Jett, J.R., Le, C.T., Lim, E., Nicholson, A.G., Shepherd, F.A. Non-small-cell lung cancer. *Lancet* 378(9804), 1727–40 (2011).

9. de Groot, P.M., Wu, C.C., Carter, B.W., Munden, R.F. The epidemiology of lung cancer. *Transl. Lung Cancer Res.* 7(3), 220 (2018).

10. Singh, C., Koduri, L.S., Singh, A., Suresh, S. Novel potential for optimization of antitubercular therapy: Pulmonary delivery of rifampicin liposperes. *Asian J. Pharm. Sci.* 10(6), 549–62 (2015).

11. Singh, C., Koduri, L.S., Dhawale, V., Bhatt, T.D., Kumar, R., Grover, V., Tikoo, K., Suresh, S. Potential of aerosolized rifampicin liposperes for modulation of pulmonary pharmacokinetics and bio-distribution. *Int. J. Pharm.* 495(2), 627–32 (2015).

12. Sung, J.C., Pulliam, B.L., Edwards, D.A. Nanoparticles for drug delivery to the lungs. *Trends Biotechnol.* 25(12), 563–70 (2007).

13. Newman, S.P. Drug delivery to the lungs: Challenges and opportunities. *Ther. Deliv.* 8(8), 647–61 (2017).

14. Tanhaei, A., Mohammadi, M., Hamishehkar, H., Hamblin, M.R. Electrospraying as a novel method of particle engineering for drug delivery vehicles. *J. Control. Release* 330, 851–61 (2020).

15. Roa, W.H., Azarmi, S., Al-Hallak, M.K., Finlay, W.H., Magliocco, A.M., Löbenberg, R. Inhalable nanoparticles, a non-invasive approach to treat lung cancer in a mouse model. *J. Control. Release* 150(1), 49–55 (2011).

16. Kalantarian, P., Najafabadi, A.R., Haririan, I., Vatranara, A., Yamini, Y., Darabi, M., Gilani, K. Preparation of 5-fluorouracil nanoparticles by supercritical antisolvents for pulmonary delivery. *Int. J. Nanomedicine* 5, 763–70 (2010).

17. Carvalho, T.C., Peters, J.I., Williams III, R.O. Influence of particle size on regional lung deposition–what evidence is there? *Int. J. Pharm.* 406(1–2), 1–10 (2011).

18. Deng, Q., Deng, L., Miao, Y., Guo, X., Li, Y. Particle deposition in the human lung: Health implications of particulate matter from different sources. *Environ. Res.* 169, 237–45 (2019).

19. Darquenne, C. Deposition mechanisms. *J. Aerosol Med. Pulm. Drug Deliv.* 33(4), 181–5 (2020).

20. Deng, Q., Ou, C., Chen, J., Xiang, Y. Particle deposition in tracheobronchial airways of an infant, child and adult. *Sci. Total Environ.* 612, 339–46 (2018).

21. Hussain, M., Madl, P., Khan, A. Lung deposition predictions of airborne particles and the emergence of contemporary diseases, Part-I. *Health* 2, 51–9 (2011).

22. Cooney, D.J., Hickey, A.J. Cellular response to the deposition of diesel exhaust particle aerosols onto human lung cells grown at the air–liquid interface by inertial impaction. *Toxicol. Vitro* 25(8), 1953–65 (2011).

23. Hofmann, W., Balásházy, I., Koblinger, L. The effect of gravity on particle deposition patterns in bronchial airway bifurcations. *J. Aerosol Sci.* 26(7), 1161–8 (1995).

24. Comer, J.K., Kleinstreuer, C., Hyun, S., Kim, C.S. Aerosol transport and deposition in sequentially bifurcating airways. *J. Biomech. Eng.* 122(2), 152–8 (2000).

25. Sznitman, J., Heimsch, T., Wildhaber, J.H., Tsuda, A., Rösgen, T. Respiratory flow phenomena and gravitational deposition in a three-dimensional space-filling model of the pulmonary acinar tree. *J. Biomech. Eng.* 131(3), 031010 (2009).

26. Darquenne, C. Aerosol deposition in the human lung in reduced gravity. *J. Aerosol Med. Pulm. Drug Deliv.* 27(3), 170–7 (2014).

27. Balashaz, I., Hofmann, W., Heistracher, T. Computation of local enhancement factors for the quantification of particle deposition patterns in airway bifurcations. *J. Aerosol Sci.* 30(2), 185–203 (1999).

28. Kleinstreuer, C., Zhang, Z., Kim, C.S. Combined inertial and gravitational deposition of microparticles in small model airways of a human respiratory system. *J. Aerosol Sci.* 38(10), 1047–61 (2007).

29. Goldberg, I.S., Lourenço, R.V. Deposition of aerosols in pulmonary disease. *Arch. Intern. Med.* 131(1), 88–91 (1973).

30. Hidy, G.M., Brock, J.R. Lung deposition of aerosols: A footnote on the role of diffusiophoresis. *Environ. Sci. Technol.* 3(6), 563–7 (1969).

31. Guha, A. Transport and deposition of particles in turbulent and laminar flow. *Annu. Rev. Fluid Mech.* 40(1), 311–41 (2008).

32. Matida, E.A., Finlay, W.H., Breuer, M., Lange, C.F. Improving prediction of aerosol deposition in an idealized mouth using large-eddy simulation. *J. Aerosol Med.* 19(3), 290–300 (2006).

33. Sharma, P., Mehta, M., Dhanjal, D.S., Kaur, S., Gupta, G., Singh, H., Thangavelu, L., Rajeshkumar, S., Tambuwala, M., Bakshi, H.A., Chellappan, D.K., Dua, K., Satija, S. Emerging trends in the novel drug delivery approaches for the treatment of lung cancer. *Chem. Biol. Interact.* 309, 108720 (2019).

34. Kulkarni, S.A., Feng, S.S. Effects of particle size and surface modification on cellular uptake and biodistribution of polymeric nanoparticles for drug delivery. *Pharm. Res.* 30(10), 2512–22 (2013).

35. Nandiyanto, A.B., Okuyama, K. Progress in developing spray-drying methods for the production of controlled morphology particles: From the nanometer to submicrometer size ranges. *Adv. Powder Technol.* 22(1), 1–9 (2011).

36. Tran, N., Bramnik, K.G., Hibst, H., Prölß, J., Mronga, N., Holzapfel, M., Scheifele, W., Novák, P. Spray-drying synthesis and electrochemical performance of lithium vanadates as positive electrode materials for lithium batteries. *J. Electrochem. Soc.* 155(5), A384 (2008).

37. Ma, Z., Gao, B., Wu, P., Shi, J., Qiao, Z., Yang, Z., Yang, G., Huang, B., Nie, F. Facile, continuous and large-scale production of core–shell HMX@ TATB composites with superior mechanical properties by a spray-drying process. *RSC Adv.* 5(27), 21042–9 (2015).

38. Jeyakumari, A., Zynudheen, A.A., Parvathy, U. Microencapsulation of bioactive food ingredients and controlled release-A review. *MoJ Food Process & Technol.* 2, 00059 (2016).

39. Noh, J., Kim, J., Kim, J.S., Chung, Y.S., Chang, S.T., Park, J. Microencapsulation by pectin for multi-components carriers bearing both hydrophobic and hydrophilic active agents. *Carbohydr. Polym.* 182, 172–9 (2018).

40. Sobel, R., Versic, R., Gaonkar, A.G. Introduction to microencapsulation and controlled delivery in foods. In *Microencapsulation in the Food Industry* 3–12 (Academic Press, 2014).

41. D'Souza, S.S., DeLuca, P.P. Methods to assess in vitro drug release from injectable polymeric particulate systems. *Pharm. Res.* 23(3), 460–74 (2006).

42. Ahmad, Z., Shah, A., Siddiq, M., Kraatz, H.B. Polymeric micelles as drug delivery vehicles. *RSC Adv.* 4(33), 17028–38 (2014).

43. Yang, L., Wu, X., Liu, F., Duan, Y., Li, S. Novel biodegradable polylactide/poly (ethylene glycol) micelles prepared by direct dissolution method for controlled delivery of anti-cancer drugs. *Pharm. Res.* 26(10), 2332–42 (2009).

44. Sant, V.P., Smith, D., Leroux, J.C. Novel pH-sensitive supramolecular assemblies for oral delivery of poorly water soluble drugs: Preparation and characterization. *J. Control. Release* 97(2), 301–12 (2004).
45. Reis, C.P., Neufeld, R.J., Ribeiro, A.J., Veiga, F., Nanoencapsulation, I. Methods for preparation of drug-loaded polymeric nanoparticles. *Nanomed. Nanotechnol. Biol. Med.* 2, 8–21 (2006).
46. Nava-Arzaluz, M.G., Piñón-Segundo, E., Ganem-Rondero, A., Lechuga-Ballesteros, D. Single emulsion-solvent evaporation technique and modifications for the preparation of pharmaceutical polymeric nanoparticles. *Recent Pat. Drug Deliv. Formul.* 6(3), 209–23 (2012).
47. Hung, L.H., Teh, S.Y., Jester, J., Lee, A.P. PLGA micro/nanosphere synthesis by droplet microfluidic solvent evaporation and extraction approaches. *Lab Chip* 10(14), 1820–5 (2010).
48. Maiolino, S., Russo, A., Pagliara, V., Conte, C., Ungaro, F., Russo, G., Quaglia, F. Biodegradable nanoparticles sequentially decorated with polyethyleneimine and hyaluronan for the targeted delivery of docetaxel to airway cancer cells. *J. Nanobiotechnology* 13, 1–3 (2015).
49. Xu, W., Ling, P., Zhang, T. Polymeric micelles, a promising drug delivery system to enhance bioavailability of poorly water-soluble drugs. *J. Drug Deliv.* 2013, 1–15 (2013).
50. Mei, D., Zhao, L., Chen, B., Zhang, X., Wang, X., Yu, Z., Ni, X., Zhang, Q. α-conotoxin ImI-modified polymeric micelles as potential nano-carriers for targeted docetaxel delivery to α7-nAChR overexpressed non-small cell lung cancer. *Drug Deliv.* 25(1), 493–503 (2018).
51. Somani, S., Laskar, P., Altwaijry, N., Kewcharoenvong, P., Irving, C., Robb, G., Pickard, B.S., Dufès, C. Pegylation of polypropylenimine dendrimers: Effects on cytotoxicity, DNA condensation, gene delivery and expression in cancer cells. *Sci. Rep.* 8(1), 1–3 (2018).
52. Nejati-Koshki, K., Mesgari, M., Ebrahimi, E., Abbasalizadeh, F., Fekri Aval, S., Khandaghi, A.A., Abasi, M., Akbarzadeh, A. Synthesis and in vitro study of cisplatin-loaded Fe_3O_4 nanoparticles modified with PLGA-PEG$_{6000}$ copolymers in treatment of lung cancer. *J. Microencapsul.* 31(8), 815–23 (2014).
53. Wu, H.C., Chang, X., Liu, L., Zhao, F., Zhao, Y. Chemistry of carbon nanotubes in biomedical applications. *J. Mater. Chem.* 20(6), 1036–52 (2010).
54. Ali-Boucetta, H., Al-Jamal, K.T., McCarthy, D., Prato, M., Bianco, A., Kostarelos, K. Multiwalled carbon nanotube–doxorubicin supramolecular complexes for cancer therapeutics. *Chem. Commun.* 459–61, (2008).
55. Zrazhevskiy, P., Sena, M., Gao, X. Designing multifunctional quantum dots for bioimaging, detection, and drug delivery. *Chem. Soc. Rev.* 39(11), 4326–54 (2010).
56. Hu, L., Zhang, C., Zeng, G., Chen, G., Wan, J., Guo, Z., Wu, H., Yu, Z., Zhou, Y., Liu, J. Metal-based quantum dots: Synthesis, surface modification, transport and fate in aquatic environments and toxicity to microorganisms. *RSC Adv.* 6(82), 78595–610 (2016).
57. Qu, Y.G., Zhang, Q., Pan, Q., Zhao, X.D., Huang, Y.H., Chen, F.C., Chen, H.L. Quantum dots immunofluorescence histochemical detection of EGFR gene mutations in the non-small cell lung cancers using mutation-specific antibodies. *Int. J. Nanomedicine* 9, 5771–8 (2014).
58. Doh, K.O., Yeo, Y. Application of polysaccharides for surface modification of nanomedicines. *Ther. Deliv.* 3(12), 1447–56 (2012).
59. Mansour, H.M., Rhee, Y.S., Wu, X. Nanomedicine in pulmonary delivery. *Int. J. Nanomedicine* 4, 299–319 (2009).
60. Rahimpour, Y., Hamishehkar, H. Lactose engineering for better performance in dry powder inhalers. *Adv. Pharm. Bull.* 2(2), 183 (2012).
61. Wu, L., Miao, X., Shan, Z., Huang, Y., Li, L., Pan, X., Yao, Q., Li, G., Wu, C. Studies on the spray dried lactose as carrier for dry powder inhalation. *Asian J. Pharm. Sci.* 9(6), 336–41 (2014).

62. Sham, J.O., Zhang, Y., Finlay, W.H., Roa, W.H., Lobenberg, R. Formulation and characterization of spray-dried powders containing nanoparticles for aerosol delivery to the lung. *Int. J. Pharm.* 269(2), 457–67 (2004).

63. Singh, D.J., Jain, R.R., Soni, P.S., Abdul, S., Darshana, H., Gaikwad, R.V., Menon, M.D. Preparation and evaluation of surface modified lactose particles for improved performance of fluticasone propionate dry powder inhaler. *J. Aerosol Med. Pulm. Drug Deliv.* 28(4), 254–67 (2015).

64. Grenha, A., Seijo, B., Remunán-López, C. Microencapsulated chitosan nanoparticles for lung protein delivery. *Eur. J. Pharm. Sci.* 25(4–5), 427–37 (2005).

65. Kundawala, A.J., Patel, V.A., Patel, H.V., Choudhary, D. Influence of formulation components on aerosolization properties of isoniazid loaded chitosan microspheres. *Int. J. Pharm. Sci. Drug Res.* 3, 297–302 (2011).

66. Focaroli, S., Mah, P.T., Hastedt, J.E., Gitlin, I., Oscarson, S., Fahy, J.V., Healy, A.M. A design of experiment (DoE) approach to optimise spray drying process conditions for the production of trehalose/leucine formulations with application in pulmonary delivery. *Int. J. Pharm.* 562, 228–40 (2019).

67. Sou, T., Kaminskas, L.M., Nguyen, T.H., Carlberg, R., McIntosh, M.P., Morton, D.A. The effect of amino acid excipients on morphology and solid-state properties of multi-component spray-dried formulations for pulmonary delivery of biomacromolecules. *Eur. J. Pharm. Biopharm.* 83(2), 234–43 (2013).

68. Li, X., Vogt, F.G., Hayes, Jr., D., Mansour, H.M. Design, characterization, and aerosol dispersion performance modeling of advanced co-spray dried antibiotics with mannitol as respirable microparticles/nanoparticles for targeted pulmonary delivery as dry powder inhalers. *J. Pharm. Sci.* 103(9), 2937–49 (2014).

69. Wang, Z., Meenach, S.A. Optimization of acetalated dextran–based nanocomposite microparticles for deep lung delivery of therapeutics via spray-drying. *J. Pharm. Sci.* 106(12), 3539–47 (2017).

70. Muddineti, O.S., Shah, A., Rompicharla, S.V., Ghosh, B., Biswas, S. Cholesterol-grafted chitosan micelles as a nano-carrier system for drug-siRNA co-delivery to the lung cancer cells. *Int. J. Biol. Macromol.* 118(A), 857–63 (2018).

71. Kudarha, R.R., Sawant, K.K. Albumin based versatile multifunctional nano-carriers for cancer therapy: Fabrication, surface modification, multimodal therapeutics and imaging approaches. *Mater. Sci. Eng. C* 81, 607–26 (2017).

72. Joshi, M., Nagarsenkar, M., Prabhakar, B. Albumin nanocarriers for pulmonary drug delivery: An attractive approach. *J. Drug Deliv. Sci. Technol.* 56, 101529 (2020).

73. Kamel, N.M., Helmy, M.W., Abdelfattah, E.Z., Khattab, S.N., Ragab, D., Samaha, M.W., Fang, J.Y., Elzoghby, A.O. Inhalable dual-targeted hybrid lipid nanocore–protein shell composites for combined delivery of genistein and all-trans retinoic acid to lung cancer cells. *ACS Biomater. Sci. Eng.* 6(1), 71–87 (2019).

74. Lakio, S., Morton, D.A., Ralph, A.P., Lambert, P. Optimizing aerosolization of a high-dose L-arginine powder for pulmonary delivery. *Asian J. Pharm. Sci.* 10(6), 528–40 (2015).

75. Rattanupatam, T., Srichana, T. Budesonide dry powder for inhalation: Effects of leucine and mannitol on the efficiency of delivery. *Drug Deliv.* 21(6), 397–405 (2014).

76. Yang, X.F., Xu, Y., Qu, D.S., Li, H.Y. The influence of amino acids on aztreonam spray-dried powders for inhalation. *Asian J. Pharm. Sci.* 10(6), 541–8 (2015).

77. Muttil, P., Prego, C., Garcia-Contreras, L., Pulliam, B., Fallon, J.K., Wang, C., Hickey, A.J., Edwards, D. Immunization of guinea pigs with novel hepatitis B antigen as nanoparticle aggregate powders administered by the pulmonary route. *AAPS J.* 12(3), 330–7 (2010).

78. Feng, A.L., Boraey, M.A., Gwin, M.A., Finlay, P.R., Kuehl, P.J., Vehring, R. Mechanistic models facilitate efficient development of leucine containing microparticles for pulmonary drug delivery. *Int. J. Pharm.* 409(1–2), 156–63 (2011).

79. Adhikari, B.R., Bērziņš, K., Fraser-Miller, S.J., Gordon, K.C., Das, S.C. Co-amorphization of kanamycin with amino acids improves aerosolization. *Pharmaceutics* 12(8), 715 (2020).

80. Li, H.Y., Seville, P.C., Williamson, I.J., Birchall, J.C. The use of amino acids to enhance the aerosolisation of spray-dried powders for pulmonary gene therapy. *J. Gene Med.* 7(3), 343–53 (2005).

81. Chao, P., Deshmukh, M., Kutscher, H.L., Gao, D., Rajan, S.S., Hu, P., Laskin, D.L., Stein, S., Sinko, P.J. Pulmonary targeting microparticulate camptothecin delivery system: Anti-cancer evaluation in a rat orthotopic lung cancer model. *Anti Cancer Drugs* 21(1), 1–24 (2010).

82. Li, M., Song, W., Tang, Z., Lv, S., Lin, L., Sun, H., Li, Q., Yang, Y., Hong, H., Chen, X. Nanoscaled poly (L-glutamic acid)/doxorubicin-amphiphile complex as pH-responsive drug delivery system for effective treatment of non-small cell lung cancer. *ACS Appl. Mater. Interfaces* 5(5), 1781–92 (2013).

83. Lv, S., Li, M., Tang, Z., Song, W., Sun, H., Liu, H., Chen, X. Doxorubicin-loaded amphi-philic polypeptide-based nanoparticles as an efficient drug delivery system for cancer therapy. *Acta Biomater.* 9(12), 9330–42 (2013).

84. Rasheed, A. Cyclodextrins as drug carrier molecule: A review. *Sci. Pharm.* 76(4), 567–98 (2008).

85. Amaro, M.I., Tewes, F., Gobbo, O., Tajber, L., Corrigan, O.I., Ehrhardt, C., Healy, A.M. Formulation, stability and pharmacokinetics of sugar-based salmon calcitonin-loaded nanoporous/nanoparticulate microparticles (NPMPs) for inhalation. *Int. J. Pharm.* 483(1–2), 6–18 (2015).

86. Morton, D., Zhou, Q., Qu, L., Larson, I., Stewart, P. Surface modification of micronized drug powders to improve aerosolization via mechanical dry powder coating. *Proceedings of the Electronic Conference on Pharmaceutical Sciences* 1–6 (2011).

87. Zhou, Q.T., Qu, L., Gengenbach, T., Larson, I., Stewart, P.J., Morton, D.A. Effect of sur-face coating with magnesium stearate via mechanical dry powder coating approach on the aerosol performance of micronized drug powders from dry powder inhalers. *AAPS PharmSciTech* 14(1), 38–44 (2013).

88. Abd Elwakil, M.M., Mabrouk, M.T., Helmy, M.W., Abdelfattah, E.Z., Khiste, S.K., Elkhodairy, K.A., Elzoghby, A.O. Inhalable lactoferrin–chondroitin nanocomposites for combined delivery of doxorubicin and ellagic acid to lung carcinoma. *Nanomed. J.* 13, 2015–35 (2018).

Spray Dried Particles for Inhalation

12

Raj Kumar, Neha Kumari, and David Oupicky

Contents

DOI: 10.1201/9781003182566-16

12.1 INTRODUCTION

Human life as we know it has significantly changed with time. The development of science and technology has played a major role in how our modern lifestyle has progressed, particularly by providing us with a wide breadth of knowledge. As our lifestyles and our environment have changed, though, a number of diseases and infections have been increasing [1]. Among the range of diseases that affect humans, lung-based diseases are very critical to prevent and treat as they are a leading global health issue with a huge economic burden. To fight such diseases and disorders, considerable progress has been made in our scientific understanding and technological response to these issues [2]. Developing new drugs and improving the efficacy of existing drugs are active areas of research, however developing new drugs is a long, expensive process and the rate of success is very low – only 1 drug molecule will enter into the market out of every 10,000 molecules developed. Hence, enhancing the efficacy or effective delivery of existing drugs is a more attractive strategy [3]. Moreover, understanding the mechanism of action of drug molecules at a deeper level further adds value. In the last decade, the development of innovative technologies has allowed researchers to characterize and understand the mode of action of several drugs.

Several strategies have been developed to enhance the performance of existing drugs. One such promising strategy has been the formulation of nanoparticles of different drugs [4]. The nanoformulation of drugs reduces the particle size and enhances the surface area of the drugs. It is well reported that nanoparticles of active pharmaceutical ingredients (APIs) showed novel physicochemical properties compared to their bulk form [5]. There is a range of nanoforomulation techniques, such as solid lipid nanoparticles, high pressure homogenization, milling, microemulsion, and antisolvent precipitation [5]. However, most techniques produce the dispersion or suspension form of the drug nanoparticles, and it is challenging to remove the large amount of solvent from the formulation to obtain dry powder for therapeutic applications. Therefore, techniques that can feasibly produce dry powder are high priority.

Among the techniques widely used to produce ultrafine dry powders of APIs, spray drying is the most promising technique because it is reproducible, affordable, timesaving, continuous, up scalable, and can produce micro- and nanoparticles of APIs [6]. Spray drying can produce nanoparticles with controlled physicochemical properties by varying the process parameters. The first time spray drying was mentioned was in 1860, followed by the registration of the first patent in 1872 [7]. The first device made was primitive and had major issues associated with its process efficiency, performance, and safety. These issues limited its use, and it was not until 1920 that this technique evolved [7]. During World War II (WW-II), spray drying technology gained a lot of attention as the transportation of large amounts of food had become a major problem [7]. Interestingly, spray drying was an ideal technique to resolve this challenge. After WW-II, pharmaceutical industries adopted this technique and it evolved, starting with the production of milk powder, the first industrial application of spray drying [8]. In the 1940s, Bullock et al. formulated ascorbic acid by spray drying [9]. Since the 1940s, spray drying has been in used in pharmaceutical industries for processing pharmaceuticals to obtain dry powders with desired properties, such as a specific size, shape, and aerosolization efficiency. Spray drying also provides an opportunity to combine a number of formulation processes, such as encapsulation, complexation, and polymerization [10–12]. Moreover, it is favorable to process heat sensitive pharmaceuticals, drugs, proteins, nucleic acids, and vaccines using spray drying techniques. Even today, spray drying has remained an important application in daily life. Currently, spray drying is widely used in the chemical, food, and pharmaceutical industries. As our understanding of spray drying has progressed, the main focus has moved from the development of this technique to producing formulations with specific characteristics, such as storage stability. Compared to powder formulations from other techniques, spray drying based formulations have better properties. Nearly 150 years of research and development into spray drying technology has proven that is a powerful tool, and thus it has become the most frequently used process of drying [7, 13]. Nevertheless, there are many interesting avenues for researchers to explore.

In this chapter, we have discussed the state-of-the-art of spray drying, the influence of various parameters on physicochemical properties of products, the formulation of drug nanoparticles for inhalation, other applications of spray drying, comparison of lab scale versus industrial scale, and we provide an overview of commercially available dry powder inhalation devices, products, and the current market.

12.2 SPRAY DRYING TECHNOLOGY

Spray drying works based on the idea of producing dry powder from a solution by spraying it into a hot air environment, which allows for evaporation of a solvent and results in the production of a dry powder (Figure 12.1) [14]. Initially, spray drying was considered a dehydration process. This technique has significantly advanced by controlling various experimental variables to produce the dry powder of targeted substances, and has even been used to induce novel drug delivery properties for precise control and targeted delivery through the presence of various foreign entities and combining different ingredients [6]. Spray drying techniques are now widely used in the formulation of hydrophilic and hydrophobic drug-encapsulated micro- and nanoparticles as systems for delivery [15, 16]. Moreover, this technique is even applicable to thermally labile substances that do not undergo thermal degradation due to heat exposure during spray drying. Spray drying mainly used for the production of amorphous solid dispersion, self-emulsifying drug delivery, and micro- and nanoparticles [17–21]. Spray dried products are highly homogenous.

The spray drying techniques are broadly classified into three phases: atomization, drying, and collection. The first phase is the atomization of a solution of a substance through a suitable device. Atomization is defined as the generation of discrete droplets from a solution in drying gas [7, 10]. This process generates droplets with very high surface areas. For example, 1 m^3 of liquid atomization into 100 μm size droplets generates 60,000 m^2 of surface area. This large change in surface area allows the transfer of heat from the gas to form droplets, resulting in the evaporation of the solvent. The process of atomization is also convenient to heat-sensitive materials/APIs. There are several well-known atomization devices, such as the rotary atomizer, hydraulic nozzles, pneumatic

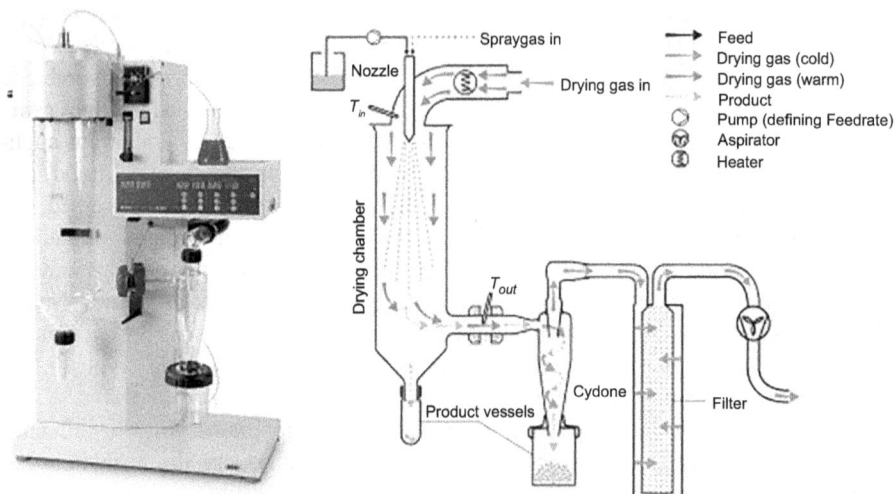

FIGURE 12.1   Mini Spray Dryer B-290 (left) with principle flow diagram (right). Reproduced with permission from ref. [14]. Copyright 2017, Elsevier.

nozzles, and ultrasonic nozzles [7, 22]. The choice of atomizing device is crucial and depends on the type of spray dryer and material to be subjected to the drying process. Different atomization devices have their own advantages and limitations.

In the second phase, when the feed droplets interact with the drying gas at an adequate temperature, it results in the evaporation of the solvent from the droplet, which produces solid particles [23]. After atomization, the droplets are exposed to drying gas or air. Based on the physicochemical properties of the drugs being created, inert gases or nitrogen are used. The movement of droplets in air is uncontrolled and hence the local conditions are different for different droplets and loose solvents in different conditions [24, 25]. It is also important to adjust the temperature to avoid burning of the product as this can affect the solvent content in the final product. The chamber of the spray dryer is in a cylinder with an inverted cone at the bottom. Based on the device used for atomization, a suitable chamber must be used, which further depends on the desired substance properties [25, 26]. Chambers are subdivided into two types, tall and small. Tall chambers have a ratio of height to diameter of 5:1, whereas for small chambers this ratio is 2:1. Moreover, the selection of the chamber type should allow for enough time for the solvent to evaporate from the droplets before moving from the top to the bottom of the chamber [27–29]. Compared to small droplets, larger droplets need more time to evaporate solvent. Thus, the process conditions decide the droplet size, and the chamber dimensions needed are based on droplet size. However, different spray dryers have different types of chambers.

In the final phase, the formed solid particles are separated from the drying gas and are collected into a dry powder. After the drying process, the product particles that settled in the bottom can be collected with the use of a proper device such as a scraper. Vibratory devices and mechanical brushes are used as scrapers [7, 30]. In other cases, product particles may leave the chamber along with the outgoing air and get separated at cyclones or bag filters. Sometimes, dry particles do not fully separate from particles which are not completely dried; to overcome this limitation, additional devices are used to supply hot air into the chamber. This is common in laboratory spray dryers. Highly effective external devices are required due to the demand of particles below 10 μm for pharmaceutical uses. Cyclones are widely used devices that separate solid particles from the air by utilizing centrifugal forces that direct the particles towards the walls of the device [31]. However, this causes an issue of buildup of solid powder on the walls of the cylinder; therefore, specialized coatings are used to help ameliorate this issue [7, 10].

12.2.1 Influence of Processing Parameters

Several spray drying apparatuses are available by changing the various parameters involved. For example, there are: different nozzles types, such as two-fluid, pressure, rotary, and vibrating; drying chambers with different shapes, sizes, heights, widths, and materials; air flow directions, types of cyclone design, types of drying gas, and scales; and there are different process parameters, such as inlet temperatures, outlet temperatures, air velocity, rate of feeding, and several others [32]. However, all three phases and experimental conditions affect the efficacy of the process and determine the properties of the final product (Figure 12.2) [7, 33, 34]. Interestingly, all these parameters are

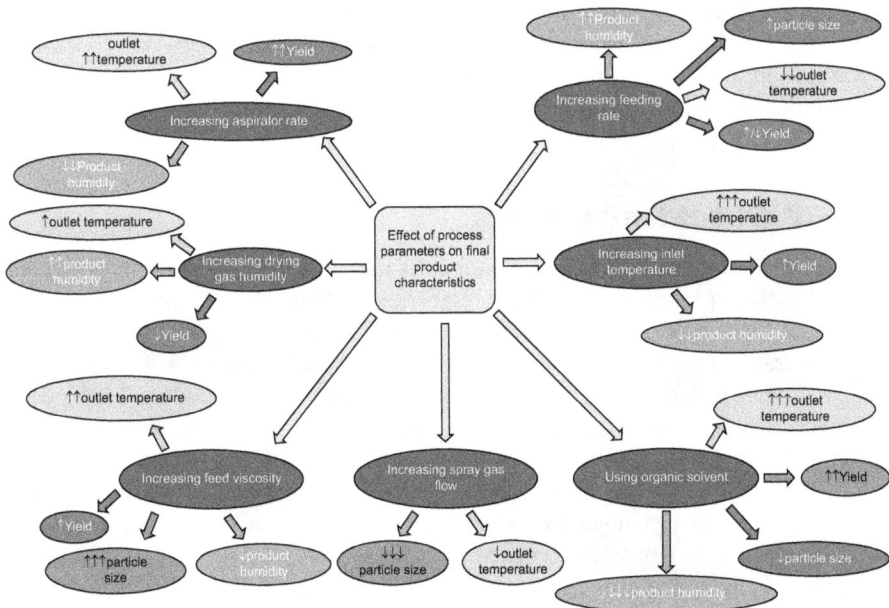

FIGURE 12.2 Effect of process parameters on the final product characteristics (www .buchi.com). ↑, ↑ ↑, and ↑ ↑ ↑ represent minor, moderate, and high influence on increase in final product characteristics, respectively, and ↓, ↓ ↓, and ↓ ↓ ↓ are minor, moderate, and high influence on decrease in final product characteristics, respectively. Reproduced with permission from Ref. [34]. Copyright 2020, Springer Nature.

interrelated. Here we have discussed the major parameters that influence on the properties of dry powder produced [33]. The most important parameters are discussed in the following section.

12.2.1.1 Inlet temperature

Inlet temperature has a significant effect on the physicochemical properties of the powder produced. The inlet temperature affects the moisture content in the product, where higher inlet temperatures reduces or removes the moisture content entirely. However, it also simultaneously affects the properties of temperature sensitive substances. There are several reports on the effect of inlet temperature on particle size. Wei et al. formulated chitosan-tripolyphosphate particles loaded with theophylline through spray drying. They found that the particle mean diameter was increased by 48 nm as the inlet temperature increased from 70 °C to 150 °C [35]. A different investigation led by Santhalakshmy et al. investigated the effect of inlet temperature on jamun fruit juice powder prepared by spray drying and found that lower inlet temperatures produced smooth surface particles, whereas higher inlet temperature produced particles with some degree of shrinkage [36]. However, the outlet temperature also depends on the inlet temperature, and thus outlet temperature is also a major factor in spray drying. Hence, inlet temperature should be set as per the required outlet temperature while still considering the thermal stability of the drug. It is good practice to use lower inlet temperatures to reduce the thermal stress on the substance [37]. However, temperatures below 10 °C of the glass transition temperature (Tg) are safer, otherwise it is difficult to process the spray drying, for example low molecular weight sugars. Such substances can be processed by combination with high molecular weight excipients such as maltodextrin [38].

12.2.1.2 Outlet temperature

Outlet temperature is another critical parameter that influences particle size, morphology, and surface properties. The outlet temperature affects the formation of droplets, how the solvent evaporates, and the drying rate, and is also directly co-related with particle temperature and the rate of droplet drying and crystallization [39, 40]. In general, low outlet temperatures produce smooth surface particles due to slower evaporation, and higher outlet temperatures produce rough surface particles due to fast evaporation of the solvent from small droplets [33, 40]. Mass et al. showed that it was possible to form particles with different surface topographies at different outlet temperatures. Moreover, increases in temperature should have caused particle size to decrease, but the authors observed larger sized particles. This may have been due to the interparticle interactions between the drug and the carrier [39].

12.2.1.3 Feed concentration and viscosity

The effect of feed concentration and viscosity of the solution on droplet size is comparatively very low. A reduction in particle size is observed at low concentrations; this is due to the different concentrations of solids and how they release their water volume during the drying process [41]. Usually, with higher concentrations particle size will slightly increase [42]. However, it is dependent on the solubility of the substance in its respective solvent. Similarly, with increases in viscosity of the feed solution, particle size also increases due to an increase of solid present in the feed. However, after the threshold limit, increases in the viscosity may inhibit the formation of droplets because of longer retention times at the atomizer [43].

12.2.1.4 Miscellaneous properties

Other parameters, such as surface tension, solvent volatility, solubility, and nozzle diameter, also influence the product properties [7]. As the surface tension increases, the size of the particles increases [44]. However, the optimum surface tension needs to be maintained to get high quality product for the desired applications. Solvent volatility is another important parameter. More volatile solvents are favorable for spray drying compared to other, less volatile solvents [45]. However, the solubility of the substance also plays a crucial role. It has been suggested to use a combination of volatile solvents with other miscible solvents to overcome this solubility issue, such as by using a mixture of ethanol and water. The widely used solvents are water, methanol, acetone, ethanol, dichloromethane, chloroform, acetonitrile, and combinations of these listed solvents [7, 10]. Nozzle diameter also has an effect on particle size. As the size of the nozzle diameter increases, it generates larger sized droplets and hence forms larger size particles [46]. However, small nozzles are limited in use to dilute solutions or low concentrations of substances. Given this limitation, medium sized nozzles are commonly used. It is good practice to use the same nozzle for every series within an experiment to avoid errors in the desired particle size. Wei et al. thoroughly investigated the influence of processing parameters on chitosan tripolyphosphate particles loaded with theophylline, which are widely used to prevent rapid drug metabolism, using spray drying technology [35]. Their results showed that temperature and air flow are the two crucial parameters that affect the particle size. As the drying air temperature increased, the feed air rate increased the size of the particles. However, nozzle diameter, concentration, choice of solvent, pump volume, and spray also effect the final particle size [35].

12.3 SPRAY DRIED PARTICLES FOR INHALATION

Nanoparticles formed during the solidifying of a nanosuspension is an effective method for the delivery of drugs to the lungs through inhalation. Several strategies have been developed to formulate nanoparticles, such as spray drying, freeze drying, spray-freeze drying, and aerosol flow reactor [47]. Among these methods, spray drying is a promising strategy that has been widely studied. Briefly, spray drying converts a liquid solution to a solid powder of micro- or nanoparticles. When a liquid solution or suspension is sprayed via a nozzle into a drying chamber, it generates droplets that encounter the hot drying gas. Solvents evaporate and dry particles are collected at bottom of the vessel

[48]. Dry powders that are generated from spray drying techniques show suitable physicochemical properties for inhalation, and many different formulations have had their efficacy tested *in vitro* and *in vivo* [49]. Inhalation is widely used for the delivery of various active substances, such as APIs, nucleic acids, vaccines, peptides, and proteins, to treat pulmonary diseases like tuberculosis, lung cancer, lung infections, asthma, COPD, cystic fibrosis, and other maladies [50–52].

In the last few decades, nanoparticles have gained a significant amount of attention, particularly for drug delivery. Nanoparticles have been studied in various routes of administration, including oral, intravenous, transdermal, ocular, and pulmonary [53]. The pulmonary route is the preferred method for the delivery of drugs for respiratory diseases, including asthma, COPD, and cystic fibrosis. The major benefit of the pulmonary delivery route is that you can circumvent the first-pass effect of hepatic metabolism and hence be able to use reduced doses to avoid adverse side effects. Furthermore, this route allows for fast absorption of the drug due to a large pulmonary surface area – human lungs contain 2,300 km of airways and around 500 million alveoli with a surface area of 75–140 m² – in addition to the thin epithelial layer and rich blood supply [54].

The mechanism of pulmonary deposition of particles can be classified into three types: inertial impaction, gravitational sedimentation, and Brownian diffusion (Figure 12.3) [55]. Particles with median mass aerodynamic diameter (MMAD) > 3 µm undergo inertial impaction while passing through the oropharynx and large conducting airways. Particles that are 0.5 to 3 µm undergo gravitational sedimentation in the smaller airways. And lastly, particles that are < 0.5 µm undergo diffusion through Brownian motion-based deposition. Nanoparticles between 1 to 5 µm are the best to achieve lung deposition [56]. Moreover, this drug delivery method boasts high patience compliance. Taken together, this is an attractive delivery route.

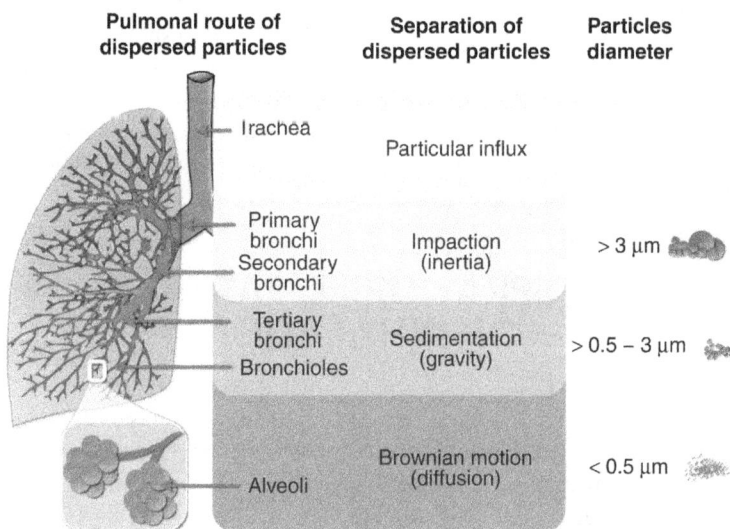

FIGURE 12.3 Pulmonary deposition of inhaled particles and their way of separation in healthy lungs is dependent on the particle size (A). Reproduced with permission from Ref. [55]. Copyright 2015, Informa.

Although extensive investigations of delivering drugs via nanoparticles have been done, their use in delivering drugs to the lungs is still rare. This is because a large number of drug molecules are poorly water-soluble. Drugs that cannot dissolve in water fall into the class II category according to the biopharmaceutical classification system. Among the newly designed and developed drug molecules, nearly 40% of drug entities are poorly water-soluble [57]. Several conventional strategies have been developed in the last 20 years to overcome this issue. By reducing the size of the particle from the scale of millimeters or microns (< 10 μm) to the nanoscale has enhanced the surface area and hence has increased aqueous solubility and bioavailability [58]. The most well-known nanotechnology-based strategies to reduce the particle size of poorly water-soluble drugs are re-precipitation [59], sonochemistry [60], the supercritical fluid process [61], milling, high pressure homogenization [62], and spray drying [32]. Most of these strategies generate the drug nanoparticles via dispersion or suspension, which then need to process further to remove the solvent to get dry powder. Then, the powder may be analyzed to determine its *in vitro* and *in vivo* efficacy. Spray drying is one of the techniques that can produce dry powdered nanoparticles of drugs with controlled sizes and shapes [32, 63]. Moreover, compared to other processes, spray drying is cost effective, simple, and efficient, and it is possible to control the product properties through tuning the process parameters mentioned earlier.

12.3.1 Excipients

To control the physicochemical properties and stability of nanoparticles, excipients are widely used with poorly water-soluble drugs during spray drying; examples include hydroxypropyl methylcellulose acetate succinate (HPMC-AS), polyvinylpyrrolidone (PVP), and mannitol. The most used excipients in inhalation drug delivery are lactose monohydrate, mannitol, leucin, sodium carboxymethylcellulose, beta-cyclodextrin, soium deoxycholate, trehalose dihydrate, and xyloglucan. All these excipients used in various drug delivery systems with combination of different drugs, siRNA and vaccines. The corresponding literature was summarized in Table 12.1. Mannitol and lactose are generally recognized as safe (GRAS) excipients. Both used in DPI delivery. Mannitol improves the lung function of cystic fibrosis patients. Leucin is hydrophobic and used with water soluble excipients in formulation of DPI. Leucin increase dispersibility through decreasing the particle cohesiveness [64]. Friesen et al. studied 139 drugs combined with a HPMC-AS polymer [65]. However, it is also important to consider the amorphous stability of the product, and hence hydrogen bonding is essential. Efavirenz, an anti-HIV drug, is formulated as an amorphous solid through spray drying using Soluplus with different concentrations; stability studies confirmed its 12 month stability at accelerated conditions of 40 °C and 75% humidity [66]. Poorly water-soluble drugs can also be combined with water-soluble excipients like sodium salicylate to enhance their aqueous solubility [67]. Researchers have also attempted to spray dry curcumin with polyvinylpyrrolidone (PVP), which produced a water-soluble amorphous form of curcumin due to enhancement of the viscosity presence of PVP [68]. Similarly, enhanced aqueous solubility was reported for piroxicam through microencapsulation into gelatin through spray drying [69]. We have summarized the literature reports of

TABLE 12.1 Literature reports of drug nanoparticles formulated through spray dried techniques for inhalation

SR. NO.	API	CARRIER	SPRAY DRYER USED	PARTICLE SIZE D=(0.5) / MM	MORPHOLOGY	STABILITY	DEVICE USED	DOSE	FPF
1	Disodium cromoglycate [77]	6% w/v Ethanol in water, lactose monohydrate	(Btichi Minispray drier type 190, F.R.G.).	1–5	Almost spherical	Drug did not decompose, however its structure changed from crystal to amorphous	J.S.F. Inhalator, Italy	40 mg	NR
2	Budesonide [78]	5% (w/v) mannitol in 25%:75% v/v ethanol:water	Buchi B-290 Mini spray dryer and inert loop B-295 organic solvents accessory	9.58	Spherical and smooth surface with deposited fine needle crystals and small particle	Stable at the conditions	Cyclohaler device	Total dose: 20±5 mg (Budesonide dose: 200±10 μg)	NR
3	Budesonide [78]	5% (w/v) mannitol in 25%:75% v/v ethanol:water (2% w/v NH4HCO3 as pore forming agent)	Buchi B-290 Mini spray dryer and inert loop B-295 organic solvents accessory	12.4	Spheroidal and irregular structure and rough surface due to the formation of large crystals on the surface	Stable at the conditions and Content of α Mannitol increased that means amorphous nature increased	Cyclohaler device	Total dose: 20±5 mg (Budesonide dose: 200±10μg)	NR
4	Tobramycin (5% w/v in isopropanol using 2% * Na glycolate surfactant [79]	No carrier used	Buchi mini spray dryer B-191a	0.2	Loose porous agglomerates of 50–200 μm in size that were less smooth, less regular, and less cohesive	Crystalline state of Tobramycin conserved. Stable at 40 °C and 75% relative humidity (RH) for 6 months	Aerolizer®, Novartis	15 mg	61%

(Continued)

TABLE 12.1 (CONTINUED) Literature reports of drug nanoparticles formulated through spray dried techniques for inhalation

SR. NO.	API	CARRIER	SPRAY DRYER USED	PARTICLE SIZE D=(0.5) / MM	MORPHOLOGY	STABILITY	DEVICE USED	DOSE	FPF
5	Tobramycin (5%, w/v) and Clarithromycin (0.5%, w/v) in isopropanol nanosuspension prepared using 2%* Na Glycocholate surfactant [80]	No carrier used	Buchi mini spray dryer B-191a	0.7	Loose agglomerates with high porosity	Clarithromycin structure changed from crystalline to amorphous, Tobramycin crystalline structure was conserved.	Axahaler, Galephar	25 mg	T=63%, C=62%
6	Urea-crosslinked hyaluronic acid (0.15% w/v) and sodium ascorbyl phosphate (0.45% w/v) in deionized water [81]	No carrier used	Buchi B-290 Mini Spray Dryer,	Dv50 of 3.4±.3 µm	Spherical Particles with smooth surface	No degradation	RS01 dry powder inhaler, Plastiape	28 mg	35.3±0.3%
7	Levofloxacin loaded Polycaprolactone nanoparticles using Pluronic F-68 as surfactant [64]	Leucin (to reduce particles cohesiveness) (conc. ratio of nanoparticle: lactose: leucine is 1:6:1)	Büchi B-290 mini spray dryer	0.23	Porous or hollow aggregates	Antimicrobial activity is retained	NR	25mg	NR
8	Salbutamol sulphate [70]	Sodium carboxymethylcellulose	Büchi B-290 mini spray dryer	Dv=6	Almost spherical and wrinkled surface	NR	Cyclohaler®, Pharmachemie BV	25 mg	45%
9	Salbutamol sulphate [70]	Beta-cyclodextrin	Büchi B-290 mini spray dryer	Dv=2.3	Almost spherical and wrinkled surface	NR	Cyclohaler, Pharmachemie BV	25 mg	40.3%

(Continued)

TABLE 12.1 (CONTINUED) Literature reports of drug nanoparticles formulated through spray dried techniques for inhalation

SR. NO.	API	CARRIER	SPRAY DRYER USED	PARTICLE SIZE D=(0.5) / MM	MORPHOLOGY	STABILITY	DEVICE USED	DOSE	FPF
10	Dexamethasone [82]	Sodiumdeoxycholate (Surfactant)	Nano Spray Dryer Advanced Model B90® (Buchi)	1	Spherical particles with a very rugged surface	Crystalline organization of Dexamethasone was conserved	Single-dose inhaler (Aerolizer®, Novartis)	11 mg	61.68 %
11	Dexamethasone [82]	Poly(ε-caprolactone),Sodiu mdeoxycholate (Surfactant)	Nano Spray Dryer Advanced Model B90® (Buchi)	1	Spherical particles with a rough surface	Crystalline organization of Dexamethasone and Polyε-caprolactone) was conserved	Single-dose inhaler (Aerolizer®, Novartis)	22 mg	59.24 %
12	Porous Sodium Cromoglycate [83]	Lactose monohydrate (ammonium bicarbonate as pore forming agent)	Mini Spray Dryer Büchi B-290	Daer.73 ± 0.03, Dv50: 6.08–7.44	Porous particles	No degradation of sample. Stable even after12 months of storage.	Breezhaler®, Novartis	12 mg	54.56%
13	No API (API added to 1% of total solids had no impact on the powder properties) [84]	Trehalose dihydrate, L-Leucine	Supercritical CO2- Assisted Spray Drying (SASD) technology	Dv50: 1	Spherical with slightly corrugated surface	Organization of amorphous Trehalose and crystalline Leucine was not changed. After 6 months, no degradation of tobramycin could be observed	Plastiape RS01 device	20 mg	76-86%
14	Lipid nanocapsules (LNC) (polyoxyl 15 hydroxystearate, hydrogenated lecithin (surfactant) and caprylic acid triglycerides. [85]	LNC-Lactose Trojan microparticles particles	Büchi Mini Spray Dryer B-290	3.71- 7.85	The Trojan-LNCs microparticles were spherical in shape with rough surfaces. The particles had holes and cracks and were hollow.	Crystalline lactose converted to amorphous form of lactose. Spray drying process did not destroy LNC.	Cyclohaler®, N.V. Medicopharma	20 mg	29%

(Continued)

TABLE 12.1 (CONTINUED) Literature reports of drug nanoparticles formulated through spray dried techniques for inhalation

SR. NO.	API	CARRIER	SPRAY DRYER USED	PARTICLE SIZE D=(0.5) / MM	MORPHOLOGY	STABILITY	DEVICE USED	DOSE	FPF
15	Montelucast sodium [86]	Xyloglucan, Lactose monohydrate	LU222, Labultima, India	MMAD: 2.53	Spherical particles with smooth surface.	No degradation of drug during spray drying due to complete encapsulation of drug. Amorphous dispersion of drug into polymer matrix.	Rotahaler®	15 mg of Montelukast sodium	43.8%

* Relative to Tobramycin weight; NR: Not reported; D=(0.5): 50% of the total particles are smaller than this size.

spray dried drug nanoparticles for inhalation therapy and their physicochemical properties in Table 12.1.

Therapeutics can also be load into the matrix of the water-soluble candidates, such as sugars, that act as a delivery vehicle during their use and at the site of action, causing the matrix to dissolve and release the loaded therapeutic nanoparticles. E-Y. Xu et al. investigated the effect of the excipient on spray dry powder inhalation by using four different saccharides, namely β-cyclodextrin, starch, sodium carboxymethylcellulose (NaCMC), and lactose. The NaCMC-based spray dried formulation showed a sustained release of the loaded drug salbutamol sulphate after an hour and had enhanced aerosolization efficiency [70]. Drug-loaded micro- and nanoparticles are frequently administered through inhalation for therapy of lung diseases. This is because APIs can be delivered to the site of action, thus making them an effective treatment modality [51]. The most promising behaviors of the formulation that require great attention for effective inhalation properties are the aerosolization efficiency and the controlled release of the drug following deposition within the lungs. The major challenges in dry powder inhaler formulation are stability of the particles in a dry state, controlling aggregation of nanoparticles in the inhaler, re-dispersion efficiency of nanoparticles in lung fluid, and the ability to retain therapeutic activity [71, 72].

12.3.2 Active Pharmaceutical Ingredients

The spray dried particles have various advantages for their application in dry powder inhalation such as storing the drug in dry powder form. The drug storage dry state offer long term stability. There are several drug molecules have been developed for the treatment of tuberculosis and lung cancer. Rifampicin is a first line, highly effective oral drug used to treat tuberculosis. Khadka et al. formulated inhalable rifampicin through spray drying. The formulated powder showed interesting solid-state properties, such as a size below 3.8 μm, fine particle fraction (FPF) above 58%, *in vitro* aerosolization, and aerosolization stability over three months in different humidity conditions. The mass percentage of drug particles with an aerodynamic diameter below 5 μm is considered as fine particle fraction. Moreover, the inhalable drug is excipient free and can be delivered at high doses of rifampicin to the lung for effective treatment of tuberculosis [73]. Rajeev Ranjan et al. formulated the dry powder inhaler of two second line anti-tuberculosis drugs, D-cycloserine and ethionamide, through spray drying for the treatment of multi-drug resistant tuberculosis. The optimum formulation had a mass median aerodynamic diameter (MMAD) of 1.776 ± 3.1 μm [74]. Kwok et al. formulated inhalable antimicrobial peptides using spray drying techniques for the treatment of tuberculosis. Antimicrobial peptides, such as D-enantiomeric AMPs (D-LAK120-HP13 and D-LAK120-A), were spray dried with mannitol. The particle size was 3 μm, and the water content was below 3% (w/w) [75]. Zhang et al. developed a liposomal curcumin dry powder inhaler with an aerodynamic diameter of 5.81 μm and fine particle fraction of 46.71% for inhalation in the treatment of lung cancer. This formulation had greater anticancer effects than curcumin powder and gemcitabine [76].

12.3.3 siRNA

Inhalation is a preferred route of administration of siRNA for respiratory diseases treatment. Spray drying technique offer advantages such as formulation of powder of siRNA suitable for inhalation with good aerodynamic properties with altering the properties of siRNA and maintain high concentration at site of action where enzymes are minimum active. Excellent dispersity, and release at site of action through degradation of excipient such as lactose, mannitol, and trehalose. Excipient used in spray drying offer a good protection for siRNA from degradation. They undergo decomposition in the ling lining fluid and releasing the siRNA. It is well known that the therapeutic efficacy of siRNA is more effective than pharmaceutical drugs. Recently, siRNA-based therapy has gained significant attention for the treatment of various diseases, including pulmonary diseases [87]. However, it is challenging to formulate siRNA based drugs to deliver at the site of action (Figure 12.4) [87]. Moreover, siRNA is sensitive to high temperatures, thus a large number of techniques have been investigated for siRNA-based formulations for pulmonary delivery [88]. Spray drying is one such strategy that can produce siRNA-loaded dry powder formulations without altering the efficacy of the siRNA. The excipients are

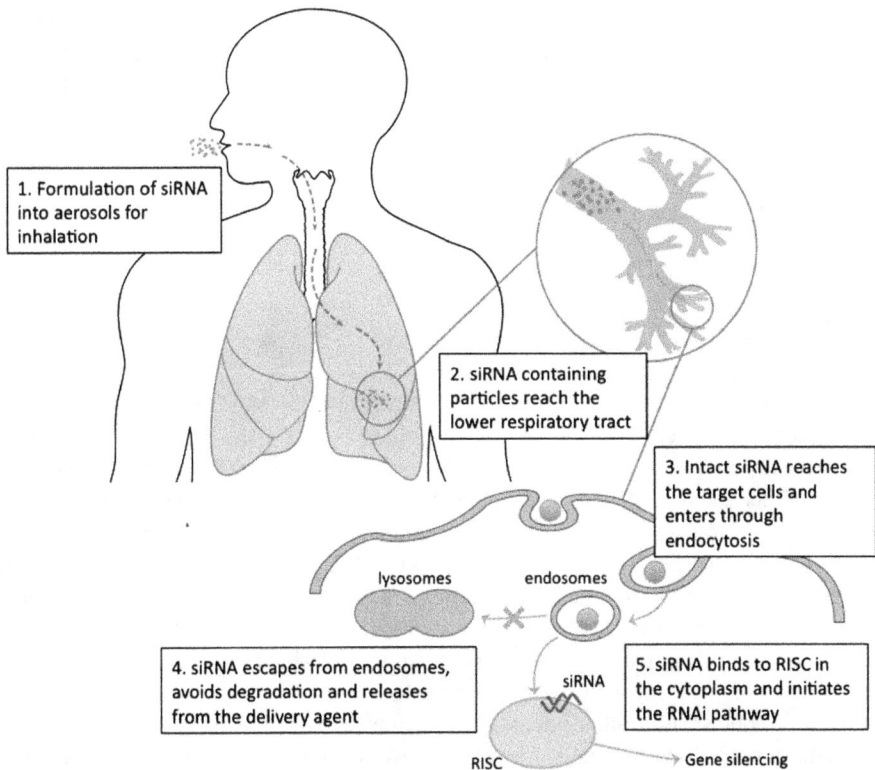

1. Formulation of siRNA into aerosols for inhalation

2. siRNA containing particles reach the lower respiratory tract

3. Intact siRNA reaches the target cells and enters through endocytosis

lysosomes   endosomes

4. siRNA escapes from endosomes, avoids degradation and releases from the delivery agent

siRNA

5. siRNA binds to RISC in the cytoplasm and initiates the RNAi pathway

RISC   Gene silencing

FIGURE 12.4 Systemic presentation of inhalation-based delivery of siRNA and mechanism of action for treatment of the lungs. Reproduced with permission from Ref. [87]. Copyright 2012, Elsevier.

added to the formulation to provide some degree of protection of the nanoparticles and the encapsulated siRNA during the process of spray drying, in particular shear forces and increased temperatures [89]. Additionally, it is suitable to deliver through inhalation. Jensen et al. formulated siRNA containing a PLGA nanoparticle intended for inhalation through a spray drying technique [89]. Local delivery of the small interfering RNA to the lungs is a promising strategy in effective therapeutics. Jensen et al. have studied the powder characteristics through statistical design of experiments by varying the formulation parameters, such as concentration, carbohydrate excipients used (trehalose, lactose, and mannitol), adjusting the ratio of nanoparticles to excipients and monitoring the effect on moisture content, size and morphology of particles, and powder yield. The results showed that characteristics such as lower water content and aerodynamic diameter were suitable for inhalation. The moisture content had to lower with mannitol compared to trehalose and lactose. Importantly, the integrity and biological activity of the siRNA were preserved during the spray drying process. This study showed the feasibility of this spray drying technique to produce micro- and nanoparticles comprising siRNA for inhalation therapy [89]. Another interesting formulation for siRNA delivery is polyplexes, a complex system of siRNA with cationic polymers through electrostatic interactions. Polyplexes can be delivered through inhalation by encapsulation into a polymer through spray drying. Keil et al. achieved delivery of siRNA-based polyplexes through spray drying [90]. Formulating polyplexes is simple, easy, and can be used to control the particle size and loading. Chow et al. formulated a naked siRNA-based inhalation powder through spray drying techniques using L-Leucine as a dispersion enhancer. Results showed that a 50% L-Leucine-based formulation showed excellent aerodynamic performance with 45% of fine particles fraction. More importantly, the siRNA retain its integrity [91]. Moreover, there are few spray dried siRNA formulation at at clinical trials [91].

12.3.4 Vaccines

Vaccines play a crucial role in public health globally by preventing two to three million deaths each year. Since 2020, vaccines have gained further attention due to the appearance of the coronavirus called SARS-CoV-2 (severe acute respiratory syndrome coronavirus 2), which led to a global pandemic and the lockdown of more than 100 countries. In order to control the spread of the virus, many researchers developed several technologies to detect, prevent, and treat COVID-19 [92]. There are several vaccines that have been formulated as liquids. The stability of a liquid vaccine is challenging because it undergoes degradation through physical and chemical pathways. Moreover, the vaccine antigens are sensitive to the aqueous environment, which limits the vaccine's shelf life. Hence, spray drying is a suitable option to produce dry vaccines. Moreover, dry vaccines provide several other advantages, such as extended shelf lives and less stringent requirements for cold chain storage. This would enable distribution of the vaccine to remote areas with poor resources and to avoid wastage as well. Recently, Preston et al. comprehensively reviewed the wide range of dry vaccine formulations through spray drying [93]. Very recently, Gomez et al. developed a platform for a spray dried inhalable tuberculosis vaccine by formulating a dry powder of ID93+GLA-SE, an adjuvant subunit TB vaccine that contains recombinant fusion protein ID93 and glucopyranosyl lipid A (GLA) in a squalene emulsion (SE), through spray drying. This formulation showed good retention of the antigen and suitable aerosol performance [94]. Saluja et al. formulated a dry powder version of the influenza subunit vaccine for inhalation through spray drying and compared it with a spray freeze drying formulation. Interestingly, the spray dried-based formulation showed better antigen integrity and stability over three years at 20 °C [95]. To the best of our knowledge, there is no spray dried inhalable vaccine for the treatment of lung diseases in the market. Several spray dried vaccines are focused on influenza and tuberculosis. Vaccines that are used to treat respiratory diseases should be administrable through inhalation as this is the most feasible manner to deliver the drug to the local site. Overall, several spray dried vaccine candidates have shown good results in preclinical studies yet only a few have been tested in clinical trials that includes an inhalable dry powder measles vaccine that contained live attenuated measles virus and could induce robust specific measles virus T-cell response in during Phase I clinical trial in India [96], and AERAS-402 Tuberculosis vaccine that contains adenovirus 35-vector expressing TB antigens Ag85A, Ag85B, and TB10.4 and was assessed as safe and immunogenic during Phase II B clinical trial in South Africa [97]. Moreover, spray drying techniques are convenient to formulate adjuvants that are freeze sensitive, for example alumina [93]. Spray drying is also often used to stabilize different type of vaccines, such as live attenuated, inactivated, and subunit vaccines. However, further research is needed to develop an all-in-one dry vaccine [98].

12.4 LAB SCALE VS INDUSTRIAL SCALE

Prototype spray dried products at a small scale can show promising properties, such as particle size distribution, mean size, shape, and moisture content. However, it is a major challenge to achieve similar particle size, morphology, fine particle fraction, and other parameters for spray dried particles on an industrial scale that match those designed on the lab scale. The process of spray drying involves several steps during which the sample may undergo complex physical transformations, and therefore it becomes difficult to predict the effects that scaling up would make at any stage. Physical transformations mainly occur during the atomization, drying, and gas-solid separation stage in spray drying. Changes made at these stages govern the droplet size, process throughput, drying kinetics, and final morphology of particles, therefore systematic scaling up of the whole process is important [99]. Improper scale up can lead to huge losses of expensive raw materials and ultimately jeopardize the whole drug development timeline [99].

The main goal during scale-up is to maintain the desired product qualities while still generating satisfactory yield. Final product characteristics are governed primarily by input variables and equipment configurations and settings. Various experimental design methods can be used to arrive at the experimental conditions suitable for achieving the required product characteristics, but such an empirical approach requires a lot of funds and time. Additionally, this process will have to be repeated every time the desired product characteristics are changed, which implies this process does not add to the fundamental knowledge of scaling up that can be reused. It has been proposed that an alternate way to maintain desired product characteristics during scale-up is by keeping key response variables similar across different scales [99]. Based on various reviews, these key response variables during scale up were identified as the size distribution of droplets, outlet temperature, relative humidity, loss in separator pressure coefficient, and collection efficiency [13, 18, 99, 100]. A very detailed road map (Figure 12.5) for scaling up a spray drying process has been proposed by Poozesh and Bilgili et al. [99] This road map describes how to maintain the key response variables across different scales to maintain the product characteristics. Briefly, first a suitable range of Sauter-mean diameter (SMD) of droplet size distribution and thermodynamic design space for the spray drying process must be identified using small/pilot scale data. Then, similar SMD of droplets across scales can be achieved by using a spray simulator to get the atomization air flow rate of the same atomizer at the scaled-up spray rate and by using semi-empirical correlations. Subsequently, similar drying

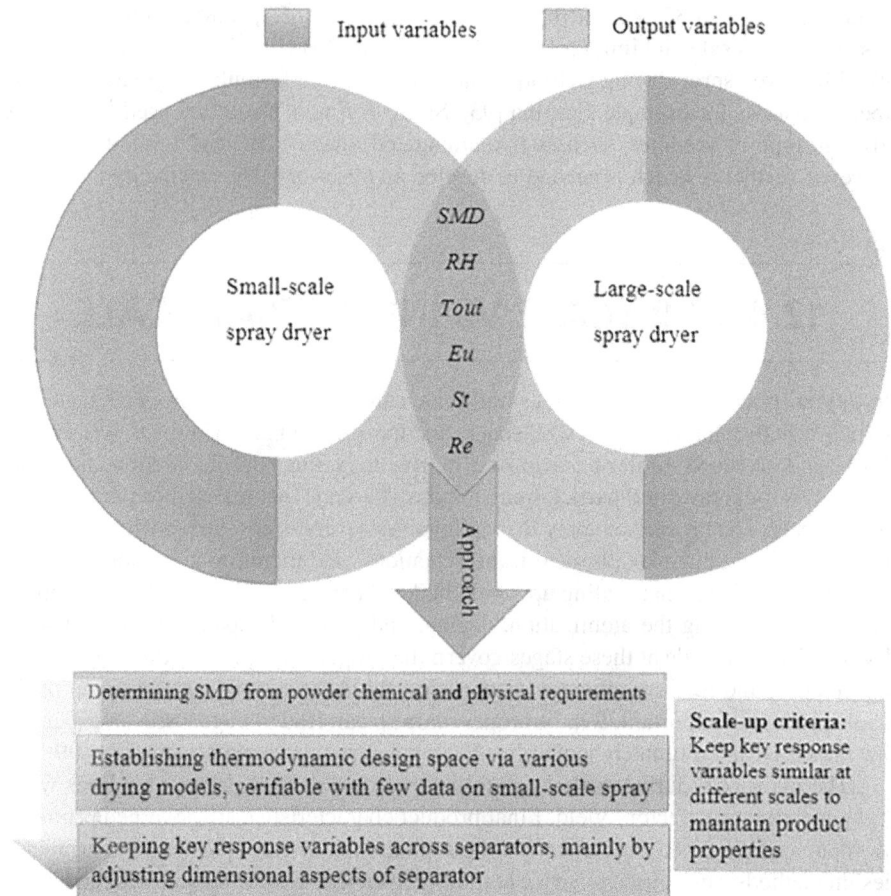

FIGURE 12.5 Proposed roadmap to scale-up a spray drying process. Reproduced with permission from Ref. [97]. Copyright 2019, Elsevier.

conditions (outlet temperature [Tout], relative humidity [RH]) across scales can be achieved by adjusting the inlet temperature and maintaining the ratio of spray rate to drying gas flow rate. Finally, similar pressure drop coefficients (Eu) and collection efficiencies, through Reynolds number (Re) and stokes number (St), can be maintained by the geometrical aspects of the separator, such as inlet and outlet diameter, along with inlet and outlet pressure differences and inlet velocity. This road map has been depicted in Figure 12.5 [99].

Successful scale up depends on yielding results that are qualitative and quantitative, and reproducible [101]. Parameters such as air inlet temperature, feed flow rate, outlet temperature, and feed solid concentration are the critical parameters that affect the quality of product at the industrial scale of spray drying. However, it is challenging to design a system for the production of specific substances at such a large scale for industrial applications because optimization of the aforementioned conditions through trial-and-error is a long process and requires many experiments. Hence, an alternative strategy is to study the system and optimize it through a computational process. Computational fluid dynamics (CFD) is a powerful tool to study spray drying to predict drying performance and design alternatives [102].

Spray drying is widely used in several industries to produce foodstuffs, detergents, pharmaceuticals, and cosmetics. One such major industrial application of spray drying is in producing dairy products. Fonterra co-op Group Ltd., is the world's largest exporter of milk powder and operates 40 spray dryers at different sites in New Zealand [102]. The capacity of spray dryers in the dairy industry ranges from 1 to 20 tons per hour. Therefore, industrial scale spray dryers require large amounts of energy and it is challenging to maintain the quality of the product produced [103]. Hence, there is a great potential to develop smart, energy efficient, and high-performance spray dryers at the industrial scale.

To conclude, scaling up of a spray drying process is complicated and very little is known about scaling spray drying up from a lab scale to the industry scale. More work needs to be done in this area to develop more mechanistic and predictive scale-up approaches by using modeling and mathematical tools in addition to limited empirical measurements. A shift from the trial-and-error approaches of the past to meaningful model-based scale-up approaches will help enhance control over product properties without much experimental effort or capital investment.

12.5 INHALATION DEVICES

Spray dried products should have suitable aerosol and particle properties to develop effective inhalers. It is possible to deliver the drug particles produced through spray drying through different devices, such as nebulizers, pressurized metered dose inhaler (pMDIs), and dry powder inhalers (DPIs). Successful delivery of drugs through inhalation depends not only on the powder characteristics but also on the performance of the inhaler device used. The design of the inhaler device extensively influences its performance in delivering the dose. Instead of depending on the patient's inspiratory flow, the majority of inhaler devices themselves aerosolize the powder formulation. This aerosolization is important for separation of the drug from the drug-carrier mixtures, or deagglomeration, and for final deposition of the drug dose into the lungs of the patients [104]. The inhaler device should assist in formation of fine particles (0.5–7 µm) such that they are able to cross the impaction barrier of the lungs. An ideal dry powder inhaler system should include most or all of the following attributes [105]:

- Convenient to use (compact in design).
- Economical to use frequently.
- Delivers reproducible emitted and fine particle dose throughout the lifespan of inhaler.
- Non-reactive and suitable for a wide range of drugs and doses.
- Leads to minimal extrapulmonary loss of drug (low oropharyngeal deposition, low device retention, and low exhaled loss).
- Powder should be protected from the external environment in all climates and protected from moist exhaled air.
- Provides overdose protection and indicates number of doses delivered and/ or remaining.

Over time, there have been steady improvements in the design and characteristics of inhalers developed. Figure 12.6 presents various DPI devices [106, 107]. The first-generation DPI devices, such as the Spinhaler (Fisons, Ipswich, UK), Handihaler (Boehringer-Ingelheim, Ingelheim am Rhein, Germany), and Rotahaler® (Glaxo, London, UK) were single unit dose devices and delivered a relatively low fine particle fraction (FPF) of approximately 10%–20% [108]. Then the second generation of DPI devices, like Turbohaler (Astra Zeneca, UK and Sweden) and Diskhaler (GlaxoSmithKline, UK), which are multi-unit dose or multiple dose DPIs, were able to deliver an FPF between 20–40% [108]. Afterwards, various novel DPI systems emerged that were able to deliver a much higher FPF and were more convenient to use. Various dry powder inhalers approved for marketing are listed in Table 12.2.

12.6 COMMERCIAL PRODUCTS AND MARKET

The spray drying process was first introduced in the food and chemical industries in the 19th century. It is one of the most rapid, cost-effective, and established ways to produce stable dry powders and has numerous applications in various industries. 40% of the market share of global spray drying equipment as of 2018, as reported by HVAC and construction, is of food and dairy industries and nearly 50% of pharmaceutical and nutraceutical industries, and chemical industries shared 25% [128]. It made its entry in the pharmaceutical industry for the production of API and excipients, and is now being widely used for taste-masking, production of amorphous solid dispersions, controlled release formulations, and advanced powder forms [119]. Figure 12.7 presents the commercially available dry powder inhaler

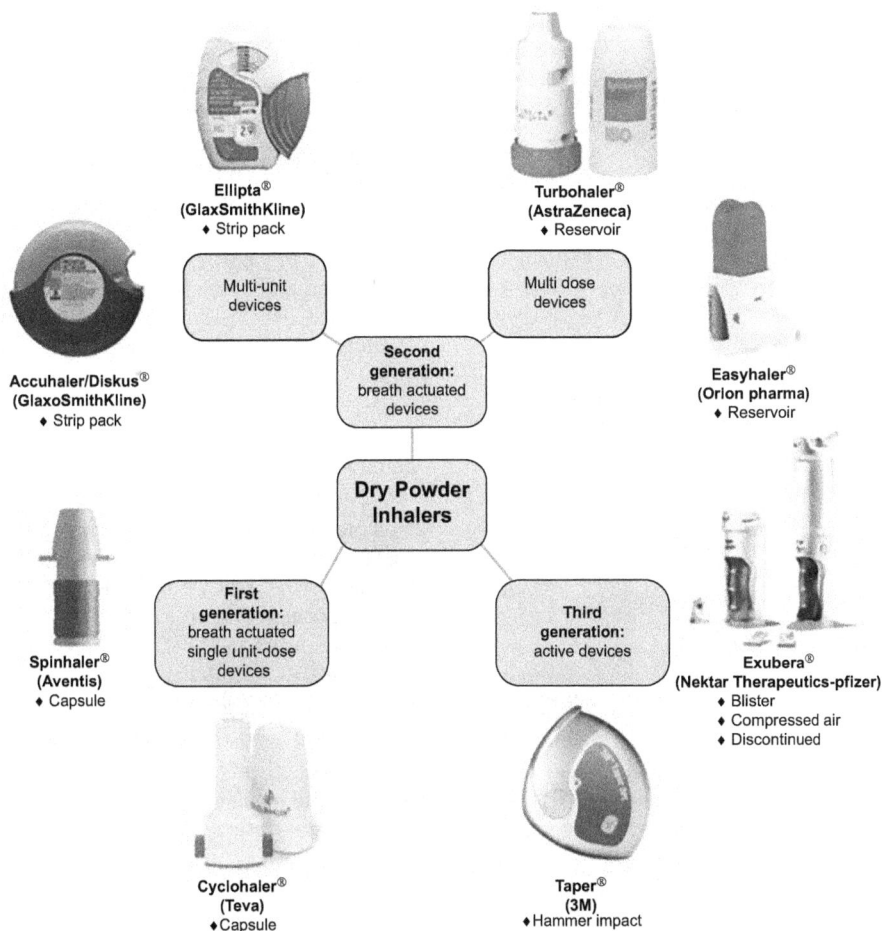

FIGURE 12.6 Different generation dry powder inhalation devices. Reproduced with permission from ref. [105]. Copyright 2016, Open access, University College London and Ref. [106]. Copyright 2020, open access, MDPI.

devices [129, 130–133]. Some examples of FDA approved pharmaceutical inhalation products processed by spray drying are:

- **Exubera:** This is the trade name for an oral inhalation insulin powder prescription medicine for diabetes. It is marketed by Pfizer and is available in 1 mg and 3 mg dose blisters which deliver an FPF of 75% and 50%, respectively, using the Exubera inhaler. Other inactive ingredients present are sodium citrate (dihydrate), mannitol, glycine, and sodium hydroxide as excipients. This was withdrawn from the market one year after it was released in 2006 due to long term safety issues [134].
- **Novopulmon Novolizer 200**: This is the trade name for Budesonide inhalation powder used for the treatment of Asthma. It is marketed by MEDA Pharma and

TABLE 12.2   Various FDA approved and commercially available dry powder inhalers

TYPE	COMPANY	DPI	DESCRIPTION
Capsule based devices	GSK/Cipla	Rotahaler	It is a completely transparent plastic inhalation device. The capsule breaks due to twisting of the device and medication is released due to patient's inhalation [109].
	Aventis	Spinhaler	It contains a tiny propeller with a cap. Pushing up and down with the cap breaks the capsule and the fan helps to push the formulation down the throat [110].
	Pharmachemie /Novartis	Cyclohaler /Aerolizer	It consists of a mouthpiece that has a mesh enclosing the capsule chamber. The air enters tangentially which leads to aerosolization due to swirling or cyclonic flow [111].
	Boehringer Ingelheim	Handihaler	It is a breath actuated inhaler. It contains a capsule chamber covered with convex metallic mesh. The capsule is inserted in vertical position and aerosolization is due to radial flow of air [111].
	Boehringer Ingelheim	Aerohaler	It contains a magazine which can hold up to 6 capsules at once and aerosolizes using patient's inspirational flow [112].
Blister based devices	GSK	Diskhaler (Rotadisk)	It is a breath-activated, Refillable and inhalation device containing sealed blister dosage pack [113].
	GSK	Diskus (Accuhaler)	It is a flat, round, multi-dose inhaler. It is breath activated. It has a dose counter window to show how many doses are left [113].
		Pro haler	It is pre-metered multi-dose DPI. It is breath triggered dose opening function [114].
	Vectura	Aspirair	Used for systemic delivery through lungs [105]
	Sandoz AG	Forspiro	The inhaler contains 60 doses of powder medication in a coiled strip of foil. It has a dose counter which indicates how many doses are left. It is non reusable [115].
	Vectura	Gyrohaler	It is a multi-unit dose dry powder inhaler designed to deliver locally to the lungs. The dry powder formulation is packaged in foil blister strips of up to 60 pre-metered doses[116]
	GSK	Ellipta	Contains two separate blister strips and requires low inspiratory flow rate [117].

(Continued)

TABLE 12.2 (CONTINUED) Various FDA approved and commercially available dry powder inhalers

TYPE	COMPANY	DPI	DESCRIPTION
Cartridge Based Device	MEDA Pharma	Novolizer	It is a multidose breath-actuated DPI. It has multiple patient feedback mechanisms to optimize dosage [118].
	Sanofi	Pulmojet	It has a breath actuator which is responsible for the protection and release of the loaded dose. It also has a de-aggregator which ensures the medication particles are the ideal size for inhalation. Formulation is kept under pressure by a spring which fixes the position of the powder [119].
	Ratiopharm	Jethaler /MAGhaler	Dose measuring by the Jethaler is independent of the inhaler position [120].
	Sanofi	Ultrahaler	It is breath actuated and does not require coordination of inhalation with the actuation of the device [121].
	MannKind	Dreamboat inhaler	It contains unit dose cartridge and uses passive aerosolization mechanism [117].
Reservoir based	Astra Zeneca	Turbuhaler	It is a plastic device containing dry powdered medication. It is breath-activated [105].
	Recipharm	Clickhaler	It is a novel passive DPI which can deliver 200 doses [122].
	AstraZeneca	Flexhaler	It is a plastic device containing dry powdered medication, and it is breath activated [123].
	Merck	Twisthaler	It is a plastic device containing dry powdered medication, and it is breath activated [124].
Other novel DPI	3M	3M™ Taper	It contains dimpled carrier tape upon which several doses of API can be coated. An impactor is triggered upon inhalation that strikes the tape and releases the API into the air stream for aerosolization and further size reduction. It eliminates the need to use carrier for inhalation formulation [125].
	3 M	3M Conix™	It uses novel reverse flow cyclone technology to improve the effectiveness of API delivery by increasing effectiveness of energy transfer from patient's inspiratory flow to aerosolize the drug. The design allows flexibility to use different formulations and provides protection to the formulation from moisture [126].

(Continued)

TABLE 12.2 (CONTINUED)   Various FDA approved and commercially available dry powder inhalers

TYPE	COMPANY	DPI	DESCRIPTION
	Novartis	Breezhaler	It offers low resistance and gives better performance. Patient can check if full dose is inhaled [117].
	Chiesi	NEXThaler	Releases extra fine particles of MMAD < 2µm [117].
	MannKind	Disposable Cricket™ Technology	Small and low-cost device for acute and short treatment durations [127].

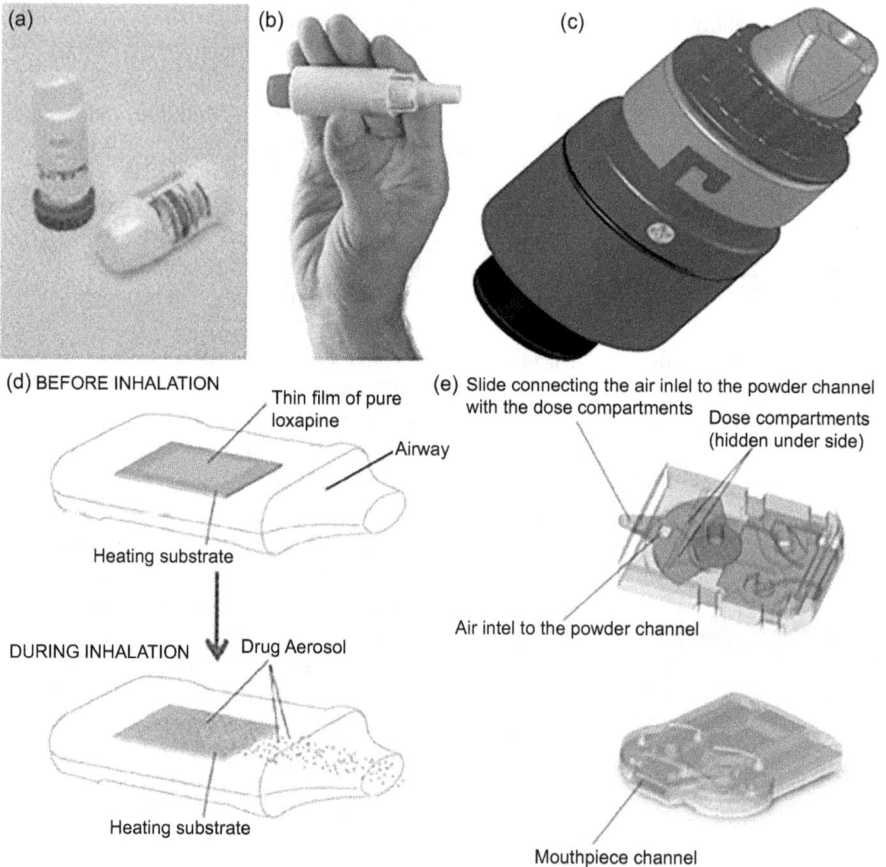

(a)

(b)

(c)

(d) BEFORE INHALATION

Thin film of pure loxapine

Airway

Heating substrate

DURING INHALATION   Drug Aerosol

Heating substrate

(e) Slide connecting the air inlet to the powder channel with the dose compartments

Dose compartments (hidden under side)

Air intel to the powder channel

Mouthpiece channel

FIGURE 12.7   Different DPI in market (a) Turbuhaler/Turbohaler [136], (b) Podhaler™ [137], (c) DPI – The University Of Western Ontario [138], (d) Staccato [139], (f) Twincer [140]. All figures are reproduced with permission from Refs. [136–140]. Copyrights, 2003 Elsevier, 2013 Springer Nature, 2012 Elsevier, 2011 Elsevier, and 2006 Elsevier, respectively.

each actuation contains 200 µg of budesonide. It contains a total of 1.09 g or 2.18 g white powder in a cartridge that provides up to 100 to 200 metered doses, respectively. The carrier used for spray drying in this case is Lactose monohydrate and it delivers an FPF of about 75% using the Novolizer inhaler [135].

- **Formatris Novolizer:** This is the trade name for formoterol inhalation powder that is used for the treatment of asthma and COPD. This is also marketed by MEDA Pharma and is available in 6 µg and 12 µg doses of formoterol with each actuation. It contains the Novolizer inhaler that contains a cartridge that can deliver 60 doses. The carrier used is also Lactose monohydrate [136]. A similar dry powder inhaler product of formoterol is Formotop, marketed by Astellas Pharma [137].
- **Ventilastin Novolizer:** This is an inhalation powder formulation containing Salbutamol (anti-asthmatic agent) with lactose as carrier. It is marketed by MEDA Pharma. Each cartridge contains about 2.308 g of powder to deliver 200 doses each containing 200 µg of Salbutamol [138]. Salbu is also a Salbutamol containing dry powder inhalation product marketed by the same company [139].
- **Aridol/Osmohale:** This is an inhalation product manufactured by Pharmaxis Ltd containing only Mannitol. This product is used to test the airway sensitivity of a patient. The mannitol powder in the capsules is supplied in blister packs that are utilized for inhalation [140].
- **TOBI Podhaler:** This is trade name for Tobramycin inhalation powder in capsules along with the Podhaler device. It is the prescribed medication for cystic fibrosis patients whose lungs contain the bacteria *Pseudomonas aeruginosa*. It is marketed by Novartis. Each capsule contains 28 mg of Tobramycin along with other inactive ingredients, namely 1,2-distearoyl-sn-glycero-3-phosphocholine (DSPC), calcium chloride, and sulfuric acid [141].

This technique is also becoming very popular in the bio-pharmaceutical industry. It is predicted that the future growth of spray drying products in the market will primarily be driven by aseptic spray

12.7 CHALLENGES AND FUTURE PERSPECTIVES

One major challenge remains in spray drying technology, and that is the collection of particles along the wall of the collector. Nearly 20–30% of the sample is lost due to the large area of the wall and a lack of an advanced instrument to collect the particles. Vacuum-based techniques may be a great option to combat this limitation. Another limitation is that the amount of substance required is in the range of tens milligrams. Therefore, it is not feasible to formulate biological materials, such as protein and siRNA, because there is a lack of enough sample availability required for biological studies in micrograms or nanograms that are too expensive. Hence, spray drying is widely used in pharmaceutical formulations, especially polymer micro- and nanoparticles loaded with drug. Spray dryers are also highly specialized devices that are very expensive. As mentioned earlier, scalability is another major limitation of spray drying techniques. Further, the powder properties need to be optimum for emptying of the capsule and dispersion. Use of adhesive may offer good flow properties but effect the dispersion behavior. Moreover, due to high flow rate may led to central and peripheral lung deposition. If we use substantial amounts of excipients, mass of powder to be administration may become too high and increases the increase the dose number. Spray dried particles may not be a suitable for designing a special patient due to their accessibility and limitation of physical conditions. All together it is clear that there is great scope to explore the spray drying technology for inhalation to achieve the more better healthcare system.

12.8 CONCLUSIONS

Spray drying is a well-established strategy to formulate particles. There is more than 150 years of research and development into this field. Significant advancements have been made in instrument design, and different designs are now available to address the various requirements of processing conditions and parameters. Spray drying is one of the most promising strategies to produce dry particles because it is simple, cost effective, time saving, and easy to operate, among many other flexibilities. Several different parameters affect the particles properties, with inlet temperature, outlet temperature, and feed concentration being the major parameters. Spray drying is now widely used in the pharmaceutical and food industries and is a promising technique for different applications. For example, spray drying can be used to enhance the aqueous solubility of poorly water-soluble drugs through the formulation of nanoparticles, improve storage stability of biologics like proteins, to produce peptides as dry powders that show enhanced shelf half-life, and it plays a key role in the production of dry vaccines to overcome the limitations of liquid vaccines. In conclusion, spray drying has a lot of potential in the pharmaceutical industry and in biomedical science overall. Because of its wide-ranging applications, several devices have been developed for inhalation of dry particles and many are now commercially available.

ACKNOWLEDGEMENTS

This work is supported in part by NIH grant.

REFERENCES

1. S. Ehlers, S.H.E. Kaufmann, Infection, inflammation, and chronic diseases: Consequences of a modern lifestyle, *Trends in Immunology*, 31(5) (2010) 184–190.

2. V. Raffa, O. Vittorio, C. Riggio, A. Cuschieri, Progress in nanotechnology for healthcare, *Minimally Invasive Therapy and Allied Technologies*, 19(3) (2010) 127–135.

3. D.C. Cipolla, I. Gonda, Formulation technology to repurpose drugs for inhalation delivery, *Drug Discovery Today: Therapeutic Strategies*, 8(3–4) (2011) 123–130.

4. L.M. Tatham, S.P. Rannard, A. Owen, Nanoformulation strategies for the enhanced oral bioavailability of antiretroviral therapeutics, *Therapeutic Delivery*, 6(4) (2015) 469–490.

5. R. Kumar, S.V. Dalvi, P.F. Siril, Nanoparticle-based drugs and formulations: Current status and emerging applications, *ACS Applied Nano Materials*, 3(6) (2020) 4944–4961.

6. M.-I. Ré, Formulating drug delivery systems by spray drying, *Drying Technology*, 24(4) (2006) 433–446.

7. K. Cal, K. Sollohub, Spray drying technique. I: Hardware and process parameters, *Journal of Pharmaceutical Sciences*, 99(2) (2010) 575–586.

8. C.W. Hall, T.I. Hedrick, *Drying milk and milk products*, Westport, CT: AVI Publ. Co., Inc., 1966.

9. K. Bullock, J.W. Lightbown, A.D. Macdonald, The spray drying of pharmaceutical products, *Journal of Pharmacy and Pharmacology*, 16 (1943) 221–226.

10. K. Sollohub, K. Cal, Spray drying technique: II. Current applications in pharmaceutical technology, *Journal of Pharmaceutical Sciences*, 99(2) (2010) 587–597.

11. D. Medarević, K. Kachrimanis, Z. Djurić, S. Ibrić, Influence of hydrophilic polymers on the complexation of carbamazepine with hydroxypropyl-β-cyclodextrin, *European Journal of Pharmaceutical Sciences*, 78 (2015) 273–285.

12. W.D. Hergeth, C. Jaeckle, M. Krell, Industrial process monitoring of polymerization and spray drying processes, *Polymer Reaction Engineering*, 11(4) (2003) 663–714.

13. A. Sosnik, K.P. Seremeta, Advantages and challenges of the spray-drying technology for the production of pure drug particles and drug-loaded polymeric carriers, *Advances in Colloid and Interface Science*, 223 (2015) 40–54.

14. C. Arpagaus, P. John, A. Collenberg, D. Rütti, 10: Nanocapsules formation by nano spray drying. In: S.M. Jafari (Ed.) *Nanoencapsulation technologies for the food and nutraceutical industries*, Academic Press, 2017, pp. 346–401.

15. K. Kadota, T. Nishimura, D. Hotta, Y. Tozuka, Preparation of composite particles of hydrophilic or hydrophobic drugs with highly branched cyclic dextrin via spray drying for dry powder inhalers, *Powder Technology*, 283 (2015) 16–23.

16. C. Arpagaus, A. Collenberg, D. Rütti, E. Assadpour, S.M. Jafari, Nano spray drying for encapsulation of pharmaceuticals, *International Journal of Pharmaceutics*, 546(1–2) (2018) 194–214.

17. M.M. Kamal, A. Salawi, M. Lam, A. Nokhodchi, A. Abu-Fayyad, K.A. El Sayed, S. Nazzal, Development and characterization of curcumin-loaded solid self-emulsifying drug delivery system (SEDDS) by spray drying using Soluplus® as solid carrier, *Powder Technology*, 369 (2020) 137–145.

18. A. Singh, G. Van den Mooter, Spray drying formulation of amorphous solid dispersions, *Advanced Drug Delivery Reviews*, 100 (2016) 27–50.

19. L.M. De Mohac, B. Raimi-Abraham, R. Caruana, G. Gaetano, M. Licciardi, Multicomponent solid dispersion a new generation of solid dispersion produced by spray-drying, *Journal of Drug Delivery Science and Technology*, 57 (2020) 101750.

20. R. Deshmukh, A. Mujumdar, J. Naik, Production of aceclofenac-loaded sustained release micro/nanoparticles using pressure homogenization and spray drying, *Drying Technology*, 36(4) (2018) 459–467.

21. A. Homayouni, F. Sadeghi, J. Varshosaz, H.A. Garekani, A. Nokhodchi, Comparing various techniques to produce micro/nanoparticles for enhancing the dissolution of celecoxib containing PVP, *European Journal of Pharmaceutics and Biopharmaceutics*, 88(1) (2014) 261–274.

22. N. Ashgriz, *Handbook of atomization and sprays: Theory and applications*, New York: Springer, 2011.

23. R. Vehring, W.R. Foss, D. Lechuga-Ballesteros, Particle formation in spray drying, *Journal of Aerosol Science*, 38(7) (2007) 728–746.

24. R. Vehring, Pharmaceutical particle engineering via spray drying, *Pharmaceutical Research*, 25(5) (2008) 999–1022.

25. Santos, D., A.C. Maurício, V. Sencadas, J. Santos, M.H. Fernandes, P.S. Gomes, Spray drying: An overview - Ch. 2. In *Biomaterials - Physics and Chemistry - New Edition*, edited by R. Pignatello & T. Musumeci, London: IntechOpen, 2017. https://doi.org/10.5772/intechopen.72247.

26. C. Arpagaus, A novel laboratory-scale spray dryer to produce nanoparticles, *Drying Technology*, 30(10) (2012) 1113–1121.

27. R. Pignatello, T. Musumeci, *Biomaterials: Physics and chemistry - New edition*, London: IntechOpen, 2018. 10.5772/intechopen.69128

28. S. Keshani, W.R.W. Daud, M.M. Nourouzi, F. Namvar, M. Ghasemi, Spray drying: An overview on wall deposition, process and modeling, *Journal of Food Engineering*, 146 (2015) 152–162.

29. A.S. Mujumdar, L.-X. Huang, X.D. Chen, An overview of the recent advances in spray-drying, *Dairy Science and Technology*, 90(2–3) (2010) 211–224.

30. J. Bögelein, G. Lee, Cyclone selection influences protein damage during drying in a mini spray-dryer, *International Journal of Pharmaceutics*, 401(1–2) (2010) 68–71.

31. S. Poozesh, S.M. Jafari, N.K. Akafuah, Interrogation of a new inline multi-bin cyclone for sorting of produced powders of a lab-scale spray dryer, *Powder Technology*, 373 (2020) 590–598.

32. M. Davis, G. Walker, Recent strategies in spray drying for the enhanced bioavailability of poorly water-soluble drugs, *Journal of Controlled Release*, 269 (2018) 110–127.

33. E.M. Littringer, A. Mescher, S. Eckhard, H. Schröttner, C. Langes, M. Fries, U. Griesser, P. Walzel, N.A. Urbanetz, Spray drying of mannitol as a drug carrier—The impact of process parameters on product properties, *Drying Technology*, 30(1) (2012) 114–124.

34. A.H. Salama, Spray drying as an advantageous strategy for enhancing pharmaceuticals bioavailability, *Drug Delivery and Translational Research*, 10(1) (2020) 1–12.

35. Y. Wei, Y.-H. Huang, K.-C. Cheng, Y.-L. Song, Investigations of the influences of processing conditions on the properties of spray dried chitosan-tripolyphosphate particles loaded with theophylline, *Scientific Reports*, 10(1) (2020) 1155.

36. S. Santhalakshmy, S.J. Don Bosco, S. Francis, M. Sabeena, Effect of inlet temperature on physicochemical properties of spray-dried jamun fruit juice powder, *Powder Technology*, 274 (2015) 37–43.

37. M. Ameri, Y.-F. Maa, Spray drying of biopharmaceuticals: Stability and process considerations, *Drying Technology*, 24(6) (2006) 763–768.

38. P. Mishra, S. Mishra, C.L. Mahanta, Effect of maltodextrin concentration and inlet temperature during spray drying on physicochemical and antioxidant properties of amla (Emblica officinalis) juice powder, *Food and Bioproducts Processing*, 92(3) (2014) 252–258.

39. S.G. Maas, G. Schaldach, E.M. Littringer, A. Mescher, U.J. Griesser, D.E. Braun, P.E. Walzel, N.A. Urbanetz, The impact of spray drying outlet temperature on the particle morphology of mannitol, *Powder Technology*, 213(1–3) (2011) 27–35.

40. Y.-F. Maa, H.R. Costantino, P.-A. Nguyen, C.C. Hsu, The effect of operating and formulation variables on the morphology of spray-dried protein particles, *Pharmaceutical Development and Technology*, 2(3) (1997) 213–223.

41. D.Q. Nguyen, T.H. Nguyen, S. Mounir, K. Allaf, Effect of feed concentration and inlet air temperature on the properties of soymilk powder obtained by spray drying, *Drying Technology*, 36(7) (2018) 817–829.

42. A.M. Goula, K.G. Adamopoulos, Spray drying of tomato pulp: Effect of feed concentration, *Drying Technology*, 22(10) (2004) 2309–2330.

43. C.A. Aguilar, G.R. Ziegler, Viscosity of molten milk chocolate with lactose from spray-dried whole-milk powders, *Journal of Food Science*, 60(1) (1995) 120–124.

44. K. Schmid, C. Arpagaus, W. Friess, Evaluation of the nano spray dryer B-90 for pharmaceutical applications, *Pharmaceutical Development and Technology*, 16(4) (2011) 287–294.

45. R. Deshmukh, P. Wagh, J. Naik, Solvent evaporation and spray drying technique for micro- and nanospheres/particles preparation: A review, *Drying Technology*, 34(15) (2016) 1758–1772.

46. R. Patel, M. Patel, A. Suthar, Spray drying technology: An overview, *Indian Journal of Science and Technology*, 2(10) (2009) 44–47.

47. F. Emami, A. Vatanara, E.J. Park, D.H. Na, Drying technologies for the stability and bioavailability of biopharmaceuticals, *Pharmaceutics*, 10(3) (2018) 131.

48. X. Li, N. Anton, C. Arpagaus, F. Belleteix, T.F. Vandamme, Nanoparticles by spray drying using innovative new technology: The Büchi nano spray dryer B-90, *Journal of Controlled Release*, 147(2) (2010) 304–310.

49. S.A. Shoyele, S. Cawthorne, Particle engineering techniques for inhaled biopharmaceuticals, *Advanced Drug Delivery Reviews*, 58(9–10) (2006) 1009–1029.

50. Q. Zhou, S.S.Y. Leung, P. Tang, T. Parumasivam, Z.H. Loh, H.-K. Chan, Inhaled formulations and pulmonary drug delivery systems for respiratory infections, *Advanced Drug Delivery Reviews*, 85 (2015) 83–99.

51. W.-H. Lee, C.-Y. Loo, D. Traini, P.M. Young, Nano- and micro-based inhaled drug delivery systems for targeting alveolar macrophages, *Expert Opinion on Drug Delivery*, 12(6) (2015) 1009–1026.

52. M.P. Timsina, G.P. Martin, C. Marriott, D. Ganderton, M. Yianneskis, Drug delivery to the respiratory tract using dry powder inhalers, *International Journal of Pharmaceutics*, 101(1–2) (1994) 1–13.

53. P. Couvreur, Nanoparticles in drug delivery: Past, present and future, *Advanced Drug Delivery Reviews*, 65(1) (2013) 21–23.

54. L. Ding, S. Tang, T.A. Wyatt, D.L. Knoell, D. Oupický, Pulmonary siRNA delivery for lung disease: Review of recent progress and challenges, *Journal of Controlled Release*, 330 (2021) 977–991.

55. M. Klinger-Strobel, C. Lautenschläger, D. Fischer, J.G. Mainz, T. Bruns, L. Tuchscherr, M.W. Pletz, O. Makarewicz, Aspects of pulmonary drug delivery strategies for infections in cystic fibrosis – Where do we stand?, *Expert Opinion on Drug Delivery*, 12(8) (2015) 1351–1374.

56. T. Praphawatvet, J.I. Peters, R.O. Williams, Inhaled nanoparticles–An updated review, *International Journal of Pharmaceutics*, 587 (2020) 119671.

57. R. Kumar, Solubility and bioavailability of fenofibrate nanoformulations, *ChemistrySelect*, 5(4) (2020) 1478–1490.

58. R. Kumar, Nanotechnology based approaches to enhance aqueous solubility and bioavailability of griseofulvin: A literature survey, *Journal of Drug Delivery Science and Technology*, 53 (2019) 101221.

59. R. Kumar, P.F. Siril, F. Javid, Unusual anti-leukemia activity of nanoformulated naproxen and other non-steroidal anti-inflammatory drugs, *Materials Science and Engineering: Part C*, 69 (2016) 1335–1344.

60. R. Kumar, A. Singh, N. Garg, P.F. Siril, Solid lipid nanoparticles for the controlled delivery of poorly water soluble non-steroidal anti-inflammatory drugs, *Ultrasonics Sonochemistry*, 40(A) (2018) 686–696.

61. P.F. Siril, M. Türk, Synthesis of metal nanostructures using supercritical carbon dioxide: A green and upscalable process, *Small*, 16(49) (2020) 2001972.

62. A.A. Thorat, S.V. Dalvi, Liquid antisolvent precipitation and stabilization of nanoparticles of poorly water soluble drugs in aqueous suspensions: Recent developments and future perspective, *Chemical Engineering Journal*, 181–182 (2012) 1–34.

63. H. Chen, C. Khemtong, X. Yang, X. Chang, J. Gao, Nanonization strategies for poorly water-soluble drugs, *Drug Discovery Today*, 16(7–8) (2011) 354–360.

64. K. Kho, W.S. Cheow, R.H. Lie, K. Hadinoto, Aqueous re-dispersibility of spray-dried anti-biotic-loaded polycaprolactone nanoparticle aggregates for inhaled anti-biofilm therapy, *Powder Technology*, 203(3) (2010) 432–439.

65. D.T. Friesen, R. Shanker, M. Crew, D.T. Smithey, W.J. Curatolo, J.A.S. Nightingale, Hydroxypropyl methylcellulose acetate succinate-based spray-dried dispersions: An overview, *Molecular Pharmaceutics*, 5(6) (2008) 1003–1019.

66. Z.M.M. Lavra, D. Pereira de Santana, M.I. Ré, Solubility and dissolution performances of spray-dried solid dispersion of efavirenz in Soluplus, *Drug Development and Industrial Pharmacy*, 43(1) (2017) 42–54.

67. Y. Kawashima, K. Matsuda, H. Takenaka, Physicochemical properties of spray-dried agglomerated particles of salicylic acid and sodium salicylate, *Journal of Pharmacy and Pharmacology*, 24(7) (1972) 505–512.

68. A. Paradkar, A.A. Ambike, B.K. Jadhav, K.R. Mahadik, Characterization of curcumin–PVP solid dispersion obtained by spray drying, *International Journal of Pharmaceutics*, 271(1–2) (2004) 281–286.

69. M.G. Piao, C.-W. Yang, D.X. Li, J.O. Kim, K.-Y. Jang, B.K. Yoo, J.A. Kim, J.S. Woo, W.S. Lyoo, S.S. Han, Y.-B. Lee, D.-D. Kim, C.S. Yong, H.G. Choi, Preparation and *in vivo* evaluation of piroxicam-loaded gelatin microcapsule by spray drying technique, *Biological and Pharmaceutical Bulletin*, 31(6) (2008) 1284–1287.

70. E.-Y. Xu, J. Guo, Y. Xu, H.-Y. Li, P.C. Seville, Influence of excipients on spray-dried powders for inhalation, *Powder Technology*, 256 (2014) 217–223.

71. S. Haque, M.R. Whittaker, M.P. McIntosh, C.W. Pouton, L.M. Kaminskas, Disposition and safety of inhaled biodegradable nanomedicines: Opportunities and challenges, *Nanomedicine: Nanotechnology, Biology and Medicine*, 12(6) (2016) 1703–1724.

72. I. d'Angelo, C. Conte, M.I. La Rotonda, A. Miro, F. Quaglia, F. Ungaro, Improving the efficacy of inhaled drugs in cystic fibrosis: Challenges and emerging drug delivery strategies, *Advanced Drug Delivery Reviews*, 75 (2014) 92–111.

73. P. Khadka, P.C. Hill, B. Zhang, R. Katare, J. Dummer, S.C. Das, A study on polymorphic forms of rifampicin for inhaled high dose delivery in tuberculosis treatment, *International Journal of Pharmaceutics*, 587 (2020) 119602.

74. R. Ranjan, A. Srivastava, R. Bharti, L. Ray, J. Singh, A. Misra, Preparation and optimization of a dry powder for inhalation of second-line anti-tuberculosis drugs, *International Journal of Pharmaceutics*, 547(1–2) (2018) 150–157.

75. P.C.L. Kwok, A. Grabarek, M.Y.T. Chow, Y. Lan, J.C.W. Li, L. Casettari, A.J. Mason, J.K.W. Lam, Inhalable spray-dried formulation of D-LAK antimicrobial peptides targeting tuberculosis, *International Journal of Pharmaceutics*, 491(1–2) (2015) 367–374.

76. T. Zhang, Y. Chen, Y. Ge, Y. Hu, M. Li, Y. Jin, Inhalation treatment of primary lung cancer using liposomal curcumin dry powder inhalers, *Acta Pharmaceutica Sinica B*, 8(3) (2018) 440–448.

77. M. Vidgren, P. Vidgren, T. Paronen, Comparison of physical and inhalation properties of spray-dried and mechanically micronized disodium cromoglycate☆, *International Journal of Pharmaceutics*, 35(1–2) (1987) 139–144.

78. F. Lyu, J.J. Liu, Y. Zhang, X.Z. Wang, Combined control of morphology and polymorph in spray drying of mannitol for dry powder inhalation, *Journal of Crystal Growth*, 467 (2017) 155–161.

79. G. Pilcer, F. Vanderbist, K. Amighi, Preparation and characterization of spray-dried tobramycin powders containing nanoparticles for pulmonary delivery, *International Journal of Pharmaceutics*, 365(1–2) (2009) 162–169.

80. G. Pilcer, R. Rosière, K. Traina, T. Sebti, F. Vanderbist, K. Amighi, New co-spray-dried tobramycin nanoparticles-clarithromycin inhaled powder systems for lung infection therapy in cystic fibrosis patients, *Journal of Pharmaceutical Sciences*, 102(6) (2013) 1836–1846.

81. A. Fallacara, L. Busato, M. Pozzoli, M. Ghadiri, H.X. Ong, P.M. Young, S. Manfredini, D. Traini, Co-spray-dried urea cross-linked hyaluronic acid and sodium ascorbyl phosphate as novel inhalable dry powder formulation, *Journal of Pharmaceutical Sciences*, 108(9) (2019) 2964–2971.

82. M.C. Fontana, T.L. Durli, A.R. Pohlmann, S.S. Guterres, R.C.R. Beck, Polymeric controlled release inhalable powder produced by vibrational spray-drying: One-step preparation and in vitro lung deposition, *Powder Technology*, 258 (2014) 49–59.

83. L. Gallo, M.V. Ramírez-Rigo, V. Bucalá, Development of porous spray-dried inhalable particles using an organic solvent-free technique, *Powder Technology*, 342 (2019) 642–652.

84. C. Moura, T. Casimiro, E. Costa, A. Aguiar-Ricardo, Optimization of supercritical CO_2-assisted spray drying technology for the production of inhalable composite particles using quality-by-design principles, *Powder Technology*, 357 (2019) 387–397.

85. A. Umerska, N.A. Mugheirbi, A. Kasprzak, P. Saulnier, L. Tajber, Carbohydrate-based Trojan microparticles as carriers for pulmonary delivery of lipid nanocapsules using dry powder inhalation, *Powder Technology*, 364 (2020) 507–521.

86. H.S. Mahajan, S.A. Gundare, Preparation, characterization and pulmonary pharmacokinetics of xyloglucan microspheres as dry powder inhalation, *Carbohydrate Polymers*, 102 (2014) 529–536.

87. J.K.-W. Lam, W. Liang, H.-K. Chan, Pulmonary delivery of therapeutic siRNA, *Advanced Drug Delivery Reviews*, 64(1) (2012) 1–15.

88. O.M. Merkel, T. Kissel, Nonviral pulmonary delivery of siRNA, *Accounts of Chemical Research*, 45(7) (2012) 961–970.

89. D.M.K. Jensen, D. Cun, M.J. Maltesen, S. Frokjaer, H.M. Nielsen, C. Foged, Spray drying of siRNA-containing PLGA nanoparticles intended for inhalation, *Journal of Controlled Release*, 142(1) (2010) 138–145.

90. T.W.M. Keil, D.P. Feldmann, G. Costabile, Q. Zhong, S. da Rocha, O.M. Merkel, Characterization of spray dried powders with nucleic acid-containing PEI nanoparticles, *European Journal of Pharmaceutics and Biopharmaceutics*, 143 (2019) 61–69.

91. M.Y.T. Chow, Y. Qiu, F.F.K. Lo, H.H.S. Lin, H.-K. Chan, P.C.L. Kwok, J.K.W. Lam, Inhaled powder formulation of naked siRNA using spray drying technology with l-leucine as dispersion enhancer, *International Journal of Pharmaceutics*, 530(1–2) (2017) 40–52.

92. J. Machhi, F. Shahjin, S. Das, M. Patel, M.M. Abdelmoaty, J.D. Cohen, P.A. Singh, A. Baldi, N. Bajwa, R. Kumar, L.K. Vora, T.A. Patel, M.D. Oleynikov, D. Soni, P. Yeapuri, I. Mukadam, R. Chakraborty, C.G. Saksena, J. Herskovitz, M. Hasan, D. Oupicky, S. Das, R.F. Donnelly, K.S. Hettie, L. Chang, H.E. Gendelman, B.D. Kevadiya, Nanocarrier vaccines for SARS-CoV-2, *Advanced Drug Delivery Reviews*, 171 (2021) 215–239.

93. K.B. Preston, T.W. Randolph, Stability of lyophilized and spray dried vaccine formulations, *Advanced Drug Delivery Reviews*, 171 (2021) 50–61.

94. M. Gomez, J. McCollum, H. Wang, M. Ordoubadi, C. Jar, N.B. Carrigy, D. Barona, I. Tetreau, M. Archer, A. Gerhardt, C. Press, C.B. Fox, R.M. Kramer, R. Vehring, Development of a formulation platform for a spray-dried, inhalable tuberculosis vaccine candidate, *International Journal of Pharmaceutics*, 593 (2021) 120121.

95. V. Saluja, J.P. Amorij, J.C. Kapteyn, A.H. de Boer, H.W. Frijlink, W.L.J. Hinrichs, A comparison between spray drying and spray freeze drying to produce an influenza subunit vaccine powder for inhalation, *Journal of Controlled Release*, 144(2) (2010) 127–133.

96. S. Agarkhedkar, P.S. Kulkarni, S. Winston, R. Sievers, R.M. Dhere, B. Gunale, K. Powell, P.A. Rota, M. Papania, S. Agarkhedkar, P.S. Kulkarni, S. Winston, R. Sievers, R.M. Dhere, B. Gunale, K. Powell, P.A. Rota, M. Papania, Safety and immunogenicity of dry powder measles vaccine administered by inhalation: A randomized controlled phase I clinical trial, *Vaccine*, 32(50) (2014) 6791–6797.

97. T.H. Jin, E. Tsao, J. Goudsmit, V. Dheenadhayalan, J. Sadoff, Stabilizing formulations for inhalable powders of an adenovirus 35-vectored tuberculosis (TB) vaccine (AERAS-402), *Vaccine*, 28(27) (2010) 4369–4375.

98. J. Machhi, F. Shahjin, S. Das, M. Patel, M.M. Abdelmoaty, J.D. Cohen, P.A. Singh, A. Baldi, N. Bajwa, R. Kumar, L.K. Vora, T.A. Patel, M.D. Oleynikov, D. Soni, P. Yeapuri, I. Mukadam, R. Chakraborty, C.G. Saksena, J. Herskovitz, M. Hasan, D. Oupicky, S. Das, R.F. Donnelly, K.S. Hettie, L. Chang, H.E. Gendelman, B.D. Kevadiya, A role for extracellular vesicles in SARS-CoV-2 therapeutics and prevention, *Journal of Neuroimmune Pharmacology* 16(2) (2021) 270–288.

99. S. Poozesh, E. Bilgili, Scale-up of pharmaceutical spray drying using scale-up rules: A review, *International Journal of Pharmaceutics*, 562 (2019) 271–292.

100. A. Al-Khattawi, A. Bayly, A. Phillips, D. Wilson, The design and scale-up of spray dried particle delivery systems, *Expert Opinion on Drug Delivery*, 15(1) (2018) 47–63.

101. K. Masters, Scale-up of spray dryers, *Drying Technology*, 12(1–2) (1994) 235–257.

102. J.R. Gabites, J. Abrahamson, J.A. Winchester, Air flow patterns in an industrial milk powder spray dryer, *Chemical Engineering Research and Design*, 88(7) (2010) 899–910.

103. Y. Jin, X.D. Chen, Entropy production during the drying process of milk droplets in an industrial spray dryer, *International Journal of Thermal Sciences*, 50(4) (2011) 615–625.

104. N. Islam, E. Gladki, Dry powder inhalers (DPIs)—A review of device reliability and innovation, *International Journal of Pharmaceutics*, 360(1–2) (2008) 1–11.

105. A.M. Healy, M.I. Amaro, K.J. Paluch, L. Tajber, Dry powders for oral inhalation free of lactose carrier particles, *Advanced Drug Delivery Reviews*, 75 (2014) 32–52.

106. M. Malamatari, *Engineering nanoparticle agglomerates as dry powders for pulmonary drug delivery*, London: UCL (University College London), 2016.

107. M. Malamatari, A. Charisi, S. Malamataris, K. Kachrimanis, I. Nikolakakis, Spray drying for the preparation of nanoparticle-based drug formulations as dry powders for inhalation, *Processes*, 8(7) (2020) 788.

108. K. Berkenfeld, A. Lamprecht, J.T. McConville, Devices for dry powder drug delivery to the lung, *AAPS PharmSciTech*, 16(3) (2015) 479–490.

109. A. Mullen, *Rotahaler®, dry powder inhaler*, Denver: National Jewish Health, November 1, 2016.

110. M. Haas, A.C. Kluppel, E.S. Wartna, F. Moolenaar, D.K. Meijer, P.E. De Jong, D. De Zeeuw, Drug-targeting to the kidney: Renal delivery and degradation of a naproxen-lysozyme conjugate in vivo, *Kidney International*, 52(6) (1997) 1693–1699.

111. J. Shur, S. Lee, W. Adams, R. Lionberger, J. Tibbatts, R. Price, Effect of device design on the in vitro performance and comparability for capsule-based dry powder inhalers, *The AAPS Journal*, 14(4) (2012) 667–676.

112. Z. Zhang, Q. Zheng, J. Han, G. Gao, J. Liu, T. Gong, Z. Gu, Y. Huang, X. Sun, Q. He, The targeting of 14-succinate triptolide-lysozyme conjugate to proximal renal tubular epithelial cells, *Biomaterials*, 30(7) (2009) 1372–1381.

113. S.P. Galant, J. van Bavel, A. Finn, G. Gross, W. Pleskow, A. Brown, A.G. Hamedani, S.M. Harding, Diskus and diskhaler: Efficacy and safety of fluticasone propionate via two dry powder inhalers in subjects with mild-to-moderate persistent asthma, *Annals of Allergy, Asthma and Immunology*, 82(3) (1999) 273–280.

114. Z.-X. Yuan, X.-K. He, X.-J. Wu, Y. Gao, M. Fan, L.-Q. Song, C.-Q. Xu, Peptide fragments of human serum albumin as novel renal targeting carriers, *International Journal of Pharmaceutics*, 460(1–2) (2014) 196–204.

115. V. Acharya, J. Olivero, The kidney as an endocrine organ, methodist Debakey, *Cardiovascular Journal*, 14(4) (2018) 305–307.

116. C. Reece, P. Swanbury, An overview of the design verification testing process for the GyroHaler® dry powder inhaler, DDL conference, (2014).

117. M. Ibrahim, R. Verma, L. Garcia-Contreras, Inhalation drug delivery devices: Technology update, *Medical Devices (Auckland, NZ)*, 8 (2015) 131.
118. C. Fenton, G.M. Keating, G.L. Plosker, Novolizer®, *Drugs*, 63(22) (2003) 2437–2445.
119. K. Doi, K. Okamoto, K. Negishi, Y. Suzuki, A. Nakao, T. Fujita, A. Toda, T. Yokomizo, Y. Kita, Y. Kihara, S. Ishii, T. Shimizu, E. Noiri, Attenuation of folic acid-induced renal inflammatory injury in platelet-activating factor receptor-deficient mice, *The American Journal of Pathology*, 168(5) (2006) 1413–1424.
120. A.H. de Boer, D. Gjaltema, P. Hagedoorn, H.W. Frijlink, Comparative in vitro performance evaluation of the Novopulmon 200 Novolizer and Budesonid-ratiopharm Jethaler: Two novel budesonide dry powder inhalers, *Pharmazie*, 59(9) (2004) 692–699.
121. A. Wischnjow, D. Sarko, M. Janzer, C. Kaufman, B. Beijer, S. Brings, U. Haberkorn, G. Larbig, A. Kübelbeck, W. Mier, Renal targeting: Peptide-based drug delivery to proximal tubule cells, *Bioconjugate Chemistry*, 27(4) (2016) 1050–1057.
122. M.T. Newhouse, N.P. Nantel, C.B. Chambers, B. Pratt, M. Parry-Billings, Clickhaler (a novel dry powder inhaler) provides similar bronchodilation to pressurized metered-dose inhaler, even at low flow rates, *Chest*, 115(4) (1999) 952–956.
123. Y. Morishita, H. Yoshizawa, M. Watanabe, K. Ishibashi, S. Muto, E. Kusano, D. Nagata, siRNAs targeted to Smad4 prevent renal fibrosis in vivo, *Scientific Reports*, 4 (2014) 1–8.
124. L.J. Stallons, R.M. Whitaker, R.G. Schnellmann, Suppressed mitochondrial biogenesis in folic acid-induced acute kidney injury and early fibrosis, *Toxicology Letters*, 224(3) (2014) 326–332.
125. D. Martin-Sanchez, O. Ruiz-Andres, J. Poveda, S. Carrasco, P. Cannata-Ortiz, M.D. Sanchez-Niño, M.R. Ortega, J. Egido, A. Linkermann, A. Ortiz, A.B. Sanz, Ferroptosis, but not necroptosis, is important in nephrotoxic folic acid–induced AKI, *Journal of the American Society of Nephrology*, 28(1) (2017) 218–229.
126. Y. Fu, C. Tang, J. Cai, G. Chen, D. Zhang, Z. Dong, Rodent models of AKI-CKD transition, *American Journal of Physiology Renal Physiology*, 315(4) (2018) F1098–F1106.
127. M. Ibrahim, R. Verma, L. Garcia-Contreras, Inhalation drug delivery devices: Technology update, *Medical Devices (Auckl)*, 8 (2015) 131–139.
128. Y.-H. Hsu, I.-J. Chiu, Y.-F. Lin, Y.-J. Chen, Y.-H. Lee, H.-W. Chiu, Lactoferrin contributes a renoprotective effect in acute kidney injury and early renal fibrosis, *Pharmaceutics*, 12(5) (2020) 434.
129. I.J. Smith, M. Parry-Billings, The inhalers of the future? A review of dry powder devices on the market today, *Pulmonary Pharmacology and Therapeutics*, 16(2) (2003) 79–95.
130. H. Stass, J. Nagelschmitz, S. Willmann, H. Delesen, A. Gupta, S. Baumann, Inhalation of a dry powder ciprofloxacin formulation in healthy subjects: A phase I study, *Clinical Drug Investigation*, 33(6) (2013) 419–427.
131. X. Zhang, Y. Ma, L. Zhang, J. Zhu, F. Jin, The development of a novel dry powder inhaler, *International Journal of Pharmaceutics*, 431(1–2) (2012) 45–52.
132. K. Dinh, D.J. Myers, M. Glazer, T. Shmidt, C. Devereaux, K. Simis, P.D. Noymer, M. He, C. Choosakul, Q. Chen, J.V. Cassella, In vitro aerosol characterization of Staccato® loxapine, *International Journal of Pharmaceutics*, 403(1–2) (2011) 101–108.
133. A.H. de Boer, P. Hagedoorn, E.M. Westerman, P.P.H. Le Brun, H.G.M. Heijerman, H.W. Frijlink, Design and in vitro performance testing of multiple air classifier technology in a new disposable inhaler concept (Twincer®) for high powder doses, *European Journal of Pharmaceutical Sciences*, 28(3) (2006) 171–178.
134. M. Ferreira, L. Barreiros, M.A. Segundo, T. Torres, M. Selores, S.A.C. Lima, S. Reis, Topical co-delivery of methotrexate and etanercept using lipid nanoparticles: A targeted approach for psoriasis management, *Colloids and Surfaces, Part B: Biointerfaces*, 159 (2017) 23–29.
135. P.R. Desai, S. Marepally, A.R. Patel, C. Voshavar, A. Chaudhuri, M. Singh, Topical delivery of Anti-TNFα siRNA and capsaicin via novel lipid-polymer hybrid nanoparticles efficiently inhibits skin inflammation in vivo, *Journal of Controlled Release*, 170(1) (2013) 51–63.

136. A. Jose, S. Labala, K.M. Ninave, S.K. Gade, V.V.K. Venuganti, Effective skin cancer treatment by topical co-delivery of curcumin and STAT$_3$ siRNA using cationic liposomes, *AAPS PharmSciTech*, 19(1) (2018) 166–175.

137. G. Sharma, Y. Yachha, K. Thakur, A. Mahajan, G. Kaur, B. Singh, K. Raza, O. Katare, Co-delivery of isotretinoin and clindamycin by phospholipid-based mixed micellar system confers synergistic effect for treatment of acne vulgaris, *Expert Opinion on Drug Delivery*, 18(9) (2021) 1291–1308.

138. C. Carbone, V. Fuochi, A. Zielińska, T. Musumeci, E.B. Souto, A. Bonaccorso, C. Puglia, G. Petronio Petronio, P.M. Furneri, Dual-drugs delivery in solid lipid nanoparticles for the treatment of Candida albicans mycosis, *Colloids and Surfaces, Part B: Biointerfaces*, 186 (2020) 110705.

139. S. Banerjee, S. Roy, K.N. Bhaumik, J. Pillai, Mechanisms of the effectiveness of lipid nanoparticle formulations loaded with anti-tubercular drugs combinations toward overcoming drug bioavailability in tuberculosis, *Journal of Drug Targeting*, 28(1) (2020) 55–69.

140. R. Pandey, S. Sharma, G. Khuller, Oral solid lipid nanoparticle-based antitubercular chemotherapy, *Tuberculosis*, 85(5–6) (2005) 415–420.

141. R. Pandey, G. Khuller, Solid lipid particle-based inhalable sustained drug delivery system against experimental tuberculosis, *Tuberculosis*, 85(4) (2005) 227–234.

Inhalation Aerosol Phospholipid Particles for Targeted Lung Delivery

13

Basanth Babu Eedara, David Encinas-Basurto, Don Hayes Jr, and Heidi M. Mansour

Contents

DOI: 10.1201/9781003182566-17

13.1 INTRODUCTION

Lung diseases are among the most common causes of death worldwide.[1] In 2019 according to the World Health Organization (WHO) and others, a total of 3.23 million deaths were due to chronic obstructive pulmonary disorder (COPD),[2] 461,000 due to asthma,[3] 1.4 million due to tuberculosis,[4] and 1.76 million due to lung cancer.[5] More recently, coronavirus disease-19 (COVID-19), caused by severe acute respiratory syndrome coronavirus-2 (SARS-CoV-2), has produced a global pandemic, contributing to even more respiratory-related mortality. As of December 29, 2021, there have been a total of 281,808,270 confirmed cases of COVID-19, including 5,411,759 deaths worldwide.[6]

Pulmonary drug delivery allows for local treatment of lung disease, including asthma, COPD, cystic fibrosis, pneumonia, pulmonary hypertension (PH), respiratory distress syndrome, and lung cancer.[7,8] Key advantages of pulmonary drug delivery locally over conventional routes of administration for the treatment of pulmonary conditions include: pain-free administration, reduced systemic side effects, higher concentrations of drug in the lungs, potentially reduced frequency of administration, and the overall dose required for effective treatment which can potentially improve patient compliance.[9-14]

The most common inhaler systems used for the pulmonary delivery of drugs include nebulizers, metered-dose inhalers (MDIs), and soft mist inhalers (SMIs) for liquid formulations, and dry powder inhalers (DPIs) for solid formulations.[15,16] DPI formulations consist of either micronized dry powder drug particles (1 μm to 5 μm) alone or mixed with inactive carrier particles.[17] DPI formulations are preferred due to their greater chemical stability. Further, DPIs are propellent-free, portable, and easy to use.[18] Excipients are added to the DPI formulations, which improve drug dosing reproducibility, aerosolization performance, physical and chemical stability, mechanical properties, and modify drug pharmacokinetics and/or dynamics.[19]

Generally, an excipient for inhalation should be pharmacologically inactive and non-toxic to lung tissue. A list of excipients approved or interesting for inhalation delivery include sugars (lactose, glucose, mannitol, trehalose), hydrophobic additives (magnesium stearate), lipids (dipalmitoylphosphatidylcholine (DPPC), distearoylphosphatidylcholine (DSPC), dimyristoyl phosphatidylcholine (DMPC), cholesterol), amino acids (leucine, trileucine), surfactants (poloxamer), absorption enhancers (hydroxypropyl-β-cyclodextrin, natural γ-cyclodextrin, bile salts, chitosan, trimethylchitosan) and biodegradable polymers (poly(lactic-co-glycolic acid), PLGA).[20] Among them, phospholipids are endogenous, biocompatible, and generally regarded as safer (GRAS) excipients for inhalation administration. Over the last decades, phospholipids have been widely used as particle engineering excipients. This chapter will describe phospholipid dry powder particles for lung delivery. It covers a summary of the anatomy and physiology of lungs, lung lining fluid and endogenous phospholipids, phospholipids used in inhalation formulations, various phospholipid-based drug delivery systems, and engineering of phospholipid microparticulate dry powder formulations.

13.2 LUNG ANATOMY AND PHYSIOLOGY

Lungs are paired organs of respiration with branching air tubes ending in compound sacs, i.e., alveoli. As shown in Figure 13.1, the airways are divided into conducting and respiratory zones with 23 bifurcations.[21] The conducting zone starts with the trachea (generation 0, i.e., G_0) and is subdivided into two main bronchi (G_1), which subdivides into bronchus (G_2), bronchioles (G_{3-15}), and terminal bronchioles (G_{16}). The respiratory zone consists of respiratory bronchioles (G_{17-19}), alveolar ducts (G_{20-22}), and alveolar sacs (G_{23}). The proximal conducting airways (tracheobronchial region) comprise

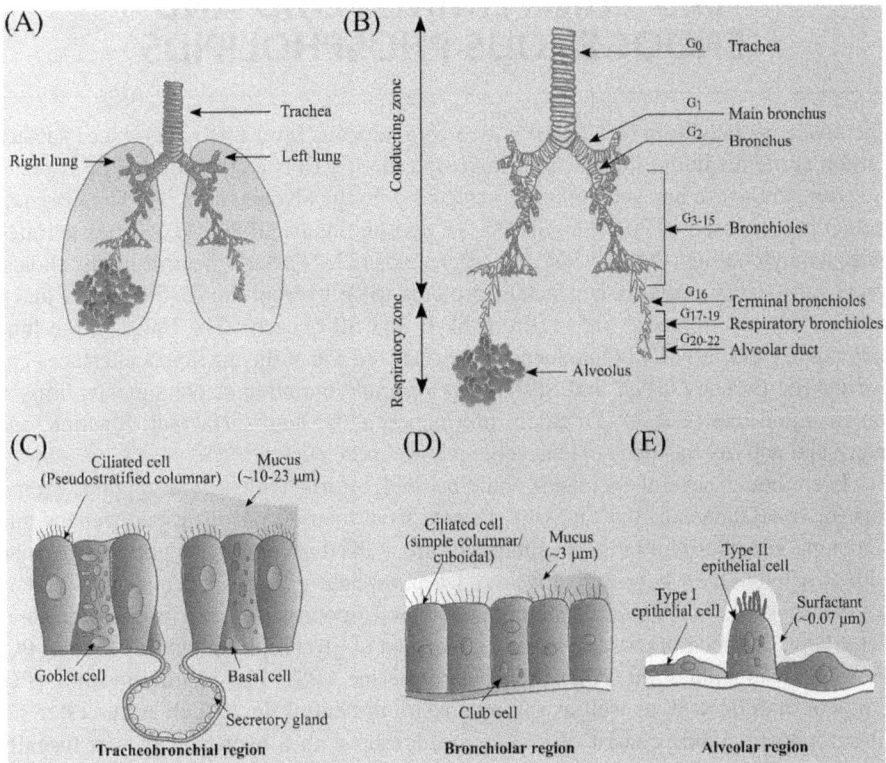

FIGURE 13.1 Schematic diagram of lungs with conducting (G_0-G_{16}) and respiratory zones (G_{17}-G_{23}) (A and B). Comparison of tracheobronchial (C), bronchiolar (D), and alveolar regions of the lungs (E).

pseudostratified columnar epithelium (~58 μm thick) composed of ciliated cells, mucus-secreting goblet cells, basal cells, and mucus-secreting glands (Figure 13.1C). The distal bronchioles (bronchiolar region) contain simple columnar or cuboidal cells without goblet cells and secretory glands (Figure 13.1D). In comparison, the alveoli (alveolar region) walls consist of extremely thin epithelium composed of type I pneumocytes (squamous epithelial cells) and type II pneumocytes (large cuboidal cells) (Figure 13.1E). The type II pneumocytes are secretive in function and produce lung surfactant.

The lungs' airway region (trachea, bronchi, and bronchioles) is covered with a mucus gel (~3–23 μm) over an area of 1–2 m^2. It is composed of 95% of water, 2–3% mucins, 0.3–0.5% lipids, 0.1–0.5% non-mucin proteins, and other cellular debris. In contrast, the alveolar region (> 100 m^2) is covered with an extremely thin (estimated thickness ~0.07 μm) film of lung surfactant.

13.3 LUNG LINING FLUID AND ENDOGENOUS PHOSPHOLIPIDS

The alveolar epithelium is covered with a thin aqueous layer and experiences surface tension at the air-liquid interface during respiration.[22] To overcome this, type II pneumocytes synthesize and secrete lung surfactant into the alveolar sacs.[23,24] The lung surfactant is composed of 90.0% lipids (85.0% phospholipids: DPPC (47.0%), unsaturated phosphatidylcholine (PC) (29.3%) and other lipids (23.7%); 5.0% neutral lipids: cholesterol) and ~10.0% proteins (surfactant proteins (SP): hydrophilic (3–5% SP-A, and < 0.5% SP-D), hydrophobic (0.5–1.0% of SP-B and SP-C each). The lipids in the lung surfactant, especially DPPC, reduces the surface tension at the air-liquid interface. The hydrophilic proteins (SP-A and SP-D) help form and maintain stable aqueous films at the air-liquid interface.[25–27] Detailed information about lung surfactant, function, and interfacial activity has been extensively reviewed previously.[23–25,28,29]

Even though several excipients could be used, efforts to identify acceptable excipients for inhalation into the lungs of patients have focused on using endogenous and biocompatible phospholipids. Phospholipids are lipids that consist of a polar head group with two long-chain acyl derivatives and a phosphate group (Figure 13.2A).[30] They are the constituents of all cell membranes, blood lipoproteins, and lung surfactant.[29] Eukaryotic cell membranes are mainly composed of glycerophospholipids such as PC, phosphatidylethanolamine (PE), phosphatidylserine (PS), phosphatidylinositol (PI), and phosphatidic acid, as well as sphingomyelin or neutral lipids such as cholesterol.[31] Glycerophospholipids consist of a polar headgroup with a hydrophobic part (usually two saturated or cis-unsaturated fatty acyl chains) which is linked to a glycerol backbone by ester linkage.[32] DPPC consists of phosphatidylcholine with two fully saturated C16:0 palmitoyl chains attached by an ester linkage to carbons 1 and 2 of the glycerol backbone.[33] Sphingomyelin is a class of phospholipids with a phosphatidylcholine headgroup attached to a ceramide linked to fatty acyl chains. Figure 13.2 shows the structures of various classes of glycerophospholipids.

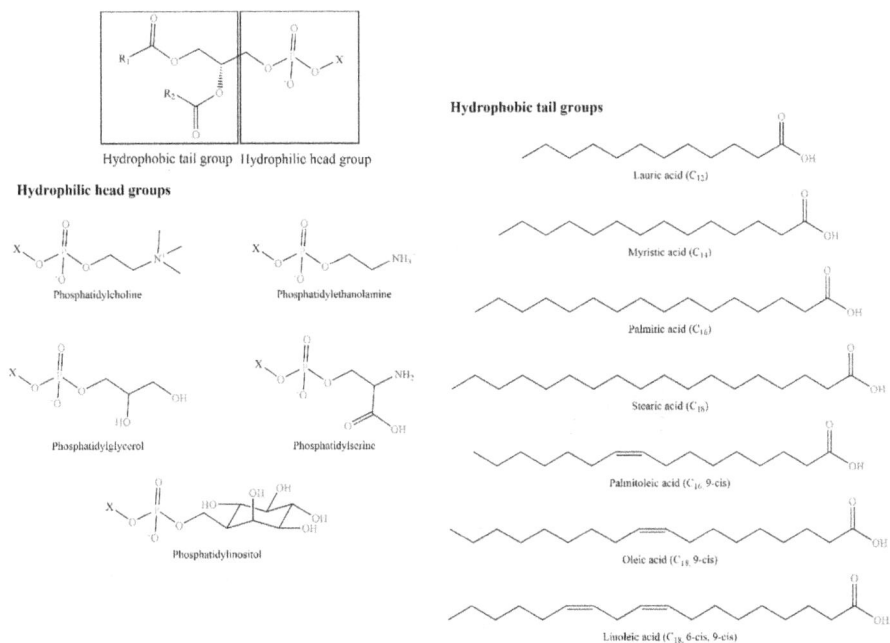

FIGURE 13.2 Chemical structures of glycerophospholipids (drawn using ChemDraw 19.1, Cambridge, MA, USA).

13.4 LUNG SURFACTANT REPLACEMENT THERAPY

Neonatal respiratory distress syndrome (NRDS) is an acute breathing disorder associated with insufficient surfactant in the peripheral lungs.[34] NRDS affects preterm infants born < 32 weeks gestation.[35,36] Physiological and anatomical immaturity of the lung and surfactant deficiency are the leading causes of respiratory distress syndrome (RDS). RDS is characterized by radiographic diffuse bilateral infiltrates, decreased respiratory compliance, small lung volumes, and severe hypoxemia. Surfactant administration decreases the surface tension and the pressure required to open atelectatic airways and collapsed alveoli, increasing respiratory capacity and improving gas exchange. Treatment for RDS includes exogenous surfactant therapy and positive pressure ventilation.[36] Table 13.1 lists the various lung surfactant preparations used to treat surfactant-related lung diseases. They are categorized into natural surfactants (animal-derived) and synthetic exogenous lung surfactants. The natural surfactants (from bovine or porcine origin) are derived from animal lungs through organic solvent extraction from either from alveolar lavage fluid or homogenized animal lung tissue. The natural surfactants contain phospholipids and proteins such as SP-A, SP-B, SP-C, and SP-D. However, synthetic surfactants lack proteins in their composition. For example, Exosurf®, a mixture

TABLE 13.1 A list of lung surfactant products used in respiratory distress syndrome (RDS).

CATEGORY	PRODUCT NAME	SOURCE	COMPOSITION (EACH ML)	DOSE
I. Natural, organic solvent extracts of lavaged animal lung surfactant	Alveofact (SF-RI1, bovactant) (Boehringer-Ingelheim Pharma, Ingelheim, Germany)	Bovine	Bovactant (bovine surfactant extract): 54 mg phospholipids as freeze dried form; a pre-filled syringe of 1.2 mL contains: sodium chloride, sodium hydrogen carbonate, water for injection	1.2 mL/kg
	Infasurf (Calfactant) (ONY, Inc., NY, USA)	Calf	Calfactant (calf lung surfactant extract): 35 mg phospholipids, 0.7 mg proteins (SP-B and SP-C), 0.9% sodium chloride	3 mL/kg
II. Natural, supplemented, or unsupplemented organic solvent extracts of animal lung tissue)	Curosurf® (poractant alfa) (Chiesi USA, Inc., Parma, Italy)	Porcine	Poractant alfa (porcine surfactant extract)- 80 mg (99% phospholipids, 1% of proteins SP-B and SP-C), 0.9% sodium chloride solution, sodium bicarbonate	Initial – 2.5 mL/kg; repeat doses – up to 2 doses of 1.25 mL/kg; maximum total dosage – 5 mL/kg
	Survanta® (beractant) (AbbVie Inc., IL, USA)	Bovine	Beractant (bovine lung extract): 25 mg/mL phospholipids, 0.5–1.75 mg/mL triglycerides, 1.4–3.5 mg/mL of free fatty acids, and < 1 mg/mL of SP (including SP-B, and SP-C), 0.9% sodium chloride, sodium chloride or hydrochloric acid	4 mL (100 mg phospholipid)
III. First-generation synthetic exogenous lung surfactants (protein-free)	Exosurf (Colfosceril palmitate) (GlaxoSmithKline Brentford, UK)	Synthetic	Colfosceril palmitate 13.5 mg/mL; tyloxapol; cetyl alcohol	5 mL/kg
IV. Second-generation synthetic humanized lung surfactants (protein-containing)	Surfaxin (lucinactant) (Discovery Laboratories, Inc., PA, USA)	Synthetic	30 mg phospholipids, 4.05 mg palmitic acid, and 0.862 mg sinapultide	5.8 mL/kg

of phospholipids that lacks surfactant proteins, is not as effective as preparations containing proteins and withdrawn from clinical use.[34,37-40] Thus, the synthetic surfactants are improved by the addition of synthetic proteins that mimic the natural surfactant protein functions.

13.5 PHOSPHOLIPIDS IN INHALATION FORMULATIONS

The saturated phosphatidylcholines such as DPPC (T_m 41 °C), DPPG (T_m 41 °C), distearoylphosphatidylcholine (DSPC, T_m 55 °C),[41] and hydrogenated soybean phosphatidylcholine (HSPC, T_m 53.7 °C),[42] with high gel-to-liquid-crystal phase transition temperatures (T_m) are generally preferred compared to the unsaturated phospholipids (T_m below 0 °C) for the preparation of free-flowing dry powder particles.[43] Figure 13.3 shows the chemical structures of phospholipids used in inhalation formulations.

DPPC and DPPG are endogenous to the lungs and are the main components of lung surfactant. The amphiphilic and lower solubility (0.18 mg/mL in 70% ethanol) nature of

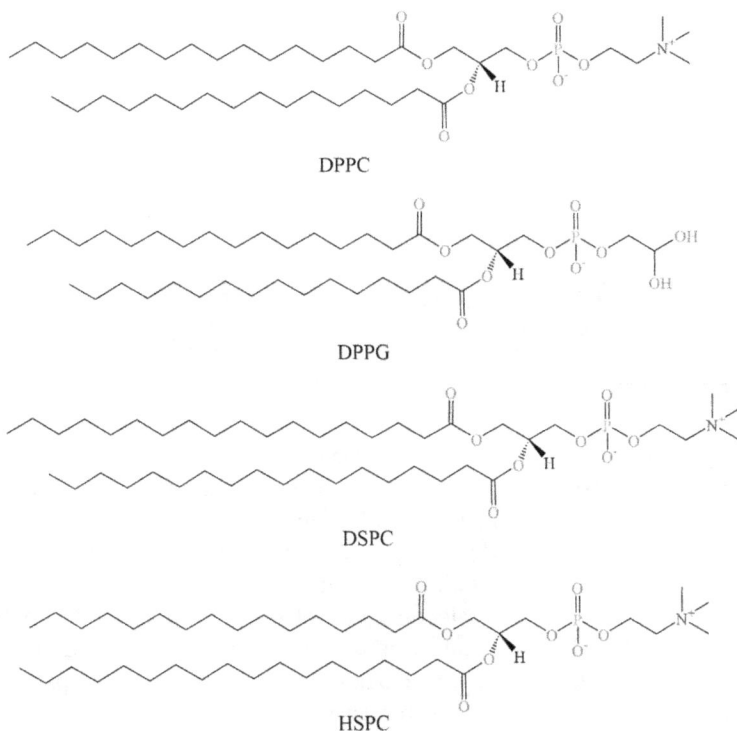

DPPC

DPPG

DSPC

HSPC

FIGURE 13.3   Chemical structures of phospholipids used in inhalation formulations (drawn using ChemDraw 19.1, Cambridge, MA, USA).

DPPC is critical in modifying the surface characteristics of particles.[44] The DPPC molecules preferentially adsorb at the droplet interface, with their aliphatic chains oriented toward the air phase during the spray drying (SD) process.[44] The aliphatic chains of the phospholipids make the particle surface hydrophobic, which reduces the surface free energy and, as a result, decreases van der Waals attractive forces and might improve the aerosolization of dry powder particles.[45-47] The surface-active DPPC also minimizes surface tension of the particle, which could possibly facilitate particle migration to the peripheral regions of the lungs.[48,49] In addition, the particles with a hydrophobic outer surface due to DPPC aliphatic chains might present a less hydrated particle surface and therefore reduce the dissolution. DSPC is another endogenous phospholipid that has been frequently used as an excipient in inhalation formulations. It is used as an emulsion stabilizer and shell-forming agent in dry powder formulations.[50] It is one of the principal excipients in the TOBI® Podhaler® formulation and produces a porous hydrophobic shell with reduced interparticle attractive forces and improved powder aerosolization.[50]

Soybean phosphatidylcholine (SPC) and HSPC are approved by FDA as excipients at a concentration up to 0.28% for inhalation use in pressurized MDI formulations.[51] They act as surfactants and improve drug solubility and wettability in the propellent. HSPC has been used in the development of several liposomal formulations. For example, Yu et al.[52] developed several liposomal formulations of ciprofloxacin and colistin using cholesterol and phospholipids, namely HSPC, 1,2-distearoyl-sn-glycero-3-ph osphoglycerol (DSPG) sodium salt, and N-(methylpolyoxyethyleneoxycarbonyl)-1,2 -distearoyl-sn-glycero-3-phosphoethanolamine sodium salt. The liposomal suspensions were transformed into dry powders via ultrasonic spray-freeze drying using mannitol and sucrose as cryoprotectants and leucine to improve the aerosolization performance of the powder.

13.6 PHOSPHOLIPID-BASED DRUG DELIVERY SYSTEMS

Phospholipids, which are solid at room temperature, can transform into solid lipid particles. They are classified as solid lipid microparticles or nanoparticles based on their size greater than or less than 1,000 nm. Solid lipid particles have several advantages, including the ability to carry a large payload of lipophilic drugs, improved drug stability, low or no toxicity, and ease of production scale-up. Furthermore, solid lipid particles could be delivered by nebulizers without causing stability issues, mixed with a standard carrier (such as lactose), or used alone as a powder for DPI delivery. For pulmonary drug delivery, solid lipid particles can be produced by spray freeze drying, spray drying, freeze-drying, supercritical fluid technologies (CO_2), etc.[53] Solid lipid particles have usually been called liposomes, lipospheres, and proliposomes; liposomes formulated as dry powders tend to form a multilamellar state that is more thermodynamically stable. Dried liposomes by freeze-drying or spray-drying increase their long-term stability during storage compared to a liposomal solution used for nebulized delivery.[54,55]

Solid-state phospholipids have been used for the replacement of commonly used dosage forms of different drugs. The dry powder has replaced tobramycin nebulized solution using DSPC phospholipids (PulmoSphere® technology), commercially available as TOBI Podhaler® designed to create porous particles with a sponge-like morphology. In addition, phospholipids in DPI have shown a faster onset of action in systemic administration after levodopa and acetylsalicylic acid inhalation with DPPC as excipient. Recently, Arcoda Therapeutics inc. developed Inbrija® showing very promising effects in patients with Parkinson's diseases. Adding DPPC as an excipient improved the flowability in the inhalation step by increasing density enhancing high dose inhalation. Another commercial product for systematic delivery is Asprihale® using DSPC for acetylsalicylic acid inhalation. The phospholipid component coats the active pharmaceutical ingredient, suppressing its bitter taste and potential for irritation when inhaled. It also acts as a viable alternative to lactose, which is commonly used to blend powders for inhalation. Asprihale® reaches maximal plasma concentration in two minutes vs 20 minutes for 162 mg non-enteric coated chewable aspirin.[56] Finally, another advantage of using phospholipids in particle-engineering for inhalation is the sustained release of the drug, reducing the frequency dosage of the patient. Phospholipids engineered in liposomes have been showing to act as a sustain release formulation after inhalation for local and systemic treatment.[57]

Many different types of delivery systems have been engineered and developed for pulmonary delivery of various therapeutics, including nanoparticles (polymeric nanoparticles, polymeric micelles), microparticles (microspheres), solid lipid nanoparticles (SLNs), nanostructured lipid carriers (NLCs), polymer-drug conjugates, macromolecules (dendrimers), and lipid vesicles (liposomes and proliposomes).

13.6.1 Liposomes for Pulmonary Delivery

Liposomes (Figure 13.4) are small composite phospholipid vesicles consisting of an aqueous compartment surrounded by a lipid bilayer (unilamellar or multilamellar).[58] Liposomes have various advantages in pulmonary applications. Liposomes will be more tolerable in the pulmonary airways if the lipids used are biodegradable, resulting in non-toxic and endogenous breakdown products. Furthermore, their small (nm) size can be easily encapsulated into particles with adequate aerosolization capabilities, allowing for satisfactory deep lung molecule deposition. In addition, liposomes adhere to the mucosal surface of the airways for a longer period than larger particles. Liposomes consist of concentrated self-assembling vesicles of the lipid bilayer, consisting of common phospholipids and cholesterols.[59,60] Liposomes are typically categorized as large unilamellar vesicles (LUVs), small unilamellar vesicles (SUVs), multilamellar vesicles (MLV) or multivesicular vesicles (MVV) according to the structure of lipid bilayers and the size of vesicles. The inner aqueous phase of liposomes is highly protected by lipid bilayers and can load hydrophilic drugs, while the hydrophobic portion can load hydrophobic drugs in the lipid bilayer. Liposomes provide the most significant advantages in terms of biomembrane biocompatibility and safety. In addition, liposomal surfaces can easily be modified by combining polymers and ligands such that the vesicles possess unique features.[61,62]

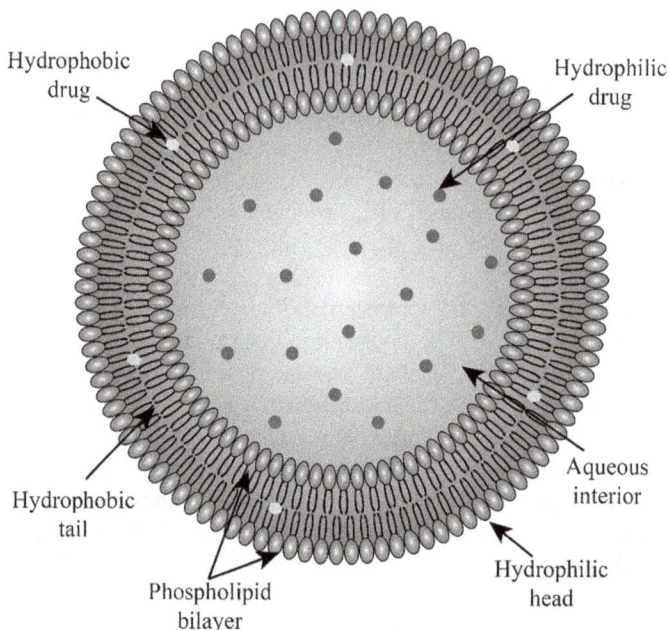

FIGURE 13.4   Schematic structure of a liposome.

Liposome particle size, adhesion, accumulation, and retention in the pulmonary airways, as well as controlled release characteristics, can contribute to enhanced therapeutic outcomes and increased patient compliance. However, one significant disadvantage of these systems is that they are easily expelled from the lungs following inhalation. However, nano-agglomeration procedures, nanoparticle-rooted microparticles, or nanoparticles-in-microparticles can be used to create particles with acceptable aerodynamic dimensions for pulmonary administration.[63]

Soy lecithin is a complex mixture of phospholipids, including phosphatidylcholine, phosphatidylethanolamine, phosphatidylinositol, phosphatidylserine, phosphatidic acid, triglycerides and other substances.[64] The other substances include carbohydrates, pigments, sterols and sterol glycosides. It has been extensively used for liposome production for solid lipid particle inhalation. For example, Tran et al.[65] produced liposomes using soy lecithin for ciprofloxacin antibiotic lung delivery; by spray-freezing dry with D-mannitol, a well-known cryoprotectant, mucolytic and bulk agent. In a more recent study, sorafenib tosylate, an antineoplastic agent for treating lung cancer, liposome solution containing mannitol was engineered by spray drying. The *in vitro* drug release pattern revealed a biphasic release pattern, with burst release in the first 6 hours followed by a sustained release for the next 72 hours.[66] Pegylated-1,2-distearoyl-sn-gl ycero-3-phosphoethanolamine also been used to synthesize liposomes for inhalation, Zhu et al.[67] co-spray dried docetaxel loaded folic acid conjugated liposomes prepared using DSPE-PEG-FA (1,2-distearoyl-sn-glycero-3-phosphophoethanolamine-N-(polye thylene glycol)-folic acid)/DSPE-PEG-COOH with mannitol and leucine. Exposure of docetaxel-loaded formulation after intratracheal administration resulted in a longer

$t_{1/2}$ and more sustainable therapeutic effect when compared with free drug. Therefore, liposome combined with commonly used carrier, bulk agent as mannitol, lactose or trehalose for inhaled dry powders production, could be used for further clinical trials to achieve higher drug co-localization and enhance drug diffusion for systemic delivery after inhalation.

13.6.2 Proliposomes for Pulmonary Delivery

Proliposomes are dry, free-flowing powders, composed of lipid component and an active pharmaceutical ingredient (API), which forms multilamellar vesicles upon hydration with an aqueous solution.[68–70] Proliposomes have higher stability profiles than other lipid solutions/suspensions because they are collected and stored in dry conditions. Because proliposomes are in dry powder form, they facilitate product transfer and storage, lowering the costs that would otherwise be required. Unlike liposomes in bulk micro/nanoparticles, proliposomes go through a fast and easy hydration step under temperature and agitation control to produce liposome structure. Proliposomes are easily hydrated in the aqueous environment of the lungs and exert their action locally or, if necessary, can be rapidly absorbed and enter the systemic circulation without the need of mannitol or trehalose carriers. The technology is based on the inherent ability of hydrated membrane lipids to form vesicles when exposed to water (Figure 13.5). The phospholipids are layered onto a finely divided particulate support, resulting in the formation of dry powders. When the dry powders are hydrated with an aqueous solution and gently mixed, the phospholipids on the solid support disperse rapidly, resulting in a liposomal suspension in an aqueous solution. Liposomes can be formed *in vivo* under physiological fluids or *in vitro* before using a suitable hydrating fluid. Several research groups have used this one-step process to produce liposomes or microparticles for lung delivery of very diverse agents and phospholipids.

Lung surfactants 1,2-dipalmitoyl-sn-glycero-3-phosphocholine (DPPC) and 1,2-d ipalmitoyl-sn-glycero-3-phosphoglycerol, sodium salt (DPPG) have been used for proliposome formulation at the same physiology ratio of 3:1.[71–73] Gomez et al.[74] developed and characterized inhalable proliposomal microparticles/nanoparticles of antifungal amphotericin B (AmB) by spray drying technique. Aerosolization of formulations showed higher local drug deposition *in vitro* (Figure 13.6), particularly in the small

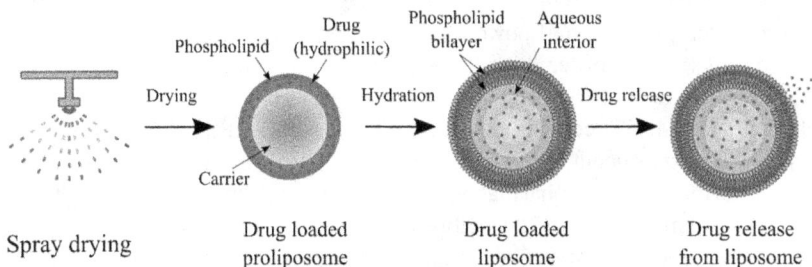

FIGURE 13.5   Proliposome synthesis and the mechanism of drug release.

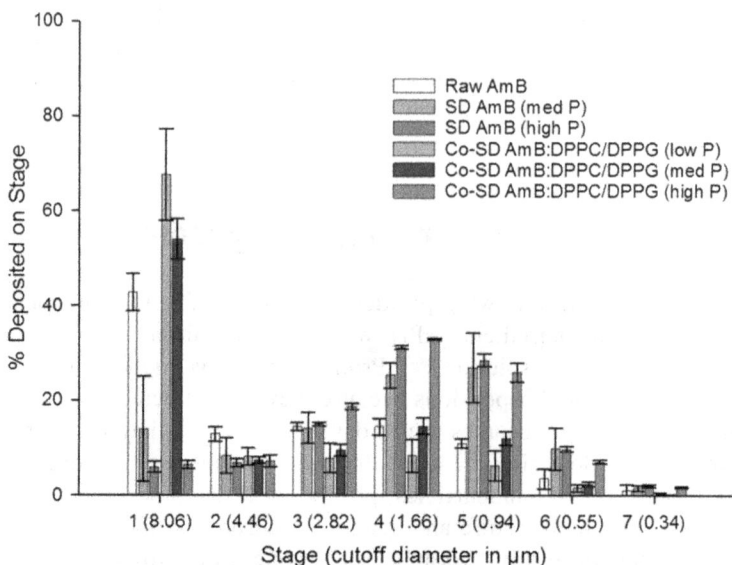

FIGURE 13.6 *In vitro* aerosol dispersion performance using the NGI® under an airflow rate (Q) of 60 L/min with the HandiHaler® human DPI device for SD AmB powders and Co-SD AmB:DPPC/DPPG (n=3, mean±SD). Different spray drying pump rates chosen for the preparation of spray dried and co-spray dried powders were: low P- 15 mL/min; med P- 22.5 mL/min; high P- 30 mL/min. Adapted with permission from Ref.[74] Copyright (2020 Elsevier).

airways and alveolar regions (lower stages) in the next generation impactor (NGI) compared to the aerosol performance of drugs without phospholipids (Fine particle fraction (FPF)=46.8 ± 5.4%). In another study, zwitterionic DSPE in combination with DPPC were used to prepare cisplatin proliposomes[75]; the addition of PEGylated excipients to the lipid fraction of these dry powder formulations was demonstrated to be feasible, potentially giving cisplatin-loaded proliposomes stealth abilities against macrophages. Furthermore, localized administration of controlled-release cisplatin at high doses, combined with appropriate deposition in the deeper lung, has the potential to improve treatment efficiency.[75] Furthermore, lecithin is also used in the production of proliposome. Adel et al.[76] used lecithin and cholesterol as lipids for the preparation of curcumin-loaded proliposomal powders for lung delivery. The optimized formulation composed of 1:1:1 ratio of lecithin:cholesterol:stearylamine and 1 g of hydroxypropyl beta-cyclodextrin as a carrier, showed an enhanced aerosolization performance with a higher FPF of 54.35% compared to curcumin powder (FPF- 16.35%). Cytotoxicity studies showed a significant reduction of proinflammatory cytokines compared to pure curcumin. Further, the lung pharmacokinetic studies confirmed the superiority of proliposomal curcumin (C_{max}- 5052.4 ng.h/mL) over curcumin drug alone (C_{max}- 1232.5 ng.h/mL). Therefore, combining a therapeutic molecule with a properly chosen lipid moiety, carrier, and technique may be an excellent strategy for creating proliposomes with good aerodynamic properties.

13.7 ENGINEERING OF PHOSPHOLIPID MICROPARTICULATE DRY POWDER FORMULATIONS

Liposomes and proliposomes for inhalation can be made using a variety of approaches. The preparation method affects many factors, including vesicle size, size distribution, encapsulation capability, and content retention. The choice of a method is based on the physicochemical properties of the drug, the desired type of phospholipid(s), the particle size range, and the ease of preparation. An ideal preparation method should use as little organic solvent as possible, avoid prolonged mechanical stress, use low temperature and pressure, be reproducible and economical, yield a high drug/lipid ratio, and be adaptable for future use. Various delivery systems have been designed, developed, and studied, for the treatment of lung diseases, such as pressurized MDIs (pMDIs), SMIs, DPIs, and nebulizers.[77,78] Because of their better physicochemical stability and ability to deliver the drug into the deeper lung compartments using the patient's respiration, DPIs are the preferred platform for inhalation therapy.

DPIs for targeted pulmonary delivery are appealing because they offer several advantages over liquids, including increased solid-state stability, reduced systemic side effects, and higher local lung-specific levels in the lung for various pulmonary conditions. In addition, when compared to immediate dissolution systems, controlled-release drug delivery may offer additional benefits such as reduced side effects, greater convenience, and higher patient compliance due to a simplified dosage schedule.[79] However, the effectiveness of clearance mechanisms in the respiratory tract (mucociliary clearance, phagocytosis by macrophages) made it challenging to develop adequate controlled-release preparations.[80,81]

For pulmonary drug delivery, solid lipid particles can be produced by spray freeze drying, spray drying, freeze-drying, supercritical fluid (SCF) technologies (CO_2), etc. (Figure 13.7)[53,82–84] and some formulations produced by these methods are listed in Table 13.2.

13.7.1 Spray Drying

Spray drying has been utilized in the pharmaceutical industry since the early 20th century when it was employed for drying blood. It has been used in a variety of pharmaceutical applications such as the formation of amorphous solid dispersions, the encapsulation of drugs and essential oils in excipient matrices, and the spray drying of biopharmaceuticals (e.g., proteins, vaccines, deoxyribonucleic acid (DNA), antibodies).[87,106]

Spray drying is a one-step drying procedure that uses less energy and is more cost-effective than freeze-drying. Compared to a dry cake generated by the freeze-drying process, spray drying creates a fine powder with superior aerosolization. As a result, spray drying is employed in various industries, including pharmaceuticals, food, and cosmetics.[107] Spray drying also enables the engineering of particles with

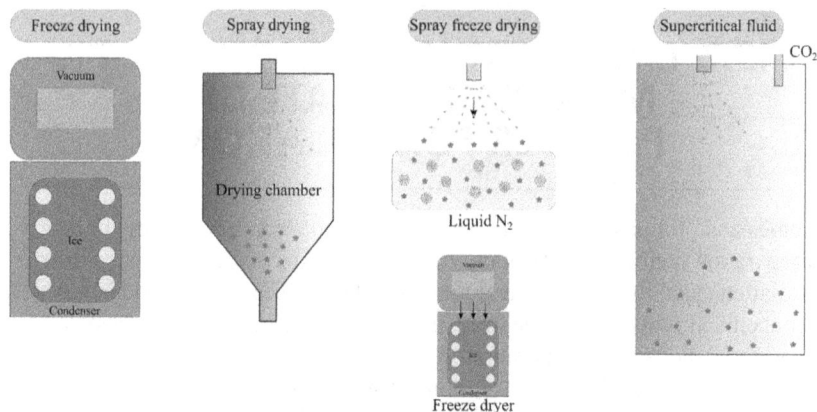

FIGURE 13.7   Illustration of techniques for dry liposome production.

desired size, shape, morphology, and surface texture for improved aerosolization performance and the large-scale manufacture of powders with excellent batch-to-batch reproducibility.[108–110]

The creation of inhalable dry powder liposomes has been examined utilizing freeze-drying of liposomes in the presence of a cryoprotectant followed by micronization; however, milling may negatively affect vesicle stability drug leakage upon rehydration. Spray-drying of liposomes distributed in carbohydrate solutions has been examined as an alternative to freeze-drying (lyophilization), with good powder "respirability" observed in several investigations.[111] The spray drying process consists of three basic steps: liquid feed atomization, dehydration, and powder collection. The feed solution (including lipid base, drug and carrier) is atomized into small droplets by a nozzle into the main drying chamber. The fine mist of liquid droplets dehydrates fast as it passes through the drying chamber with heated air, producing dry powder particles.[112]

Proliposome formulations for inhalation have been created as an alternative to standard liposome powders. Proliposomes can use diluted carbohydrate carriers coated with phospholipids that form liposomes when combined with an aqueous phase. In the context of this chapter, proliposomes are phospholipid and drug blends with carbohydrate carriers to generate liposomes upon contact with the pulmonary physiological fluid. Sugar carriers are commonly avoided in the process. Gomez et al.[74] developed and characterized inhalable proliposomal microparticles/nanoparticles of antifungal amphotericin B by spray drying technique without a sugar carrier. Proliposomes feed solution consisted of lipids (DPPC and DPPG,1:3) and were formulated using a range of lipid-to-drug ratios. The resultant proliposome powders showed smooth surface and spherical morphology (Figure 13.8) with a geometric size range of 1.10 μm–1.31 μm. Particles were thoroughly characterized using a next-generation impactor (NGI), the drug's deposition was assessed following proliposome delivery from an FDA-approved human DPI. Aerosolization of formulations showed high local drug deposition *in vitro*, particularly in the small airways and alveolar regions (lower stages) in the NGI with 46% FPF, 93.6% RF and 2.2 μm MMAD.

TABLE 13.2   Developed liposomes formulations with phospholipids in lung delivery.

PHOSPHOLIPID	DRUG	TECHNIQUE	REFERENCE
Soy lecithin (Phosphatidylcholines 8–20% content)	Sorafenib tosylate	Spray drying	[66]
	Itraconazole	Spray drying	[85]
	Rifapentine	Spray drying	[86]
	Salbutamol sulphate	Spray drying	[87]
	Curcumin	Spray drying	[76]
	Ciprofloxacin	Spray-freeze dry	[65]
	Clarithromycin	Spray-freeze dry	[88]
	Insulin	Spray-freeze dry	[89]
	Budesonide	Freeze-dry	[90]
	Budesonide	Freeze-dry	[91]
	Bovine serum albumin	Supercritical fluid	[92]
	Lutein	Supercritical fluid	[93]
	Berberine HCl	Supercritical fluid	[94]
1,2-Distearoyl-sn-glycero -3-phosphorylethanol amine (DSPE)	Docetaxel	Spray drying	[67]
	Cisplatin	Spray drying	[75]
	Beclomethasone dipropionate	Freeze-dry	[95]
1,2-dipalmitoyl-sn- glycero-3- phosphatidylcholine (DPPC)	Vancomycin and clarithromycin	Spray drying	[96]
	Pyrazinamide	Spray drying	[97,98]
	Moxifloxacin	Spray drying	[98]
	Combination of pyrazinamide and moxifloxacin	Spray drying	[99]
	Paclitaxel	Spray drying	[100,101]
	Tacrolimus	Spray drying	[102]
	Amphotericin B	Spray drying	[74]
	Erlotinib	Freeze-dry	[103]
1,2-Distearoyl-sn-glycero -3-phospho-rac-glycerol, sodium salt (DSPG)	Gemcitabine HCl	Freeze-dry	[104]
	Amphotericin B	Freeze-dry	[105]

13.7.2 Spray Freeze-Drying

Spray freeze-drying method (SFD) is recommended over traditional spray-drying or freeze-drying (FD) as a method for easing the development of dosage forms for alternate distribution paths for a variety of reasons. First, SFD approaches can improve the apparent solubility of weakly water-soluble pharmaceuticals, which is a common issue

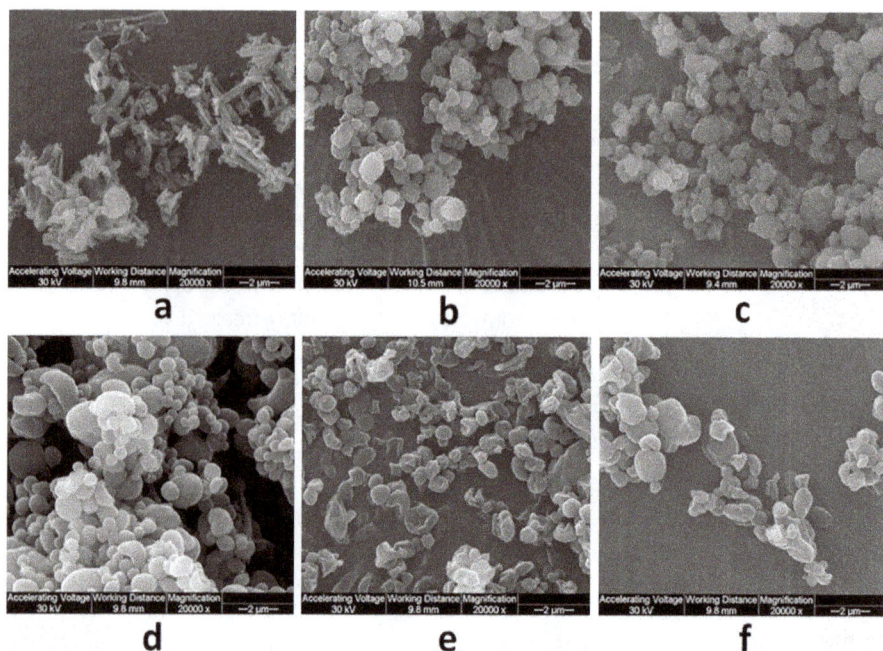

FIGURE 13.8 Scanning electron microscopy images of raw AmB, SD Particles, and co-SD particles: (a) raw amphotericin B (AmB); (b) SD AmB (med P); (c) SD AmB (high P), (d) co-SD AmB:DPPC/DPPG (low P); (e) co-SD AmB:DPPC/DPPG (med P); and (f) co-SD AmB:DPPC/DPPG (high P). Magnifications for all micrographs were 20,000x. Different spray drying pump rates chosen for the preparation of spray dried and co-spray dried powders were: low P- 15 mL/min; med P- 22.5 mL/min; high P- 30 mL/min. Adapted with permission from Ref.[74] Copyright (2020 Elsevier).

with freshly developed API. Furthermore, the drug is embedded amorphously in the excipient due to an ultra-fast freezing process, reducing the potential of phase separation between the drug and excipients and resulting in a molecular distribution of the drug in the excipient material. The main advantage of the SD procedure is the generation of defined and powdery particle shapes; however, heat can destroy loaded active chemicals. Although the FD technique is ideal for storing thermolabile chemicals, it is time-intensive and, depending on the nature of the ingredients, the final products dry cake shape can be very hygroscopic. The technique of SFD involves three important steps: atomization, freezing and FD.[113] Atomization is the first step when the prepared feed solution is converted into spherical droplets via an atomizer. The freezing and FD processes are then done to solidify the droplets with a cryogenic agent (or cold fluid) and sublimate the ice at low temperatures and pressure.[114] The particle size, particle morphology, density, and porosity of the final product following SFD have been observed to vary depending on the kind of atomizer, freezing period, and the composition and concentration of the feed solution.

The droplets are supercooled by liquid nitrogen, which facilitates small ice crystals, which are then sublimated at low temperatures and pressures. Sublimation produces a product with a high porosity feature. The amount of solids in the feed solution is also critical for maintaining the shape of the produced droplets particles.[115] Ye et al.[88] synthesize liposomes using soybean phosphatidylcholine (SPC) by the thin lipid film hydration technique for clarithromycin lung delivery. To improve their aerosolization performance as dry powder formulation, liposomal engineering by ultrasonic SFD with two different bulk carriers, mannitol and sucrose as co-cryoprotectants, was carried. The formulation featured a porous structure with micronsized particles and good drug recovery. Co-cryoprotectants may be able to prevent liposomal powder from absorbing moisture. NGI data suggest a good lung deposition after aerosolization with emitted dose > 85% and fine particle fraction in the range of 43%–50%. SFD, as opposed to FD, enables the creation of flowable powders with varying particle sizes and densities ideal for nasal, pulmonary (low density), and needle-free epidermal applications (high density).

13.7.3 Freeze Drying

This is one of the most extensively utilized methods for improving the long-term stability of liposomes and preventing the degradation of sensitive compounds enclosed in the liposome structure.[116] The removal of water via the freeze-drying process, on the other hand, may have various negative impacts on the liposomes, including changes in vesicle size, loss of membrane integrity, loss of the encapsulated material, and changes in rheological properties. The formation of liposome bilayers is generated by the interaction of water molecules with the hydrophilic head groups of phospholipids.[117]

By replacing water and forming hydrogen bonds, stabilizers can guard against these changes during freezing (cryoprotectants) and lyophilization (lyoprotectants).[118] The formation of liposome bilayers is generated by the interaction of water molecules with the hydrophilic head groups of phospholipids. Furthermore, excipients can generate a glassy matrix, reducing phospholipid mobility in a solid dosage form[119]; among the most commonly employed cryoprotectants are trehalose, dextran, mannitol, glycerine, PEG, and others.[117] Liposome FD typically consists of three steps: freezing of the liposome solution, primary drying (sublimation), and secondary drying (desorption). Freezing is a critical phase in determining the ice nucleation process and the shape of the frozen materials. Primary drying removes most of the free water through sublimation, whereas secondary drying removes the bound water, resulting in low residual water content of the freeze-dried cakes.[120]

Investigations are still necessary to improve the liposome lyophilization, optimizing the formulation and technological parameters to improve the lyoprotective impact. The lipid composition of the bilayer is a prerequisite for determining the protective effect for lyoprotectants, the addition of cholesterol can reduce encapsulated solvent leak and vesicle adding/fusion, vesicle size and cryoprotective distribution on two sides of the two layers have an effect.[121,122]

The researchers used DPPC phospholipid for liposome synthesis using a thin-film hydration standard approach and another freeze-dried process with mannitol as a cryoprotectant to generate a free-flowing powder. Erlotinib freeze-dried liposomal powder was manually combined with inhalable grade lactose at various molar ratios to create a DPI. Twin Stage Impinger examined in vitro lung deposition, revealing a percent ED and a percent FPF of 79% and 39%, respectively. The pharmacodynamic efficacy of this DPI formulation was subsequently assessed using an in-vivo hypoxic model of PH. Studies *in vivo* lung biodistribution showed that the pulmonary formulation for erlotinib liposomal DPI administered by pulmonary delivery was better biodistributed than oral administration. The direct distribution of drug in target tissue through the pulmonary route was attributed to this increased deposition of the medicament into the lungs. This delivery on-site causes the formulation to immediately enter lung tissue and the drugs permanent release.[103]

13.7.4 Supercritical Anti-Solvent Technique

Traditional liposome preparation methods, such as thin-film hydration or ethanol injection, have numerous drawbacks, including poor monodispersion, poor stability, excessive residual organic solvent, and side effects.[123]

Liposomes made using the SCF CO_2 method had higher intactness, sphericity, and uniformity than liposomes made using the thin film hydration approach. Moreover, one of the most SCF techniques used is the supercritical antisolvent (SAS) technology. Phospholipid is coated on the surface of sugar moiety, generating a thin layer that when hydrated yields multilamellar liposomes.

Phospholipid aggregates can be processed into nano/microparticles using dense phase CO_2. Their properties can be modified by adjusting the processing parameters. The size of the resultant liposomes is determined by the rate of decompression and the opening diameter of the nozzle.[124,125]

In addition to the crucial temperature and pressure, SCF uses ethylene, methanol, and carbon dioxide. A liquids critical temperature is when the vapor is not liquidated, regardless of the pressure. At its critical temperature, the pressure required to condense a gas defines its critical pressure. SCF shows the appropriate gas and liquid characteristics, including gas penetration and liquid solubility. Supercritical fluid deposition (SCFD) is a versatile approach that can change the density of SCF and the solubility of a solute by varying the pressures and temperatures employed. The organic solvent is separated from supercritical CO_2 using a separator. On the filter, the produced phospholipids are collected.

Karn et al.[126] prepared multilamellar liposomal for delivery of cyclosporine A by SCF CO_2 technique. Soybean phosphatidylcholine, lactose and cyclosporine A were dissolved in ethanol, a syringe pump delivered supercritical CO_2 to the suspension vessel. The reaction vessel conditions were studied at temperatures ranging from 35 °C to 50 °C and pressures ranging from 8 to 25 MPa. After around 30 minutes of stirring at equilibrium to wash out any leftover solvent. The vessel was then gradually depressurized to atmospheric pressure, and liposomes formed a thin coating on the surface of the lactose particles. The present work shows that the SCF-CO_2 approach allows the manufacture of liposomes with typically lower size and better morphology, combined with improved entrapment efficiency (%EE) and drug loading (%DL) (uniform in size and shape).

13.8 CONCLUSION

Among the various excipients approved to use in the inhalation formulations, phospholipids are endogenous and generally regarded as safer (GRAS) excipients for inhalation administration. They are biocompatible, biodegradable and well tolerated by the lower airways. Phospholipids are used as the main components in the liposomal formulations. Liposomes in DPI formulated with endogenous lung surfactants (e.g. liposomes and proliposomes) offer a unique advantage in pulmonary nanomedicine delivery while offering controlled release and improved stability. A large number of versatile liposomes are designed and developed using phospholipids and investigated as drug delivery carriers for treating various lung diseases. The FDA-approved inhalation products composed of phospholipids are: Arikace™ (Insmed), an amikacin liposome suspension to treat *Mycobacterium avium* infection in adults, Inbrija® (Acorda Therapeutics, Inc.) to deliver levodopa dry powder for patients with Parkinson's disease, and TOBI® Podhaler™ (Novartis), an antibacterial aminoglycoside indicated for the management of cystic fibrosis patients with Pseudomonas aeruginosa. Further, dry liposomes have the potential to be effective drug carriers with improved stability, bioavailability, and solubility of poorly soluble drugs. Furthermore, phospholipids have been used as particle engineering excipients to design particles with very low density and improve aerosolization behavior. For example, in PulmoSpheres™ technology, the particles are produced by spray drying of an emulsion composed of phospholipids which hinder the coalescence when the droplet shrinks due to the evaporation of the continuous phase.

REFERENCES

1. Forum of International Respiratory Societies. *The global impact of respiratory disease.* 2nd edn. Sheffield: European Respiratory Society, 2017.
2. Chronic Obstructive Pulmonary Disease (COPD). World Health Organization (2021). https://www.who.int/news-room/fact-sheets/detail/chronic-obstructive-pulmonary-disease-(copd).
3. Asthma. World Health Organization (2021). https://www.who.int/news-room/fact-sheets/detail/asthma.
4. Global Tuberculosis Report 2020. World Health Organization (2020). https://www.who.int/teams/global-tuberculosis-programme/tb-reports/global-tuberculosis-report-2020.
5. Guadagno, A. World lung cancer day 2019: Facts & figures. *Cure,* (2019). https://www.curetoday.com/view/world-lung-cancer-day-2019-facts--figures.
6. WHO. Coronavirus Disease (COVID-19) Dashboard: World Health Organization, (2021). Website: https://covid19.who.int/.
7. Ungaro, F. & Vanbever, R. Improving the efficacy of inhaled drugs for severe lung diseases: Emerging pulmonary delivery strategies. *Adv. Drug Deliv. Rev.* 75, 1–2 (2014).
8. Eedara, B.B. *et al.* Inhalation delivery for the treatment and prevention of COVID-19 infection. *Pharmaceutics* 13(7), 1077 (2021).

9. Rau, J.L. The inhalation of drugs: Advantages and problems. *Respir. Care* 50(3), 367–382 (2005).

10. Eedara, B.B., Tucker, I.G. & Das, S.C. In vitro dissolution testing of respirable size antitubercular drug particles using a small volume dissolution apparatus. *Int. J. Pharm.* 559, 235–244 (2019).

11. Rangnekar, B., Momin, M.A.M., Eedara, B.B., Sinha, S. & Das, S.C. Bedaquiline containing triple combination powder for inhalation to treat drug-resistant tuberculosis. *Int. J. Pharm.* 570, 118689 (2019).

12. Eedara, B.B. *et al.* Crystalline adduct of moxifloxacin with trans-cinnamic acid to reduce the aqueous solubility and dissolution rate for improved residence time in the lungs. *Eur. J. Pharm. Sci.* 136, 104961 (2019).

13. Muralidharan, P. *et al.* Design and comprehensive characterization of tetramethylpyrazine (TMP) for targeted lung delivery as inhalation aerosols in pulmonary hypertension (PH): In vitro human lung cell culture and in vivo efficacy. *Antioxidants (Basel)* 10(3), 427 (2021).

14. Eedara, B.B. *et al.* Chapter 7: Pulmonary drug delivery. In *Organelle and molecular targeting,* (eds. L.S. Milane & M.M. Amiji) 227–278 (Boca Raton, FL: CRC Press, 2022). ISBN 9781003092773

15. Hickey, A.J. & Mansour, H.M. *Modern pharmaceutics*, Vol. 2, 5th edn. (eds. A.T. Florence & J. Siepmann) 191–219 (New York: Taylor and Francis, Inc, 2009).

16. Acosta, M.F. *et al.* Advanced therapeutic inhalation aerosols of a Nrf2 activator and RhoA/Rho kinase (ROCK) inhibitor for targeted pulmonary drug delivery in pulmonary hypertension: Design, characterization, aerosolization, in vitro 2D/3D human lung cell cultures, and in vivo efficacy. *Ther. Adv. Respir. Dis.* 15, 1753466621998245 (2021).

17. Xu, Z., Mansour, H.M. & Hickey, A.J. Particle interactions in dry powder inhaler unit processes: A review. *J. Adhes. Sci. Technol.* 25(4–5), 451–482 (2011).

18. Rogliani, P. *et al.* Optimizing drug delivery in COPD: The role of inhaler devices. *Respir. Med.* 124, 6–14 (2017).

19. Zillen, D., Beugeling, M., Hinrichs, W.L.J., Frijlink, H.W. & Grasmeijer, F. Natural and bioinspired excipients for dry powder inhalation formulations. *Curr. Opin. Colloid Interface Sci.* 56, 101497 (2021).

20. Pilcer, G. & Amighi, K. Formulation strategy and use of excipients in pulmonary drug delivery. *Int. J. Pharm.* 392(1–2), 1–19 (2010).

21. Weibel, E.R. Morphological basis of alveolar-capillary gas exchange. *Physiol. Rev.* 53(2), 419–495 (1973).

22. Garcia-Mouton, C., Hidalgo, A., Cruz, A. & Pérez-Gil, J. The lord of the lungs: The essential role of pulmonary surfactant upon inhalation of nanoparticles. *Eur. J. Pharm. Biopharm.* 144, 230–243 (2019).

23. Parra, E. & Pérez-Gil, J. Composition, structure and mechanical properties define performance of pulmonary surfactant membranes and films. *Chem. Phys. Lipids* 185, 153–175 (2015).

24. Lopez-Rodriguez, E. & Pérez-Gil, J. Structure-function relationships in pulmonary surfactant membranes: From biophysics to therapy. *Biochim. Biophys. Acta Rev. Biomembr.* 1838(6), 1568–1585 (2014).

25. Perez-Gil, J. & Weaver, T.E. Pulmonary surfactant pathophysiology: Current models and open questions. *Physiol.* 25(3), 132–141 (2010).

26. Orgeig, S. *et al.* Recent advances in alveolar biology: Evolution and function of alveolar proteins. *Respir. Physiol. Neurobiol.* 173, S43–S54 (2010).

27. Serrano, A.G. & Pérez-Gil, J. Protein–lipid interactions and surface activity in the pulmonary surfactant system. *Chem. Phys. Lipids* 141(1–2), 105–118 (2006).

28. Pérez-Gil, J. Structure of pulmonary surfactant membranes and films: The role of proteins and lipid–protein interactions. *Biochim. Biophys. Acta Rev. Biomembr.* 1778(7–8), 1676–1695 (2008).

29. Bernhard, W. Lung surfactant: Function and composition in the context of development and respiratory physiology. *Ann. Anat.* 208, 146–150 (2016).

30. Li, J. *et al.* A review on phospholipids and their main applications in drug delivery systems. *Asian J. Pharm. Sci.* 10(2), 81–98 (2015).

31. van Meer, G., Voelker, D.R. & Feigenson, G.W. Membrane lipids: Where they are and how they behave. *Nat. Rev. Mol. Cell Biol.* 9(2), 112–124 (2008).

32. Notter, R.H. *Lung surfactants: Basic science and clinical applications.* (Boca Raton, FL: CRC Press, 2000).

33. Wauthoz, N. & Amighi, K. Phospholipids in pulmonary drug delivery. *Eur. J. Lipid Sci. Technol.* 116(9), 1114–1128 (2014).

34. Yeates, D.B. Chapter 21: Surfactant aerosol therapy for nRDS and ARDS. In *Inhalation aerosols* (eds. A.J. Hickey & H.M. Mansour) 327–342 (Boca Raton, FL: CRC Press, 2019). ISBN 9781315159768

35. Jeenakeri, R. & Drayton, M. Management of respiratory distress syndrome. *Paediatr. Child Health* 19(4), 158–164 (2009).

36. Mansour, H.M., Droopad, D. & Ledford, J.G. Chapter 20: Overview of lung surfactant and respiratory distress syndrome. In *Inhalation aerosols*, (eds. A.J. Hickey & H.M. Mansour) 323–326 (Boca Raton, FL: CRC Press, 2019). ISBN 9781315159768

37. Walther, F.J., Hernández-Juviel, J.M., Gordon, L.M. & Waring, A.J. Synthetic surfactant containing SP-B and SP-C mimics is superior to single-peptide formulations in rabbits with chemical acute lung injury. *PeerJ* 2, e393 (2014).

38. Schürch, D., Ospina, O.L., Cruz, A. & Pérez-Gil, J. Combined and independent action of proteins SP-B and SP-C in the surface behavior and mechanical stability of pulmonary surfactant films. *Biophys. J.* 99(10), 3290–3299 (2010).

39. Spragg, R.G. *et al.* Recombinant surfactant protein C-based surfactant for patients with severe direct lung injury. *Am. J. Respir. Crit. Care Med.* 183(8), 1055–1061 (2011).

40. Seehase, M. *et al.* New surfactant with SP-B and C analogs gives survival benefit after inactivation in preterm lambs. *PLOS ONE* 7(10), e47631 (2012).

41. Silvius, J.R. Thermotropic phase transitions of pure lipids in model membranes and their modifications by membrane proteins. *Lipid-Protein Interact.* 2, 239–281 (1982).

42. Chen, J. *et al.* Influence of lipid composition on the phase transition temperature of liposomes composed of both DPPC and HSPC. *Drug Dev. Ind. Pharm.* 39(2), 197–204 (2013).

43. Weers, J.G. & Miller, D.P. Formulation design of dry powders for inhalation. *J. Pharm. Sci.* 104(10), 3259–3288 (2015).

44. Cuvelier, B. *et al.* Minimal amounts of dipalmitoylphosphatidylcholine improve aerosol performance of spray-dried temocillin powders for inhalation. *Int. J. Pharm.* 495(2), 981–990 (2015).

45. Chew, N.Y. *et al.* Effect of amino acids on the dispersion of disodium cromoglycate powders. *J. Pharm. Sci.* 94(10), 2289–2300 (2005).

46. Lechuga-Ballesteros, D. *et al.* Trileucine improves aerosol performance and stability of spray-dried powders for inhalation. *J. Pharm. Sci.* 97(1), 287–302 (2008).

47. Lucas, P., Anderson, K., Potter, U.J. & Staniforth, J.N. Enhancement of small particle size dry powder aerosol formulations using an ultra low density additive. *Pharm. Res.* 16(10), 1643 (1999).

48. Ganguly, S. *et al.* Phospholipid-induced in vivo particle migration to enhance pulmonary deposition. *J. Aerosol Med. Pulm. Drug Deliv.* 21(4), 343–350 (2008).

49. Mansour, H., Wang, D.-S., Chen, C.-S. & Zografi, G. Comparison of bilayer and monolayer properties of phospholipid systems containing dipalmitoylphosphatidylglycerol and dipalmitoylphosphatidylinositol. *Langmuir* 17(21), 6622–6632 (2001).

50. McShane, P.J. *et al.* Ciprofloxacin dry powder for inhalation (ciprofloxacin DPI): Technical design and features of an efficient drug–device combination. *Pulm. Pharmacol. Ther.* 50, 72–79 (2018).

51. Inactive ingredient search for approved drug products. U.S. FDA and Drug Administration. https://www.accessdata.fda.gov/scripts/cder/IIG/index.cfm?event=BasicSearch.page.

52. Yu, S. *et al.* Inhalable liposomal powder formulations for co-delivery of synergistic ciprofloxacin and colistin against multi-drug resistant gram-negative lung infections. *Int. J. Pharm.* 575, 118915 (2020).

53. Gradon, L. & Sosnowski, T.R. Formation of particles for dry powder inhalers. *Adv. Powder Technol.* 25(1), 43–55 (2014).

54. Willis, L., Hayes, D. & Mansour, H.M. Therapeutic liposomal dry powder inhalation aerosols for targeted lung delivery. *Lung* 190(3), 251–262 (2012).

55. Cipolla, D., Gonda, I. & Chan, H.-K. Liposomal formulations for inhalation. *Ther. Deliv.* 4(8), 1047–1072 (2013).

56. Standsfield, M. & Yadidi, K. Advancing Asprihale® to pivotal PK/PD study. *ONdrugDelivery*, 106, 54–55 (2020).

57. van Hoogevest, P., Tiemessen, H., Metselaar, J.M., Drescher, S. & Fahr, A. The use of phospholipids to make pharmaceutical form line Extensions. *Eur. J. Lipid Sci. Technol.* 123(4), 2000297 (2021).

58. Muralidharan, P., Mallory, E., Malapit, M., Hayes, D. & Mansour, H.M. Inhalable pegylated phospholipid nanocarriers and pegylated therapeutics for respiratory delivery as aerosolized colloidal dispersions and dry powder inhalers. *Pharmaceutics* 6(2), 333–353 (2014).

59. van der Meel, R. *et al.* Extracellular vesicles as drug delivery systems: Lessons from the liposome field. *J. Control. Release* 195, 72–85 (2014).

60. Rideau, E., Dimova, R., Schwille, P., Wurm, F.R. & Landfester, K. Liposomes and polymersomes: A comparative review towards cell mimicking. *Chem. Soc. Rev.* 47(23), 8572–8610 (2018).

61. Tagami, T. & Ozeki, T. Recent trends in clinical trials related to carrier-based drugs. *J. Pharm. Sci.* 106(9), 2219–2226 (2017).

62. He, H. *et al.* Adapting liposomes for oral drug delivery. *Acta Pharm. Sin. B* 9(1), 36–48 (2019).

63. Mehta, P.P., Ghoshal, D., Pawar, A.P., Kadam, S.S. & Dhapte-Pawar, V.S. Recent advances in inhalable liposomes for treatment of pulmonary diseases: Concept to clinical stance. *J. Drug Deliv. Sci. Technol.* 56, 101509 (2020).

64. Badens, E., Magnan, C. & Charbit, G. Microparticles of soy lecithin formed by supercritical processes. *Biotechnol. Bioeng.* 72(2), 194–204 (2001).

65. Tran, T.-T. *et al.* An evaluation of inhaled antibiotic liposome versus antibiotic nanoplex in controlling infection in bronchiectasis. *Int. J. Pharm.* 559, 382–392 (2019).

66. Patel, K., Bothiraja, C., Mali, A. & Kamble, R. Investigation of sorafenib tosylate loaded liposomal dry powder inhaler for the treatment of non-small cell lung cancer. *Part. Sci. Technol.* 39(8), 1–10 (2021).

67. Zhu, X. *et al.* Inhalable dry powder prepared from folic acid-conjugated docetaxel liposomes alters pharmacodynamic and pharmacokinetic properties relevant to lung cancer chemotherapy. *Pulm. Pharmacol. Ther.* 55, 50–61 (2019).

68. Gangishetty, H., Eedara, B.B. & Bandari, S. Development of ketoprofen loaded proliposomal powders for improved gastric absorption and gastric tolerance: In vitro and in situ evaluation. *Pharm. Dev. Technol.* 20(6), 641–651 (2015).

69. Mansour, H.M., Rhee, Y.-S., Park, C.-W. & DeLuca, P.P. Chapter 9: Lipid nanoparticulate drug delivery and nanomedicine. In *Lipids in nanotechnology* (ed. M.U. Ahmad) 221–268 (Urbana, IL: AOCS Press, 2012).

70. Nalla, P., Bagam, S., Eedara, B.B. & Dhurke, R. Formulation and evaluation of domperidone oral proliposomal powders. *Int. J. Pharm. Tech. Res.* 7, 108–118 (2015).

71. Duan, J., Vogt, F.G., Li, X., Hayes Jr, D. & Mansour, H.M. Design, characterization, and aerosolization of organic solution advanced spray-dried moxifloxacin and ofloxacin dipalmitoylphosphatidylcholine (DPPC) microparticulate/nanoparticulate powders for pulmonary inhalation aerosol delivery. *Int. J. Nanomedicine* 8, 3489 (2013).

72. Wu, X., Zhang, W., Hayes Jr, D. & Mansour, H.M. Physicochemical characterization and aerosol dispersion performance of organic solution advanced spray-dried cyclosporine A multifunctional particles for dry powder inhalation aerosol delivery. *Int. J. Nanomedicine* 8, 1269 (2013).

73. Meenach, S.A. *et al.* Design, physicochemical characterization, and optimization of organic solution advanced spray-dried inhalable dipalmitoylphosphatidylcholine (DPPC) and dipalmitoylphosphatidylethanolamine poly (ethylene glycol)(DPPE-PEG) microparticles and nanoparticles for targeted respiratory nanomedicine delivery as dry powder inhalation aerosols. *Int. J. Nanomedicine* 8, 275 (2013).

74. Gomez, A.I. *et al.* Advanced spray dried proliposomes of amphotericin B lung surfactant-mimic phospholipid microparticles/nanoparticles as dry powder inhalers for targeted pulmonary drug delivery. *Pulm. Pharmacol. Ther.* 64, 101975 (2020).

75. Levet, V. *et al.* Development of controlled-release cisplatin dry powders for inhalation against lung cancers. *Int. J. Pharm.* 515(1–2), 209–220 (2016).

76. Adel, I.M. *et al.* Design and characterization of spray-dried proliposomes for the pulmonary delivery of curcumin. *Int. J. Nanomedicine* 16, 2667 (2021).

77. Sorino, C., Negri, S., Spanevello, A., Visca, D. & Scichilone, N. Inhalation therapy devices for the treatment of obstructive lung diseases: The history of inhalers towards the ideal inhaler. *Eur. J. Intern. Med.* 75, 15–18 (2020).

78. Labiris, N.R. & Dolovich, M.B. Pulmonary drug delivery. Part II: the role of inhalant delivery devices and drug formulations in therapeutic effectiveness of aerosolized medications. *Br. J. Clin. Pharmacol.* 56(6), 600–612 (2003).

79. Liang, Z., Ni, R., Zhou, J. & Mao, S. Recent advances in controlled pulmonary drug delivery. *Drug Discov. Today* 20(3), 380–389 (2015).

80. Bustamante-Marin, X.M. & Ostrowski, L.E. Cilia and mucociliary clearance. *Cold Spring Harb. Perspect. Biol.* 9(4), a028241 (2017).

81. Janssen, W.J., Stefanski, A.L., Bochner, B.S. & Evans, C.M. Control of lung defence by mucins and macrophages: Ancient defence mechanisms with modern functions. *Eur. Respir. J.* 48(4), 1201–1214 (2016).

82. Eedara, B.B., Encinas-Basurto, D., Alabsi, W., Polt, R. & Mansour, H.M. Applications of surface analytical techniques in characterization of dry powder formulations. *Inhalation* 1–9 (2021).

83. Muralidharan, P., Malapit, M., Mallory, E., Hayes, D. & Mansour, H.M. Inhalable nanoparticulate powders for respiratory delivery. *Nanomed. Nanotechnol. Biol. Med.* 11(5), 1189–1199 (2015).

84. Li, X., Vogt, F.G., Hayes Jr, D. & Mansour, H.M. Design, characterization, and aerosol dispersion performance modeling of advanced spray-dried microparticulate/nanoparticulate mannitol powders for targeted pulmonary delivery as dry powder inhalers. *J. Aerosol Med. Pulm. Drug Deliv.* 27(2), 81–93 (2014).

85. Duret, C. *et al.* Pharmacokinetic evaluation in mice of amorphous itraconazole-based dry powder formulations for inhalation with high bioavailability and extended lung retention. *Eur. J. Pharm. Biopharm.* 86(1), 46–54 (2014).

86. Patil-Gadhe, A. & Pokharkar, V. Therapeutics single step spray drying method to develop proliposomes for inhalation: A systematic study based on quality by design approach. *Pulm. Pharmacol.* 27, 197–207 (2014).

87. Omer, H.K. *et al.* Spray-dried proliposome microparticles for high-performance aerosol delivery using a monodose powder inhaler. *AAPS PharmSciTech* 19(5), 2434–2448 (2018).

88. Ye, T., Yu, J., Luo, Q., Wang, S. & Chan, H.-K. Inhalable clarithromycin liposomal dry powders using ultrasonic spray freeze drying. *Powder Technol.* 305, 63–70 (2017).

89. Bi, R., Shao, W., Wang, Q. & Zhang, N. Spray-freeze-dried dry powder inhalation of insulin-loaded liposomes for enhanced pulmonary delivery. *J. Drug Target.* 16(9), 639–648 (2008).

90. Chennakesavulu, S. *et al.* Pulmonary delivery of liposomal dry powder inhaler formulation for effective treatment of idiopathic pulmonary fibrosis. *Asian J. Pharm. Sci.* 13(1), 91–100 (2018).

91. Zhang, T. *et al.* Inhalation treatment of primary lung cancer using liposomal curcumin dry powder inhalers. *Acta Pharm. Sin. B* 8(3), 440–448 (2018).

92. Campardelli, R. *et al.* Efficient encapsulation of proteins in submicro liposomes using a supercritical fluid assisted continuous process. *J. Supercrit. Fluids* 107, 163–169 (2016).

93. Martino, M., Mouahid, A., Trucillo, P. & Badens, E. Elaboration of lutein-loaded nanoliposomes using supercritical CO_2. *Eur. J Lipid Sci.* 123(4), 2000358 (2021).

94. Jia, J. *et al.* Berberine-loaded solid proliposomes prepared using solution enhanced dispersion by supercritical CO_2: Sustained release and bioavailability enhancement. *J. Drug Deliv. Sci. Technol.* 51, 356–363 (2019).

95. Sahib, M.N., Abdulameer, S.A., Darwis, Y., Peh, K.K. & Tan, Y.T.F. Solubilization of beclomethasone dipropionate in sterically stabilized phospholipid nanomicelles (SSMs): Physicochemical and in vitro evaluations. *Drug Des. Devel. Ther.* 6, 29 (2012).

96. Park, C.-W. *et al.* Advanced spray-dried design, physicochemical characterization, and aerosol dispersion performance of vancomycin and clarithromycin multifunctional controlled release particles for targeted respiratory delivery as dry powder inhalation aerosols. *Int. J. Pharm.* 455(1–2), 374–392 (2013).

97. Eedara, B.B., Tucker, I.G. & Das, S.C. Phospholipid-based pyrazinamide spray-dried inhalable powders for treating tuberculosis. *Int. J. Pharm.* 506(1–2), 174–183 (2016).

98. Eedara, B.B., Rangnekar, B., Doyle, C., Cavallaro, A. & Das, S.C. The influence of surface active l-leucine and 1,2-dipalmitoyl-sn-glycero-3-phosphatidylcholine (DPPC) in the improvement of aerosolization of pyrazinamide and moxifloxacin co-spray dried powders. *Int. J. Pharm.* 542(1–2), 72–81 (2018).

99. Eedara, B.B. *et al.* Development and characterization of high payload combination dry powders of anti-tubercular drugs for treating pulmonary tuberculosis. *Eur. J. Pharm. Sci.* 118, 216–226 (2018).

100. Meenach, S.A., Anderson, K.W., Hilt, J.Z., McGarry, R.C. & Mansour, H.M. High-performing dry powder inhalers of paclitaxel DPPC/DPPG lung surfactant-mimic multifunctional particles in lung cancer: Physicochemical characterization, in vitro aerosol dispersion, and cellular studies. *AAPS PharmSciTech* 15(6), 1574–1587 (2014).

101. Meenach, S.A., Anderson, K.W., Zach Hilt, J., McGarry, R.C. & Mansour, H.M. Characterization and aerosol dispersion performance of advanced spray-dried chemotherapeutic pegylated phospholipid particles for dry powder inhalation delivery in lung cancer. *Eur. J. Pharm. Sci.* 49(4), 699–711 (2013).

102. Brousseau, S., Wang, Z., Gupta, S.K. & Meenach, S.A. Development of aerosol phospholipid microparticles for the treatment of pulmonary hypertension. *AAPS PharmSciTech* 18(8), 3247–3257 (2017).

103. Dhoble, S., Ghodake, V., Peshattiwar, V. & Patravale, V. Site-specific delivery of inhalable antiangiogenic liposomal dry powder inhaler technology ameliorates experimental pulmonary hypertension. *J. Drug Deliv. Sci. Technol.* 62, 102396 (2021).

104. Gandhi, M. *et al.* Inhalable liposomal dry powder of gemcitabine-HCl: Formulation, in vitro characterization and in vivo studies. *Int. J. Pharm.* 496(2), 886–895 (2015).

105. Yeganeh, E.M., Bagheri, H. & Mahjub, R. Preparation, statistical optimization and in-vitro characterization of a dry powder inhaler (DPI) containing solid lipid nanoparticles encapsulating amphotericin B: Ion paired complexes with distearoyl phosphatidylglycerol. *Iran. J. Pharm. Res.* 19(3), 45 (2020).

106. Malamatari, M., Charisi, A., Malamataris, S., Kachrimanis, K. & Nikolakakis, I. Spray drying for the preparation of nanoparticle-based drug formulations as dry powders for inhalation. *Processes* 8(7), 788 (2020).

107. Sarabandi, K., Gharehbeglou, P. & Jafari, S.M. Spray-drying encapsulation of protein hydrolysates and bioactive peptides: Opportunities and challenges. *Dry. Technol.* 38(5–6), 577–595 (2020).

108. Telko, M.J. & Hickey, A.J. Dry powder inhaler formulation. *Respir. Care* 50(9), 1209–1227 (2005).

109. Alabsi, W. *et al.* Synthesis, physicochemical characterization, in vitro 2D/3D human cell culture, and in vitro aerosol dispersion performance of advanced spray dried and co-spray dried angiotensin (1–7) peptide and PNA5 with trehalose as microparticles/nanoparticles for targeted respiratory delivery as dry powder inhalers. *Pharmaceutics* 13(8), 1278 (2021).

110. Alabsi, W., Al-Obeidi, F.A., Polt, R. & Mansour, H.M. Organic solution advanced spray-dried microparticulate/nanoparticulate dry powders of lactomorphin for respiratory delivery: Physicochemical characterization, in vitro aerosol dispersion, and cellular studies. *Pharmaceutics* 13(1), 26 (2021).

111. Lo, Y.-L., Tsai, J.-C. & Kuo, J.-H. Liposomes and disaccharides as carriers in spray-dried powder formulations of superoxide dismutase. *J. Control. Release* 94(2–3), 259–272 (2004).

112. Eedara, B.B., Alabsi, W., Encinas-Basurto, D., Polt, R. & Mansour, H.M. Spray-dried inhalable powder formulations of therapeutic proteins and peptides. *AAPS PharmSciTech* 22(5), 1–12 (2021).

113. Adali, M.B., Barresi, A.A., Boccardo, G. & Pisano, R. Spray freeze-drying as a solution to continuous manufacturing of pharmaceutical products in bulk. *Processes* 8(6), 709 (2020).

114. Chaurasiya, B. & Zhao, Y.-Y. Dry powder for pulmonary delivery: A comprehensive review. *Pharmaceutics* 13(1), 31 (2021).

115. Ishwarya, S.P. & Anandharamakrishnan, C. Spray-freeze-drying approach for soluble coffee processing and its effect on quality characteristics. *J. Food Eng.* 149, 171–180 (2015).

116. van Winden, E.C. Freeze-drying of liposomes: Theory and practice. *Methods Enzymol.* 367, 99–110 (2003).

117. Lopez-Polo, J. *et al.* Effect of lyophilization on the physicochemical and rheological properties of food grade liposomes that encapsulate rutin. *Food Res. Int.* 130, 108967 (2020).

118. Cacela, C. & Hincha, D.K. Low amounts of sucrose are sufficient to depress the phase transition temperature of dry phosphatidylcholine, but not for lyoprotection of liposomes. *Biophys. J.* 90(8), 2831–2842 (2006).

119. Costantino, H.R. *et al.* Protein spray freeze drying. 2. Effect of formulation variables on particle size and stability. *J. Pharm. Sci.* 91(2), 388–395 (2002).

120. Arakawa, T., Prestrelski, S.J., Kenney, W.C. & Carpenter, J.F. Factors affecting short-term and long-term stabilities of proteins. *Adv. Drug Deliv. Rev.* 46(1–3), 307–326 (2001).

121. Chen, C., Han, D., Cai, C. & Tang, X. An overview of liposome lyophilization and its future potential. *J. Control. Release* 142(3), 299–311 (2010).

122. Susa, F., Bucca, G., Limongi, T., Cauda, V. & Pisano, R. Enhancing the preservation of liposomes: The role of cryoprotectants, lipid formulations and freezing approaches. *Cryobiology* 98, 46–56 (2021).

123. Khan, D.R., Rezler, E.M., Lauer-Fields, J. & Fields, G.B. Effects of drug hydrophobicity on liposomal stability. *Chem. Biol. Drug Des.* 71(1), 3–7 (2008).

124. Zhao, L. & Temelli, F. Preparation of anthocyanin-loaded liposomes using an improved supercritical carbon dioxide method. *Innov. Food Sci. Emerg. Technol.* 39, 119–128 (2017).

125. Maja, L., Željko, K. & Mateja, P. Sustainable technologies for liposome preparation. *J. Supercrit. Fluids*, 165, 104984 (2020).

126. Karn, P.R., Cho, W., Park, H.-J., Park, J.-S. & Hwang, S.-J. Characterization and stability studies of a novel liposomal cyclosporin a prepared using the supercritical fluid method: Comparison with the modified conventional Bangham method. *Int. J. Nanomedicine* 8, 365 (2013).

Nebulizers

14

Ariel Berlinski

Contents

14.1 INTRODUCTION

Nebulizers are medical devices that convert a suspension or solution into an inhalable aerosol.[1] Liquid medications are placed into a reservoir and later delivered to the aerosol generator producing the inhalable mist. The first nebulization devices were reported as early as 1860 with a report of Siegel's device that used the Venturi principle to generate aerosols.[2] However, it was not until 1911 that modern inhalation began with successful nebulization of adrenaline. Two decades later early compressor nebulizers were used. Today, nebulizers are used to deliver multiple medications. Table 14.1 shows a list of drugs formulated for nebulization that are currently commercially available in

DOI: 10.1201/9781003182566-18

TABLE 14.1 Drugs formulated for nebulization commercially available in the United States

DRUG CATEGORY	DRUG NAME	AVAILABILITY IN OTHER PLATFORMS
Short acting bronchodilator	Albuterol sulfate	pMDI, DPI
	Lev-albuterol	pMDI
	Ipratropium bromide	pMDI
	Ipratropium bromide and albuterol sulfate	SMI
Long acting bronchodilator	Arformoterol	
	Formoterol	DPI
	Glycopyrrolate*	DPI
Corticosteroids	Budesonide	DPI
Mucoactive drug	Dornase alfa*	
	3 and 7% Hypertonic saline	
Antibiotic	Tobramycin*	DPI
	Aztreonam*	
	Amikacin*	
Antiviral	Ribavirin*	
	Pentamidine*	
Pulmonary vasodilator	Iloprost*	
	Treprostinil*	

pMDI = pressurized metered dose inhaler, SMI = soft mist inhaler, DPI = dry powder inhaler.
*These drugs were approved by the Food and Drug Administration as drug-device combinations.

the United States. Availability of the drug in other delivery platforms is also noted. Although most devices are considered open-source devices, many newly approved inhaled drugs are approved by the regulatory agencies as drug-device combinations. Many drugs not approved for inhalation therapy are used in clinical care. Table 14.2 shows a list of drugs delivered via nebulizers that are used off-label. This list includes many drug classes: antibiotic, antifungal, immunosuppressant, opioid, sedative, mucoactive and pulmonary vasodilator.

Like any delivery platform, nebulizers have advantages and disadvantages (Table 14.3). Some of the advantages are that nebulizers can be used by patients of any age, they can be adapted to be used in patients who either have artificial airways (tracheostomy tube, endotracheal tube) or are receiving noninvasive respiratory support (noninvasive ventilation, heated high-flow nasal cannula), and they can be used in cooperative or uncooperative patients. In addition, nebulizers allow the delivery of larger drug doses than other platforms, they are the only platform that can deliver drugs that have not been formulated for inhalation, they do not require difficult breathing maneuvers, and they are typically less expensive than other platforms. Due to the open nature of the reservoir, nebulizers allow aerosolization of drug admixtures and allow modification of drug dose and concentration. Disadvantages include bigger size than other platforms,

TABLE 14.2 Off-label use of medications delivered via nebulizer

DRUG CATEGORY	DRUG NAME
Antibiotic	Colistin
	Ceftazidime
	Amikacin
	Tobramycin
	Gentamycin
Antifungal	Amphotericin
Immunosuppressant	Cyclosporine
Opiod	Fentanyl
	Morphine
Sedative	Midazolam
	Dexmedetomidine
	Ketamine
Mucoactive	N-acetyl cysteine
Pulmonary vasodilator	Epoprostenol
	Alprostadil
Anticoagulant	Heparin
Antifibrinolytic	Tranexamid acid

Intravenous formulations of these drugs are placed in the nebulizer's reservoir for nebulization.

high variability of the quality of aerosol among different nebulizer brands, and different quality of aerosols generated by different combinations of compressors and nebulizers. In addition, nebulizers require cleaning and disinfection to avoid contamination, they typically have longer treatment times than other platforms, and they require a power source that is often noisy.

14.2 CONDITIONS TREATED WITH NEBULIZER THERAPY

Nebulizers are used to treat a large variety of medical conditions throughout the lifespan. Some of these medications are used off-label especially in the pediatric population.[3] It was not until recently when the regulatory agencies offered incentives to manufacturers that pediatric indications began to be pursued more frequently. Many medications are used off-label for the treatment of different conditions in adult patients as well.

During the neonatal period bronchodilators (albuterol and ipratropium bromide) are used to treat wheezing. Nebulized corticosteroids (budesonide) are used in patients with bronchopulmonary dysplasia.[4] Nebulized racemic epinephrine is used to treat post-extubation stridor. During the pediatric age bronchodilators (albuterol, lev-albuterol

TABLE 14.3   Comparative advantages and disadvantages of different types of nebulizers

ADVANTAGES	DISADVANTAGES
Inexpensive (Jet)	Expensive (US and MN)
Small footprint (US and MN)	Large footprint due to compressor (Jet)
Noiseless aerosol production (US and MN)	Require a generally noisy power source (Jet)
Short treatment times (MN)	Generally require longer treatment times (US and Jet)
Can have an adherence monitor (MN)	Lack of adherence monitor (US and Jet)
Allows for use of drug admixtures (All)	Some admixtures could be incompatible (All)
Allows delivery of large drug doses (All)	Large intra-lot and inter-brand variability (Jet)
Can be used with all ages (All)	Risk of electrical malfunction (US and MN)
Can be used in patients unable to follow instructions (All)	Risk for contamination (All)
Can be adapted to be used with artificial airways (All)	Not all medications allowed (US)
Can be adapted to be used in patients receiving respiratory support (noninvasive ventilation or heated high-flow nasal cannula) (MN and Jet)	

Jet = jet nebulizers, US = ultrasonic nebulizers, MN = mesh nebulizers, All = all devices.

and ipratropium bromide) and corticosteroids (budesonide) are used for the treatment of asthma.[5] Budesonide and racemic epinephrine are used to treat laryngotracheitis. Hypertonic saline and albuterol have been used for the treatment of bronchiolitis.

Patients with cystic fibrosis are treated with inhaled short- and long-acting bronchodilators as well as inhaled corticosteroids. They are also treated with inhaled mucoactive drugs such as hypertonic saline and dornase alfa. Patients with cystic fibrosis are prescribed inhaled antibiotics to eradicate or suppress *Pseudomonas Aeruginosas's* growth.[6] Patients with primary ciliary dyskinesia use inhaled hypertonic saline, inhaled bronchodilators, and inhaled antibiotics. Patients with chronic pulmonary obstructive disease are treated with inhaled long-acting bronchodilators (arformoterol, formoterol, glycopyrrolate) and inhaled corticosteroids.[7] Patients with pulmonary hypertension are treated with inhaled pulmonary vasodilators.[8] Patients who have undergone lung transplant are prescribed inhaled antifungal, and inhaled anti-rejection medications. These and other immunocompromised patients may use inhaled antivirals for *Pneomocystis jirovesi* pneumonia prophylaxis. Patient with ventilator associated pneumonia and those with tracheitis may be treated with inhaled antibiotics. Inhaled opioids are used for pain control for certain procedures and in terminal patients.[9]

Administration of traditional vaccines via nebulization has been studied but results showed lower seroconversion rates than the subcutaneous ones.[10] Newer messenger ribonucleic acid vaccines using lipid nanoparticle technology are being developed. Nebulized alpha 1 antitrypsin has been studied for the treatment of patients with alpha 1 antitrypsin deficiency presenting with chronic obstructive pulmonary disease exacerbations.[11] Nebulized insulin is currently undergoing clinical trials for the treatment of diabetes. Nebulized surfactant delivered through continuous pressure devices is currently undergoing clinical trials for the treatment of surfactant deficiency in premature newborns.[12] Inhaled oncologic agents have been studied for the treatment of lung cancer without much success.[13] Nebulization is also being evaluated for delivery of phages and gene therapy in patients with cystic fibrosis.[14–15]

Nebulized medications are also used for diagnostic purposes including measuring bronchodilator response (albuterol, lev-albuterol, and ipratropium bromide) and evaluation of bronchial hyperresponsiveness (methacholine and histamine). Nebulized hypertonic is used to induce sputum for diagnosis of tuberculous and nontuberculous mycobacteria. It is also used to obtain respiratory cytology as part of the evaluation of asthma research.

It is crucial that drug and device developers keep in mind the clinical and physiological characteristics of the intended recipient. Section 14.5 discusses patient factors affecting drug delivery from nebulizers. These factors should be considered even during preclinical work. In addition, patient preferences play an important role in adherence to therapy. Therefore, ease of use and cleaning, and portability are to be considered during design development. Evaluation of patient acceptability and ability to successfully operate new devices is crucial.

14.3 OPERATING PRINCIPLES

Nebulizers can be classified according to their operating principle: jet, ultrasonic, and mesh. Furthermore, jet nebulizers can be classified into continuous output (small and large volume), breath-enhanced, and breath-actuated.

14.3.1 Jet Nebulizers

Jet nebulizers are operated by forcing gas through a small orifice in the device. This results in a decrease in pressure at the sides of the high velocity jet stream (Bernoulli effect) then sucking the liquid medication present in the reservoir.[1] Figure 14.1 shows a diagram of the mechanism of aerosol production of jet nebulizers specifically for the continuous output type. The aerosol impacts into baffles thus reducing the size of the emitted aerosol with large particles being recycled. Table 14.4 includes a list of formulation and device related variables that influence drug delivery efficiency and aerosol characteristics of jet nebulizers. Jet nebulizers are manufactured as disposable or durable devices. The gas source in hospitals is either central oxygen or compressed air (50 pounds per square inch). Nebulizers are typically operated between 6 and 10 liters/minute.[16] Nebulizers could also be powered by helium-oxygen combinations (heliox)

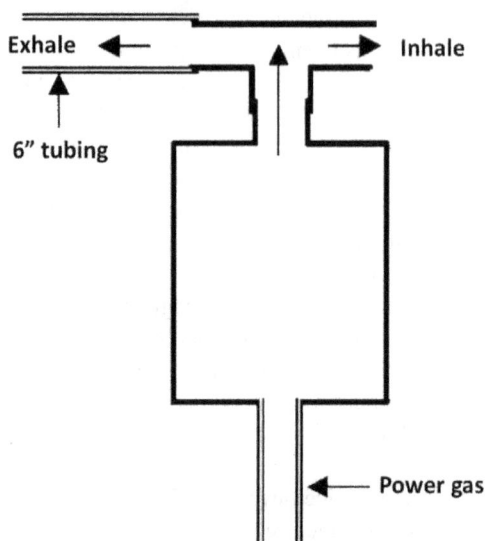

FIGURE 14.1 Aerosol production from a continuous output nebulizer. Modified with permission from Rau J.L., Ari A., Restrepo R.D. Performance comparison of nebulizer designs: constant-output, breath-enhanced, and dosimetric. *Respir Care* **49**, 174-179 (2004).

TABLE 14.4 Device and drug formulation variables that influence drug delivery efficiency and aerosol characteristics of jet nebulizers

VARIABLE
Fill volume
Residual volume
Nebulizer position
Use of extension or conserver devices
Gas pressure and flow
Gas density
Nebulizer medication characteristics (solutions vs. suspension, viscosity, and surface tension)

resulting in smaller size aerosol and decreased drug delivery.[17] Therefore, heliox driving gas flow has to be increased two-fold to produce aerosols of similar characteristics to those generated with oxygen. Electric compressors are typically used for home care. In general, compressors generate gas at low flows (3–9 liters/minute) and pressures (15–30 pounds per square inch). While air compressors generate a wet gas, medical gases are dry. Compressor characteristics vary significantly among different brands and models.[18] Compressors also suffer decay over time especially if used many hours a day like in cystic fibrosis.[19] This explains in part why so many patients who do not obtain relief from the inhaled bronchodilator delivered by compressor report significant improvement when the nebulizer is powered by high pressure gases at a health care facility.

Nebulizers are at significant risk for contamination and cleaning and disinfection after each use is recommended.[20] Once nebulizers are cleaned either cold or heat disinfection methods can be used. The latter include submerging units in boiling water for five minutes, placing in a dishwasher (top rack) for 30 minutes as long as the temperature is hotter than 70 Celsius, microwaving for five minutes in submerged water, or using a baby bottle sterilizer. Cold methods include submersion in 70% isopropyl alcohol for five minutes or submersion in 3% hydrogen peroxide for 30 minutes. Nebulizers should be rinsed with distilled water if disinfected with a cold method before they can be used. More recently ozone-based and ultraviolet-C-based methods are being evaluated as alternatives.

14.3.1.1 Continuous output

Continuous output jet nebulizers are the most common nebulizer type used due to their low cost. Several variables influence the amount and characteristics of the emitted aerosol (Table 14.2). These devices show significant inter-brand and intra-lot variability.[21] Continuous output jet nebulizers are the most inefficient type of nebulizer due to the fact that they generate and release aerosol during patient's inspiration and expiration, and because they typically have a high residual volume (Figure 14.1).[22] The latter is defined as the amount of aerosol that remains in the nebulizer cup at the end of nebulization. This is unique to each nebulizer cup and it typically ranges between 0.5 and 3 milliliters. This is important to keep in mind when dose adjustments are considered for special populations. Decreasing the loading dose from 3 to 1.5 milliliters in a nebulizer with a residual volume of 1 milliliter will result in a 75% dose reduction rather than the intended 50% dose reduction. Continuous output jet nebulizers also result in aerosol exposure to the caregivers. Some literature suggests that this exposure is responsible for an increase in respiratory problems among respiratory therapists.[23] Moreover, environmental exposure concerns have recently resurfaced during the coronavirus-19 (COVID-19) pandemic.[24] The nebulizer is typically connected to a T-piece that has an extension tube in one end and a mouthpiece in the other end. The extension tube, made of corrugated tubing (15 centimeters long and volume of 50 milliliters), acts as a reservoir. Other devices incorporate a reservoir with a one-way valve to enhance drug delivery. Patients who cannot produce a seal around the mouthpiece use face masks. The use of this type of interface results in facial and ocular exposure.[25] Face masks are designed with holes that prevent carbon dioxide rebreathing and should not be occluded. Conversely to valved holding chambers, the dead space of the mask does not affect drug delivery.[26]

Small volume nebulizers typically hold 5–20 milliliters of solution/suspension. The position of the nebulizer could affect aerosol production with most devices having to be operated vertically. A higher loading volume results in higher drug output by overcoming the loss due to residual volume.[16] However, high loading volumes also result in prolonged nebulization time. Increasing loading volume from 3 to 5 milliliters resulted in doubling nebulization time.[16] This phenomenon is more evident when nebulizers are operated at low gas flows.[16] This could have a negative impact on adherence to inhaled therapies that is an area of major importance for treatment success. The flow of the gas source is inversely related to the size of the emitted aerosol and the nebulization time.[16] The magnitude of reduction of nebulization time that occurs when flow is increased is inversely related to the loading volume. Jet nebulizers are typically operated until sputtering when most of the aerosol has been already released.

Drug characteristics also affect nebulizer performance.[27] Viscous medications decrease output rate and generate aerosols of smaller particle size when aerosolized with jet nebulizers. In one study a six-fold increase in viscosity without changes in surface tension resulted in 30% decrease in mass median aerodynamic diameter and 35% decrease in drug output.[27] Medications of high surface tension generate aerosols of larger particle size. In one study a 35% decrease in surface tension without changes in viscosity resulted in 50% decrease in mass median aerodynamic diameter and no change in drug output.[27] Suspensions tend to have larger particle size than solutions that are more uniformly distributed.

Large volume nebulizers are mostly used to deliver bronchodilators and typically hold 200–240 milliliters of solution. These devices could be operated for up to 8 hours without needing to change the nebulizer solution.[28] However, some of the characteristics might change after 4–5 hours.[28,29] Albuterol concentration in the reservoir increases between 140 and 250% of loading concentration after the fourth to fifth hour of use.[28] These devices are popular for the treatment of status asthmaticus because they require less contact time of the respiratory therapist with the patient. The devices are typically connected to a 50 pounds per square inch oxygen source, and some models allow concomitant use of heliox. The emitted dose is controlled by modifying the admixture of albuterol and saline solutions, the gas flow, and type of gas used. Large volume nebulizers are also used to provide humidity to patients with artificial airways. Devices are operated at high flows (greater than 10 liters/minute) to avoid carbon dioxide rebreathing.

14.3.1.2 Breath-enhanced

Breath-enhanced nebulizers incorporate one-way valves into the device design.[1] An inspiratory valve opens during inhalation increasing the amount of aerosol delivered to the patient and closes during exhalation. An expiratory valve placed on the mouthpiece opens during exhalation and some models allow the placement of an expiratory filter to minimize environmental exposure. A diagram of the operating principle of these devices can be seen in Figure 14.2. These systems increase drug delivery and decrease environmental exposure. These devices continue producing aerosol during expiration. These devices have been extensively used to deliver treatments for patients with cystic fibrosis including dornase alfa, hypertonic saline, and tobramycin. The Food and Drug Administration approved dornase alfa and tobramycin for use with specific nebulizer-compressor combinations.

14.3.1.3 Breath-actuated

Breath-actuated nebulizers generate aerosol only during inhalation by use of a spring-loaded one-way valve.[30] A diagram of the operating principle of these devices can be seen in Figure 14.3. Drug delivery is more precise than with other nebulizers and was recently recommended for its use during methacholine challenge procedure.[31] Since the drug is produced and released during inhalation, dose adjustments might be necessary

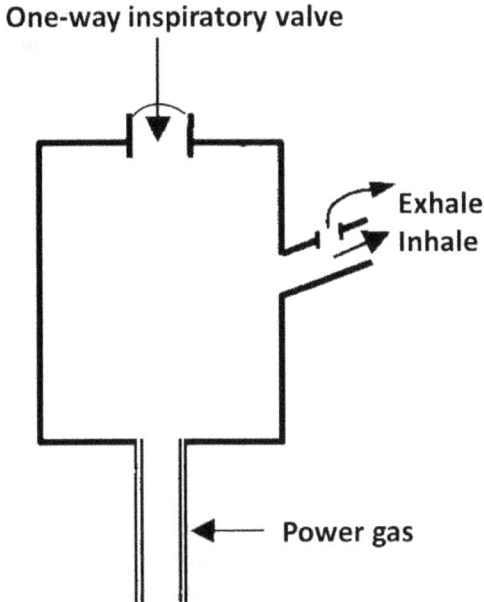

FIGURE 14.2 Aerosol production from a breath-enhance nebulizer. Modified with permission from Rau J.L., Ari A., Restrepo R.D. Performance comparison of nebulizer designs: constant-output, breath-enhanced, and dosimetric. *Respir Care* **49**, 174-179 (2004).

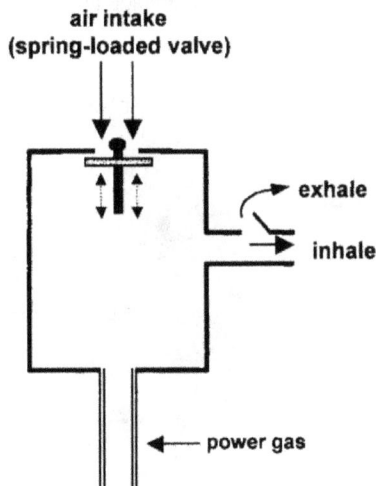

FIGURE 14.3 Aerosol production from a breath-actuated nebulizer. Modified with permission from Rau J.L., Ari A., Restrepo R.D. Performance comparison of nebulizer designs: constant-output, breath-enhanced, and dosimetric. *Respir Care* **49**, 174-179 (2004).

to avoid overdosing especially with drugs that have a narrow therapeutic index. These devices also minimize environmental exposure. There is minimum flow necessary to trigger the valve, so practitioners need to verify the patient's ability to do it. This could be a problem for the young pediatric population, geriatric population, and those with cognitive impairment.

14.3.2 Ultrasonic Nebulizers

Ultrasonic nebulizers were introduced in the form of humidifiers in 1949.[32] These nebulizers utilize a piezoelectric crystal that vibrates at high frequency (1 to 3 megahertz).[1] These vibrations are transmitted to the liquid present in the reservoir resulting in aerosol formation. A diagram of the operating principle of these devices can be seen in Figure 14.4. Some devices use a medication cup that is submerged in the liquid that is in contact with the piezoelectric crystal. This design change results in a lower risk for superinfection than when the medication is in contact with the piezo-electric crystal. The particle size of the aerosols is inversely proportional to the vibration frequency of the device and directly proportional to the surface tension and density of the formulation.[27] The effect of drug characteristics on generated aerosols is different for ultrasonic nebulizers than for jet nebulizers.[27] A four-fold increase in viscosity without changes in surface tension resulted in a 35% increase in mass median aerodynamic diameter and a 90% decrease in drug output. A 28% reduction in surface tension without changes in viscosity resulted in a 10% decrease in mass aerodynamic diameter and 50% increase in drug output. Ultrasonic nebulizers are not suitable for the delivery of suspensions like budesonide or liquids with high viscosity or surface tension.[27,33] The aerosols generated

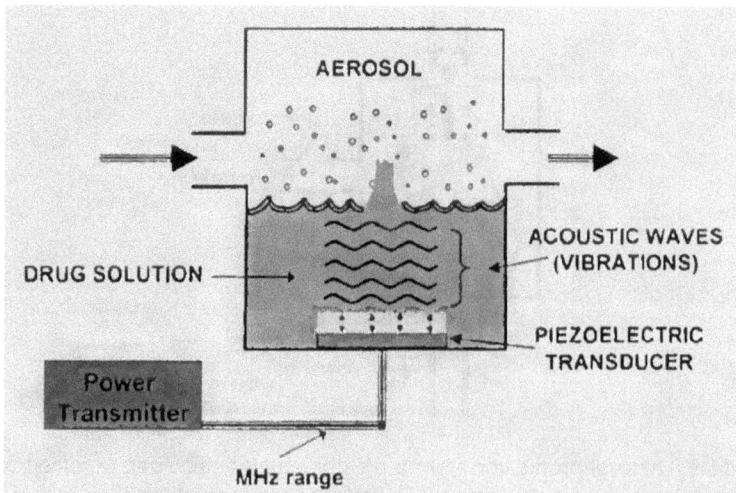

FIGURE 14.4   Aerosol production from an ultrasonic nebulizer. Reproduced with permission from Rau J.L. Design principles of liquid nebulization devices currently in use. *Respir Care* **47**; 1257-1275 (2002).

by ultrasonic nebulizers are generally larger than those generated by jet nebulizers. Opposite to jet nebulizers that progressively cool the generated mist, ultrasonic nebulizers heat the solutions left in the reservoir as much as 20 Centigrades. The latter makes them not suitable as delivery devices for drug formulations whose structure could be affected by heat (i.e. proteins). Although once popular due to their noiseless operation, they became less used since the introduction of mesh nebulizers.

14.3.3 Mesh Nebulizers

Mesh nebulizers generate aerosols by forcing liquids through a membrane with laser-drilled holes.[34] The number and size of the holes vary with the different devices and intended drug to be delivered. Mesh nebulizers can be classified into active (vibrating) or passive based on their mechanism of aerosol production. Figure 14.5 shows the mechanism of aerosol production of mesh nebulizers. In passive devices, the piezo-electric crystal vibrates an ultrasonic horn what results in fluid being pushed through a mesh. The I-neb (Philips Respironics, Murraysville, Pennsylvania) and the open-source NEU-22 (Omron, Kyoto, Japan) are examples of passive devices.[35] The latter began to be marketed in 1993. In active devices, the piezoelectric crystal vibrates the plate resulting in fluid being pushed through the membrane with 1000–4000 funnel-shape holes. The following devices are examples of active vibrating mesh technology: eFlow nebulizer platform (Pari, Midlothian, Virginia), Aeroneb Pro and Solo nebulizers (Aerogen, Inc, Galway, Ireland), InnoSpire and NIVO nebulizers (Philips Respironics, Murraysville, PA), and FOX (Vectura group plc, Wiltshire, United Kingdom).[36]

Mesh nebulizers produce a slow aerosol without additional airflow and are able to nebulize drug volumes in the microliter range. The aerosol generated during the patient's inspiratory time can be stored in a chamber and released during inhalation. Device manufacturers work jointly with drug developers to modify the size of these holes to optimize drug delivery of a formulation of specific characteristics (surface tension and viscosity). This is the rationale behind some drugs being approved by the regulatory agencies as drug-device formulations. Aztreonam (Cayston™), amikacin

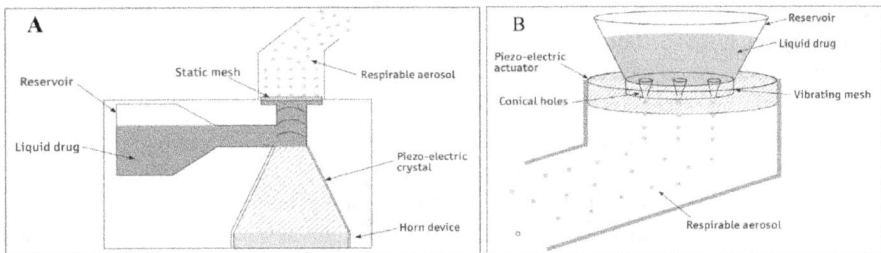

FIGURE 14.5 Aerosol production from mesh nebulizers. Figure A represents a passive mesh nebulizers. Figure B represents an active mesh nebulizers. Reproduced with permission of the ©ERS 2022. Breathe 2 (3) 252-260; DOI: 10.1183/18106838.0203.252 Published 1 March 2006.

(Arikayce®) and glycopyrrolate (Lonhala Magnair™) are examples of this process. The latter is different than the other two because it is a closed system nebulizer that requires unique vials to load the medication.[37] Most devices, except FOX® and I-neb, consist of a controller and a handset connected by a cord, and can be powered by batteries or AC/DC adapters.

Mesh technology can be used to deliver a variety of formulations except suspensions with drug particles larger than the size of the mesh holes.

In contrast to jet nebulizers, mesh nebulizers have a low residual volume. Using the same unit doses in these devices that have low residual volume could result in overdosing the patient. The eRapid® introduced design modifications (larger capacity reservoir and smaller aerosol chamber) to the Trio® thus matching the characteristics of their predicate devices. Therefore, no dose adjustment was required. Some devices, such as eRapid and FOX nebulizers, are affected by the inclination of the device.[35]

Conversely to jet and ultrasonic nebulizers, mesh ones neither change the temperature of the fluid being nebulized nor progressively concentrate the remaining liquid medication. Proper care of the mesh is of utmost importance for proper drug delivery. Poor cleaning and disinfection could result in bacterial superinfection and clogging of the holes. The latter will result in prolonged treatment times. Touching the mesh during the cleaning process will result in damage to the unit. Steam disinfection of the mesh with a baby bottle sterilizer has shown effectiveness without affecting its function.[38]

The cost of the open-source devices and the replacement mesh is a limiting factor for the increase of the market share of this technology. Devices approved as a drug-device combination are dispensed with the drug as well as the replacement headsets.

14.4 SMART NEBULIZERS

Smart nebulizers utilize microprocessors and algorithms to interact with the patient, resulting in drug delivery optimization. They also coach the patient with a goal of improving drug delivery. These devices are also capable of recording patient adherence (occurrence and duration of treatments), thus overcoming a limitation of the nebulizer technology as a group. These devices are more precise in delivering a specified dose than other nebulizer types, therefore are ideal for delivering drugs with narrow therapeutic index and/or expensive ones.

The Akita® Jet nebulizer (Vectura Group plc, United Kingdom) is a breath-actuated device that guides the inhalation maneuver and provides real-time feedback.[39] The device controls the inhalation flow (12–15 liters/minute) and volume (60–70% of inspiratory capacity) thus decreasing upper airways deposition and minimizing variability in drug delivery. The device allows for more peripheral deposition than traditional nebulizers. The device can be programmed to deliver the aerosol bolus at the beginning or in the middle of the inspiratory maneuver. This allows the device to target distal and central airways respectively. The device has monitoring capabilities (date and duration of treatments). The cost and size of the unit are significant drawbacks to using this technology. A small vibrating mesh handheld device, FOX®, is also manufactured by the same group.[36] The device can also target more central or peripheral deposition as a result of varying the timing of the release of aerosol. Both devices have 510(k) premarket authorizations for marketing in the United States. The FOX nebulizer is commercialized in Europe as a drug-device combination for the delivery of inhaled Iloprost for the treatment of pulmonary hypertension.

The I-Neb AAD system is a portable, battery-operated, breath-actuated passive mesh nebulizer.[35] It is commercialized in the United States for the delivery of an inhaled pulmonary vasodilator (Iloprost). The device can be operated in two different modes: tidal breathing and targeted inhalation. During tidal breathing mode, the device monitors the three previous breaths to predict the duration of the following tidal breath and release the medication during the first half. The targeted inhalation mode utilizes a flow restrictor, auditory and tactile feedback to coach the patient to take slow and deep breaths. The use of this mode results in higher lung deposition than with the tidal breathing mode by significantly increasing the duration of the inspiratory time. The device allows the personalization of drug delivery and has auditory feedback to inform the patient that he/she has inhaled the prescribed dose.

The eFlow platform also has adherence monitoring capabilities that are mostly used in the context of clinical research. However, they are now being evaluated as an integral part of the delivery of telehealth.[40]

14.5 PATIENT FACTORS AFFECTING DRUG DELIVERY FROM NEBULIZERS

There are many patient-related factors that influence the efficiency of drug delivery from nebulizers (Table 14.5). The patient's age, behavior, and degree of cooperation with the treatment are crucial. Infants and children who cry while receiving nebulizer therapy receive significantly less drug than those who do not irrespective of the presence of lung disease. The reduction in aerosol deposition can reach magnitudes of 80%.

TABLE 14.5 Patient variables that influence drug delivery efficiency and aerosol characteristics of jet nebulizers

VARIABLE
Patient's age
Patient's cooperation and cognitive status
Inhalation maneuver
Disease state
Concomitant use with airway clearance device
Use in conjunction with ventilatory support (invasive, noninvasive, and heated high-flow cannula systems)

This can be explained in part by the fact that crying results in high inspiratory flows that facilitate drug impaction in the upper airway. Breathing patterns of pediatric patients are responsible for dose-adjustment of inhaled doses. Pediatric breathing patterns typically have lower tidal volumes, higher respiratory rates, and shorter inspiratory times than adult ones. If the patient's inspiratory flow is larger than the one generated by the nebulizer the inhaled aerosol is diluted with entrained air. This typically occurs after six months of age. In general, a slow inhalation maneuver results in higher pulmonary deposition than a fast one. This can be used to target aerosol delivery to peripheral or central airways respectively when aerosols of small mass median aerodynamic diameter are inhaled.[41] One study compared inhaled aerosols of mass median aerodynamic diameter of 3.68 and 1.1 microns inhaled at slow and fast rate. They reported no change in distribution of deposition (central vs. peripheral) for the larger size aerosol with different inhalation flows (12 and 31 liters/minute respectively). However, the smaller aerosol was deposited more peripherally with slow inhalation (18 liters/minute) and more centrally with faster inhalation (38 liters/minute). In addition, nasal breathing results in the reduction of intrapulmonary deposition due to a filtering effect. Upper airway deposition decreases with older age and larger tidal volume but could represent up to 50% in infants. This can be explained in part by anatomical and physiological differences between pediatric and adult patients. Patients with more preserved lung function have a more uniform distribution of drugs deposited in the lungs. Many patients who suffer suppurative lung diseases are treated with inhaled aerosols and airway clearance techniques/devices. Some devices allow for concomitant inhalation while the device is being used. Minimal changes to the aerosol characteristics occur when the aerosol generator is placed between the airway clearance device (positive expiratory pressure device) and the mouth. However, the use of the device requires altering the breathing pattern by using prolonged expiratory times thus reducing inhaled drug delivery. When the aerosol generator is placed before the airway clearance device the resulting aerosol is small and the delivered mass is low. In one study the mass median aerodynamic diameter decreased from 4.13 to 1.22 microns and delivered mass decreased by 65 to 80%. This occurs mainly through a filtering phenomenon that occurs when the aerosol travels through the device.

Patients unable to cooperate and those of young or advanced age need a mask to be able to receive a nebulizer treatment. The material of the mask and the tightness of the fit to the patient's face is crucial. Mask made of hard materials are typically uncomfortable to wear are result in leaks. The latter is important because it can not only result in ocular deposition but also in increased caregiver exposure. Masks that have a straight aerosol path (front loaded) are more efficient than those that have a vertical path (bottom loaded). In one study the difference of deposition between front and bottom loaded aerosols was in the order of two- to three-fold. This is exaggerated when a gap is introduced between the face and the mask. In another study moving the mask 2 centimeters away from the face resulted in a reduction in drug delivery of 55 and 17% for the bottom and front-loaded interface respectively. The use of facemask results in equivalent outcomes when compared to the use of a mouthpiece. Patient and health care workers' education about assembly and care of the nebulizers is necessary for achieving treatment success. Unfortunately, knowledge about nebulizers remains low among healthcare practitioners and consequently among their patients.

14.6 DRUG DELIVERY IN PATIENTS RECEIVING VENTILATORY SUPPORT

Patients receiving ventilatory support often require concomitant administration of inhaled medications. Bronchodilators, corticosteroids, antibiotics, pulmonary vaso-dilators, and mucolytics are typically delivered to these patients. There are different modalities of ventilatory support: heated high-flow nasal cannula, noninvasive mechanical ventilation, tracheostomy, and invasive mechanical ventilation. It is important to understand the variation of efficiency of the inhaled drug under the different types of ventilatory support because patients may transition from one system to the other. Patients might need escalating support moving from heated high-flow nasal cannula to noninvasive mechanical ventilation and then to invasive mechanical ventilation. Once improving they will de-escalate to noninvasive ventilation, then to heated high-flow nasal cannula, and finally to not receiving ventilatory support. Therefore, understanding drug delivery variation will help practitioners avoid under or overdosing their patients.

14.6.1 Heated High-Flow Nasal Cannula

The use of heated high-flow nasal cannula systems to treat hypoxemic respiratory failure has become more prevalent in the past decade. This technology is being used by neonates to the geriatric population. These systems provide heated and humidified gases of varying oxygen fractions.

There has been a growing interest in the use of heated high-flow nasal cannula systems to concomitantly deliver inhaled medications (bronchodilators and pulmo-nary vasodilators) and provide ventilator support. The system consists of a flow/oxygen source, a heater-humidifier chamber, a circuit, and different size cannulas. Figure 14.6 shows a picture of a heated high-flow nasal cannula system. The aerosol generator can be placed before the humidifier (preferred), right after the humidifier (not recommended), or between the circuit and the nasal cannula (not preferred). When heated high-flow systems are used they impair drug delivery from a nebulizer with a face mask.[42,43] Thus, in order to increase delivery efficiency in patients receiving heated high-flow nasal cannula support aerosols can be delivered in different modalities: 1) through the heated high-flow system operated at low flows, 2) through the heated high-flow system operated at high-flows that are transiently reduced, or 3) through a face mask provided the flow of the heated high-flow nasal cannula system is reduced. Several factors affect aerosol delivery efficiency including flow (cannula and patient), cannula size, type of aerosol generator, type of heated high- flow cannula system. There is an inversely proportional relationship between the cannula flow and delivery efficiency. The mass median aero-dynamic diameter of aerosols released by the cannulas is typically below 2 microns. In addition, delivery efficiency increases when the patient's inspiratory flow is lower than the cannula flow. Also, there is a directly proportional relationship between cannula size and drug delivery efficiency. An increase in drug losses in the equipment due to

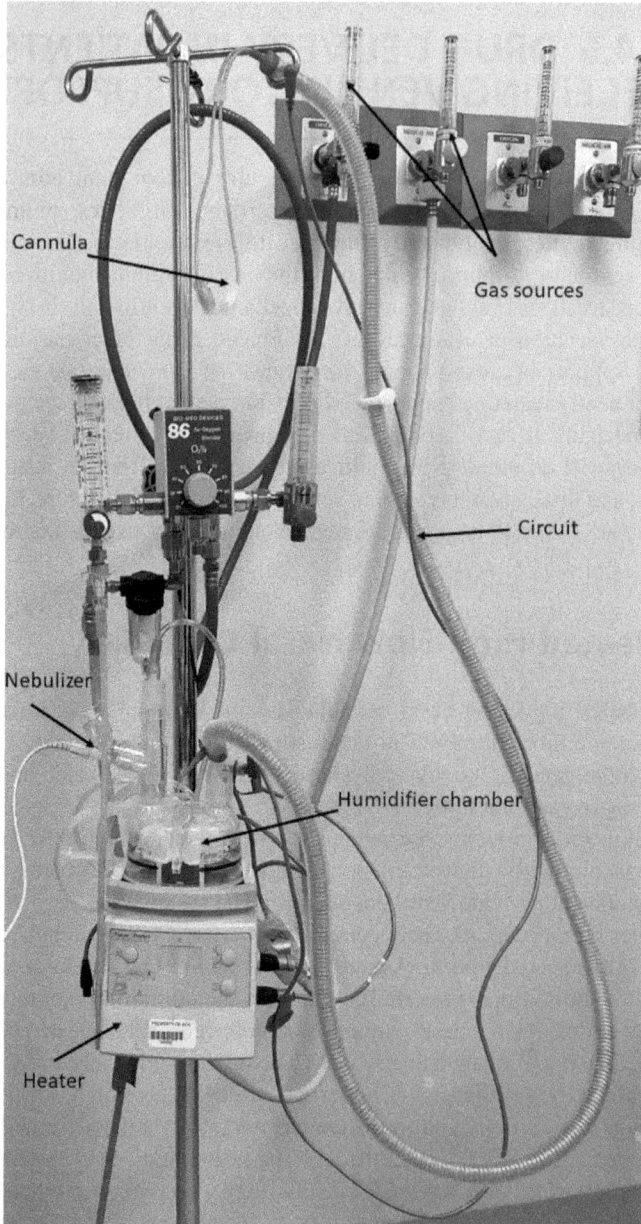

FIGURE 14.6   Heated high-flow nasal cannula system with mesh nebulizer.

impaction is responsible for these phenomena. Although some devices allow placement before the humidifier, other only allow placement between the circuit and the cannula. The former allows a reduction of the size of the aerosol as it travels through the system thus minimizing impaction losses. However, when the nebulizer is placed right before the cannula impaction loss increases. Although jet and vibrating mesh nebulizers can be used, the latter have been more extensively studied and favored mostly due to the fact that they don't add flow to the system. The high cost of the disposable vibrating mesh devices significantly limits the uptake in the use of these technologies.

The use of transnasal systems could be an option for overnight drug delivery. This modality would reduce some of the treatment burdens of these patients. In addition, younger children seem to tolerate better the cannula that a face mask.

In addition to in vitro studies evaluating delivery efficiency, other studies demonstrated good lung deposition using radiolabeled aerosols and positive clinical response to bronchodilators and pulmonary vasodilators.

14.6.2 Noninvasive Mechanical Ventilation

Noninvasive ventilation can be delivered either with single-limb or double-limb ventilator circuits attached to a tightly fit face mask.[44] Figure 14.7 shows diagrams of single and double-limb noninvasive ventilator systems. Face mask leaks severely impair drug delivery efficiency during noninvasive ventilation. When a double-limb circuit is used a mask without leak is utilized and the exhaled air goes through the expiratory limb. Placing the nebulizer at the end of the inspiratory limb or before the mask is more efficient than placing it before the humidifier. Increasing the difference between inspiratory and expiratory pressure does not have an effect on drug delivery in pediatric models but leads to improvement in adult models. When a single-limb ventilator circuit is used an exhalation

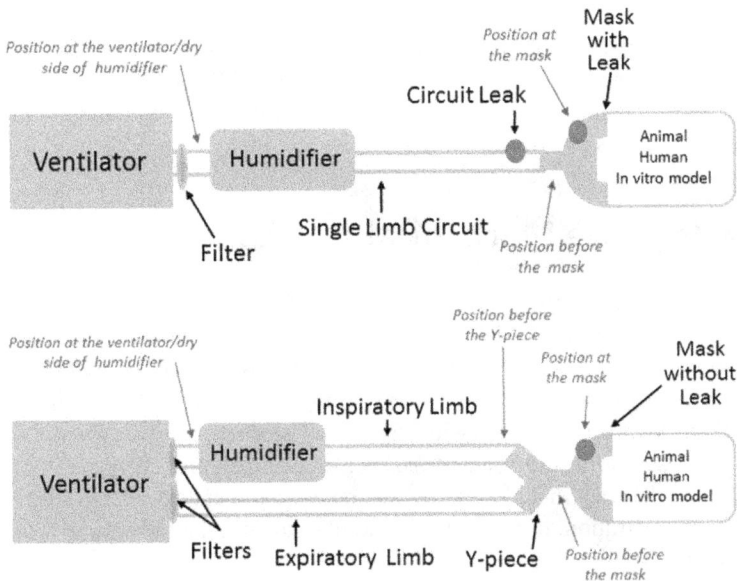

FIGURE 14.7 Diagrams of single and double-limb circuit noninvasive ventilator systems. Figure A Corresponds to single-limb circuit system. Figure B corresponds to a double-limb circuit system. Reproduced with permission from Berlinski A. Inhalation Aerosols: Physical and Biological Basis for Therapy: Neonatal & Pediatric Inhalation Drug Delivery Ch.8 (New York, NY. CRC Press, 2019).

valve is incorporated. If the nebulizer is placed before the humidifier a significant loss of aerosol occurs through the exhalation valve. This explains a four-fold increase in aerosol delivery efficiency that occurs when the nebulizer is placed after the exhalation valve.

Vibrating mesh nebulizers are two- to three-fold more efficient than jet nebulizers. Nebulizer loading volume directly correlates with the amount of delivered aerosol. The use of humidification does not seem to affect drug delivery from nebulizers.

14.6.3 Tracheostomy

Pediatric patients undergo tracheostomy due to the presence of airway malformations or for need chronic ventilatory support. Adults in general, receive tracheostomies when needing prolonged mechanical ventilation. Pediatric and adult patients undergoing mechanical ventilation via tracheostomy can be divided into those who can be removed from the ventilator to receive the aerosol treatment and those who cannot. The latter behave like those who are intubated and receive mechanical ventilation except that drug delivery is higher due to difference in length between the endotracheal and the tracheostomy tubes.

Several factors affect drug delivery in spontaneously breathing tracheostomized patients.[45] Tracheostomy internal diameter directly correlates with drug delivery efficiency. This becomes critical in the neonatal/pediatric tracheostomy sizes. Tracheostomy tubes need to be suctioned before being used. A T-piece connector is more efficient than a tracheostomy mask interface. Vibrating mesh nebulizers are more efficient than jet nebulizers in this population. The use of bias flows decreases drug delivery efficiency. The use of resuscitation bag to assist drug delivery results in a high deposition in the large airways. Treatment strategies using inhaled antibiotics for tracheitis take advantage of this phenomenon. Changing the delivery route of nebulized therapy from tracheostomy to oral results in a decrease in lung dose.

14.6.4 Invasive Mechanical Ventilation

Many factors influence the delivery efficiency of nebulized drugs given in line to patients who are receiving invasive mechanical ventilation. Figure 14.8 shows a diagram of invasive mechanical ventilation system.[44] Most of the information regarding delivery efficiency has been obtained through in vitro studies with the limitation that most studies have been conducted with albuterol. Therefore, drug developers should not extrapolate these findings to solutions/suspensions of different characteristics. Factors affecting drug delivery include internal diameter of the endotracheal tube, bias flow, timing of administration, nebulizer type and placement, type of ventilator, and circuit size/diameter.

There is a direct relationship between the internal diameter of the endotracheal tube and drug delivery efficiency. This becomes more evident with smaller sizes used by infants and children. The mass median aerodynamic diameter of aerosol released by endotracheal tubes is typically below 3 microns. There is an inverse relationship between the bias flow of ventilator and drug delivery efficiency. Studies on the timing

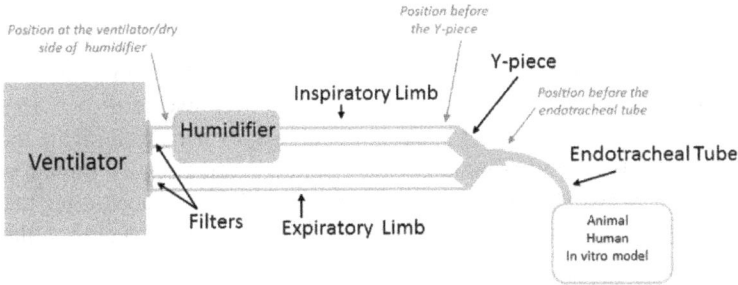

FIGURE 14.8 Diagram of invasive mechanical ventilation system. Reproduced with permission from Berlinski A. Inhalation Aerosols: Physical and Biological Basis for Therapy: Neonatal & Pediatric Inhalation Drug Delivery Ch.8 (New York, NY. CRC Press, 2019).

of administration (continuous, expiratory, or inspiratory time) have yielded conflicting results. Ultrasonic and vibrating mesh nebulizers are more efficient than continuous output jet nebulizers irrespective of their placement in the ventilator circuit.[46] The effect of device placement is quite complex.[46,47] Placing the vibrating mesh nebulizers before the humidifier is several fold more efficient than placing them before the Y-piece when an adult-type circuit is used in a conventional ventilator. However, the opposite occurs when a neonatal circuit is used. Increasing the tidal volume does not result in increase of delivery efficiency. During high frequency oscillatory ventilation, the use of jet nebulizers should be avoided and vibrating mesh nebulizers have to be placed right before the endotracheal tube. Studies on the effect of the ventilator mode on drug delivery efficiency have yielded conflicting results.

14.7 PRECAUTIONS FOR USE OF NEBULIZERS IN THE ERA OF COVID-19

The high morbidity and mortality associated with COVID-19 infections and the realization that the virus was not only transmitted by contact and droplets but also by aerosols led to several changes in the way nebulizer therapy is now administered. Although uncontaminated nebulizers are not a source of bio-aerosols, the patient's exhale breathing is. Patient interfaces (mouthpiece or face mask) are at higher risks of contamination than the nebulizer unit itself. Careful and clean assembly of the nebulizer is necessary to avoid potential contamination. These changes in practice affected all patients irrespective if they were receiving any type of ventilator support. The first change was to try to shift patients to pressurized metered dose inhalers, soft mist inhalers, and dry powder inhalers if the drug was available in that platform and the patient was able to use the device. However, it should be noticed that the use of some dry powder inhalers may result in cough, therefore, defeating in part the reasoning for the change in devices. In these situations, an exhalation filter could be added as well as one-way valves that prevent contact of patient's breath with the nebulizer unit.[48] Careful evaluation of the need for nebulization therapy should occur in every patient.

Placement of a surgical face mask covering mouth and nose in patients receiving heated high flow nasal cannula reduced the amount of fugitive aerosols.[49] Health care practitioners should be aware that some of the strategies used to mitigate the risk of exposure in patients receiving noninvasive ventilatory support may impair ventilator functioning.[49] The use of a double-limb circuit with a filter placed after the expiratory limb reduces the risk of malfunction. If not available, placement of a filter on the exhaust valve of a single-limb circuit is recommended.

The strategies to reduce fugitive emissions in patients receiving invasive mechanical ventilation are several-fold. These strategies include placement of high efficiency particulate air filters on the expiratory intake of the ventilator and minimizing disconnection of the circuit from the patient for delivery of aerosols. This can be achieved by using inline suction catheter systems, and vibrating mesh nebulizers and jet nebulizers with spring-loaded T-piece connectors. Health care workers should be aware that larger tidal volumes generate higher fugitive aerosols.

It is of utmost importance the use of proper personal protective equipment and reducing the number of potentially exposed personnel irrespective of the presence and type, or absence of ventilatory support. It is important to closely monitor the filter to prevent impairment of the ventilators. Proper ventilation of the room is also very important to minimize exposure risk. Negative pressure rooms provide the best protection. Rooms with high air exchange/hour should be used when the former are not available.

14.8 UNMET NEEDS

Nebulizer cost is a significant public health problem that disproportionately affects minorities and low-income countries. Reimbursement problems in the United States health care system result in lack of incentives for manufacturing companies to develop affordable, high efficiency compressors. Breath-actuated nebulizers that could be triggered by infants and children are needed. As a group, nebulizers present a major disadvantage compared to other delivery systems (pressurized metered dose inhalers and dry powder inhalers): lack of affordable systems that provide reminders, biofeedback, and monitoring.

REFERENCES

1. O'Callaghan C. & Barry P.W. The science of nebulised drug delivery. *Thorax* 52, S31–S44 (1997).
2. Sanders M. Inhalation therapy: An historical review. *Prim Care Respir J* 16(3), 71–81 (2007). Erratum in: *Prim Care Respir J* 16(3), 196 (2007).
3. Schmiedl S. *et al.* Utilisation and off-label prescriptions of respiratory drugs in children. *PLoS One* 9(9), e105110 (2014).

4. Michael Z. *et al*. Bronchopulmonary dysplasia: An update of current pharmacologic therapies and new approaches. *Clin Med Insights Pediatr* 12, 1179556518817322 (2018).
5. Global Initiative for Asthma. *Global strategy for asthma management and prevention*, 2021. Available from www.ginasthma.org. Last accessed on 11/16/2021.
6. Flume P.A. *et al*. Cystic fibrosis pulmonary guidelines: Chronic medications for maintenance of lung health. *Am J Respir Crit Care Med* 176(10), 957–969 (2007).
7. Barjaktarevic I.Z. & Milstone A.P. Nebulized therapies in COPD: Past, present, and the future. *Int J Chron Obstruct Pulmon Dis* 15, 1665–1677 (2020).
8. Olschewski H. *et al*. Inhaled prostacyclin and iloprost in severe pulmonary hypertension secondary to lung fibrosis. *Am J Respir Crit Care Med* 160(2), 600–607 (1999).
9. Afolabi T.M., Nahata M.C. & Pai V. Nebulized opioids for the palliation of dyspnea in terminally ill patients. *Am J Health Syst Pharm* 15(14), 1053–1061 (2017).
10. Low N. *et al*. A randomized, controlled trial of an aerosolized vaccine against measles. *N Engl J Med* 372(16), 1519–1529 (2015).
11. Stolk J. *et al*. Efficacy and safety of inhaled α1-antitrypsin in patients with severe α1-antitrypsin deficiency and frequent exacerbations of COPD. *Eur Respir J* 54(5), 1900673 (2019).
12. Sood B.G. *et al*. Aerosolized beractant in neonatal respiratory distress syndrome: A randomized fixed-dose parallel-arm phase II trial. *Pulm Pharmacol Ther* 66, 101986 (2021).
13. Wauthoz N., Rémi Rosière R. & Amighi K. Inhaled cytotoxic chemotherapy: Clinical challenges, recent developments, and future prospects. *Expert Opin Drug Deliv* 18(3), 333–354 (2021).
14. Law N. *et al*. Successful adjunctive use of bacteriophage therapy for treatment of multidrug-resistant pseudomonas aeruginosa infection in a cystic fibrosis patient. *Infection* 47(4), 665–668 (2019).
15. Chow M.Y.T., Chang R.Y.K. & Chan H.K. Inhalation delivery technology for genome-editing of respiratory diseases. *Adv Drug Deliv Rev* 168, 217–228 (2021).
16. Hess D. *et al*. Medication nebulizer performance: Effects of diluent volume, nebulizer flow, and nebulizer brand. *Chest* 110(2), 498–505 (1996).
17. Corcoran T. Carrier gases and their effects on aerosol drug delivery. *J Aerosol Med Pulm Drug Deliv* 34(2), 71–78 (2021).
18. Smith E.C., Denyer J. & Kendrick A.H. Comparison of twenty three nebulizer/compressor combinations for domiciliary use. *Eur Respir J* 8(7), 1214–1221 (1995).
19. Awad S., Williams D.K. & Berlinski A. Longitudinal evaluation of compressor/nebulizer performance. *Respir Care* 59(7), 1053–1061 (2014).
20. Saiman L. *et al*. Infection prevention and control guideline for cystic fibrosis: 2013 update. *Infect Control Hosp Epidemiol* 35, S1–S67 (2014).
21. Alvine G.F. *et al*. Disposable jet nebulizers: How reliable are they? *Chest* 101(2), 316–319 (1992).
22. Kradjan W.A. & Lakshminarayan S. Efficiency of air compressor-driven nebulizers. *Chest* 87(4), 512–516 (1985).
23. Christiani D.C. & Kern D.G. Asthma risk and occupation as a respiratory therapist. *Am Rev Respir Dis* 148(3), 671–674 (1993).
24. Centers for Disease Control and Prevention. Interim infection prevention and control recommendations for healthcare personnel during the coronavirus disease 2019 (COVID-19) pandemic. Updated September 10 2021. https://www.cdc.gov/coronavirus/2019-ncov/hcp/infection-control-recommendations.html#.
25. Geller D.E. Clinical side effects during aerosol therapy: Cutaneous and ocular effects. *J Aerosol Med* 20, S100–S108 (2007); discussion S109.
26. Berlinski A. Effect of mask dead space and occlusion of mask holes on delivery of nebulized albuterol. *Respir Care* 59(8), 1228–1232 (2014).
27. McCallion O.N.M. *et al*. Nebulization of fluids of different physicochemical properties with air-jet and ultrasonic nebulizers. *Pharm Res* 12(11), 1682–1688 (1995).

28. Berlinski A., Willis J.R. & Leisenring T. In-vitro comparison of 4 large-volume nebulizers in 8 hours of continuous nebulization. *Respir Care* 55(12), 1671–1679 (2010).

29. Berlinski A. & Waldrep J.C. Four hours of continuous albuterol nebulization. *Chest* 114(3), 847–853 (1998).

30. Rau J.L., Ari A. & Restrepo R.D. Performance comparison of nebulizer designs: Constant-output, breath-enhanced, and dosimetric. *Respir Care* 49(2), 174–179 (2004).

31. Dean J. *et al*. Methacholine challenges: Comparison of different tidal breathing challenge methods. *ERJ Open Res* 7(4), 00282-2021 (2021).

32. Dessanges J.F. A history of nebulization. *J Aerosol Med* 14(1), 65–71 (2001).

33. Berlinski A. & Waldrep J. Effect of aerosol delivery system and formulation on nebulized budesonide output. *J Aerosol Med* 10(4), 307–318 (1997).

34. Vecellio L. The mesh nebuliser: A recent technical innovation for aerosol delivery. *Breathe* 2(3), 252–260 (2006).

35. Hardaker L.E. & Hatley R.H. In vitro characterization of the I-neb adaptive aerosol delivery (AAD) system. *J Aerosol Med Pulm Drug Deliv* 23, S11–S20 (2010).

36. Pritchard J.N. *et al*. Mesh nebulizers have become the first choice for new nebulized pharmaceutical drug developments. *Ther Deliv* 9(2), 121–136 (2018).

37. Pham S. *et al*. In vitro characterization of the eFlow closed system nebulizer with glycopyrrolate inhalation solution. *J Aerosol Med Pulm Drug Deliv* 31(3), 162–169 (2018).

38. Hohenwarter K. *et al*. An evaluation of different steam disinfection protocols for cystic fibrosis nebulizers. *J Cyst Fibros* 15(1), 78–84 (2016).

39. Fischer A. *et al*. Novel devices for individualized controlled inhalation can optimize aerosol therapy in efficacy, patient care and power of clinical trials. *Eur J Med Res* 14, 71–77 (2009).

40. Thee S. *et al*. A multi-centre, randomized, controlled trial on coaching and telemonitoring in patients with cystic fibrosis: conneCT CF. *BMC Pulm Med* 21(1), 131 (2021).

41. Laube B.L. *et al*. Targeting aerosol deposition in patients with cystic fibrosis: Effects of alterations in particle size and inspiratory flow rate. *Chest* 118(4), 1069–1076 (2000).

42. Dugernier J. *et al*. Nasal high-flow nebulization for lung drug delivery: Theoretical, experimental, and clinical application. *J Aerosol Med Pulm Drug Deliv* 32(6), 341–351 (2019).

43. Réminiac F. *et al*. Nasal high flow nebulization in infants and toddlers: An in vitro and in vivo scintigraphic study. *Pediatr Pulmonol* 52(3), 337–344 (2017).

44. Berlinski A. *Inhalation aerosols: Physical and biological basis for therapy: Neonatal & pediatric inhalation drug delivery Ch.8*. (New York: CRC Press, 2019).

45. Berlinski A. *et al*. Workshop report: Aerosol delivery to spontaneously breathing tracheostomized patients. *J Aerosol Med Pulm Drug Deliv* 30(4), 207–222 (2017).

46. Berlinski A. & Willis J.R. Effect of tidal volume and nebulizer type and position on albuterol delivery in a pediatric model of mechanical ventilation. *Respir Care* 60(10), 1424–1430 (2015).

47. DiBlasi R.M. *et al*. Iloprost drug delivery during infant conventional and high-frequency oscillatory ventilation. *Pulm Circ* 6(1), 63–69 (2016).

48. Lavorini F., Usmani O.S. & Dhand R. Aerosol delivery systems for treating obstructive airway diseases during the SARS-CoV-2 pandemic. *Intern Emerg Med* 16(8), 2035–2039 (2021).

49. Leonard S. *et al*. Preliminary findings on control of dispersion of aerosols and droplets during high-velocity nasal insufflation therapy using a simple surgical mask: Implications for the high-flow nasal cannula. *Chest* 158(3), 1046–1049 (2020).

Protein and Peptide Delivery to the Lung via Inhalation

15

Xiaofei Xin, Qiyue Wang, Virender Kumar,
Ajit S. Narang, and Ram I Mahato

Contents

DOI: 10.1201/9781003182566-19

15.1 INTRODUCTION

Biomacromolecules like proteins and peptides are a diverse group of therapeutic agents which are generally large and complex molecules produced through biotechnology. Unlike chemically synthesized small molecule drugs which have well-defined large molecular size biopharmaceuticals are immunogenic and sensitive to external conditions with and high polarity. Thus, the permeability of biologics through the intestinal epithelium is low or even negligible. In addition, enzymatic degradation by peptidases and proteinases in the gastrointestinal tract, pH variability, first-pass hepatic metabolism, and intestinal flora could deactivate these biologics when delivered orally [1]. Injection and infusion are suitable for liquid biologic formulations, but specific storing and handling instructions are required to be followed, and people may develop needle phobia during long-term administration.

The pulmonary drug delivery system is a needle free technique and has been widely used in various disease conditions like asthma, diabetes, cancer, migraine, tuberculosis, acute lung injury, and many other diseases. The pulmonary route has been considered as a tremendous scientific and biomedical importance in recent years due to its unique

Resistance to aerosolization depends on:
- nature of biotherapeutics
- drug formulation (taking into account the limited range of approved excipients)
- aerosol device

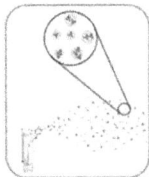

Optimal site of deposition depends on:
- type of drug (vaccine, Ab,...)
- site of infection/immune effectors
- device performance

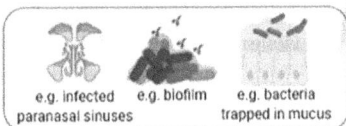

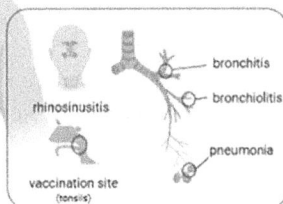

bronchitis
bronchiolitis
rhinosinusitis
pneumonia
vaccination site (tonsils)

e.g. infected paranasal sinuses   e.g. biofilm   e.g. bacteria trapped in mucus

Pharmacological effect depends on:
- quantity depositied in the region of interest
- target accessibility (biological barriers)
- clearance and metabolic degradation
- mucosal immune response
- compliance/adherence of patients

FIGURE 15.1   The multifaceted features from the development of inhaled biopharmaceuticals [11].

properties such as a large drug absorption area and good blood supply. However, the preparation of inhalation formulation of large molecules has its own limitations. This chapter discusses the challenges in developing protein therapeutics for pulmonary delivery and targeting of protein and peptide drugs, advancements in devices, different types of biopharmaceuticals, and advancements in the formulation of proteins peptides (Figure 15.1).

15.2 CHALLENGES IN THE DEVELOPMENT OF PROTEIN THERAPEUTICS FOR PULMONARY DELIVERY

Although the pulmonary delivery of peptides and proteins with advantages such as a large surface area for absorption, low thickness of the alveolar epithelium, and lack of enzyme activity [2], it is not easy to deliver formulated bioactive drugs deep into the lung that be able to penetrate circulation. The lung is one of the most complex organs in the body. Each lung is divided into lobes: three in the right lung and two in the left lung. The functional units of the lungs includes the respiratory bronchioles, alveolar ducts, sacs, and alveoli. Several generations of bronchioles are differentiated from bronchi by the absence of cartilage in their walls, connecting the small bronchi to the alveolar ducts and alveoli. The bronchi themselves branch many times into smaller airways, ending in the narrowest airways (bronchioles), which are as small as one-half of a millimeter across. Large airways are held open by semiflexible, fibrous connective tissue. The walls

TABLE 15.1   Current clinical trials and approved products for the inhalation delivery of biologics

NAME	DELIVERY APPROACH	BIOLOGIC	APPLICATION/ INDICATION	CLINICAL TRIAL
AP301	Orally inhaled	Animal blood cells derived from hygienically collected porcine or bovine blood	Primary Graft Dysfunction After Lung Transplantation	NCT02095626
Dance 501	Inhaler	Human insulin	Mild to moderate asthma or COPD	NCT02713831
MVA85A (Oxford University)	Aerosol	Recombinant modified vaccinia virus Ankara expressing antigen 85A (MVA85A)	Tuberculosis vaccine	NCT01954563
PUR003 (Pulmatrix)	Nebulizer	Not listed	Flu vaccine	NCT00947687
Ad5Ag85A (McMaster University)	Aerosol	Recombinant replication-deficient human adenoviral tuberculosis vaccine containing immunodominant antigen Ag85A	Tuberculosis vaccine	NCT02337270
Exubera (Pfizer)	Inhaled through mouth	Human insulin	Diabetes mellitus	NCT00359801
Afrezza (MannKind)	Inhaled through mouth	Human insulin	Diabetes mellitus	NCT03313960

of smaller airways have a thin, circular layer of smooth muscle. The airway muscle can relax or contract, thus changing airway size. In mammals, the lung is made up of conducting airways that carry air to the alveoli, the gas-exchange units of the lung. Several anatomical barriers determine the delivery efficiency of inhaled protein and peptide, including the airway epithelium, alveolar epithelium, endocytosis types, mucociliary clearance, enzymatic degradation, and the innate immune system (Table 15.1).

15.2.1 Airway Epithelium

Lung epithelial cells are intimately connected by several proteins forming tight junctions and presenting a paracellular barrier to drug absorption. Therefore, it is a challenge to achieve a sufficient dose of protein and peptide in the lung. For systemically acting biological drugs, the drug molecules need to gain access to the systemic circulation in addition to proper lung deposition and dissolution. The pulmonary epithelium is the primary barrier for the transportation of protein drugs to the bloodstream. Transportation of biological drugs across the respiratory epithelium is size-dependent. Compounds essentially hydrophilic and $\leq$ 40 kDa are principally transported across biological membranes by means of diffusion-limited paracellular pathways. Non-specific pinocytosis and receptor-mediated transcytosis via albumin, alpha-1 antitrypsin, and transferrin can become significant for macromolecules > 40 kDa.

15.2.2 Alveolar Epithelium

Thousands of small alveoli are at the end of each bronchiole. Together, the millions of alveoli form a surface of more than 100 square meters. Within the alveolar walls is a dense network of tiny blood vessels called capillaries. The extremely thin barrier between air and capillaries allows oxygen to move from the alveoli into the blood and allows carbon dioxide to move from blood in the capillaries into the air in the alveoli. There are two types of epithelial cells here: terminally differentiated squamous type I cells cover most of the alveolar surface but the cuboidal type II cells, which are more in numbers. Typical features of the thin alveolar epithelium coating the inner surface of the lungs include high permeability and significant vascularization, which can facilitate drug absorption. However, alveolar macrophages (AM) which resides on the surface of alveolar epithelium comprise a major "barrier" to the transport of macromolecules from the lungs into the bloodstream. Alveolar macrophages rapidly take up small insoluble particles that deposit in the alveoli by means of phagocytosis or "cell eating". Alveolar macrophages are a barrier to the transport of large proteins from the airway lumen into the bloodstream. In contrast, alveolar macrophages have no impact on pulmonary absorption of small proteins and peptides ($\leq$ 25 kDa), which are cleared from the airspaces within minutes. Therefore, there is significant potential for noninvasive systemic administration of peptides and smaller molecular weight protein therapeutics.

The specific uptake mechanisms of biologics by alveolar epithelial cells is highly dependent on the interaction of inhaled biologics with the pulmonary surfactant layer. this layer is composed of phospholipids and surfactant proteins A, B, C, and D. For instance, interactions between particle of biologics and pulmonary surfactants may lead its translocation across the epithelium via receptor-mediated recycling of pulmonary surfactant components by type II pneumocytes [3]. On the other hand, biologics may also be cleared from the alveolar space by surfactant protein-A and surfactant protein-D-mediated macrophage phagocytosis [4].

The mechanism of endocytosis of bioactive cargo across endothelial cells include clathrin-dependent, caveolae-mediated, and caveolae/clathrin-independent endocytosis as well as micropinocytosis. Clathrin- and caveolae-mediated endocytoses result in similar size endosomes, but caveolae-mediated endocytosis appears to be a slower process and involves a complex signaling pathway. Micropinocytosis is generally an actin-independent process, including a membrane protrusion that extends around biologics and the protrusion rejoins the cell membrane after engulfing the cargo [5]. Identification of specific receptors for uptake of proteins and peptides is important for the development of efficient pulmonary delivery strategies. Albumin, alpha-1 antitrypsin, and transferrin can facilitate transcytosis of biologics to permeate the alveolar epithelium. Neonatal Fc receptor (FcRn) is a major IgG Fc receptor capable of facilitating IgG translocation like cetuximab with high affinity at low pH in sorting endosomes, which either recycle or transcytose to the plasma membrane [6].

15.2.3 Mucociliary Clearance

Low absorption of protein or peptide therapeutics is also attributed to the mucociliary clearance [7,8]. The mucociliary clearance is a critical and physiologically regulated protective function of the airways and lungs that is essential for the clearance of respiratory pathogens [9]. Proteins deposited in the ciliated airways are disposed by the mucociliary escalator, usually within 24–48 h, leading to low bioavailability of those therapeutics [10]. When peptide and protein drugs are formulated as nanoparticles, the influence of these clearance mechanisms could lead to insufficient efficacy in vivo, whereas large microparticles may overcome the clearance and achieve more efficient absorption and a sustained therapeutic effect [8].

15.2.4 Dissolution Rate and Enzyme Degradation in the Lung Fluid

The dissolution rate of biologics in lung tissue dominates cellular uptake, absorption, deposition, and clearance efficiency. Water-soluble proteins may rapidly be absorbed by airway epithelium and reach the blood circulation, which could decrease their potency local in respiratory diseases. In the case of poorly water-soluble protein and peptide, the slow dissolution rate due to limited lung lining fluid could prolong their retention but may lead to macrophage clearance at the same time. This hypothesis was tested to increase the bioavailability of insulin via respiratory route. It is well known that the monomeric or dimeric form of insulin could convert to a hexamer in the presence of zinc ions, affording an insoluble complex. The hexamer of insulin is gradually depolymerized into absorbable monomer form of insulin and increase the absorption time in the lungs [12].

A wide range of pulmonary protease and peptidases have been found for in the lung fluid, including elastase, collagenase, chymotrypsin, prolyl endopeptidase, aminopeptidase P, some species of carboxypeptidase, angiotensin-converting enzyme (ACE), neutral endopeptidase (enkephatinase), cathepsin B, mast cell proteases and neutrophil proteases [13]. Alveolar macrophages and other inflammatory cells, including neutrophils, are the main sources of those enzymes. Unlike large peptides (6–50 kDa), peptides containing less than 30 amino acids generally are more vulnerable to pulmonary peptidases. The development of sheath formulations can improve drug absorbance and bioavailability. Conjugation of one or more hydrophilic polyethylene glycol (PEG) chains to peptides and proteins has been shown to increase the molecular weight and provide shielding effect to the conjugated molecules [14].

15.3 MECHANISM FOR PULMONARY DELIVERY

The deposition behavior of aerosol particles in the respiratory system is the key factor that affect bioavailability [15, 16]. The deposition behavior of particles depends on physical, chemical, and physiological factors [16]. Based on the continuous research progress in aerosol technology in recent decades, the deposition mechanism of aerosol particles has been well established. Herein, we will introduce the several deposition mechanisms of aerosol particles and describe the parameters determining particle deposition in the deep lung.

15.3.1 Aerosol Deposition Mechanisms

After aerosol administration in the pulmonary airway, the deposition mechanisms of particles are mainly based on the following four categories: i) impaction (inertial deposition), ii) sedimentation (gravitational deposition), iii) diffusion and iv) electrostatic precipitation and interception [17]. All the four mechanisms occur simultaneously during the bio-drug deposition (Figure 15.2). However, while the impaction and sedimentation are mainly mechanisms in the tracheal and bronchus, the other mechanisms are closely related with specific particle size, shape, and charge [18].

15.3.1.1 Impaction (inertial deposition)

The impaction is the primary mechanism of deposition of drug-loaded nanoparticles in the respiratory tract with an aerodynamic diameter larger than 5 μm. The likelihood of impaction also depends on the air velocity. The impaction occurs when the airflow direction sudden change due to the bifurcate of the respiratory tract. The particles in the airflow keep their initial trajectories followed by impact and adhesion on the airway walls. The estimated deposition of particles by inertial impaction is expressed by Yeh [19] using Equation (1):

$$f_I = 1 - \frac{2}{\pi} cos^{-1}(\theta \cdot Stk) + \frac{1}{\pi} sin[2cos^{-1}(\theta \cdot Stk)]$$

Where f_I is the fraction of aerosol that deposits in the airway by impaction, Stk is the Stokes number and θ is the bending angle which means the change in the direction of the flow.

The deposition by inertial impaction is increase with the increasing particle size and flow velocity, indicating the particles deposition by impaction mostly happens in the upper respiratory tract, such as the oral cavity and throat.

15.3.1.2 Sedimentation (gravitational deposition)

The sedimentation, also known as gravitational deposition, is another main mechanism for particles deposited in the respiratory tract. The particles in the aerodynamic diameter range 2 to 8 μm is mainly impacted by this deposition mechanism. The gravitational

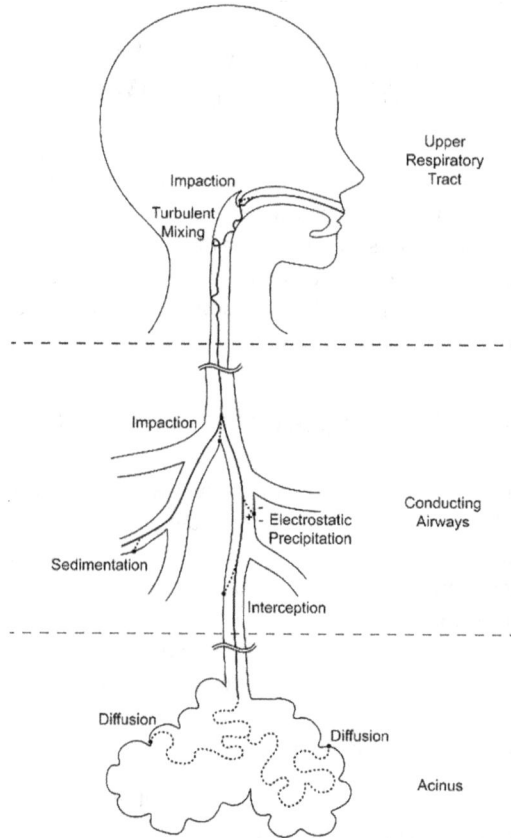

FIGURE 15.2   Schematic illustration of typical aerosol-generation and deposition mechanisms [17].

forces and air resistance of particles in the airflow overcome the buoyancy and induce particles setting in the bronchi or bronchioles. The estimated deposition of particles by sedimentation is expressed by Pich [20] using Equation (2):

$$f_s = \frac{2}{\pi}\left[2\varepsilon\sqrt{1-\varepsilon^{\frac{2}{3}}} - \varepsilon^{\frac{1}{3}}\sqrt{1-\varepsilon^{\frac{2}{3}}} + \arcsin\left(\varepsilon^{\frac{1}{3}}\right)\right]$$

where $\varepsilon = (3vsl)/(4ud)$ and l is the airway length.

The deposition increases with increasing particle size and particle residence time in airspaces, indicating the possible deposition by sedimentation mostly happens for large particles in upper respiratory tract and for the small particles with high residence time in the small airways or alveoli.

15.3.1.3 Diffusion

When the aerodynamic diameter is lower than 0.5 μm, the movement of particles like gas molecules which is known as "Brownian motion". As particles are in random motion, they deposit on the small respiratory tract, and alveolus is mostly by chance. Brownian diffusion increased with decreasing particle size; therefore, this is the main deposition mechanism of small particles (< 0.5 µm). Gormley and Kennedy [21] provide the exact solution of particle diffusion to the walls (simulating the absorption) in a fluid in laminar flow in a cylinder using Equation (3):

$$f_D = 1 - 0.819 \cdot e^{-7.315h} - 0.0976 \cdot e^{-44.61h} - 0.0325 \cdot e^{-114h}$$

$$D_B = \frac{ckT}{3\pi\mu d_p}$$

Where $h = (2l\,D_B)/(ud^2)$, k is Boltzmann's constant, T is the absolute temperature, and c is the Cunningham correction factor.

The deposition by diffusion increases with the decreasing of particle size. The diffusion mainly occurs in the acinar region and also in the upper respiratory tract.

15.3.1.4 Interception

The deposition of particles is not only affected by the aerodynamic diameter but also caused on their specific shapes. The particles such as fibers could easily touch the surface of the respiratory tract when they travel close to the airway, which is followed by interception and deposition on the tract. This mechanism is increased with fiber length and the irregularity of particle shapes, indicating the equivalent spherical diameter is not the only key factor for fiber deposition [22]. It has been proven that the total deposition of fibers in the lung is smaller than the spherical particles with the same mass. For example, a fiber with length of 40 µm and diameter of 0.5 µm has an equivalent spherical diameter of 1.3 µm, while the deposition of the fiber has a lower deposition efficiency in lower respiratory tract compared to the spherical particles with same diameter.

15.3.1.5 Electrostatic precipitation

Compared to impaction, sedimentation, and diffusion, electrostatic precipitation is a less important mechanism of particle deposition. However, there are limited data that suggest surface charge of particles may potentially affect their deposition in airways. Although human airways are normally neutral, some surface area still has opposite polarity charges to the particles and may induce electrostatic precipitation, especially in small airways. Charging of particles will occur during contact or friction to the inhaler or between themselves when dispersion. Liquid droplets also carry charges when the electrical double layer is disrupted. Key parameters such as formulation component, device construction, and relative humidity can affect the surface charges of particles [23]. Majid et al. found that charged particles in the alveolar region are five times higher than in the tracheobronchial region [24]. Also, the different breathing conditions also affect the deposition of charged particles. The higher deposition in bronchial occurs under sitting conditions than light exercise breathing conditions, and the pause time during the inhalation also improves the ratio of effective deposition. Based on the knowledge of electrostatic precipitation mechanism effects on particles deposition, optimizing the charges on particles could help to increase the percentage of the targeted deposition of particles in the lung and reduce the possible toxic particles deposition in the sensitive regions.

15.3.2 Mechanism of Protein Release from Particles

Due to their low stability and limited penetration through biological barriers application of peptide drugs in clinics is limited [25]. Therefore, carriers such as micro- and nanoparticles have been proposed to administer proteins and peptides for high delivery, effective controlled release profile, and safety. There are limited processes, such as emulsion polymerization, freeze drying, and spray freeze drying, that can be used to prepare protein or peptides loaded formulations as they are sensitive to light, heat, moisture and pH environment [26, 27]. Many theoretically possible mechanisms may be considered for the release of proteins and peptides from micro and nanoparticles.

15.3.2.1 Diffusion-controlled release

Diffusion-controlled drug release occurs in the delivery systems such as micelles and nanoparticles where the drug is dispersed in a core or evenly dispersed in the polymer matrix [28]. The diffusion process is always through aqueous channels created by peptide dissolution [29]. The concentration gradient between core and release medium is driving the diffusion process. Although polymer matrix has no membrane as a physical barrier to control the diffusion, the micelles and nanoparticles always exhibit a high initial release, also called burst release, followed by release rate keeps decreasing as drug molecule needs diffusion longer distance inside the matrix.

15.3.2.2 Solvent-controlled release

Solvent transport into drug carriers may affect drug release profiles. Solvent-controlled release mechanism mostly happens in swelling controlled release of hydrogels [30]. When the polymeric hydrogel system comes in contact with an aqueous liquid such as body fluids, the water starts diffusing into the polymeric system's space, followed by hydrogel swelling and peptide release. The drug release rate is consistent with water diffusion and the relaxation rate of the polymer chain [31]. The chain swelling in the hydrogel forms a three-dimensionally crosslinked network. The pore size in this hydrogel network plays a vital role in the drug release and depends on degree of polymerization (DP) and molecular chain length of the polymer [32].

15.3.2.3 Degradation-controlled release

Peptide-loaded solid micro- or nanoparticles are always prepared using biodegradable polymers such as polyesters, polyamides, poly (amino acids), or lipid-based polymers [33, 34]. The hydrolytic and enzymatic degradation of the ester bond and amide bond in backbones leads to the release of peptide. The drug release kinetics depends on polymers' degradation rate, which is affected by the molecular weight, monomer component composition, and crystallinity polymers [35]. Polyesters such as poly(lactic-co-glycolicacid)

(PLGA), polylactic acid (PLA), and poly-caprolactone (PCL) mainly undergo bulk degradation, which leads to degradation of the entire matrix, while the poly(orthoesters) and poly anhydrides always degrade starting from the surface of the particles into the core [36].

15.3.2.4 Permeation controlled release

Microcapsules formed via layer-by-layer adsorption of oppositely charged carriers are proven to be an effective reservoir for protein and peptide delivery with controlled-release ability. The release of loaded drugs is driven by the concentration difference between the capsule interior and the external medium. The single or multi-layers of the polymeric shell act as a physical barrier for diffusion of compounds, which leads the layered membrane to play a key role in the drug release process. Han and coworkers demonstrated that the drug release behavior from chitosan and alginate glutaraldehyde crosslinked microcapsules were affected by the concentration of gradient across the capsule shell based on the highly permeable network [37]. The number of layers, thickness, and composition of shells are significantly affecting drug release. Hamishehkar et al. prepared respirable and biodegradable PLGA microcapsules to load insulin by oil in the emulsification/solvent evaporation method. The insulin loaded PLGA dry powder inhalers (DPI) illustrated a sustained release profile after pulmonary administration, which confirms the encapsulation of peptides and proteins into PLGA microcapsules technique could be a promising controlled delivery system for pulmonary administration.

15.3.2.5 Stimuli-controlled release

Except for the common drug release mechanism, the environment stimulating drug release also provides a new release mechanism used for peptide and protein release [38]. Stimuli-responsive nanocarriers provide target-specific ability for the delivery system, such as pH-sensitive release in the tumor microenvironment. pH-sensitive release was also developed to increase the intracellular drug release while minimizing extracellular release, which improves efficiency and reduces side effects [39]. Glucose-sensitive delivery system has also been investigated for the smart release of insulin for type II diabetes [40]. Pleural fluid pH usually is about 7.6 because bicarbonate accumulation in the pleural cavity is higher than in blood. The insulin dry powder inhaler Afrezza® manufactured by Mankind company uses fumaryl diketopiperazine (FDKP) microparticles to load insulin for pulmonary administration. After deposition in the lung, FDKP could rapidly dissolve into the pleural fluid with a neutral pH environment and release all the loaded insulin to achieve fast uptake [41].

15.3.3 Manufacturing Techniques of Making Particulate Matter for Lung Delivery

The selection of inhaler type is a crucial step to modulate the efficiency of protein and peptide delivery. Although DPI development has been rapid in the last few decades, over 50% of inhaled protein formulations in clinical research are still liquids. Nebulizers, pressured metered dose inhalers (pMDIs), DPIs and soft mist inhalers (SMIs) are the

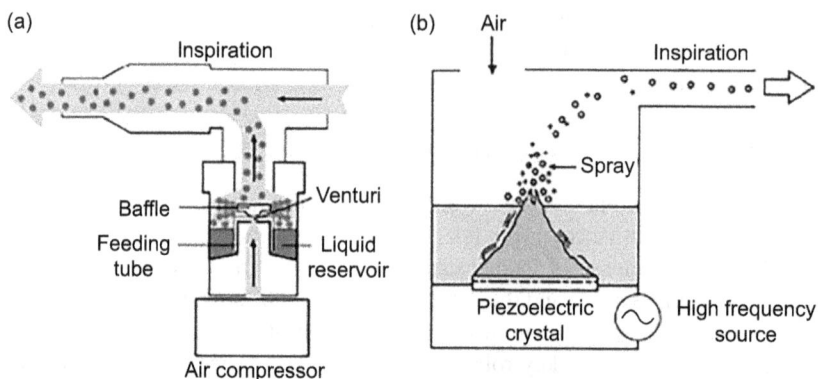

FIGURE 15.3   Schematic illustration of a typical (a) jet nebulizer; (b) ultrasonic nebulizer [44].

most commonly used devices for inhaled drug delivery. Insufficient stability of proteins and peptides during aerosolization remains the main obstacle for their pulmonary delivery. Dry powder formulation is suitable dosage form for pulmonary delivery of proteins and peptides, while new nebulizers with less shear stress are also being investigated for their pulmonary delivery.

15.3.3.1 Nebulizers

Nebulizers are widely available to treat respiratory diseases for many years. The drug for nebulization needs to be dispersed in an aqueous medium to form aerosol droplets, followed by inhalation and deposition in the lungs. According to different atomization principles, nebulizers are divided into air-jet nebulizers and ultrasonic nebulizers (Figure 15.3).

Air-jet nebulizers used compressed gas to spray drug solutions and micronized them to form droplets [42]. A jet of high-pressure air stream rapidly travels through a narrow hole and decreases the pressure on the top of the drug solution, which is aerosolized through the narrow capillary tube. Most of the currently marketed nebulized inhalants use jet mist Carburizers, such as budesonide inhalation suspension (Pulmicort®, AstraZeneca). The nebulization process requires only simple and tidal breathing for drug delivery. However, a large and bulky blower is needed to generate aerosol with a loud noise which is not convenient for patient use [43].

Ultrasonic nebulizers generate aerosols using the vibration of a piezoelectric crystal in a drug solution [45]. The droplets produced by this type of nebulizer will draw out of the device by the patient's inhalation or pushed out by an airflow through the device generated by a small compressor such as in the iloprost aerosol inhaler (Ventavis®, Bayer). Although the particles in aerosols have uniform size and the atomization process is not affected by the patient's breathing behavior, the device is much more expensive and fragile than the jet device. In addition, the ultrasonic nebulizer may cause drug degradation due to the strong ultrasonic power and may not nebulize suspensions and viscous solution well [46].

In summary, spray inhalants are easy to use and can be applied to young and elderly patients, but nebulizers are expensive, require external power supplies, and have poor portability, which limits their use.

15.3.3.2 Pressurized metered-dose inhalers (pMDIs)

Pressurized metered-dose inhalers, also known as metered-dose inhalers (MDIs), are popular respiratory devices to deliver drugs such as bronchodilator agents due to their portability and simple operation. The pressurized drugs or drug-loaded particles are formed and dispersed as suspension or solution in a liquefied propellant system in micron size. Pharmaceutical excipients such as surfactants are also mixed in the formulation to reduce particle agglomeration. After actuating the container's bottom, the metered dose of the drug is released in the actuator seating and generated aerosol spray during the expansion and vaporization of propellant [47].

Although there are many advantages of convenient use and precise dose, the major benefits of pMDIs device are that expelled aerosol spray is independent of the patient's respiratory effort because of the atomizing force of the propellant with high volatility [48]. However, to obtain the best efficiency, the specific breathing technique is needed, requiring patients to adjust their breathing behavior such as appropriate coordination between actuation and inspiration, steady and slow inspiration, and a breath hold. At the same time, Freon (chlorofluorocarbon, CFC) commonly used as propellants, such as: CFC-11, CFC-12, CFC-114, and CFC-115 are easy to cause damage to the atmospheric ozone layer, so switch to non-hydrofluoroalkane propellants (HFA-134a, HFA-227, etc.) [49]. Moreover, the "cold Freon" effects might induce stop inhaling of patients by the cold blast of propellants.

How to improve the stability of proteins and peptides, especially to maintain their conformational stability, in the environment within pMDI formulation is a challenge for biologics pulmonary delivery by pMDI. Despite this, some successes have been reported for preparing biologics formulation in pMDI. To prepare biologics into a crystal form to improve the stability, some researchers developed a crystalline insulin zinc (CFC as propellant) pMDI formulations which could keep insulin stable for several months [50]. More, using water in oil emulsion method to formulate HFA134a and cineole into a pMDI could maintain primary, secondary and tertiary insulin structures and give an extra-fine particle fraction of around 45% [51]. The use of porous microparticles has also been reported as potential carriers to protect the stability of proteins and have also been reported as potential carriers to protect protein stability in pMDI formulations [52].

15.3.3.3 Dry powder inhalers (DPIs)

Dry powder inhalers (DPIs) carry capsules, vesicles or other multi-dose medicine reservoirs loaded with micronized drugs only or combined with effective excipients as carriers. Followed by setting the drug loaded capsules in the device, the dry powder is atomized to form an aerosol through the active respiration of patients and then inhaled into the lungs.

Drug inhaled into lungs do not need hand-breath coordination. The device is designed with compactness and portability to carry out without auxiliary devices and propellants to drive the atomization of the powder. Drugs stored as dry powder form in capsules or other multi-dose reservoirs to increase stability with precise drug dose. Although most drugs delivered currently by DPI are in microgram quantities, it is possible to develop formulations for DPIs that can be delivered in very high doses.

The DPIs device is key factor in the development of DPI products [53]. In present, over 20 DPI devices are available on the market and more than 25 are still in development [54, 55]. Even though such more successful product, there are still no device could meet all of the requirements of an ideal DPI device such as simple use, accurate deliver dose, suitability for a wide range of drugs and doses with minimum adhesion between drug formulation and devices, and highly drug stability. A list of current DPI devices with delivery mechanism has been presented in Table 15.2.

DPIs need to disperse individual doses into capsules or self-dose form bulk powder [56]. The certain limitation of these devices is their high susceptibility to moisture. There are limited biologics products on market like Exubera® and Affreza® insulin [57], while several peptides such as anti-IL-13 monoclonal antibody fragment VR942 (Abrezekimab), Cyclohaler® for administration of DAS181 (Fludase®), and Concept1 for administration of the anti-thymic stromal lymphopoietin (TSLP) monoclonal antibody Fab fragment (CSJ117) have been investigating in clinical trials to confirm the optimized formulation can successfully be administered to patients using dry powder inhaler [58] (Table 15.2).

15.3.3.4 Soft mist inhaler (SMI)

Soft mist inhalers (SMIs) are propellant-free mechanical devices that are slightly larger than a conventional pMDI. The device functions by forcing a metered dose of drug solution through a unique engineered nozzle, producing two fine jets of liquid [59]. The collision of these two jets generates the soft mist. SMIs contain a higher fine particle fraction (over 65%) than aerosol clouds from conventional portable inhaler devices, such as pMDIs and DPIs. In addition, the relatively long generation time of the aerosol cloud (approximately 1.5 s) facilitates coordination of inhalation and actuation which significantly overcome drawbacks of pMDIs [60]. These features, together with the slow velocity of the soft mist, result in larger amounts of the drug reaching the lungs and less being deposited in the oropharynx compared with either pMDIs or DPIs [61].

15.3.4 Types of Carriers Used for Pulmonary Delivery

15.3.4.1 Lactose and other Sugars

Lactose is the most commonly used excipient in commercial DPIs (Beclophar®, Flixotide®, Relenza®, Seretide®, Spiriva®, and Symbicort®). Manufacturers using different physical forms of lactose for DPI inhalation such as α-lactose monohydrate (prepared by milling) or anhydrous β-lactose (prepared by spray drying) with a wide range of particle-size distribution to load small molecules [62, 63]. Due to the reducibility of lactose, it is not suitable for protein delivery. Other sugars such as mannitol, glucose monohydrate, trehalose, dextrose, maltose, sorbitol, maltitol and xylitol also been investigated as carrier for pulmonary delivery. Mannitol was used in a drug formulation for DPI insulin delivery (Exubera®, Pfizer) [64].

TABLE 15.2 Summary of capsule-based inhaler devices, blister-based inhaler devices and reservoir/cartridge-based inhaler devices

CAPSULE BASED INHALER DEVICES		BLISTER BASED INHALER DEVICES		RESERVOIR/CARTRIDGE BASED INHALER DEVICES	
DEVICE NAME	PATENT NUMBER	DEVICE NAME	PATENT NUMBER	DEVICE NAME	PATENT NUMBER
Aerohaler	US7284553	Vortran DPI	US5533502	3M Conix 1 DPI	US8820324
Aerolizer	US3991761	Acu-Breathe	US6550477	Aespironics DPI	US20100139655
ARCUS	US7278425	Acu-Breathe single dose	US6561186	Bespak Unit dose	US6945953
Axahaler	US201003000440	Acu-Breathe Twin DPI	US7931022	C-Haler	US6422236
Braunform DPI	WO2007093149	Aspirair	US7845349	Clickhaler	US5924417
Breezhaler	US8479730	Bang Olufsen DPI	EP1522325	Cricket	US8424518
Cipla Rotahaler	WO2005113043	Blister inhaler	US5881719	Dreamboat	US8499757
DOTT DPI	US7275538	Diskhaler	US5860419	Duohaler	US2011120464
Eclipse	US6470884	Diskus/ Accuhaler	US5860419	Easyhaler	US8550070
FlowCaps	US5673686	ElpenHaler	EP1467787	E-flex	US6892727
Rotahaler	AU6512580	Forspiro	US7069929	Genuair	US8567394
Handihaler	WO2005044353	GSK resuable electronic DPI	WO03092575	Jethaler	US6054082
Hanmi dry powder inhaler	KR20140046935	Gyrohaler	US7069929	LRRI DPI	US6003512
Plastiape MonoDose DPI	US7284552	Manta Multi Dose DPI	US8763605	MedTone	WO0107107
Podhaler	US2003150454	Manta single dose	US2013291865	Miat-Haler	US5033463
RediHaler DPI	WO2009091780	MeadWestvaco	WO2011071845	NEXThaler	US7854226
resQhaler	US9056173	Microdose DPI	US5694920	Novartis MultiDose DPI	WO2011073306
Revolizer	US8006695	MultiHaler	US2010126507	Novolizer	US6071498
Rexam metered dose DPI	US5651359	Nektar Deep-lung DPI	US5740794	Otsuka DPI for freeze dried formulations	US7448379
SpinHaler	GB1122284	Prohaler	US8261740	PADD	US6482391
Turbospin	US20040025876	ProHaler	US20080035143	Pulmolet	US20130092161
Twister	US9242055	Sanovel DPI	EP2239002	Pulvinal	US5351683
Vectura unit dose	US20080190424	Solis	US6889690	SkyeHaler	US7131441
XCaps	US8677992	SunHaler	WO2005110519	Spiromax	US5503144

15.3.4.2 Lipids

As the surfactant present in the lungs is mainly composed by lipid which weight of approximately 90%. The lipids are characterized by an unusually high level of saturated fatty acid chains such as the predominant dipalmitoyl phosphatidylcholine (DPPC), which represents 40% by weight of lung surfactant, unsaturated PC (35%), phosphatidylglycerol (10%), phosphatidylinositol (2%), phosphatidylethanolamine (3%) and sphingomyelin (2.5%). There is also a small amount of neutral lipid composed of mainly cholesterol [65]. Therefore, lipid materials are been considered as the potential carriers for protein or peptides pulmonary delivery. Lipids such as egg PC, distearoyl PC (DSPC) and DPPC can be used to prepare liposomes or lipid nanoparticles to encapsulate drugs. After pulmonary administration, liposomes could increase in drug retention time and reduce the toxicity with controlled release behavers of drugs, which could significantly improve the treatment efficiency [66].

15.3.4.3 Biodegradable polymers

Large numbers of carriers have been developed to prepare a potential controlled drug delivery platform for the pulmonary delivery of lung. As polymer degradation affect drug accumulation and delivery platform clearance, the non-biodegradable polymers is prohibited to be used as carriers for lung delivery. Poly(d,l-lactide-co-glycolide) (PLGA) is the most widely used biodegradable materials that has been used to produce microspheres/nanoparticles. Long-acting inhalable chitosan-coated PLGA nanoparticles containing hydrophobically modified exendin-4 for treating type 2 diabetes [67, 68]. PLGA microspheres have been investigated in pulmonary delivery for the controlled release of different types of drugs such as anti-asthmatic drugs, antibiotics, and proteins. However, because the degradation rate of PLGA is extremely slow, this polymer many not be suitable for pulmonary delivery of proteins and peptides. Chitosan has also been widely used as carriers for proteins and peptides to improve their absorption when formulated with PLGA [69, 70]. Chitosan can significantly improve the cellular uptake and absorption of proteins due to its positive charges, however it could also induce a significant pulmonary inflammatory response after pulmonary administration.

15.4 EXPERIMENTAL MODELS FOR TESTING INHALED PARTICLE TRANSPORT IN LUNG AIRWAYS

15.4.1 Cell Culture Models

Cell culture systems of isolated airway and alveolar epithelial cells have been developed, which provide a means to study the mechanisms of binding and transport processes at the level of the pulmonary epithelium of interest, without the influence of other tissues. Cell monolayer models can be utilized for permeability measurements, tissue retention can be measured with tissue slices, and the dissolution rate can be based on solubility measures. Primary cell culture monolayer models such as alveolar epithelial cells and type 2 pneumocytes, are costly, time-consuming with short life-time, but extremely useful for pulmonary drug transport studies. Air-interface cultures (AIC) are models that allow aerosol particles to deposit directly onto semi-dry apical cell surface. The Calu-3 cell line was derived from human bronchial epithelium and apparent permeability coefficients in Calu-3 cells correlated well with permeability values obtained in primary culture. The tight polarized monolayer formed by Calu-3 cells appears to be a reproducible and potential model to screen protein and peptide candidates or formulations for pulmonary delivery with high TEER value and similarity to in vivo physiology [71]. Although the applications of Calu-3 cells include pulmonary drug absorption, metabolism, drug interactions, disease pathophysiology and toxicity, in vitro in vivo comparisons of drug permeability using Calu-3 airway cell model is still limited [72]. Calu-3 monolayer lacks a mucociliary clearance mechanism, and intact structure and full absorptive pathway. Additionally, the use of such reconstructed monolayer cell barriers cannot satisfactorily be reproduced to represent the complex tissue kinetics of absorption and disposition found in vivo.

15.4.2 Ex Vivo Isolated Perfused Lung Model

The ex vivo isolated perfused lung (IPL) model is well suited for many kinds of physiological, pharmacological, and surgical studies, when the physiological and biochemical conditions in the lung can be maintained near to those in vivo. IPL has also been applied for drug absorption and disposition in pulmonary delivery [73]. The procedure for establishing the model requires a skilled operator, a validated technique for intratracheal drug delivery and a system for maintenance and monitoring of the preparation. The value of the IPL model is in discerning lung-specific drug absorption and disposition kinetics that may be difficult to interpolate from in vivo data and cannot be modelled with physiological relevance using reductive in vitro techniques such as cell culture. In simulated physiological and biochemical conditions, IPL can be applied to the uptake and distribution of anticancer drugs in lung tumors and in normal lung tissue [74].

15.4.3 Preclinical Model

Small rodents such as mice, rats and guinea pigs are common animal models for initial studies for pulmonary drug delivery. Rat model is more suitable model for pharmacokinetic studies for pulmonary research than mouse model due to larger size helps in handling and dosing. Allergic asthma and infectious disease of guinea pig models have been widely used and evaluated due to their similarity to human cases. However, there are significant upper airway differences among human infants, adults and rodents. The inability to inhale via the mouth limits the relevance of lung deposition data obtained through preclinical rodent models that utilize whole-body and nose-only exposures.

In addition, intravascular macrophages in human, that can attack pathogens entering the lungs through the bloodstream, are absent in rodents. These notable differences between humans and the most commonly employed rodent-based animal models call for a more cautious approach in extrapolating pulmonary drug delivery and disposition results from preclinical studies to humans [75].

Non-human primates appear to constitute a particularly relevant preclinical model for respiratory infectious diseases, as their pathogenesis more closely resembles that in human patients, and treatments found to be effective in them can more easily be translated into clinical trial for humans. Apes and chimpanzees in particular, were historically used as research models for studies of infectious diseases [76].

15.5 PEPTIDE AND PROTEIN IN PULMONARY DELIVERY

Effective biologics delivery systems can potentially lower the administration cost, thus enhancing patient's and healthcare system's affordability. The unique structure and characteristics of biological drugs such as proteins and peptides separate them as a special group of therapeutics. Delivery of most peptide and protein drugs by pulmonary route display their pharmacological effect by interacting with cell surface receptors or extracellular ligands. Therefore, the objective of biological drug delivery is to maintain the drug concentration at extracellular sites within the therapeutic window for sufficient period of time. However, still some biologics drugs delivered for systemic treatment by pulmonary route to avoid first-pass metabolism. Include peptides, cytokines, enzymes, vaccines, monoclonal antibodies, clotting factors, aptamers, RNA, siRNA, miRNA, and ribozymes [77]. Various approaches have been applied to enhance their pulmonary absorption and maintain in vivo stability. Herein, we summarize the pulmonary delivery of peptides and proteins for the treatment of various diseases.

15.5.1 Suitable Conditions for Pulmonary Delivery

15.5.1.1 Diabetes mellitus

Diabetes mellitus (DM) is a metabolic disorder characterized by relative or absolute deficiency of insulin, resulting in hyperglycemia. Subcutaneous insulin and oral hypoglycemic agents (OHA) constitute the main treatment option for DM. Pulmonary route is one of the most desired route for insulin delivery. Inhaled insulin could completely eliminate the psychological barriers associated with subcutaneous insulin delivery, such as needle phobia and incorrect injection. Inhaled insulin can be applied in both Type I and Type II diabetic patients. Exubra was the first inhaled insulin approved by the FDA in 2006, but withdrawn by Pfizer in October 2007 due to economic reasons [78]. Afrezza® (insulin human) inhalation powder approved by the FDA in 2014, is a rapid-acting Technosphere® insulin administered via a small breath-powered oral inhaler to diabetic patients. Apart from that, a novel nebulizer-compatible liposome for aerosol pulmonary drug delivery of insulin was invented to achieve encapsulation of insulin to liposomal carriers and reduction in pulmonary side effects [79]. Peptide tyrosine-tyrosine (PYY3-36) is an endogenous 36-amino acid peptide found in the endocrine L cells of the intestinal mucosa, and has been shown to suppress appetite and body weight gain in animals and humans with diabetes and obesity issues, when given by injection [80]. Needle-free pulmonary delivery of PYY3-36 in an aerosol formulation with inhaler device technology has been explored via either intratracheal or orotracheal instillation in rats, rabbits, rhesus macaques, etc. [81, 82]. PYY3-36 caused dose-dependent and 4–6 h food intake suppression following pulmonary delivery with 12–14% of lung absorption and hypothalamic arcuate nucleus interaction, leading to reduced body weight gain in rats [83].

15.5.1.2 Hormone disorder

Hormone deficiency (HD) is a condition caused by insufficient amounts of hormone in the body. Dry powder inhalers may be particularly suitable devices for pulmonary administration of proteins like human growth hormone (hGH, 22 kDa), follicle stimulating hormone (FSH, 36 kDa), thyrotropin stimulating hormone (TSH, 24–30 kDa), and human chorionic gonadotropin (HCG, 45 kDa), because of their facility of use and the improved drug stability provided by the dry state of the formulation. Recombinant hGH (pI 5.2) is currently delivered via subcutaneous injection to children due to growth hormone deficiency. DPPC, which is a principal component of lung surfactant, can be applied to the formation of large porous particles. Cynthia et al. studied a more effective dry powder aerosol prepared with hGH, lactose and DPPC than the intratracheal instillation of a solution [84]. FSH is a glycoprotein hormone that is crucial in the development and maturation of ovarian follicles and secretion of gonadal hormones [85]. TSH is a pituitary hormone and regarded as the primary biomarker for evaluating thyroid function[86]. It has been shown that the bioavailability of TSH and FSH delivered in alkaline solution were 30-fold greater than those in neutral pH conditions. Meanwhile, the bioavailability of TSH and FSH when given intratracheally as dry powder were 1.6 and 0.6%, respectively [87].

15.5.1.3 Osteoporosis

Osteoporosis is a debilitating metabolic bone disease characterized by low bone mass and architectural deterioration of bone tissue that leads to enhanced bone fragility. Salmon calcitonin (sCT) is a 32 amino acid cyclic poly-peptide with a molecular weight of approximately 3,450 Da and displays the highest affinity for receptors in bones [88]. Calcitonin inhibits bone resorption by decreasing the number of osteoclasts and their resorptive activities and limiting osteocytic osteolysis. However, sCT has a short half-life around 16.9–57.3 min can be degraded by intestinal enzymes and stomach acids when given orally [89, 90]. Leonie et al. and Sato et al. described PEG-lipid micelles and PLGA microspheres prepared by the fine droplet drying, which has been demonstrated as promising carriers for enhanced pulmonary delivery of sCT [91, 92].

15.5.1.4 Multiple sclerosis

Inteferon beta (IFN-β), a type 1 interferon, is an anti-inflammatory cytokine and was the first available disease modifying therapies for the treatment of multiple sclerosis. Proteinaceous molecules can be linked to the Fc fragment of IgG to produce Fc-conjugated or Fc-fusion proteins. These hybrid biomacromolecules have prolonged plasma half-life because of FcRn-mediated recycling in the blood vessel endothelium [93]. SNG001 (Synairgen, Southampton, UK) is an inhaled formulation containing IFN-β, a natural protein controls viral infection in the body. Phase II studies showed that inhaled SNG001 boosted antiviral defense in both asthmatic and COPD subjects.

15.5.2 For Respiratory Diseases

15.5.2.1 Infection for Viral Infections

Since influenza virus infect the body mainly though respiratory system, flu vaccines should ideally be administered via the pulmonary route to achieve the goals to active immune response and prevent viral infection. An influenza monovalent vaccine (A Panama/2007/99) was spray dried or spray-freeze dried to formulate as inhalable dry powder. Both vaccines formulations could significantly improve the pulmonary immunization with higher IgG titers compare to i.m. immunization [94].

At the same times, pulmonary delivery of biologicals has been developed to prevent and against respiratory viral infections. DAS181 (Fludase®, Ansun BioPharma) is a sialidase fusion protein composed of the catalytic domain of Actinomyces viscosus sialidase and the epithelial anchoring domain of human amphiregulin. DAS181 is designed to bind the respiratory epithelial cells and then removes cell-surface sialic acid residues to reduce influenza virus attachment to lung epithelium and inhibit infection. For pulmonary delivery, DAS181 was formulated as dry powder composed of microparticles and delivered using DPI (Cyclohalcr®). A Phase II clinical study recruited 177 participants infected with influenza B, H3N2, or H1N1 to evaluate DAS181 antivirus effects. Significant effects were observed on decreased change from baseline viral load and viral shedding in the multiple-dose group, which confirm the inhibitory activity against seasonal influenza strains and a highly pathogenic avian influenza strain [95].

Interferon-β (INF-β) is one of the first cytokines induced by viral infection of a cell. The INF-β is a key cytokine to active the innate response during antiviral immune response by both potent antiviral and immunomodulatory functions. Therefore, SNG001 as a formulation of recombinant IFN-β in aqueous solution was developed for inhalation delivery by nebulizer to investigate treatment efficiency on of virus-induced lower respiratory tract illnesses. A phase II study shown the boosted antiviral defense in patients with asthmatic or COPD which potentially improved the asthmatic symptom induce by the infection [96].

COVID-19 is a contagious disease caused by severe acute respiratory syndrome coronavirus 2 (SARS-CoV-2). Several clinical trials are undergoing to develop effective treatment drugs against viral infection. DAS181 is a sialidase fusion protein and SNG001, which is an inhaled IFN-β1a formulation. Since DAS181 and SNG001 exhibit hose-directed anti-viral effects with wide antiviral spectrum, they could also to inhibit COVID-19 infection. There are already two clinical trials undergoing to evaluate the effects of DAS181 and SNG001 on COVID-19 infection treatment. Patients who received nebulized SNG001 exhibit higher chance to relieve symptom and improve the recover form SARS-CoV-2 infection compare the patients who received placebo. This positive result provides the new strategy to prevention and against the COVID-19 pandemics infection [97].

Respiratory syncytial virus (RSV) is a common respiratory tract pathogen to cause lower respiratory tract infections in infants. Palivizumab (Synagis®) is a monoclonal antibody used to prevent severe disease caused by respiratory syncytial virus (RSV) infections by intramuscular injection. The recent study from Aunshi et al. confirmed the potential of nebulized palivizumab on RSV infection treatment by pulmonary delivery [98]. They use both HYDRA and AeroNeb Go® device to produced palivizumab aerosols with similar median aerosol droplet diameters. Over 88% of palivizumab aerosols was deposited in the lungs. Compare to intramuscular injection, pulmonary delivery may rapidly produce the therapeutic benefits for high-risk infants.

ALX-0171 is designed as a trivalent nanobody directed towards the RSV fusion protein. ALX-0171 could inhibit RSV replication by directly binding the F-protein on the surface of virus and reduce RSV entry into host cells followed by clearing the virus though immune system. For the lower respiratory tract deposit, ALX-0171 was developed for delivery directly into lungs by nebulization for RSV treatment. Research form Alejandro et al. suggests that nebulized ALX-0171 was able to reduce viral load in airway secretions and improve clinical symptoms and lung pathology in a newborn lamb model infected with human RSV [99]. The same conclusions were also confirmed by Laurent et al. in cotton rats [100]. An undergoing phase II study confirms ALX-0171 nebulizer was able to rapidly reduce the RSV viral load in nasal mid turbinate specimens. However, reduced viral loading in upper respiration system is not reciprocated by significant improvement in clinical outcomes [101]. Steve et al. suggest that future studies should focus on the earlier intervention as antivirals agents might be unable to improve clinical outcomes once RSV infection is established in lower respiratory tract.

15.5.2.2 Cystic Fibrosis

Inhaled proteins also have been investigated as an effective therapy approach of inherited disorders including cystic fibrosis (CF). CF is caused by the presence of mutations in both copies of the gene for the cystic fibrosis transmembrane conductance regulator (CFTR) protein, leading to symptom such as excessive mucus secretion and recurrent infection in the respiratory tract followed by decrease in lung function. Airway mucus secretions produced by individuals with CF have higher viscosity and elasticity than mucus from individuals without lung disease. The mucus barrier has been increasingly recognized as a major hurdle to airway protein and peptide delivery. Suk et al. developed a mucolytics/nanoparticle-coating strategy, in which the N-acetyl cysteine (NAC) treatment of CF mucus can greatly increase the mesh spacing, thereby allowing large fractions of polymeric nanoparticles (NPs) to rapidly penetrate NAC-treated CF mucus. This non-mucoadhesive NPs were comprised of polystyrene with carboxyl-modification, mucolytic as the adjuvants and/ or low molecular weight PEG as the dense brush layer [102]. Mucus-penetrating solid lipid nanoparticles (SLNPs) of different surface properties have also been investigated for crossing pulmonary mucus barriers. Poloxamer-coated SLNs showed faster diffusion rate in mucus followed by Tween-coated SLNs, whereas PVA coating ensured very weak mucus penetration [103, 104].

ALX-009 is a fixed combination of hypothiocyanite (OSCN⁻) and bovine lactoferrin (bLF), both are deficient in the airway surface liquid of CF patients. OSCN⁻ could oxidize free thiol radicals of proteins to created disulfide bonds which disturb the bacterial physiology. LF act by direct interaction with bacterial cell membranes and/or depriving bacteria of iron. By providing both molecules, ALX-009 will contribute to restore the natural capacity of the lung to fight against infections and relieve CF symptoms.

Dornase alfa (Pulmozyme®) is recombinant human deoxyribonuclease I (rhDNase) solution which could selectively cleave DNA, which is the first inhaled protein approved by the FDA for the CF treatment. It acts as a mucolytic agent to reduce the viscosity of mucus in the airway and promoting improved clearance of secretions [105]. A research from Henry et al. performed a randomized, double-blind, placebo-controlled study to determine the effects of pulmonary administration of rhDNase on pulmonary function. Daily inhaled rhDNase I improved the lung function and reduction in the incidence of exacerbations in CF patients [106].

Although dornase alfa has been successfully marketed for respiratory diseases, the activity of DNase I is substantially inhibited by actin which found existed in CF sputum. Alidornase alfa (PRX-110) is a modified of DNase I was developed to resist the inhibition activity of actin. The safety and efficacy of inhaled Alidornase alfa was investigated in a Phase II switchover trial in CF patients. Interim analysis indicated that Alidornase alfa could potentially improve the lung function in CF patients without side effects.

Several studies have shown that inhaled alpha1-proteinase inhibitor (PI), commonly known as alpha(1)-antitrypsin (AAT), could reduce neutrophil elastase burden in some patients with CF. Aerosolized delivery of human AAT to the respiratory tract and has been shown to reduce neutrophil elastase burden and inflammation in respiratory secretions of AAT–deficient patients [107]. Gaggar et al. determined the effects of AA on CF patients in a randomized, double-blinded placebo-controlled clinical trial. In this study, AKITA2® APIXNEB™ electronically regulated nebulizer system was used to nebulize drug solution with increased drug deposition compared to older nebulizer systems and allows for accurate dosing that is independent of lung function impairment [108]. The pulmonary delivery of AAT is well tolerated, accepted, and effective in raising the alpha1-PI levels in the sputum of CF patients. Brand et al. also evaluated lung deposition of alpha1-PI using same device. The drug deposition was around 70% of the filling dose which no different all treatment groups, with no adverse effect on lung function or any influence of disease severity on total lung deposition [109].

15.5.3 Immunotherapy

Granulomatosis with polyangiitis (GPA) is a systemic necrotizing vasculitis, which affects small- and medium-sized blood vessels and is often associated with cytoplasmic antineutrophil cytoplasmic antibody (ANCA) [110]. Rituximab (RTX), a chimeric human-mouse monoclonal antibody targeting CD20, has reportedly achieved successful remission of GPA and microscopic polyangiitis (MPA) in 80%–100% of patients with severe and/or refractory diseases [111]. Terrance et al. has successfully applied the ex vivo lung perfusion model to deliver monoclonal antibody rituximab, which led to targeted depletion of allograft B-cells [112].

Eosinophilic granulomatosis with polyangiitis (EGPA) closely associated with asthma and eosinophilia, is autoimmune disorder, belonging to the small vessel ANCA-associated vasculitis, and necrotizing vasculitis predominantly affecting small to medium-sized vessels [113]. Mepolizumab a humanized, immunoglobulin G1 (IgG1), anti-interleukin (IL)-5 monoclonal antibody, can actively bind to circulating IL-5 to prevent it from binding to alpha chain of IL-5 receptor (IL-5 Rα) on the surface of eosinophils, and further block the activation of eosinophils resulting in decreased eosinophilic airway inflammation and reduced eosinophil survival [114]. Mepolizumab is a humanized antibody used and has shown to reduce exacerbation frequency, decrease oral corticosteroid dependence, and improve health-related quality of life and lung function, compared with placebo [115]. Mepolizumab branded as Nucala® has been used in adults to help control symptoms and reduce flares of eosinophilic granulomatosis with polyangiitis (EPGA).

15.6 APPROACHES TO ENHANCE THE INHALATION AND LUNG DEPOSITION OF PROTEIN THERAPEUTICS

The use of dry powder formulations for inhalation drug delivery is illustrated in Figure 15.4. Polymeric NPs and liposomes can be used for controlled drug release at the target site and to maintain their therapeutic concentrations for a longer duration in the

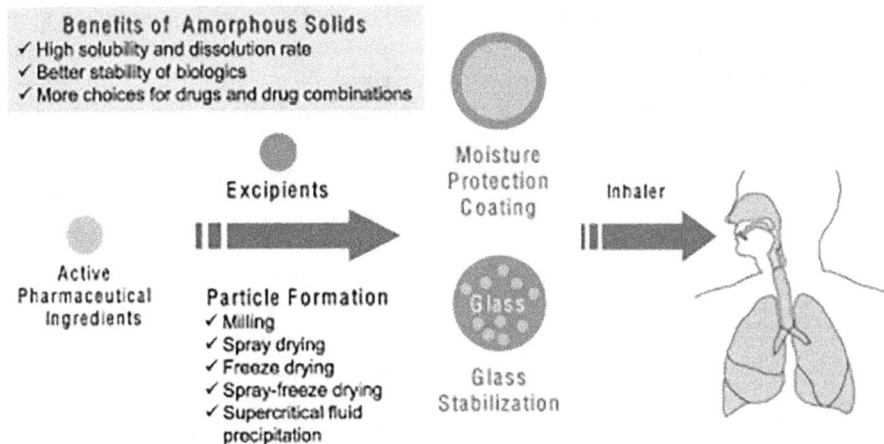

Benefits of Amorphous Solids
✓ High solubility and dissolution rate
✓ Better stability of biologics
✓ More choices for drugs and drug combinations

Excipients

Moisture Protection Coating

Inhaler

Active Pharmaceutical Ingredients

Particle Formation
✓ Milling
✓ Spray drying
✓ Freeze drying
✓ Spray-freeze drying
✓ Supercritical fluid precipitation

Glass Stabilization

FIGURE15.4 Dry powder formulation for inhalation drug delivery.

lungs. Passive targeting in the lung is mainly achieved by changing the characteristics of the delivery vehicle to influence localization and uptake based on various manufacturing techniques as discussed in Section 15.3. A nanoformulation was developed and achieved suitable aerodynamic properties to reach the alveolar zone, using spray-drying for preparing NPs in mannitol microspheres [116]. Alginate, an anionic polysaccharide, has a strong ability to form hydrogen bonds with mucin layer of mucosa and is widely used to obtain mucoadhesive drug delivery systems [117]. Amore et al. developed a novel mucoadhesive polymer-coated solid lipid microparticles with suitable characteristics for controlled release of fluticasone propionate to treat COPD.

Active targeting can increase the concentration of therapeutic macromolecules at the desired location by targeting specific cell types. This approach involves the conjugation of the carrier or macromolecule to a targeting ligand such as protein and peptides, polysaccharides, glycolipids, glycoproteins, or antibodies. The human polymeric immunoglobulin receptor on the lung epithelial cells also can be used for protein and peptide targeting for the treatment of cystic fibrosis [118]. Although there are a extensive number of identified targets for various cells involved in lung pathologies, very few have been investigated for efficacy after pulmonary delivery.

The administration of drugs with immunogenicity such as polysaccharides, proteins or peptides to the lungs may stimulate an immune response in the lungs, and subsequently produce anti-drug antibodies, which can significantly reduce the efficacy of these therapeutic molecules [119]. Therefore, the long-term adverse effects of inhaled proteins and peptides remain uncertain. To maintain the pharmacological efficiency of the inhaled drugs in deep lung, good excipients should be selected for pulmonary administration. Endogenous lipids such as PC can be applied to avoid unwanted immune response [120]. When using dry powder formulations, natural and bio-inspired excipients are applied to improve dosing reproducibility and aerosolization performance. Amino acids, especially L-leucine and its tripeptide trileucine, can improve powder dispersibility and decrease moisture uptake. Sugars, particularly lactose, are used as drug-carrying diluents, flow enhancers, biopharmaceuticals stabilizers, microparticulate matrices for nanoparticles and surface enrichers. Lipids like magnesium stearate can reduce interparticle adhesive forces and phospholipids are used to compose of liposomal drug delivery systems for generating liposomal inhalation of dry powders [121]. Frequently used biodegradable polymer PLGA and mucoadhesive polymer chitosan are used to facilitate sustained release and targeted drug delivery [122].

15.7 CONCLUDING REMARKS

Pulmonary delivery offers several advantages over systemic delivery such as it is noninvasive, applies higher concentrations of drugs directly to the disease site, minimizes the systemic side effects, and avoids first-pass metabolism for the treatment of respiratory disorders. Moreover, the slow mucociliary clearance in the lungs results in prolonged drug residence and is independent of dietary complications. There are a number of specialized needs for these aerosol formulations that must be addressed. Only a small percentage of the dose is deposited in the lung in most of the current inhaled formulations. The aerodynamic particle size between 1 and 5 μm and high porosity exhibit better penetration to the lung periphery. Advancements in the design of inhaled particles and their respective devices over the past decades resulted in highly reliable delivery of the therapeutic aerosol with lung deposition reaching up to 60%. The predominant mechanism of drug absorption into the lungs is by simple diffusion and the absorption rate primarily depends on the physicochemical properties of the molecule.

Proteins and peptides find many applications in treating various diseases due to their high potency and specificity; however, there are several challenges that impede optimum efficacy. These include the physical and chemical stresses that the protein faces during manufacturing/aerosolization, the requirement of special handling and storage conditions, the need to overcome mucociliary clearance and other disease-related physical barriers to reach target sites within the lung, the need to stay stable in the presence of abundant proteases, and the need to avoid reticuloendothelial system (RES) clearance, among others. The lung epithelia also pose a crucial barrier to the absorption of inhaled drugs and proteins. It has a variable thickness of 50–60 μm in the trachea to 0.2 μm in the alveoli. Therefore, most of the protein and peptides dose deposited stays in the lung and minimizes systemic exposure. It is beneficial when the target site is the lung itself (i.e., airway epithelium, alveolar macrophages and neutrophils). However, strategies are needed to optimize the bioavailability of the peptides for systemic action (including insulin). The rational modifications of proteins, absorption enhancers, or proteinase inhibitors could accomplish systemic delivery and are emerging techniques for pulmonary drug delivery.

The stability of inhaled proteins is critical during formulation development for successful therapeutics. Protein aggregation is although a major cause of instability, studies should also be focused on other instability issues such as specific chemical modifications. Further, the selection of excipients could have a significant effect on formulation stability. For example, in protein-containing formulations intended for nebulization, the addition of Polysorbate 80 could exert a protective effect since protein degradation mostly takes place at air-liquid interfaces.

Nanotechnology has emerged as a powerful technique for advancing the development of inhalation pharmaceuticals for respiratory diseases. The innovative nanocarrier approaches could not only enhance the stability and pharmacokinetic profile of proteins, they could also provide sustained release, reduce toxicity, and enhance the deposition of active drugs locally. Further, NPs could be easily surface modified to target the drug to specific cells o the lungs. Several proteins and enzymes have recently been encapsulated in NPs to increase their pulmonary delivery, including catalase, glutathione, and superoxide dismutase. However, nebulizers were used to administer these drugs intratracheally. The use of nebulization to deliver nanocarriers may cause long-term stability complications and lead to drug leakage.

Therefore, dry powders formulations for drug delivery to the lungs because of the unmatched stability are being developed. Drugs alone or in combination with excipients that serve as a carrier for delivery to the lungs are used in dry powder products. Freeze-drying and spray-drying are among the leading techniques that have been prepared for aerosol delivery. For example, to test respirable characteristics, superoxide dismutase was encapsulated in spray-dried liposomes. To minimize the immunogenicity of protein drugs such as heparin, insulin, aminoglycosides, ergotamine, and ribavirin inhalation drug delivery have been successfully reported. Further, the current delivery systems are quite effective in delivering the cargo into the lungs, irrespective of the different epithelial surfaces.

There are still several overarching obstacles in the path of successful protein inhalation drugs. For example, there is a lack of FDA-approved excipients for this category of drugs. The physicochemical properties of each protein drug as well as its compatibility with carriers need special emphasis for a high efficacy formulation. This could be a rate-limiting factor in product development and in large-scale production. Therefore, expanding the list of approved excipients through increased toxicological testing would provide more options for formulation design. The majority of in vivo efficacy and toxicity studies described to date have been preclinical and are still in the early stages of testing, thus their therapeutic effects must be confirmed. Future research should concentrate on the effects of therapeutic nanomedicine on performance, molecular mechanisms, and potential toxicity during the treatment process. These methods would be extremely beneficial to the field of pulmonary drug delivery, allowing more inhaled protein therapies to reach the clinic in the future. However, the knowledge in this field is continually progressing and we expect inhalation will become a convenient administration method for proteins and peptides in the future.

REFERENCES

1. R.I. Mahato, A.S. Narang, L. Thoma, D.D. Miller, Emerging trends in oral delivery of peptide and protein drugs, *Crit. Rev. Ther. Drug Carrier Syst.* 20(2–3) (2003) 153–214.
2. J.S. Patton, P.R. Byron, Inhaling medicines: Delivering drugs to the body through the lungs, *Nat. Rev. Drug Discov.* 6(1) (2007) 67 74.
3. R. Guagliardo, J. Perez-Gil, S. De Smedt, K. Raemdonck, Pulmonary surfactant and drug delivery: Focusing on the role of surfactant proteins, *J. Control. Release* 291 (2018) 116–126.
4. X. Murgia, C. de Souza Carvalho, C. Lehr, Overcoming the pulmonary barrier: New insights to improve the efficiency of inhaled therapeutics, *Eur. J. Nanomed.* 6(3) (2014) 157–169.
5. P. Rees, Uptake and toxicology of nanoparticles, *Front. Nanosci.* 5 (2013) 123–138.
6. S. Guo, Y. Zhang, Z. Wu, L. Zhang, D. He, X. Li, Z. Wang, Synergistic combination therapy of lung cancer: Cetuximab functionalized nanostructured lipid carriers for the co-delivery of paclitaxel and 5-Demethylnobiletin, *Biomed. Pharmacother.* 118 (2019) 109225.
7. A. Patel, K. Cholkar, A.K. Mitra, Recent developments in protein and peptide parenteral delivery approaches, *Ther. Deliv.* 5(3) (2014) 337–365.
8. R.U. Agu, M.I. Ugwoke, M. Armand, R. Kinget, N. Verbeke, The lung as a route for systemic delivery of therapeutic proteins and peptides, *Respir. Res.* 2(4) (2001) 198–209.
9. J.D. Londino, J.F. Collawn, S. Matalon, Regulation of airway lining fluid in health and disease, in: *Anonymous comparative biology of the normal*, R.A. Parent ed., Lung, Elsevier, 2015, pp. 467–477.

10. H. Tandel, K. Florence, A. Misra, Protein and peptide delivery through respiratory pathway, in: *Anonymous challenges in delivery of therapeutic genomics and proteomics*, A. Misra ed., Mumbai, Elsevier, 2011, pp. 429–479.

11. T. Secher, A. Mayor, N. Heuze-Vourc'h, Inhalation of immuno-therapeutics/-Prophylactics to fight respiratory tract infections: An appropriate drug at the right place!, *Front. Immunol.* 10 (2019) 2760.

12. R. Vanbever, A. Ben-Jebria, J.D. Mintzes, R. Langer, D.A. Edwards, Sustained release of insulin from insoluble inhaled particles, *Drug Dev. Res.* 48(4) (1999) 178–185.

13. P.C.L. Kwok, H. Chan, Pulmonary delivery of peptides and proteins, in: *Anonymous peptide and protein delivery*, C. Van Der Walle ed., Glasgow, Elsevier, 2011, pp. 23–46.

14. J.S. Suk, Q. Xu, N. Kim, J. Hanes, L.M. Ensign, PEGylation as a strategy for improving nanoparticle-based drug and gene delivery, *Adv. Drug Deliv. Rev.* 99(A) (2016) 28–51.

15. H. Douafer, V. Andrieu, J.M. Brunel, Scope and limitations on aerosol drug delivery for the treatment of infectious respiratory diseases, *J. Control. Release* 325 (2020) 276–292.

16. P. Muralidharan, M. Malapit, E. Mallory, D. Hayes, H.M. Mansour, Inhalable nanoparticulate powders for respiratory delivery, *Nanomedicine* 11(5) (2015) 1189–1199.

17. C. Darquenne, Deposition mechanisms, *J. Aerosol Med. Pulm. Drug Deliv.* 33(4) (2020) 181–185.

18. C. Bosquillon, C. Lombry, V. Preat, R. Vanbever, Influence of formulation excipients and physical characteristics of inhalation dry powders on their aerosolization performance, *J. Control. Release* 70(3) (2001) 329–339.

19. H.C. Yeh, Use of a heat transfer analogy for a mathematical model of respiratory tract deposition, *Bull. Math. Biol.* 36(2) (1974) 105–116.

20. J. Pich, Theory of gravitational deposition of particles from laminar flows in channels, *J. Aerosol Sci.* 3(5) (1972) 351–361.

21. P. Gormley, M. Kennedy, Diffusion from a stream flowing through a cylindrical tube 52 (1948) 163–169.

22. M. Lippmann, Effects of fiber characteristics on lung deposition, retention, and disease, *Environ. Health Perspect.* 88 (1990) 311–317.

23. P.C.L. Kwok, H. Chan, Electrostatics of pharmaceutical inhalation aerosols, *J. Pharm. Pharmacol.* 61(12) (2009) 1587–1599.

24. H. Majid, P. Madl, W. Hofmann, K. Alam, Implementation of charged particles deposition in stochastic lung model and calculation of enhanced deposition, *Aerosol Sci. Technol.* 46(5) (2012) 547–554.

25. D. Ghosh, X. Peng, J. Leal, R.P. Mohanty, Peptides as drug delivery vehicles across biological barriers, *J. Pharm. Investig.* 48(1) (2018) 89–111.

26. F. Emami, A. Vatanara, E.J. Park, D.H. Na, Drying technologies for the stability and bioavailability of biopharmaceuticals, *Pharmaceutics* 10(3) (2018) http://doi.org/10.3390/pharmaceutics10030131.

27. E. Swider, O. Koshkina, J. Tel, L.J. Cruz, I.J.M. de Vries, M. Srinivas, Customizing poly(lactic-co-glycolic acid) particles for biomedical applications, *Acta Biomater.* 73 (2018) 38–51.

28. E. Cauchetier, M. Deniau, H. Fessi, A. Astier, M. Paul, Atovaquone-loaded nanocapsules: Influence of the nature of the polymer on their in vitro characteristics, *Int. J. Pharm.* 250(1) (2003) 273–281.

29. R. Bawa, R.A. Siegel, B. Marasca, M. Karel, R. Langer, An explanation for the controlled release of macromolecules from polymers, *J. Control. Release* 1(4) (1985) 259–267.

30. F. Khan, M. Atif, M. Haseen, S. Kamal, M.S. Khan, S. Shahid, S.A.A. Nami, Synthesis, classification and properties of hydrogels: Their applications in drug delivery and agriculture, *J. Mater. Chem. B* 10(2) (2022) 170–203.

31. N.A. Peppas, P. Bures, W. Leobandung, H. Ichikawa, Hydrogels in pharmaceutical formulations, *Eur. J. Pharm. Biopharm.* 50(1) (2000) 27–46.

32. C.C. Lin, A.T. Metters, Hydrogels in controlled release formulations: Network design and mathematical modeling, *Adv. Drug Deliv. Rev.* 58(12–13) (2006) 1379–1408.
33. S.H. Lee, H. Mok, Y. Lee, T.G. Park, Self-assembled siRNA-PLGA conjugate micelles for gene silencing, *J. Control. Release* 152(1) (2011) 152–158.
34. M. Prabaharan, J.J. Grailer, S. Pilla, D.A. Steeber, S. Gong, Amphiphilic multi-arm-block copolymer conjugated with doxorubicin via pH-sensitive hydrazone bond for tumor-targeted drug delivery, *Biomaterials* 30(29) (2009) 5757–5766.
35. S. Fredenberg, M. Wahlgren, M. Reslow, A. Axelsson, The mechanisms of drug release in poly(lactic-co-glycolic acid)-based drug delivery systems–A review, *Int. J. Pharm.* 415(1–2) (2011) 34–52.
36. F. von Burkersroda, L. Schedl, A. Gopferich, Why degradable polymers undergo surface erosion or bulk erosion, *Biomaterials* 23(21) (2002) 4221–4231.
37. B. Han, B. Shen, Z. Wang, M. Shi, H. Li, C. Peng, Q. Zhao, C. Gao, Layered microcapsules for daunorubicin loading and release as well as in vitro and in vivo studies, *Polym. Adv. Technol.* 19(1) (2008) 36–46.
38. S.A. Abouelmagd, H. Hyun, Y. Yeo, Extracellularly activatable nanocarriers for drug delivery to tumors, *Expert Opin. Drug Deliv.* 11(10) (2014) 1601–1618.
39. M. Talelli, M. Iman, A.K. Varkouhi, C.J. Rijcken, R.M. Schiffelers, T. Etrych, K. Ulbrich, C.F. van Nostrum, T. Lammers, G. Storm, W.E. Hennink, Core-crosslinked polymeric micelles with controlled release of covalently entrapped doxorubicin, *Biomaterials* 31(30) (2010) 7797–7804.
40. M.J. Webber, D.G. Anderson, Smart approaches to glucose-responsive drug delivery, *J. Drug Target.* 23(7–8) (2015) 651–655.
41. Q. Wang, Y. Shen, G. Mi, D. He, Y. Zhang, Y. Xiong, T.J. Webster, J. Tu, Fumaryl diketopiperazine based effervescent microparticles to escape macrophage phagocytosis for enhanced treatment of pneumonia via pulmonary delivery, *Biomaterials* 228 (2020) 119575.
42. T.C. Carvalho, J.T. McConville, The function and performance of aqueous aerosol devices for inhalation therapy, *J. Pharm. Pharmacol.* 68(5) (2016) 556–578.
43. L. Golshahi, R.L. Walenga, P.W. Longest, M. Hindle, Development of a transient flow aerosol mixer-heater system for lung delivery of nasally administered aerosols using a nasal cannula, *Aerosol Sci. Technol.* 48(10) (2014) 1009–1021.
44. L.M.P. de Araújo, P.J. Abatti, W.D. de Araújo, R.F. Alves, Performance evaluation of nebulizers based on aerodynamic droplet diameter characterization using the direct laminar incidence (DLI), *Res. Biomed. Eng.* 33(2) (2017) 105–112.
45. A. Ari, Aerosol therapy in pulmonary critical care, *Respir. Care* 60(6) (2015) 858–874; discussion 874.
46. A. Ari, Jet, ultrasonic, and mesh nebulizers: An evaluation of nebulizers for better clinical outcomes, *Eurasian. J. Pulmonol.* 16 (2014) 1–7.
47. F. Lavorini, G.A. Fontana, O.S. Usmani, New inhaler devices - The good, the bad and the ugly, *Respiration* 88(1) (2014) 3–15.
48. P.K. Deb, S.N. Abed, H. Maher, A. Al-Aboudi, A. Paradkar, S. Bandopadhyay, R.K. Tekade, Aerosols in pharmaceutical product development, in: *Anonymous drug delivery systems*, R.K. Tekade ed., Elsevier, 2020, pp. 521–577.
49. G.W. Ewart, W.N. Rom, S.S. Braman, K.E. Pinkerton, From closing the atmospheric ozone hole to reducing climate change. Lessons learned, *Ann. Am. Thorac. Soc.* 12(2) (2015) 247–251.
50. S.W. Lee, J.J. Sciarra, Development of an aerosol dosage form containing insulin, *J. Pharm. Sci.* 65(4) (1976) 567–572.
51. B.K. Nyambura, I.W. Kellaway, K.M. Taylor, Insulin nanoparticles: Stability and aerosolization from pressurized metered dose inhalers, *Int. J. Pharm.* 375(1–2) (2009) 114–122.

52. E. Cocks, S. Somavarapu, O. Alpar, D. Greenleaf, Influence of suspension stabilisers on the delivery of protein-loaded porous poly (DL-lactide-co-glycolide) (PLGA) microparticles via pressurised metered dose inhaler (pMDI), *Pharm. Res.* 31(8) (2014) 2000–2009.
53. N. Islam, E. Gladki, Dry powder inhalers (DPIs)–A review of device reliability and innovation, *Int. J. Pharm.* 360(1–2) (2008) 1–11.
54. K. Berkenfeld, A. Lamprecht, J.T. McConville, Devices for dry powder drug delivery to the lung, *AAPS PharmSciTech* 16(3) (2015) 479–490.
55. S. Xiroudaki, A. Schoubben, S. Giovagnoli, D.M. Rekkas, Dry powder inhalers in the digitalization era: Current status and future perspectives, *Pharmaceutics* 13(9) (2021) http://doi.org/10.3390/pharmaceutics13091455.
56. R.A. Pleasants, D.R. Hess, Aerosol delivery devices for obstructive lung diseases, *Respir. Care* 63(6) (2018) 708–733.
57. S.P. Newman, Drug delivery to the lungs: Challenges and opportunities, *Ther. Deliv.* 8(8) (2017) 647–661.
58. E. Frohlich, S. Salar-Behzadi, Oral inhalation for delivery of proteins and peptides to the lungs, *Eur. J. Pharm. Biopharm.* 163 (2021) 198–211.
59. R. Dalby, M. Spallek, T. Voshaar, A review of the development of Respimat® Soft Mist™ Inhaler, *Int. J. Pharm.* 283(1–2) (2004) 1–9.
60. D. Hochrainer, H. Hölz, C. Kreher, L. Scaffidi, M. Spallek, H. Wachtel, Comparison of the aerosol velocity and spray duration of Respimat® Soft Mist™ inhaler and pressurized metered dose inhalers, *J. Aerosol Med.* 18(3) (2005) 273–282.
61. T. Iwanaga, Y. Tohda, S. Nakamura, Y. Suga, The Respimat® soft mist inhaler: Implications of drug delivery characteristics for patients, *Clin. Drug Investig.* 39(11) (2019) 1021–1030.
62. F. Vanderbist, B. Wery, I. Moyano-Pavon, A.J. Moës, Optimization of a dry powder inhaler formulation of nacystelyn, a new mucoactive agent, *J. Pharm. Pharmacol.* 51(11) (1999) 1229–1234.
63. S. Zellnitz, D. Lamešić, S. Stranzinger, J.T. Pinto, O. Planinšek, A. Paudel, Spherical agglomerates of lactose as potential carriers for inhalation, *Eur. J. Pharm. Biopharm.* 159 (2021) 11–20.
64. P. Falcetta, M. Aragona, A. Bertolotto, C. Bianchi, F. Campi, M. Garofolo, S. Del Prato, Insulin discovery: A pivotal point in medical history, *Metab. Clin. Exp.* 127 (2022) 154941.
65. F. Possmayer, K. Nag, K. Rodriguez, R. Qanbar, S. Schürch, Surface activity in vitro: Role of surfactant proteins, *Comp. Biochem. Physiol. A Mol. Integr. Physiol.* 129(1) (2001) 209–220.
66. S. Chono, R. Fukuchi, T. Seki, K. Morimoto, Aerosolized liposomes with dipalmitoyl phosphatidylcholine enhance pulmonary insulin delivery, *J. Control. Release* 137(2) (2009) 104–109.
67. Y. Su, B. Zhang, R. Sun, W. Liu, Q. Zhu, X. Zhang, R. Wang, C. Chen, PLGA-based biodegradable microspheres in drug delivery: Recent advances in research and application, *Drug Deliv.* 28(1) (2021) 1397–1418.
68. M.H. Elkomy, R.A. Khallaf, M.O. Mahmoud, R.R. Sayed, A.M. El-Kalaawy, A.H. Abdel-Razik, H.M. Aboud, Intratracheally inhalable nifedipine-loaded chitosan-PLGA nanocomposites as a promising nanoplatform for lung targeting: Snowballed protection via regulation of TGF-β/β-catenin pathway in bleomycin-induced pulmonary fibrosis, *Pharmaceuticals (Basel)* 14(12) (2021) 1225.
69. N. Sivadas, D. O'Rourke, A. Tobin, V. Buckley, Z. Ramtoola, J.G. Kelly, A.J. Hickey, S. Cryan, A comparative study of a range of polymeric microspheres as potential carriers for the inhalation of proteins, *Int. J. Pharm.* 358(1–2) (2008) 159–167.
70. A. Grenha, C. Remuñán-López, E.L. Carvalho, B. Seijo, Microspheres containing lipid/chitosan nanoparticles complexes for pulmonary delivery of therapeutic proteins, *Eur. J. Pharm. Biopharm.* 69(1) (2008) 83–93.

71. K.A. Foster, M.L. Avery, M. Yazdanian, K.L. Audus, Characterization of the Calu-3 cell line as a tool to screen pulmonary drug delivery, *Int. J. Pharm.* 208(1–2) (2000) 1–11.

72. H.X. Ong, D. Traini, P.M. Young, Pharmaceutical applications of the Calu-3 lung epithelia cell line, *Expert Opin. Drug Deliv.* 10(9) (2013) 1287–1302.

73. M.A. Selo, J.A. Sake, K. Kim, C. Ehrhardt, In vitro and ex vivo models in inhalation biopharmaceutical research—Advances, challenges and future perspectives, *Adv. Drug Deliv. Rev.* 177 (2021) 113862.

74. A. Linder, G. Friedel, P. Fritz, K. Kivistö, M. McClellan, H. Toomes, The ex-vivo isolated, perfused human lung model: Description and potential applications, *Thorac. Cardiovasc. Surg.* 44(3) (1996) 140–146.

75. D.N. Price, N.K. Kunda, P. Muttil, Challenges associated with the pulmonary delivery of therapeutic dry powders for preclinical testing, *KONA Powder Part. J.* 36 (2019) 129–144.

76. J. Lemaitre, T. Naninck, B. Delache, J. Creppy, P. Huber, M. Holzapfel, C. Bouillier, V. Contreras, F. Martinon, N. Kahlaoui, Q. Pascal, S. Tricot, F. Ducancel, L. Vecellio, R. Le Grand, P. Maisonnasse, Non-human primate models of human respiratory infections, *Mol. Immunol.* 135 (2021) 147–164.

77. N. Osman, K. Kaneko, V. Carini, I. Saleem, Carriers for the targeted delivery of aerosolized macromolecules for pulmonary pathologies, *Expert Opin. Drug Deliv.* 15(8) (2018) 821–834.

78. C.J. Bailey, A.H. Barnett, Why is Exubera being withdrawn? *BMJ* 335(7630) (2007) 1156.

79. Y. Huang, C. Wang, Pulmonary delivery of insulin by liposomal carriers, *J. Control. Release* 113(1) (2006) 9–14.

80. R. Pittner, C. Moore, S. Bhavsar, B. Gedulin, P. Smith, C. Jodka, D. Parkes, J. Paterniti, V. Srivastava, A. Young, Effects of PYY [3–36] in rodent models of diabetes and obesity, *Int. J. Obes. Relat. Metab. Disord.* 28(8) (2004) 963–971.

81. F.H. Koegler, P.J. Enriori, S.K. Billes, D.L. Takahashi, M.S. Martin, R.L. Clark, A.E. Evans, K.L. Grove, J.L. Cameron, M.A. Cowley, Y.Y. Peptide, (3–36) inhibits morning, but not evening, food intake and decreases body weight in rhesus macaques, *Diabetes* 54(11) (2005) 3198–3204.

82. J. Shao, M. Chen, P.J. Kuehl, G. Hochhaus, Pharmacokinetic and pharmacodynamic modeling of gut hormone peptide YY (3–36) after pulmonary delivery, *Drug Dev. Ind. Pharm.* 45(7) (2019) 1101–1110.

83. P. Nadkarni, R. Costanzo, M. Sakagami, Pulmonary delivery of peptide YY for food intake suppression and reduced body weight gain in rats, *Diabetes Obes. Metab.* 13(5) (2011) 408–417.

84. C. Bosquillon, V. Préat, R. Vanbever, Pulmonary delivery of growth hormone using dry powders and visualization of its local fate in rats, *J. Control. Release* 96(2) (2004) 233–244.

85. B. Kim, E. Kang, M. Fava, D. Mischoulon, B. Soskin, B. Yu, D. Lee, D. Lee, H. Park, H.J. Jeon, Follicle-stimulating hormone (FSH), current suicidal ideation and attempt in female patients with major depressive disorder, *Psychiatry Res.* 210(3) (2013) 951–956.

86. S. Razvi, S. Bhana, S. Mrabeti, Challenges in interpreting thyroid stimulating hormone results in the diagnosis of thyroid dysfunction, *J. Thyroid Res.* 2019 (2019).

87. R.U. Agu, M.I. Ugwoke, M. Armand, R. Kinget, N. Verbeke, The lung as a route for systemic delivery of therapeutic proteins and peptides, *Respir. Res.* 2(4) (2001) 198–209.

88. C. Sinsuebpol, J. Chatchawalsaisin, P. Kulvanich, Preparation and in vivo absorption evaluation of spray dried powders containing salmon calcitonin loaded chitosan nanoparticles for pulmonary delivery, *Drug Des. Dev. Ther.* 7 (2013) 861.

89. J.S. Patton, Pulmonary delivery of drugs for bone disorders, *Adv. Drug Deliv. Rev.* 42(3) (2000) 239–248.

90. K. Song, S. Chung, C. Shim, Preparation and evaluation of proliposomes containing salmon calcitonin, *J. Control. Release* 84(1–2) (2002) 27–37.

91. L. Baginski, O.L. Gobbo, F. Tewes, J.J. Salomon, A.M. Healy, U. Bakowsky, C. Ehrhardt, In vitro and in vivo characterisation of PEG-lipid-based micellar complexes of salmon calcitonin for pulmonary delivery, *Pharm. Res.* 29(6) (2012) 1425–1434.

92. H. Sato, A. Tabata, T. Moritani, T. Morinaga, T. Mizumoto, Y. Seto, S. Onoue, Design and characterizations of inhalable poly (lactic-co-glycolic acid) microspheres prepared by the fine droplet drying process for a sustained effect of salmon calcitonin, *Molecules* 25(6) (2020) 1311.

93. S. Vallee, S. Rakhe, T. Reidy, S. Walker, Q. Lu, P. Sakorafas, S. Low, A. Bitonti, Pulmonary administration of interferon beta-1a-fc fusion protein in non-human primates using an immunoglobulin transport pathway, *J. Interferon Cytokine Res.* 32(4) (2012) 178–184.

94. V. Saluja, J. Amorij, J. Kapteyn, A. De Boer, H. Frijlink, W. Hinrichs, A comparison between spray drying and spray freeze drying to produce an influenza subunit vaccine powder for inhalation, *J. Control. Release* 144(2) (2010) 127–133.

95. J.M. Nicholls, R.B. Moss, S.M. Haslam, The use of sialidase therapy for respiratory viral infections, *Antiviral Res.* 98(3) (2013) 401–409.

96. R. Djukanović, T. Harrison, S.L. Johnston, F. Gabbay, P. Wark, N.C. Thomson, R. Niven, D. Singh, H.K. Reddel, D.E. Davies, R. Marsden, C. Boxall, S. Dudley, V. Plagnol, S.T. Holgate, P. Monk, INTERCIA Study Group, The effect of inhaled IFN-β on worsening of asthma symptoms caused by viral infections. A randomized trial, *Am. J. Respir. Crit. Care Med.* 190(2) (2014) 145–154.

97. P.D. Monk, R.J. Marsden, V.J. Tear, J. Brookes, T.N. Batten, M. Mankowski, F.J. Gabbay, D.E. Davies, S.T. Holgate, L. Ho, T. Clark, R. Djukanovic, T.M.A. Wilkinson, Inhaled Interferon Beta COVID-19 Study Group, Safety and efficacy of inhaled nebulised interferon beta-1a (SNG001) for treatment of SARS-CoV-2 infection: A randomised, double-blind, placebo-controlled, phase 2 trial, *Lancet Respir. Med.* 9(2) (2021) 196–206.

98. A.E. Rajapaksa, L.A.H. Do, D. Suryawijaya Ong, M. Sourial, D. Veysey, R. Beare, W. Hughes, W. Yang, R.J. Bischof, A. McDonnell, P. Eu, L.Y. Yeo, P.V. Licciardi, E.K. Mulholland, Pulmonary deposition of radionucleotide-labeled palivizumab: Proof-of-concept study, *Front. Pharmacol.* 11 (2020) 1291.

99. A. Larios Mora, L. Detalle, J.M. Gallup, A. Van Geelen, T. Stohr, L. Duprez, M.R. Ackermann, Delivery of ALX-0171 by inhalation greatly reduces respiratory syncytial virus disease in newborn lambs, *mAbs* 10(5) (2018) 778–795.

100. L. Detalle, T. Stohr, C. Palomo, P.A. Piedra, B.E. Gilbert, V. Mas, A. Millar, U.F. Power, C. Stortelers, K. Allosery, J.A. Melero, E. Depla, Generation and characterization of ALX-0171, a potent novel therapeutic nanobody for the treatment of respiratory syncytial virus infection, *Antimicrob. Agents Chemother.* 60(1) (2015) 6–13.

101. S. Cunningham, P.A. Piedra, F. Martinon-Torres, H. Szymanski, B. Brackeva, E. Dombrecht, L. Detalle, C. Fleurinck, RESPIRE Study Group, Nebulised ALX-0171 for respiratory syncytial virus lower respiratory tract infection in hospitalised children: A double-blind, randomised, placebo-controlled, phase 2b trial, *Lancet Respir. Med.* 9(1) (2021) 21–32.

102. J.S. Suk, S.K. Lai, N.J. Boylan, M.R. Dawson, M.P. Boyle, J. Hanes, Rapid transport of muco-inert nanoparticles in cystic fibrosis sputum treated with N-acetyl cysteine, *Nanomedicine (Lond)* 6(2) (2011) 365–375.

103. N. Nafee, K. Forier, K. Braeckmans, M. Schneider, Mucus-penetrating solid lipid nanoparticles for the treatment of cystic fibrosis: Proof of concept, challenges and pitfalls, *Eur. J. Pharm. Biopharm.* 124 (2018) 125–137.

104. H.K. Ibrahim, I.S. El-Leithy, A.A. Makky, Mucoadhesive nanoparticles as carrier systems for prolonged ocular delivery of gatifloxacin/prednisolone bitherapy, *Mol. Pharm.* 7(2) (2010) 576–585.

105. E. Bodier-Montagutelli, A. Mayor, L. Vecellio, R. Respaud, N. Heuze-Vourc'h, Designing inhaled protein therapeutics for topical lung delivery: What are the next steps? *Expert Opin. Drug Deliv.* 15(8) (2018) 729–736.

106. H.J. Fuchs, D.S. Borowitz, D.H. Christiansen, E.M. Morris, M.L. Nash, B.W. Ramsey, B.J. Rosenstein, A.L. Smith, M.E. Wohl, Effect of aerosolized recombinant human DNase on exacerbations of respiratory symptoms and on pulmonary function in patients with cystic fibrosis. The Pulmozyme Study Group, *N. Engl. J. Med.* 331(10) (1994) 637–642.

107. H. Abusriwil, R.A. Stockley, Alpha-1-antitrypsin replacement therapy: Current status, *Curr. Opin. Pulm. Med.* 12(2) (2006) 125–131.

108. A. Gaggar, J. Chen, J.F. Chmiel, H.L. Dorkin, P.A. Flume, R. Griffin, D. Nichols, S.H. Donaldson, Inhaled alpha1-proteinase inhibitor therapy in patients with cystic fibrosis, *J. Cyst. Fibros.* 15(2) (2016) 227–233.

109. P. Brand, M. Schulte, M. Wencker, C.H. Herpich, G. Klein, K. Hanna, T. Meyer, Lung deposition of inhaled alpha1-proteinase inhibitor in cystic fibrosis and alpha1-antitrypsin deficiency, *Eur. Respir. J.* 34(2) (2009) 354–360.

110. C. Comarmond, P. Cacoub, Granulomatosis with polyangiitis (Wegener): Clinical aspects and treatment, *Autoimmun. Rev.* 13(11) (2014) 1121–1125.

111. C. Roubaud-Baudron, C. Pagnoux, N. Meaux-Ruault, A. Grasland, A. Zoulim, J.L.E. Guen, A. Prud'homme, B. Bienvenu, M. de Menthon, S. Camps, V.L.E. Guern, A. Aouba, P. Cohen, L. Mouthon, L. Guillevin, French Vasculitis Study Group, Rituximab maintenance therapy for granulomatosis with polyangiitis and microscopic polyangiitis, *J. Rheumatol.* 39 (2012) 125–130.

112. T.J.Y. Ku, R.V.P. Ribeiro, V.H. Ferreira, M. Galasso, S. Keshavjee, D. Kumar, M. Cypel, A. Humar, Ex-vivo delivery of monoclonal antibody (rituximab) to treat human donor lungs prior to transplantation, *EBioMedicine* 60 (2020) 102994.

113. A. Gioffredi, F. Maritati, E. Oliva, C. Buzio, Eosinophilic granulomatosis with polyangiitis: An overview, *Front. Immunol.* 5 (2014) 549.

114. T. Mkorombindo, M.T. Dransfield, Mepolizumab in the treatment of eosinophilic chronic obstructive pulmonary disease, *Int. J. Chron. Obstruct. Pulmon. Dis.* 14 (2019) 1779–1787.

115. S. Shabbir, I.J. Pouliquen, J.H. Bentley, E.S. Bradford, M.C. Kaisermann, M. Albayaty, The pharmacokinetics and relative bioavailability of mepolizumab 100 mg liquid formulation administered subcutaneously to healthy participants: A randomized trial, *Clin. Pharmacol. Drug Dev.* 9(3) (2020) 375–385.

116. J.F. Pontes, A. Grenha, Multifunctional nanocarriers for lung drug delivery, *Nanomaterials (Basel)* 10(2) (2020) http://doi.org/10.3390/nano10020183.

117. E. Amore, M. Ferraro, M.L. Manca, M. Gjomarkaj, G. Giammona, E. Pace, M.L. Bondi, Mucoadhesive solid lipid microparticles for controlled release of a corticosteroid in the chronic obstructive pulmonary disease treatment, *Nanomedicine (Lond)* 12(19) (2017) 2287–2302.

118. A.M. Collin, M. Lecocq, S. Noel, B. Detry, F.M. Carlier, F. Aboubakar Nana, C. Bouzin, T. Leal, M. Vermeersch, V. De Rose, L. Regard, C. Martin, P.R. Burgel, D. Hoton, S. Verleden, A. Froidure, C. Pilette, S. Gohy, Lung immunoglobulin A immunity dysregulation in cystic fibrosis, *EBioMedicine* 60 (2020) 102974.

119. Y. Guo, H. Bera, C. Shi, L. Zhang, D. Cun, M. Yang, Pharmaceutical strategies to extend pulmonary exposure of inhaled medicines, *Acta Pharm. Sin. B* 11(8) (2021) 2565–2584.

120. G. Pilcer, K. Amighi, Formulation strategy and use of excipients in pulmonary drug delivery, *Int. J. Pharm.* 392(1–2) (2010) 1–19.

121. V. Kumar, B. Sethi, E. Yanez, D.H. Leung, Y.Y. Ghanwatkar, J. Cheong, J. Tso, A.S. Narang, K. Nagapudi, R.I. Mahato, Effect of magnesium stearate surface coating method on the aerosol performance and permeability of micronized fluticasone propionate, *Int. J. Pharm.* (2022) 121470.

122. D. Sacks, B. Baxter, B.C. Campbell, J.S. Carpenter, C. Cognard, D. Dippel, M. Eesa, U. Fischer, K. Hausegger, Multisociety consensus quality improvement revised consensus statement for endovascular therapy of acute ischemic stroke, *Int. J. Stroke* 13 (2018) 612–632.

Exosomes-Based Drug Delivery for Lung Cancer Treatment

16

Rajagopal Ramesh and Anupama Munshi

Contents

16.1 INTRODUCTION

Lung cancer remains a major health challenge in the United States. An estimated 236,740 new cases of lung cancer will be diagnosed each year accounting for over 130,180 deaths (54.9%) annually in the United States [1]. The incidence of lung cancer-related deaths is more than the estimated total numbers of deaths due to cancers of the breast, prostate, colon, and rectum combined [2]. Lung cancer now affects men and women nearly equally and accounts for more deaths than breast cancer among American women. Early detection of lung cancer is difficult because symptoms often do not appear until the disease is advanced. While damaged lung

DOI: 10.1201/9781003182566-20

tissue often returns to normal in those who stop smoking, unfortunately, only a minority of patients quit. Approximately, 80% of lung cancers will have a non-small cell carcinoma (NSCLC) histology [3] and once diagnosed, the type and stage of cancer determines the treatment options [4]. However, this staging system does not accurately determine an individual patient's prognosis. Thus, the ability to detect the disease early and have effective therapies to eradicate lung cancer will make a significant impact on patient survival.

Recent progress in treatment strategies has resulted in the development and testing of molecularly targeted therapeutics for lung cancer [5, 6]. However, complete elimination of tumor cells remains unresolved and the overall five-year survival rate of patients diagnosed with lung cancer remaining at 18% [7]. Factors contributing to treatment failure and poor survival rate include: dose-limiting toxicity, drug resistance, off-target effects, and inefficient drug delivery to local as well as distant metastatic tumor sites. Therefore, there is an urgent to need to develop and test novel forms of therapeutic agents and systemic treatment modalities for treating loco-regional and distant lung cancer metastasis.

Conventional therapy for lung cancer is surgery, chemotherapy and radiation therapy often given in combination. Platinum-based drugs such as cisplatin, carboplatin, and oxaliplatin serve as front-line chemotherapeutic drugs for lung cancer treatment [8–10]. Despite the efforts made in chemotherapy-based treatments, development of resistance is common, thereby limiting their efficacy. Factors contributing to resistance are multifactorial and include poor drug solubility and inefficient intracellular drug accumulation in the tumor; efficient drug efflux [11]; increased activity of DNA repair enzymes [12]; and loss of apoptotic activation and/or function [13]. Additionally, treatment-related non-specific toxicity to normal cells and tissues limits the dose and continued use of chemotherapy to achieve therapeutic efficacy [14, 15]. For example, nephrotoxicity and neurotoxicity is common with platinum-based drugs, especially cisplatin [16]. Despite this wealth of knowledge and testing of treatment strategies to overcome these limitations, therapeutic efficacy and survival outcomes in the clinic has not improved. The net outcome is disease relapse and metastasis, culminating in patient death.

To overcome some of the limitations of chemotherapy and improving treatment outcomes, numerous nanoparticle (NP) formulations targeted for cancer treatment have been reported [17–19]. Administration of the NPs carrying different anticancer drugs, while demonstrating therapeutic efficacy, has also revealed poor pharmacokinetics (PK) and pharmacodynamics (PD) [20–23]. The impediment for the NPs in having poor PK is its rapid opsonization and clearance by the mononuclear phagocyte system [24, 25]. While inclusion of polyethylene glycol (PEG) in the NP resulted in improved pharmacokinetic (PK) profiles, the formation of protein corona around the NPs hinders its binding and uptake by target cells resulting in reduced therapeutic efficacy [26–28]. Further, the presence of anti-PEG antibodies in the NP-treated host reduces efficacy [29, 30]. Although testing of polysialic acid (PSA) as an alternate to PEG has shown encouraging results, PSA-coated NPs have had limitations [31–33]. Recently, NPs eliciting autoimmune disease have been reported. Therefore, it is imperative to develop and test new and improved drug delivery systems for reducing mortality, and increasing the survival of lung cancer patients.

16.2 EXTRACELLULAR VESICLES

The term extracellular vesicles (EVs) broadly refers to particles naturally produced and released by cells into their surrounding environment. The EVs, based on their size, are classified, and referred to as small (< 100–200 nm) and medium-to-large (< 200 nm) EVs. Based on the biogenesis, EVs are classified into apoptotic bodies, microvesicles, exosomes, exomeres, migrasomes, and oncosomes [34, 35]. Each EV subtype irrespective of their size and shape plays a role in the normal biological and physiological processes [36]. In recent years, the publication on "Minimal Information for Studies of Extracellular Vesicles" ("MISEV") by the International Society of Extracellular Vesicles (ISEV) recommends the use of the term "small" or "medium-to-large EVs" *in lieu* of "exosomes" [37]. This recommendation is made to ensure rigor and consensus among laboratories studying EVs as the EV population is heterogeneous in size and purification into sub-size fraction remains a challenge. However, since the term "exosomes" has been used for the past several years, several laboratories including our own have continued to use the term "exosomes" which correspond to the small size EVs (<200 nm). Thus, the reference to exosomes in this chapter is interchangeable to small EVs.

16.3 EXOSOMES

Exosomes constitute the major component of the EV fraction. They are endosome-derived lipid containing vesicles that are 30–150 nm in size and are actively secreted by exocytosis by living cells [38–40]. Exosomes are spherical in shape, and their cup shaped structure often reported in the literature is attributed to sample distortion during processing [41]. The lumen of the exosomes is enriched with nucleic acids (miRNA, DNA fragments, RNA), proteins, and lipids while their surface is highly enriched with lipids and proteins. Exosomes have pleiotropic functions and play important roles in normal and pathological conditions [42, 43]. In parallel, exosomes isolated from normal cells (e.g. fibroblast, macrophage, dendritic cells among others) are being tested as drug delivery vehicles [44, 45]. The unique features of exosomes that make them attractive as drug carriers are their small size; membranotropic outer layer derived from the cells of origin that contains various adhesive proteins (e.g. tetraspanins) allowing cell-cell interaction and fusion; diminished potential for activating the immune response [46, 47]; ability to incorporate multiple therapeutics (e.g. chemotherapy, siRNA, miRNA) and imaging (e.g. iron oxide, gold) [48–55] into the lumen for use as a therapeutic, imaging agent or theranostics; ability to incorporate ligands on the surface of exosomes for achieving tumor-targeted delivery without affecting the exosome function; ability to scale-up in large scale; inherent property to freely circulate and traverse across cell membrane including the blood brain barrier (BBB); use of allogeneic cells as source of exosomes without eliciting immune response; and long-term stability and shelf-life when stored under appropriate conditions. These unique features support their testing as drug delivery vehicles for cancer therapy.

16.3.1 Exosomes as Drug Carrier

The unique properties of exosomes described above favors their development as drug carriers for cancer therapy. An added advantage of exosomes as drug carriers is their ability to escape the lysosome/endosomal trapping thereby enabling efficient drug delivery [56]. Thus, exosomes are endowed with properties that can overcome the barriers in drug delivery and some of the limitations encountered with previously tested biological and non-biological-based drug carriers.

As a first step in developing exosome-based cancer therapeutics, it is important to identify a cell source for producing exosomes. Some of the basic requirements of the cells that will be used for exosome production, hereafter referred to as "producer" cells include: easy to grow the cells; minimal growth condition requirements; not susceptible to subtle temperature or growth conditions variation that restrict or reduce exosome production; and ability to produce high numbers exosomes per milliliter of growth medium.

Initial studies focused on testing tumor-derived exosomes (TDE) as drug carriers due to the "self-recognition" concept that drives the movement of exosomes towards the cell of origin (cancer cells) from which they were derived [57]. However, a consensus in the EV and drug delivery field is that tumor-derived exosomes (TDE) are undesirable for cancer treatment due to their tumor growth promoting potential [58–60]. As an alternate, studies have resorted to using exosomes isolated from normal cells (e.g.: fibroblast, dendritic cells, stem cells) as drug carrier [54, 61, 62]. Yim et al. [63] demonstrated exosomes derived from human embryonic kidney (HEKT) cells can be efficiently loaded with designer therapeutics and tailored for treatment of specific cancers. Kim et.al. [64] demonstrated macrophage-derived exosomes encapsulated with paclitaxel (exoPTX) overcomes multidrug resistance (MDR) in Lewis Lung Carcinoma (LL/2) and produces therapeutic efficacy, with no demonstrable non-specific toxicity towards normal tissue. Another study by the same group showed that surface modification of exoPTX with pegylated aminoethylanisamide (AA-PEG) targeting sigma receptor overexpressed in lung cancer, produced profound antitumor efficacy [65]. Oral delivery of milk-derived exosomes containing paclitaxel showed efficacy against human A549 lung cancer cells [66]. Tian et al. [67] demonstrated doxorubicin (Dox) containing exosomes decorated with iRGD successfully targeted integrin alphaV expressing breast cancer cells and produced antitumor activity. Kamerkar et al. [68] elegantly demonstrated fibroblast-like mesenchymal cell-derived exosomes loaded with miRNA specific to oncogenic $KRas^{G12D}$ specifically targeted KRas mutant pancreatic cancer cells and inhibited tumor growth both *in vitro* and *in vivo*. Additional benefit of using exosomes as drug delivery vehicle is that they can exert a bystander therapeutic effect on neighboring cells. Roma-Rodriques et al. [69] showed that treatment of breast cancer cells with gold nanoparticles (GNP) functionalized with anti-RAB27A resulted in packaging of GNP-anti-RAB27A exosomes and their release from the treated tumor cells that exerted a suppressive effect on neighboring cells. Similar findings on exosome-mediated bystander effect have been reported [70–72]. Qi et al. [73] showed exosomes carrying Dox can be endowed with magnetic and tumor-targeting properties for cancer therapy. More recently, Tian et al. [74] demonstrated surface functionalized exosomes specifically and efficiently delivered drugs to cerebral ischemia. The results from all of these studies demonstrate the safety of exosomes derived from plethora of normal cells for use as drug carriers and the ability to manipulate them without affecting their antitumor efficacy.

While reports using exosomes from various cell sources as drug carrier have been reported, it is unclear whether autologous or allogeneic cells should be used as exosome source in the context of host-immunogenicity and toxicity is debated [75–77]. Early clinical studies used autologous dendritic cell-based exosomes [78–81]. However, more recent preclinical and clinical studies support the use of allogeneic cells as exosome source [82, 83]. Mendt et al. [84] demonstrated that clinical grade exosomes from allogeneic cells exhibited potent antitumor activity against pancreatic cancer. Immunotherapy studies showed exosomes from allogeneic cells were as effective as exosomes from autologous cells in eliciting a robust immune response which occurred independent of MHC molecules on exosomes [82, 83]. Additionally, improved activation of B- and T-cells was observed when exosomes from allogeneic cells were used compared to autologous cells [85, 86]. Lu et al. [87] showed exosomes from allogeneic cells exhibited antitumor activity against a broad spectrum of liver tumors. Finally, repeated injection of exosomes from allogeneic HEK293T cells in immunocompetent mice produced no toxicity [76]. The results from these studies demonstrate exosomes from allogeneic cells can be effectively used as drug delivery vehicles for cancer therapy and thus eliminates the dependency on procuring and growing autologous cells for exosome production.

16.3.2 Exosomes-Based Drug Delivery for Lung Cancer

Testing of exosomes as drug carrier for lung diseases, including lung cancer, is relatively new and limited. However, better understanding of the biology and biogenesis of exosomes as well as improvement in drug loading methods will lead to increased testing of exosomes-based therapy for lung cancer. Herein, results from various *in vitro* and *in vivo* studies, demonstrating the antitumor activity produced by exosomes loaded with various therapeutics against lung cancer, are discussed.

Some of the initial studies testing exosomes-based therapy for lung cancer involved the use of bovine milk-derived exosomes [88]. In the study, exosomes were loaded with celastrol (ExoCEL) by simple incubation and administered by oral gavage to mice bearing A549 lung tumors on the flank. Results showed ExoCEL treatment inhibited tumor growth with no treatment-related toxicity observed when compared to treatment with celastrol alone. Agrawal et al. [66] observed significant tumor growth inhibition with no treatment-related toxicity when paclitaxel-loaded exosomes (ExoPAC) was administered by oral gavage to mice bearing subcutaneous A549 lung tumors. In contrast, administration of free paclitaxel showed no significant growth inhibition but produced significant systemic toxicity. The results from these two studies, in addition to demonstrating the therapeutic efficacy of exosomes against lung cancer also revealed two important concepts: use of bovine milk-derived exosomes and the ease of isolating exosomes in large scale by procuring milk from commercial vendors; ease of loading hydrophobic and poorly soluble drugs (celastrol and paclitaxel) onto exosomes by simple incubation. In another study, milk exosomes loaded with different siRNAs were tested against a panel of human cancers including lung cancer [89]. SiRNAs were loaded onto exosomes by a combination of electroporation and chemical transfection. Further, the siRNA loaded exosomes were functionalized with folic acid (FA) ligand for achieving tumor-targeted siRNA delivery. *In vitro* studies showed increased siRNA uptake and cytotoxicity by lung cancer cells treated with FA-conjugated exosomes compared to treatment with siRNA-exosomes alone. *In vivo* studies showed treatment of subcutaneous A549 lung tumors with FA-exosomes loaded with siRNA against KRAS^{G12S} resulted in tumor cell cytotoxicity and significant suppression of tumor growth compared to treatment with vehicle control.

Kim et al. [65] using macrophage-derived exosomes loaded with paclitaxel and surface functionalized with a ligand (AA; aminoethylanisamide) targeted towards the sigma receptor showed efficient uptake of the exosomes (AA-PEG-exo-PTX) by lung cancer cells both *in vitro* and *in vivo* resulting in effective suppression of lung metastases and increased animal survival. In the study by Wang et al. [90], exosomes isolated from A549 lung tumor cells were loaded with docetaxel (Exo-DTX) by electroporation and tested for their antitumor activity *in vitro* and *in vivo*. Study results showed oral administration of Exo-DTX treatment daily for nineteen-days induced tumor cell death and inhibited tumor growth with no gross pathological changes indicating safety for cancer treatment. In another study, Nie et al. tested the organotropism of exosomes using lung cancer as a model [91]. In this study, the authors tested the organotropic effect of human breast cancer (MDA-MB-231)-derived exosomes on lung metastasis. Exosomes were transfected with miRNA-126 (miRNA-231-Exo) and administered intravenously to mice bearing human A549 lung cancer metastasis. Seven treatments over a three-week period resulted in significant reduction in the number of lung tumor nodules demonstrating treatment-related inhibitory effects on metastasis. The study revealed tumor homing properties of the breast cancer derived exosomes was due to the high expression of integrin beta 4 (ITGβ$_4$) on the exosomes and its interaction with the surfactant protein C (SPC) that is highly expressed on lung cancer cells. This study showed the cross-reactivity and homing properties of the exosomes and brings a new approach for exosome-based cancer therapy.

While the studies described have applied physical and/or chemical methods to load therapeutics onto exosomes, other studies have engineered cells to produce exosomes preloaded with the therapeutic of interest. Hao et al. [92] transfected human embryonic kidney (HEK293T) cells with a plasmid expressing soluble fms-like tyrosine kinase-1 (sFlt1) and purified exosomes from the transfected cells. Treatment of human umbilical vein endothelial (HUVEC) cells resulted in antiangiogenic activity *in vitro*. *In vivo*, intratumoral administration of the exosomes inhibited tumor growth with no change in body weight indicating treatment is safe and produced no adverse effects. While the study findings are interesting, one caveat of the study is that intratumoral treatment is not clinically translatable, in particular for treating metastatic disease. Jeong et al. [93] used exosomes from HEK293T cells transfected with microRNA-497 (miRNA-497-exo) to test against HUVECs and A549 cells in a microfluidic system. The study results showed miRNA-497-exo treatment reduced vascular endothelial growth factor -A (VEGF-A) induced HUVEC angiogenic sprouting and inhibited A549 cell proliferation. The study demonstrated the utility of the microfluidic system for rapidly screening cancer therapeutics using exosomes as a drug carrier. For overcoming drug resistance in lung cancer cells, exosomes from bone-marrow derived mesenchymal stem cells (MSCs) were transfected with miRNA-193a and an siRNA against leucine-rich repeat-containing protein 1 (LRCC1) and tested against human A549 and H1299 lung cancer cells, isogenic for cisplatin (CDDP) sensitivity. CDDP resistant A549/DDP and H1299/DDP cells exhibited sensitivity towards CDDP upon treatment with BMSC-exo *in vitro*. Additionally, inhibitory effects on cell migration and invasion and increased apoptotic cell death was observed. *In vivo*, intratumoral administration of BMSC-exo containing both miRNA-193a and siRNA-LRCC1 exhibited maximum tumor growth suppression compared to treatments carrying miRNA-193a or siRNA-LRCC1 [94]. These results indicated that exosomes can be loaded with multiple therapeutics to suppress tumor growth and/or restore chemosensitivity.

Designer approaches to generate unique and specialized cell targeted exosomes have also been developed and tested. In the study by Zhou et al. [95], HEK293T cells were co-transfected with two plasmid DNAs expressing KRAS siRNA and Lamp2b-iRGD to produce exosomes that contained the siRNA and expressing iRGD on the exosomes surface. The expression of iRGD on the surface was accomplished by fusing iRGD with the exosomal membrane protein, Lamp2b. The system offered tumor-targeted delivery of KRAS siRNA to lung cancer cells. *In vitro* studies showed iRGD exosomes carrying the KRAS siRNA (siRNA-KRAS/iRGD-exosome) significantly inhibited cell proliferation of A549 lung cancer cells compared to treatment with scrambled siRNA contained in non-targeted exosomes (scrRNA/WT-exosome). *In vivo* studies showed intravenous administration of fluorescently labeled siRNA-KRAS/iRGD-exosome had a greater accumulation in the actively growing subcutaneous A549 tumor compared to scrRNA/WT-exosome. Accumulation of the siRNA-KRAS/iRGD-exosomes in the liver and kidney was also significantly reduced compared to accumulation of scrRNA/WT-exosomes in these organs. Efficacy studies showed three systemic treatments with siRNA-KRAS/iRGD-exosomes greatly suppressed subcutaneous A549 tumor growth compared to scrRNA/WT-exosome treatment. In another study, exosomes were engineered to express a membrane penetrating peptide, tLyp1 on their surface by recombinant DNA technology. The t-Lyp1 gene sequence and Lamp2b sequence were first artificially synthesized and inserted into a plasmid DNA expression vector. Subsequently, HEK293T cells were stably transfected with the t-Lyp1 expressing plasmid DNA for producing tLyp1 expressing exosomes. The t-Lyp1 expressing exosomes purified from the culture medium of HEK293T cells were loaded with SOX2 siRNA by electroporation and tested for their antitumor activity against lung tumor and cancer stem cells (CSCs). SOX2 is a transcriptional factor overexpressed in lung cancer and CSCs and plays an important role in epithelial-mesenchymal transition (EMT) and drug resistance [96, 97]. Treatment of A549 CSCs with t-Lyp1-SOX2 siRNA exosomes resulted in the inhibition of SOX2 expression and consequently loss of stem cell like features as evidenced by the reduced number of $CD44^+/CD24^-$ cells [98]. Zhou et al. [99] undertook a different engineering approach to enrich exosomes with the tumor suppressive miR-449a. The authors used the unique properties of the transcriptional transactivator protein (TAT) and the transactivating response (TAR) element for enriching miRNA-449a in the exosomes. A549 tumor cells were co-transfected with a plasmid expression vector carrying the TAT sequence fused to ADC membrane localization protein and another plasmid vector carrying the TAR sequence fused with the 5' end of the miRNA-449a. The exosomes (miR-449a-Exo) produced from the stably transfected A549 cells demonstrated expression of TAT and enrichment of miRNA-449a. *In vitro* studies showed miR-449a-Exo specifically inhibited A549 tumor cell growth but not growth of liver (HepG2) and cervical (HeLa) cancer cells. Additionally, miR-449a-Exo treatment reduced the expression of the anti-apoptotic protein Bcl2; inhibited cell migration and invasion; and induced apoptotic cell death. Finally, *in vivo* studies showed that intravenous administration of miR-449a-Exo to mice bearing subcutaneous A549 tumor resulted in a significant inhibition of tumor growth but increased tumor growth upon treatment with PBS, empty exosomes or exosomes with scrambled miRNA sequence. Additionally, molecular studies showed marked reduction in Bcl2 protein expression in the miR-449a-Exo treated tumor tissues compared to control groups. These findings demonstrated a method for enriching tumor suppressive miRNAs in exosomes and their use in cancer therapy.

In another approach, RNA nanotechnology was combined with exosome technology to generate EGFR targeted exosomes for lung cancer treatment [100]. In the study, purified exosomes from HEK293T cells were loaded with a siRNA against Survivin by transfection and decorated on the surface with an EGFR RNA aptamer by simply mixing siRNA loaded exosomes with RNA aptamer nanoparticles. Survivin is anti-apoptotic protein that plays a role in drug resistance [101, 102]. *In vitro* studies showed treatment of human lung cancer cells (H596, H1568) with EGFR-targeted siRNA containing exosomes (EGFRapt/Exo/Survivin) reduced Survivin expression, activated the caspase death signaling pathway and inhibited cell growth. Additionally, enhanced tumor cell killing was demonstrated when EGFRapt/Exo/Survivin treatment was combined with CDDP treatment. *In vivo* studies showed a significant reduction in tumor growth of H596 subcutaneous tumors upon treatment with six doses (40 nmol/Kg of siRNA per dose) of EGFRapt/Exo/Survivin over a two-week period. The greatest inhibitory effect observed on tumor growth was in the EGFRapt/Exo/Survivin treated mice compared to mice treated with non-targeted exosomes containing Survivin siRNA (EV/siSurvivin), scrambled siRNA (EGFRapt/Exo/siCtr) and TES buffer. EV/siSurvivin treatment also showed tumor suppressive activity and delayed growth of H596 tumors when compared to tumor growth in the control groups. The main feature of this study was the incorporation of RNA nanotechnology with exosomes and establishing a proof-of-concept for combinatorial therapies with chemodrugs for cancer treatment. These study results are of great importance to the EV/exosome field. However, testing of EGFRapt/Exo/Survivin efficacy in an experimental lung metastasis model mimicking the clinical setting would have added strength.

Studies from our laboratory have exploited nanotechnology and combined them with exosome technology to produce hybrid multifunctional theranostic exosomes for cancer therapy and imaging. Initial studies focused on using spherical gold nanoparticle (GNP) for dual purpose: *first*, GNP served as a substrate for conjugating doxorubicin (Dox) *via* a pH-sensitive linker; *second*, it is well known that colloidal gold exhibits localized surface plasmon resonance that contributes to absorbing the light at specific wavelength resulting in photothermal properties that can be applied for hyperthermic cancer treatments [103, 104]. For achieving the goal, GNP was synthesized and conjugated to Dox via a pH sensitive hydrazone linker (NanoDox) to ensure selective drug release under acidic conditions that are prevalent in the tumor (pH 3.0–5.5) especially under hypoxc conditions compared to normal tissue (pH 6.0–7.2; Figure 16.1) [62]. This approach minimizes the potential for any non-specific drug toxicity on the normal cells and tissues. Next, NanoDox was loaded onto exosomes derived from normal human lung fibroblast (MRC-9) cell line. The NanoDox-loaded exosomes, referred to as "nanosomes", were subjected to physicochemical characterization for size, shape, charge potential and drug release kinetics to ensure they met set criteria prior to their testing in biological studies. Although Dox is not the appropriate drug for lung cancer treatment, the objective of the study was to establish proof-of-concept for developing multifunctional nanoparticles. Added advantage of Dox is its inherent fluorescence property which makes it easy to conduct fluorescence-based studies to track exosome uptake and movement inside the cells. As shown in Figure 16.2, nanosomes were efficiently taken up by the H1299 lung cancer cells although to lesser extent when compared to free Dox. The uptake of Dox in the decreasing order was free Dox>nanosomes>nanoDox. Cells treated with empty exosomes and receiving no treatment served as controls. Functional studies showed nanosomes, effectively and significantly, inhibited proliferation of A549 and H1299 tumor cells, induced cell-cycle arrest, mitochondrial perturbation, and DNA damage leading to apoptotic cell death (Figures 16.3 and 16.4). In normal MRC-9 lung

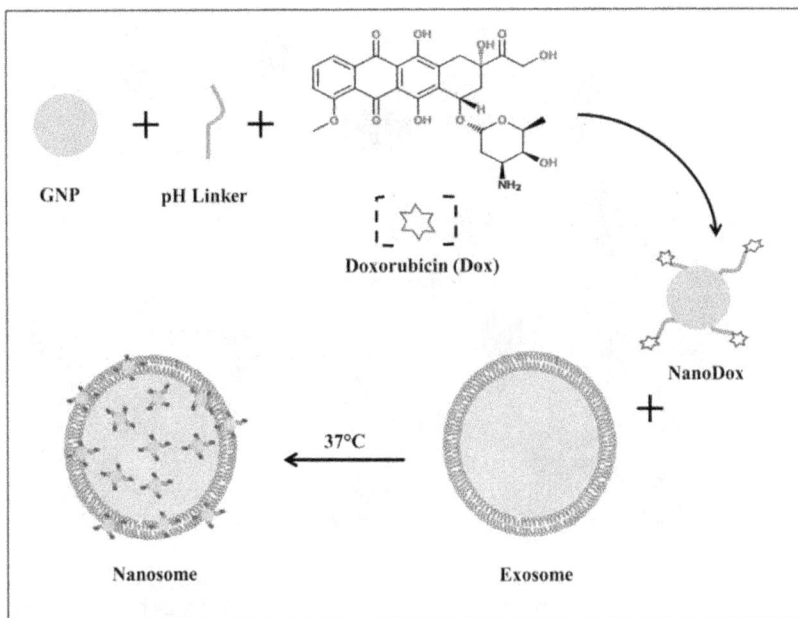

FIGURE 16.1 Schematic representation of nanosome (exosome-based hybrid delivery system consisting of cell-derived exosomes and gold nanoparticles carrying doxorubicin) synthesis for lung cancer treatment. Image was reproduced from Srivastava et al. (2016) under an open access Creative Commons CC BY 4.0 license.

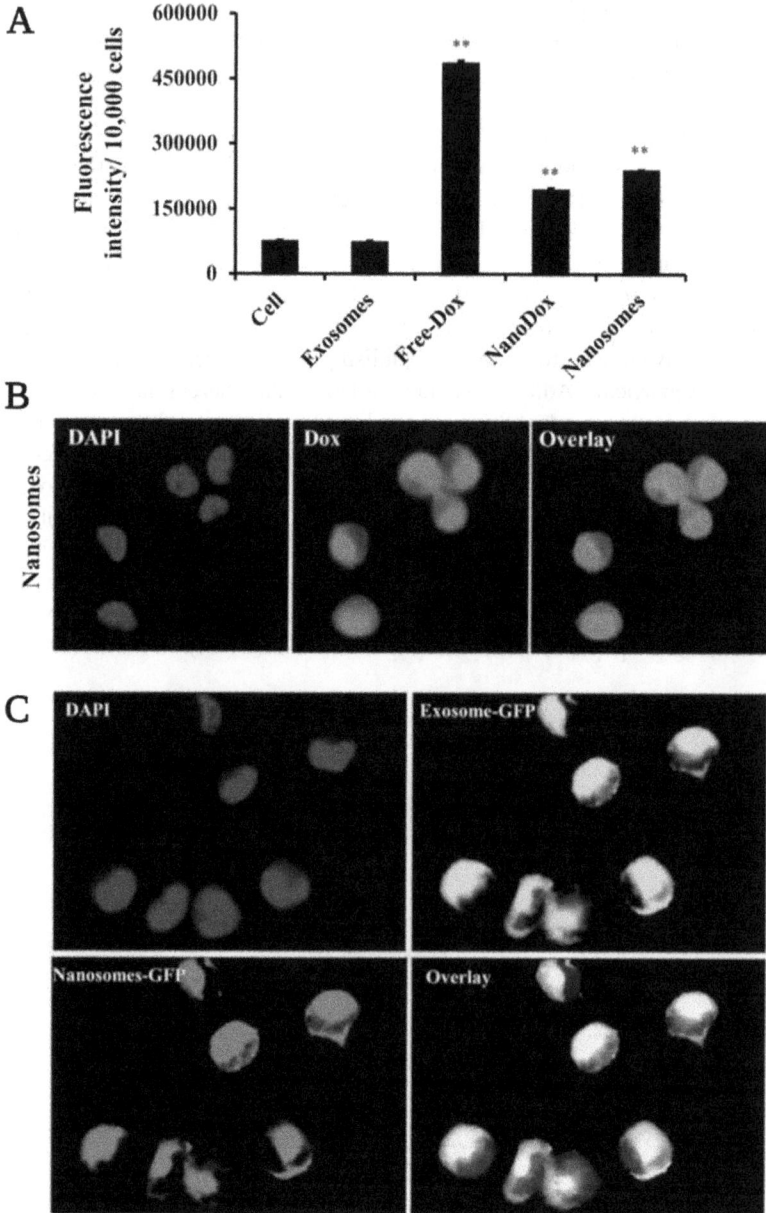

FIGURE 16.2 Representative images showing cellular uptake of nanosomes (A) Fluorescence intensity measuring Doxorubicin (Dox) uptake after 24h of treatment of H1299 cells with free-Dox, NanoDox and nanosomes, compared with untreated control cells and exosomes. (B) Epifluorescence images of nanosomes-treated H1299 cells showed colocalization of Dox to the nucleus that were stained with DAPI. (C) Epifluorescence images showing GFP-labeled exosomes (upper right panel) loaded with NanoDox (nanosomes; lower left panel) are efficiently taken up by H1299 cells (lower right panel). Top left panel shows DAPI stained nuclei. Image reproduced from Srivastava et al. (2016) under an open access Creative Commons CC BY 4.0 license.

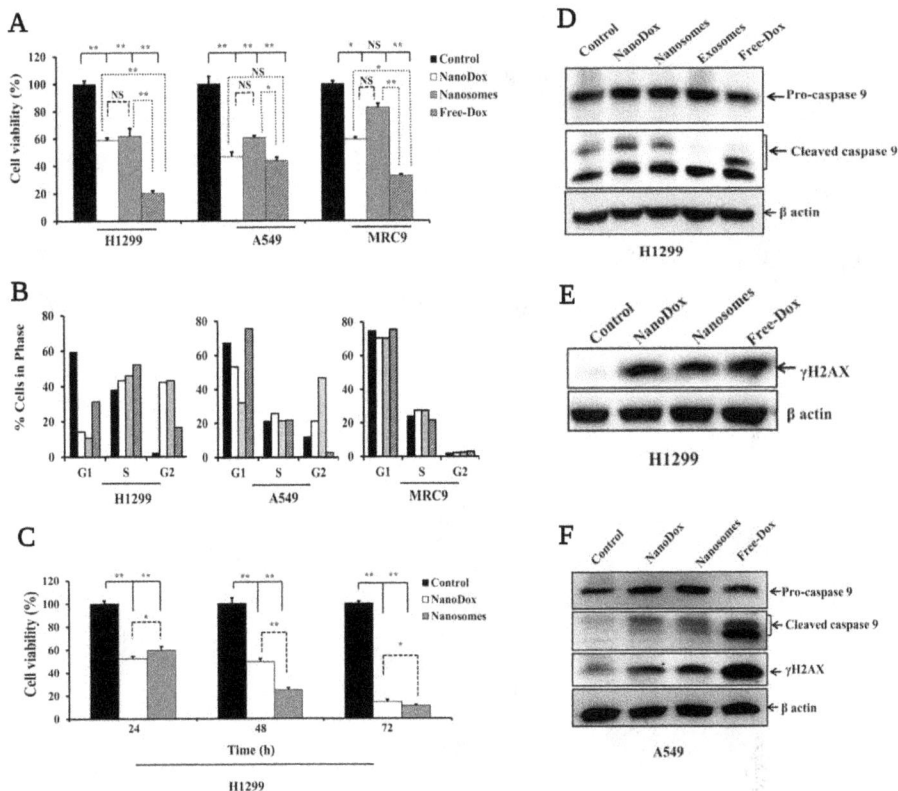

FIGURE 16.3 Nanosomes exhibit selective cytotoxicity to lung cancer cells but normal cells. (A) Cell viability, (B) Cell-cycle analysis of two lung cancer (H1299 and A549), and normal (MRC9) lung fibroblast cell lines after 24 h treatment with NanoDox, nanosome, and free-Dox, shows induction of G2 phase cell-cycle arrest in NanoDox and nanosome-treated H1299 and A549 cells but not MRC9 cells. (C) Viability of H1299 cells after treatment with NanoDox and nanosomes. (D) Western blotting analysis for caspase-9 in H1299 cells after 24 h. (E) NanoDox, nanosome and free-Dox-treated H1299 cells show increased γH2AX expression compared to control. (F) Activation of caspase-9 and increased γH2AX expression in A549 cells treated with NanoDox, nanosomes and free-Dox compared to controls. Image reproduced from Srivastava et al. (2016) under an open access Creative Commons CC BY 4.0 license.

fibroblast cells, nanosome treatment did not produce any significant inhibitory activity on proliferation nor measurable changes in cell-cycle, DNA damage or mitochondria was observed. In contrast, free Dox exhibited profound cytotoxicity to MRC-9 cells indicating nanosome treatment was safe and less harmful to normal cells. Additionally, since Dox is known to cause cardiotoxicity and limits its prolonged use in the clinic, we tested whether nanosomes would mitigate the drug-induced toxicity. For this purpose, human coronary aortic smooth muscle (HCASM) cells when treated with free Dox showed marked reduction in cell number. In contrast, nanosome treatment showed minimal-to-no toxicity towards HCASM cells compared to untreated cells demonstrating the safety of nanosome-based Dox treatment and its applicability for cancer therapy.

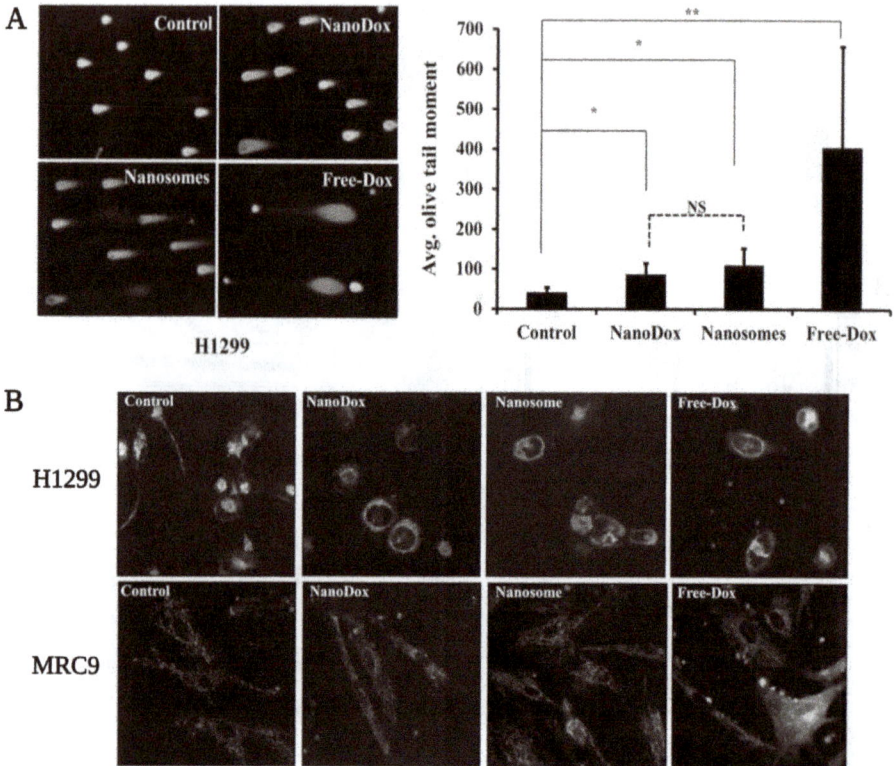

FIGURE 16.4 Nanosome-treatment produces DNA damage and induces mitochondrial perturbation and ROS. (A) Photomicrographs showing DNA damage as visualized by the extent of the tail length of the comet in NanoDox-, nanosome-, and free-Dox-treated cells. The quantitative representation of the Olive tail moment showing significant DNA damage (right panel). (B) H1299 and MRC9 cells treated with NanoDox-, nanosome-, and free Dox were analyzed for changes in mitochondrial potential using JC1 stain. Nanosome treatment markedly perturbed the mitochondrial potential in H1299 cells compared to NanoDox and control cells. Image reproduced from Srivastava et al. (2016) under an open access Creative Commons CC BY 4.0 license.

Since Dox is not a clinically relevant drug for lung cancer treatment, recent studies in our laboratory have embarked on testing CDDP, which is the first line of chemotherapy for lung cancer. In the ongoing study, CDDP conjugated to GNP via a pH sensitive ester linkage is loaded onto exosomes and decorated on the surface with transferrin to achieve tumor-targeted drug delivery. This new tumor-targeted multifunctional exosome serves as a theranostic, enables in *in vivo* monitoring of exosome accumulation in the actively growing tumor and measure tumor response to therapy by optical imaging. Additionally, the ability of photothermal therapy to increase the anticancer efficacy exists. In another study, our laboratory is developing and testing iron-oxide-based theranostic for lung cancer. While the studies are in their early stages, upon completion the results of the study will demonstrate the utility of tumor-targeted multifunctional exosomes for lung cancer therapy and their use in combinatorial therapies.

Based on the studies conducted in various laboratories and described above it is becoming clear that exosomes hold great promise as drug carriers. However, additional preclinical studies with rigor in exosome validation and testing in appropriate tumor models that mimic human disease are needed prior to advancing for clinical testing.

16.4 CHALLENGES IN ADVANCING EXOSOME-BASED THERAPEUTICS

Exosome-based drug delivery system for cancer treatment is attractive and their testing in the clinic holds promise. However, the challenges encountered while developing exosome-based cancer therapeutics as a clinical product need to be addressed.[105] The challenges center on exosomes and cancer. In the context of exosomes, there is a real need for rigor in EV characterization, and this has been strongly emphasized by the international society of extracellular vesicles (ISEV). Similarly, the National Cancer Institute (NCI) has urged investigators conducting EV-based studies to ensure rigor and reproducibility in their studies. This is because the definition of EVs and exosomes and their naming based on size has created confusion. Another issue is the lack of technology currently available to sub-fractionate EVs to homogeneity and hence the impact of size on drug delivery remains unclear. While majority of the studies have used a broad panel of established normal cell lines as a source for exosome production, there is lack of cross-validation and consensus in using a single cell source across laboratories. Studies investigating the influence of growth conditions, temperature and several other parameters that affect EV production and secretion by the producer cells are limited. Discussion on the use of autologous versus allogeneic cells for exosome production remains under debate. While use of autologous cells for exosome production and their use as drug carrier is favored for precision medicine, obtaining large number of cells (cancer or normal) from patients and expanding them for clinical application is a huge endeavor with no guarantee of success. Finally, scale-up of exosome production along with the complex steps involved in developing multifunctional exosomes poses challenges for approval by the Food and Drug Administration (FDA).

In the context of cancer, the major challenge lies in the heterogeneity of the tumor supported by a tumor growth favoring microenvironment and dense stroma that acts as a barrier to allow the drug to penetrate and reach the tumor cells. Whole genome and exome analysis shows that tumor cells are heterogeneous at the molecular level and responsible for the incomplete response observed towards molecularly targeted cancer therapeutics. Additionally, intercellular genetic variations complicate the treatment outcomes. Phenotypic and genotypic differences in the primary tumor versus metastatic tumor also play a role in treatment failure. To overcome some of these challenges the use of appropriate *in vitro* 3D and 4D models for testing drug efficacy, drug transport, and determining transfection efficiency among others are recommended. For *in vivo* studies, appropriate animal and tumor models need to be used. Often, cancer related studies use subcutaneous tumor models as exemplified in the earlier sections of this chapter. However, the use of orthotopic and transgenic tumor models is better suited for conducting anticancer therapeutic studies. Finally, in recent years, the use of patient derived xenograft (PDX) and circulating tumor cell-derived xenograft (CDX) have gained recognition as they accurately recapitulate the clinical and histopathological characteristics of the patient from whom they were derived and established.[106] However, issues related to using PDX and CDX models exist. For example, they are expensive to obtain from commercial vendors and academic institutions do not have the resources for establishing PDX/CDX facilities. Finally, contamination of host mouse DNA with the human DNA in the xenograft, as high as 47%, was reported that affected studies focused on oncogenesis and the associated downstream molecular pathways.[107] While there is no perfect animal model available for each cancer type, nevertheless using the most relevant tumor model that can closely mimic the clinical setting is important.

16.5 CONCLUSIONS

The EV field is relatively new and continues to grow exponentially. While we have a reasonably good understanding of the EVs biology, there is still a dearth of knowledge in other areas that include: EV biogenesis; cellular cues that distinguish general versus preferential packaging of cargo into the EV's lumen; availability of specific markers that can distinguish EVs from different cell source, in particular when biological samples such as blood, urine, and amniotic fluid are used. Equally challenged is the area of instrumentation technology for EVs isolation, purification and characterization at single EV level as well as industrial scale production and manufacturing (Figure 16.5). Despite these challenges, significant advances have been made in using EVs, in particular exosomes, for cancer diagnosis and treatment. While there are large number of laboratories testing EV-based drug delivery and reporting therapeutic efficacy against a broad-spectrum of cancers in preclinical studies, there are very few EV-based cancer therapies currently in Phase I clinical testing (www.clinicaltrials.org). A phase I clinical study testing mesenchymal stromal cells-derived exosomes carrying siRNA against KRASG12D for pancreatic cancer patients is in progress. Similarly, investigation on plant-derived exosomes loaded with curcumin for treatment of colorectal cancer patients is in clinical testing. For lung cancer, only one Phase 1 clinical trial focused on dendritic cell-derived exosome-based vaccination has been conducted. The study was completed in 2018 and study results are not yet available. Thus, advancing EV-based cancer therapy to the clinic has been slow. However, continued progress in the EV field will result in the testing of a larger number of EV-based cancer therapeutics in the clinic over the next few years.

ACKNOWLEDGEMENTS

This study was supported by grants received from National Institutes of Health (NIH; R01 CA167516, R01 CA233201, R01 CA254192); a Merit Grant (101BX003420A1)

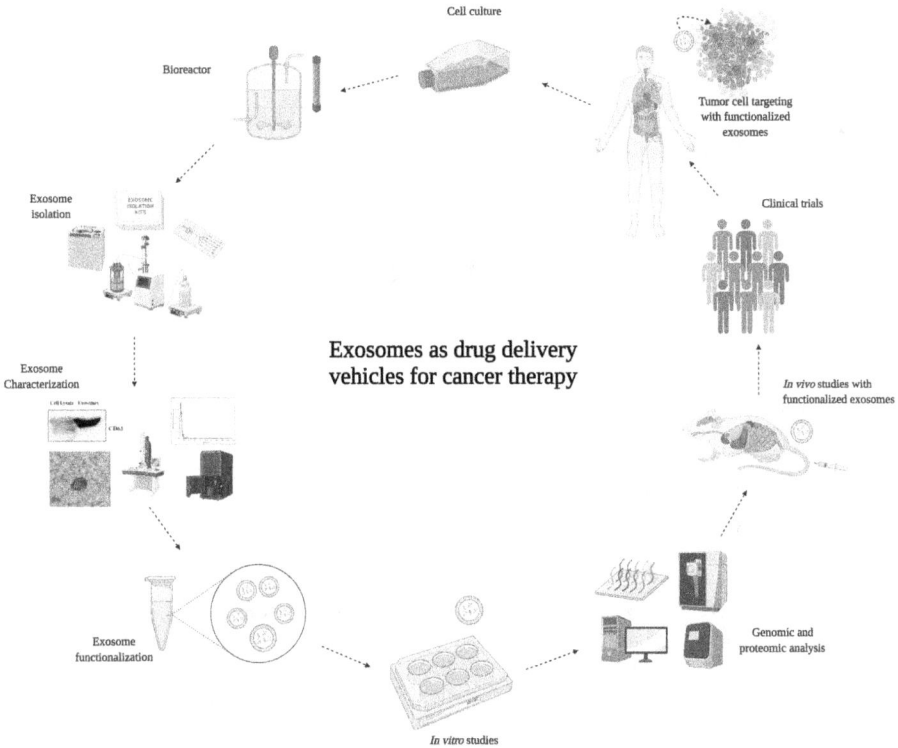

FIGURE 16.5 Schematic shows the numerous physical, biological, and functional characterization and optimization steps required for advancing exosomes-based drug delivery for cancer treatment to the clinic. The example shown is for lung cancer but similar steps are required for using exosomes as drug carrier in other cancer indications.

from the Department of Veterans Affairs; a Team Science Grant and a Pilot Grant funded by the National Cancer Institute Cancer Center Support Grant P30CA225520 awarded to the University of Oklahoma Stephenson Cancer Center; from the Department of Defense through the Lung Cancer Research Program (LCRP) under award no. W81XWH-19-1-0647; a grant (HR18-088) from the Oklahoma Center for Advanced Science and Technology (OCAST); a Team Science Grant, a Seed Grant and a Bridge Grant received from the Presbyterian Health Foundation (PHF); and funds received from the Jim and Christy Everest Endowed Chair in Cancer Developmental Therapeutics.

Rajagopal Ramesh is an Oklahoma TSET Research Scholar and holds the Jim and Christy Everest Endowed Chair in Cancer Developmental Therapeutics.

The content presented is solely the responsibility of the authors. The opinions, interpretations, conclusions and recommendations are those of the author and not necessarily endorsed by or representative of the official views of NIH, DOD, Department of Veterans Affairs, OCAST, or PHF.

CONFLICT OF INTEREST

The authors report no conflict of interest in this work.

REFERENCES

1. American Cancer Society. *Cancer facts and figures 2022*. Atlanta: American Cancer Society; 1–77, 2022.
2. Greenlee R, Murray T, Bolden S, Wingo PA. Cancer statistics, 2000. *CA Cancer J Clin* 50(1):7–33, 2000.
3. Travis W, Travis LB, Devesa SS. Lung cancer incidence and survival by histologic type. *Cancer* 75:191–202, 1995.
4. Mountain CF, Lukeman JM, Hammar SP, Chamberlain DW, Coulson WF, Page DL, Victor TA, Weiland LH. Lung cancer classification: The relationship of disease extent and cell type to survival in a clinical trials population. *J Surg Oncol* 35(3):147–156, 1987.
5. Pao W, Miller VA. Epidermal growth factor receptor mutations, small-molecule kinase inhibitors,and non-small-cell lung cancer: Current knowledge and future directions. *J Clin Oncol* 23(11):2556–2568, 2005.
6. Paez JG, Janne PA, Lee JC, Tracy S, Greulich H, Gabriel S, Herman P, Kaye FJ, Lindeman N, Boggon TJ, Naoki K, Sasaki H, Fujii Y, Eck MJ, Sellers WR, Johnson BE, Meyerson M. EGFR mutations in lung cancer: Correlation with clinical response to gefitinib therapy. *Science* 304(5676):1497–1500, 2004.
7. Siegel RL, Miller KD, Fuchs HE, Jemal A. Cancer statistics, 2022. *CA Cancer J Clin* 72(1):7–33, 2022.
8. Atmaca A, Al-Batran SE, Werner D, Pauligk C, Güner T, Koepke A, Bernhard H, Wenzel T, Banat AG, Brueck P, Caca K, Prasnikar N, Kullmann F, Günther Derigs H, Koenigsmann M, Dingeldein G, Neuhaus T, Jäger E. A randomised multicentre phase II study with cisplatin/docetaxel vs oxaliplatin/docetaxel as first-line therapy in patients with advanced or metastatic non-small cell lung cancer. *Br J Cancer* 108(2):265–270, 2013.
9. Gridelli C, Bennouna J, de Castro J, Dingemans AM, Griesinger F, Grossi F, Rossi A, Thatcher N, Wong EK, Langer C. Randomized phase IIIb trial evaluating the continuation of bevacizumab beyond disease progression in patients with advanced non-squamous non-small-cell lung cancer after first-line treatment with bevacizumab plus platinum-based chemotherapy: Treatment rationale and protocol dynamics of the AvaALL (MO22097) trial. *Clin Lung Cancer* 12(6):407–411, 2011.
10. Spigel DR, Hainsworth JD, Shipley DL, Ervin TJ, Kohler PC, Lubiner ET, Peyton JD, Waterhouse DM, Burris HA 3rd, Greco FA. A randomized phase II trial of pemetrexed/gemcitabine/bevacizumab or pemetrexed/carboplatin/bevacizumab in the first-line treatment of elderly patients with advanced non-small cell lung cancer. *J Thorac Oncol* 7(1):196–202, 2012.
11. Shanker M, Willcuts D, Roth JA, Ramesh R. Drug resistance in lung cancer. *Lung Cancer Targets Ther* 1:1–14, 2010.
12. Knipp M. Metallothioneins and platinum (II) *Anti-tumor compounds*. *Curr Med Chem* 16(5):522–537, 2009.
13. Srivastava AK, Han C, Zhao R, Cui T, Dai Y, Mao C, Zhao W, Zhang X, Yu J, Wang QE. Enhanced expression of DNA polymerase eta contributes to cisplatin resistance of ovarian cancer stem cells. *Proc Natl Acad Sci U S A* 112(14):4411–4416, 2015.

14. Chabner BA, Roberts TG, Jr. Timeline: Chemotherapy and the war on cancer. *Nat Rev Cancer* 5(1):65–72, 2005.

15. Zabernigg A, Gamper EM, Giesinger JM, Rumpold G, Kemmler G, Gattringer K, Sperner-Unterweger B, Holzner B. Taste alterations in cancer patients receiving chemotherapy: A neglected side effect? *Oncologist* 15(8):913–920, 2010.

16. McWhinney SR, Goldberg RM, McLeod HL. Platinum neurotoxicity pharmacogenetics. *Mol Cancer Ther* 8(1):10–16, 2009.

17. Pirollo KF, Rait A, Zhou Q, Hwang SH, Dagata JA, Zon G, Hogrefe RI, Palchik G, Chang EH. Materializing the potential of small interfering RNA via a tumor-targeting nanodelivery system. *Cancer Res* 67(7):2938–2943, 2007.

18. Ma Z, Zhang J, Alber S, Dileo J, Negishi Y, Stolz D, Watkins S, Huang L, Pitt B, Li S. Lipid-mediated delivery of oligonucleotide to pulmonary endothelium. *Am J Respir Cell Mol Biol* 27(2):151–159, 2002.

19. Wang Z, Chui WK, Ho PC. Nanoparticulate delivery system targeted to tumor neovasculature for combined anticancer and antiangiogenesis therapy. *Pharm Res* 28(3):585–596, 2011.

20. Laverman P, Carstens MG, Storm G, Moghimi SM. Biochim recognition and clearance of methoxypoly(ethyleneglycol)2000-grafted liposomes by macrophages with enhanced phagocytic capacity. Implications in experimental and clinical oncology. *Biophys Acta* 1526:227–229, 2001.

21. Manjunath K, Venkateswarlu V. Pharmacokinetics, tissue distribution and bioavailability of clozapine solid lipid nanoparticles after intravenous and intraduodenal administration. *J Control Release* 107(2):215–228, 2005.

22. Huang M, Wu W, Qian J, Wan DJ, Wei XL, Zhu JH. Body distribution and in situ evading of phagocytic uptake by macrophages of long-circulating poly (ethylene glycol) cyanoacrylate-co-n-hexadecyl cyanoacrylate nanoparticles. *Acta Pharmacol Sin* 26(12):1512–1518, 2005.

23. Kettiger H, Schipanski A, Wick P, Huwyler J. Engineered nanomaterial uptake and tissue distribution: From cell to organism. *Int J Nanomedicine* 8:3255–3269, 2013.

24. Dams ET, Laverman P, Oyen WJ, Storm G, Scherphof GL, van Der Meer JW, Corstens FH, Boerman OC. Accelerated blood clearance and altered biodistribution of repeated injections of sterically stabilized liposomes. *J Pharmacol Exp Ther* 292(3):1071–1079, 2000.

25. Ishida T, Kashima S, Kiwada H. The contribution of phagocytic activity of liver macrophages to the accelerated blood clearance (ABC) phenomenon of PEGylated liposomes in rats. *J Control Release* 126(2):162–165, 2008.

26. Corbo C, Molinaro R, Parodi A, Toledano Furman NE, Salvatore F, Tasciotti E. The impact of nanoparticle protein corona on cytotoxicity, immunotoxicity and target drug delivery. *Nanomedicine (Lond)* 11(1):81–100, 2016.

27. Cheng X, Tian X, Wu A, Li J, Tian J, Chong Y, Chai Z, Zhao Y, Chen C, Ge C. Protein corona influences cellular uptake of gold nanoparticles by phagocytic and nonphagocytic cells in a size-dependent manner. *ACS Appl Mater Interfaces* 7(37):20568–20575, 2015.

28. Lesniak A, Fenaroli F, Monopoli MP, Åberg C, Dawson KA, Salvati A. Effects of the presence or absence of a protein corona on silica nanoparticle uptake and impact on cells. *ACS Nano* 6(7):5845–5857, 2012.

29. Armstrong JK, Hempel G, Koling S, Chan LS, Fisher T, Meiselman HJ, Garratty G. Antibody against poly(ethylene glycol) adversely affects PEG-asparaginase therapy in acute lymphoblastic leukemia patients. *Cancer* 110(1):103–111, 2007.

30. Verhoef JJ, Carpenter JF, Anchordoquy TJ, Schellekens H. Potential induction of anti-PEG antibodies and complement activation toward PEGylated therapeutics. *Drug Discov Today* 19(12):1945–1952, 2014.

31. Gregoriadis G, Mccormack B, Wang Z, Lifely R. Polysialic acids: Potential in drug delivery. *FEBS Lett* 315(3):271–276, 1993.

32. Fernandes AI, Gregoriadis G. The effect of polysialylation on the immunogenicity and antigenicity of asparaginase: Implication in its pharmacokinetics. *Int J Pharm* 217(1–2):215–224, 2001.
33. Mohamed BM, Verma NK, Davies AM, McGowan A, Crosbie-Staunton K, Prina-Mello A, Kelleher D, Botting CH, Causey CP, Thompson PR, Pruijn GJ, Kisin ER, Tkach AV, Shvedova AA, Volkov Y. Citrullination of proteins: A common post-translational modification pathway induced by different nanoparticles in vitro and in vivo. *Nanomedicine (Lond)* 7(8):1181–1195, 2012.
34. Srivastava A, Amreddy N, Pareek V, Chinnappan M, Ahmed R, Mehta M, Razaq M, Munshi A, Ramesh R. Progress in extracellular vesicle biology and their application in cancer medicine. *Wiley Interdiscip Rev Nanomed Nanobiotechnol* 12(4):e1621, 2020.
35. Srivastava A, Rathore S, Munshi A, Ramesh R. Organically derived exosomes as carriers of anticancer drugs and imaging agents for cancer treatment. *Semin Cancer Biol* S1044-579X(22)00047-5, 2022. https://doi.org/10.1016/j.semcancer.2022.02.020 (online ahead of print)
36. Abels ER, Breakefield XO. Introduction to extracellular vesicles: Biogenesis, RNA cargo selection, content, release, and uptake. *Cell Mol Neurobiol* 36(3):301–312, 2016.
37. Thery C, Witwer KW, Aikawa E, Alcaraz MJ, Anderson JD, Andriantsitohaina R, et al. Minimal information for studies of extracellular vesicles 2018 (MISEV2018): A position statement of the international society for extracellular vesicles and update of the MISEV2014 guidelines. *J Extracell Vesicles* 7:1535750, 2018.
38. Kourembanas S. Exosomes: Vehicles of intercellular signaling, biomarkers, and vectors of cell therapy. *Annu Rev Physiol* 77:13–27, 2015.
39. Théry C, Zitvogel L, Amigorena S. Exosomes: Composition, biogenesis and function. *Nat Rev Immunol* 2(8):569–579, 2002.
40. Chinnappan M, Srivastava A, Amreddy N, Razaq M, Pareek V, Ahmed R, Peterson JE, Mehta M, Munshi A, Ramesh R. Exosomes as a drug delivery vehicle and contributor to treatment resistance. *Cancer Lett* 486:18–28, 2020.
41. Emelyanov A, Shtam T, Kamyshinsky R, Garaeva L, Verlov N, Miliukhina I, Kudrevatykh A, Gavrilov G, Zabrodskaya Y, Pchelina S, Konevega A. Cryo-electron microscopy of extracellular vesicles from cerebrospinal fluid. *PLoS One* 15(1):e0227949, 2020.
42. Andre F, Schartz NE, Movassagh M, Flament C, Pautier P, Morice P, Pomel C, Lhomme C, Escudier B, Le Chevalier T, Tursz T, Amigorena S, Raposo G, Angevin E, Zitvogel L. Malignant effusions and immunogenic tumour-derived exosomes. *Lancet* 360(9329):295–230, 2002.
43. Li XB, Zhang ZR, Schluesener HJ, Xu SQ. Role of exosomes in immune regulation. *J Cell Mol Med* 10(2):364–375, 2006.
44. Zitvogel L, Regnault A, Lozier A, Wolfers J, Flament C, Tenza D, Ricciardi-Castagnoli P, Raposo G, Amigorena S. Eradication of established murine tumors using a novel cell-free vaccine: Dendritic cell-derived exosomes. *Nat Med* 4(5):594–600, 1998.
45. Dai S, Wei D, Wu Z, Zhou X, Wei X, Huang H, Li G. Phase I clinical trial of autologous ascites-derived exosomes combined with GM-CSF for colorectal cancer. *Mol Ther* 16(4):782–790, 2008.
46. Srivastava A, Filant J, Moxley KM, Sood A, McMeekin S, Ramesh R. Exosomes: A role for naturally occurring nanovesicles in cancer growth, diagnosis and treatment. *Curr Gene Ther* 15(2):182–192, 2015.
47. Hemler ME. Tetraspanin proteins mediate cellular penetration, invasion, and fusion events and define a novel type of membrane microdomain. *Annu Rev Cell Dev Biol* 19:397–422, 2003.
48. Srivastava A, Babu A, Filant J, Moxley KM, Ruskin R, Dhanasekaran D, Sood A, McMeekin S, Ramesh R. Exploitation of exosomes as nanocarriers for gene-, drug-, and immune-therapy of cancer. *J Biomed Nanotechnol* 12:1174–1182, 2016.

49. Kooijmans SA, Vader P, van Dommelen SM, van Solinge WW, Schiffelers RM. Exosome mimetics: A novel class of drug delivery systems. *Int J Nanomedicine* 7:1525–1541, 2012.
50. Hoo JL, Wickline SA. A systematic approach to exosome-based translational medicine. *Wires Nanomed Nanobiotechnol* 4(4):458–467, 2012.
51. Alvarez-Erviti L, Seow Y, Yin H, Betts C, Lakhal S, Wood MJ. Delivery of siRNA to the mouse brain by systemic injection of targeted exosomes. *Nat Biotechnol* 29(4):341–345, 2011.
52. Momen-Heravi F, Bala S, Bukong T, Szabo G. Exosome-mediated delivery of functionally active miRNA-155 inhibitor to macrophages. *Nanomedicine* 10(7):1517–1527, 2014.
53. Ohno SI, Takanashi M, Sudo K, Ueda S, Ishikawa A, Matsuyama N, Fujita K, Mizutani T, Ohgi T, Ochiya T, Gotoh N, Kuroda M. Systemically injected exosomes targeted to EGFR deliver antitumor microRNA to breast cancer cells. *Mol Ther* 2:185–191, 2012.
54. O'Brien KP, Khan S, Gilligan KE, Zafar H, Lalor P, Glynn C, O'Flatharta C, Ingoldsby H, Dockery P, De Bhulbh A, Schweber JR, St John K, Leahy M, Murphy JM, Gallagher WM, O'Brien T, Kerin MJ, Dwyer RM. Employing mesenchymal stem cells to support tumor-targeted delivery of extracellular vesicle (EV)-encapsulated microRNA-379. *Oncogene* 37(16):2137–2149, 2018.
55. Qiao L, Hu S, Huang K, Su T, Li Z, Vandergriff A, Cores J, Dinh PU, Allen T, Shen D, Liang H, Li Y, Cheng K. Tumor cell-derived exosomes home to their cells of origin and can be used as Trojan horses to deliver cancer drugs. *Theranostics* 10(8):3474–3487, 2020.
56. Heath N, Osteikoetxea X, de Oliveria TM, Lázaro-Ibáñez E, Shatnyeva O, Schindler C, Tigue N, Mayr LM, Dekker N, Overman R, Davies R. Endosomal escape enhancing compounds facilitate functional delivery of extracellular vesicle cargo. *Nanomedicine (Lond)* 14(21):2799–2814, 2019.
57. Smyth TJ, Redzic JS, Graner MW, Anchordoquy TJ. Examination of the specificity of tumor cell derived exosomes with tumor cells in vitro. *Biochim Biophys Acta* 1838(11):2954–2965, 2014.
58. Figueroa J, Phillips LM, Shahar T, Hossain A, Gumin J, Kim H, Bean AJ, Calin GA, Fueyo J, Walters ET, Kalluri R, Verhaak RG, Lang FF. Exosomes from glioma-associated mesenchymal stem cells increase the tumorigenicity of glioma stem-like cells via Transfer of miR-1587. *Cancer Res* 77(21):5808–5819, 2017.
59. Bourkoula E, Mangoni D, Ius T, Pucer A, Isola M, Musiello D, Marzinotto S, Toffoletto B, Sorrentino M, Palma A, Caponnetto F, Gregoraci G, Vindigni M, Pizzolitto S, Falconieri G, De Maglio G, Pecile V, Ruaro ME, Gri G, Parisse P, Casalis L, Scoles G, Skrap M, Beltrami CA, Beltrami AP, Cesselli D. Glioma-associated stem cells: A novel class of tumor-supporting cells able to predict prognosis of human low-grade gliomas. *Stem Cells* 32(5):1239–1253, 2014.
60. Ringuette Goulet C, Bernard G, Tremblay S, Chabaud S, Bolduc S, Pouliot F. Exosomes induce fibroblast differentiation into cancer-associated fibroblasts through TGFβ signaling. *Mol Cancer Res* 16(7):1196–1204, 2018.
61. Tai YL, Chen KC, Hsieh JT, Shen TL. Exosomes in cancer development and clinical applications. *Cancer Sci* 109(8):2364–2374, 2018.
62. Srivastava A, Amreddy N, Babu A, Panneerselvam J, Mehta M, Muralidharan R, Chen A, Zhao YD, Razaq M, Riedinger N, Kim H, Liu S, Wu S, Abdel-Mageed AB, Munshi A, Ramesh R. Nanosomes carrying doxorubicin exhibit potent anticancer activity against human lung cancer cells. *Sci Rep* 6:38541, 2016. 10.1038/srep38541.
63. Yim N, Ryu SW, Choi K, Lee KR, Lee S, Choi H, Kim J, Shaker MR, Sun W, Park JH, Kim D, Heo WD, Choi C. Exosome engineering for efficient intracellular delivery of soluble proteins using optically reversible protein-protein interaction module. *Nat Commun* 7:12277, 2016.
64. Kim MS, Haney MJ, Zhao Y, Mahajan V, Deygen I, Klyachko NL, Inskoe E, Piroyan A, Sokolsky M, Okolie O, Hingtgen SD, Kabanov AV, Batrakova EV. Development of exosome-encapsulated paclitaxel to overcome MDR in cancer cells. *Nanomedicine* 12(3):655–664, 2016.

65. Kim MS, Haney MJ, Zhao Y, Yuan D, Deygen I, Klyachko NL, Kabanov AV, Batrakova EV. Engineering macrophage-derived exosomes for targeted paclitaxel delivery to pulmonary metastases: In vitro and in vivo evaluations. *Nanomedicine* 14(1):195–204, 2018.
66. Agrawal AK, Aqil F, Jeyabalan J, Spencer WA, Beck J, Gachuki BW, Alhakeem SS, Oben K, Munagala R, Bondada S, Gupta RC. Milk-derived exosomes for oral delivery of paclitaxel. *Nanomedicine* 13(5):1627–1636, 2017.
67. Tian Y, Li S, Song J, Ji T, Zhu M, Anderson GJ, Wei J, Nie G. A doxorubicin delivery platform using engineered natural membrane vesicle exosomes for targeted tumor therapy. *Biomaterials* 35(7):2383–2390, 2014.
68. Kamerkar S, LeBleu VS, Sugimoto H, Yang S, Ruivo CF, Melo SA, Lee JJ, Kalluri R. Exosomes facilitate therapeutic targeting of oncogenic KRAS in pancreatic cancer. *Nature* 546(7659):498–503, 2017.
69. Roma-Rodrigues C, Pereira F, Alves de Matos AP, Fernandes M, Baptista PV, Fernandes AR. Smuggling gold nanoparticles across cell types - A new role for exosomes in gene silencing. *Nanomed Nanotechnol Biol Med* 13(4):1389–1398, 2017.
70. He C, Zheng S, Luo Y, Wang B. Exosome theranostic: Biology and translational medicine. *Theranostics* 8(1):237–255, 2018.
71. Cai S, Shi GS, Cheng HY, Zeng YN, Li G, Zhang M, Song M, Zhou PK, Tian Y, Cui FM, Chen Q. Exosomal miR-7 mediates bystander autophagy in lung after focal brain irradiation in mice. *Int J Biol Sci* 13(10):1287–1296, 2017.
72. Xu S, Wang J, Ding N, Hu W, Zhang X, Wang B, Hua J, Wei W, Zhu Q. Exosome-mediated microRNA transfer plays a role in radiation-induced bystander effect. *RNA Biol* 12(12):1355–1363, 2015.
73. Qi H, Liu C, Long L, Ren Y, Zhang S, Chang X, Qian X, Jia H, Zhao J, Sun J, Hou X, Yuan X, Kang C. Blood exosomes endowed with magnetic and targeting properties for cancer therapy. *ACS Nano* 10(3):3323–3333, 2016.
74. Tian T, Zhang HX, He CP, Fan S, Zhu YL, Qi C, Huang NP, Xiao ZD, Lu ZH, Tannous BA, Gao J. Surface functionalized exosomes as targeted drug delivery vehicles for cerebral ischemia therapy. *Biomaterials* 150:137–149, 2018.
75. Gilligan KE, Dwyer RM. Extracellular vesicles for cancer therapy: Impact of host immune response. *Cells* 9(1):224, 2020.
76. Zhu X, Badawi M, Pomeroy S, Sutaria DS, Xie Z, Baek A, Jiang J, Elgamal OA, Mo X, Perle K, Chalmers J, Schmittgen TD, Phelps MA. Comprehensive toxicity and immunogenicity studies reveal minimal effects in mice following sustained dosing of extracellular vesicles derived from HEK293T cells. *J Extracell Vesicles* 6(1):1324730, 2017.
77. Gehrmann U, Näslund TI, Hiltbrunner S, Larssen P, Gabrielsson S. Harnessing the exosome-induced immune response for cancer immunotherapy. *Semin Cancer Biol* 28:58–67, 2014.
78. Morse MA, Garst J, Osada T, Khan S, Hobeika A, Clay TM, Valente N, Shreeniwas R, Sutton MA, Delcayre A, Hsu DH, Le Pecq JB, Lyerly HK. A phase I study of dexosome immunotherapy in patients with advanced non-small cell lung cancer. *J Transl Med* 3(1):9, 2005.
79. Besse B, Charrier M, Lapierre V, Dansin E, Lantz O, Planchard D, Le Chevalier T, Livartoski A, Barlesi F, Laplanche A, Ploix S, Vimond N, Peguillet I, Théry C, Lacroix L, Zoernig I, Dhodapkar K, Dhodapkar M, Viaud S, Soria JC, Reiners KS, Pogge von Strandmann E, Vély F, Rusakiewicz S, Eggermont A, Pitt JM, Zitvogel L, Chaput N. Dendritic cell-derived exosomes as maintenance immunotherapy after first line chemotherapy in NSCLC. *Oncoimmunology* 5(4):e1071008, 2015.
80. Dai S, Wei D, Wu Z, Zhou X, Wei X, Huang H, Li G. Phase I clinical trial of autologous ascites-derived exosomes combined with GM-CSF for colorectal cancer. *Mol Ther* 16(4):782–790, 2008.
81. Escudier B, Dorval T, Chaput N, André F, Caby MP, Novault S, Flament C, Leboulaire C, Borg C, Amigorena S, Boccaccio C, Bonnerot C, Dhellin O, Movassagh M, Piperno S, Robert C, Serra V, Valente N, Le Pecq JB, Spatz A, Lantz O, Tursz T, Angevin E,

Zitvogel L. Vaccination of metastatic melanoma patients with autologous dendritic cell (DC) derived-exosomes: Results of thefirst phase I clinical trial. *J Transl Med.* 3(1):10, 2005. https://doi.org/10.1186/1479-5876-3-10.

82. Hiltbrunner S, Larssen P, Eldh M, Martinez-Bravo MJ, Wagner AK, Karlsson MC, Gabrielsson S. Exosomal cancer immunotherapy is independent of MHC molecules on exosomes. *Oncotarget* 7(25):38707–38717, 2016.

83. Larssen P, Veerman RE, Akpinar GG, Hiltbrunner S, Karlsson MCI, Gabrielsson S. Allogenicity boosts extracellular vesicle-induced antigen-specific immunity and mediates tumor protection and long-term memory in vivo. *J Immunol* 203(4):825–834, 2019.

84. Mendt M, Kamerkar S, Sugimoto H, McAndrews KM, Wu CC, Gagea M, Yang S, Blanko EVR, Peng Q, Ma X, Marszalek JR, Maitra A, Yee C, Rezvani K, Shpall E, LeBleu VS, Kalluri R. Generation and testing of clinical-grade exosomes for pancreatic cancer. *JCI Insight* 3(8):e99263, 2018.

85. Näslund TI, Gehrmann U, Gabrielsson S. Cancer immunotherapy with exosomes requires B-cell activation. *Oncoimmunology* 2(6):e24533, 2013.

86. Näslund TI, Gehrmann U, Qazi KR, Karlsson MC, Gabrielsson S. Dendritic cell-derived exosomes need to activate both T and B cells to induce antitumor immunity. *J Immunol* 190(6):2712–2719, 2013.

87. Lu Z, Zuo B, Jing R, Gao X, Rao Q, Liu Z, Qi H, Guo H, Yin H. Dendritic cell-derived exosomes elicit tumor regression in autochthonous hepatocellular carcinoma mouse models. *J Hepatol* 67(4):739–748, 2017.

88. Aqil F, Kausar H, Agrawal AK, Jeyabalan J, Kyakulaga AH, Munagala R, Gupta R. Exosomal formulation enhances therapeutic response of celastrol against lung cancer. *Exp Mol Pathol* 101(1):12–21, 2016.

89. Aqil F, Munagala R, Jeyabalan J, Agrawal AK, Kyakulaga AH, Wilcher SA, Gupta RC. Milk exosomes - Natural nanoparticles for siRNA delivery. *Cancer Lett* 449:186–195, 2019.

90. Wang Y, Guo M, Lin D, Liang D, Zhao L, Zhao R, Wang Y. Docetaxel-loaded exosomes for targeting non-small cell lung cancer: Preparation and evaluation *in vitro* and *in vivo*. *Drug Deliv* 28(1):1510–1523, 2021.

91. Nie H, Xie X, Zhang D, Zhou Y, Li B, Li F, Li F, Cheng Y, Mei H, Meng H, Jia L. Use of lung-specific exosomes for miRNA-126 delivery in non-small cell lung cancer. *Nanoscale* 12(2):877–887, 2020.

92. Hao D, Li Y, Zhao G, Zhang M. Soluble fms-like tyrosine kinase-1-enriched exosomes suppress the growth of small cell lung cancer by inhibiting endothelial cell migration. *Thorac Cancer* 10(10):1962–1972, 2019.

93. Jeong K, Yu YJ, You JY, Rhee WJ, Kim JA. Exosome-mediated microRNA-497 delivery for anti-cancer therapy in a microfluidic 3D lung cancer model. *Lab Chip* 20(3):548–557, 2020.

94. Wu H, Mu X, Liu L, Wu H, Hu X, Chen L, Liu J, Mu Y, Yuan F, Liu W, Zhao Y. Bone marrow mesenchymal stem cells-derived exosomal microRNA-193a reduces cisplatin resistance of non-small cell lung cancer cells via targeting LRRC1. *Cell Death Dis* 11(9):801, 2020.

95. Zhou Y, Yuan Y, Liu M, Hu X, Quan Y, Chen X. Tumor-specific delivery of KRAS siRNA with iRGD-exosomes efficiently inhibits tumor growth. *ExRNA* 1(1):28, 2019.

96. Karachaliou N, Rosell R, Viteri S. The role of SOX2 in small cell lung cancer, lung adenocarcinoma and squamous cell carcinoma of the lung. *Transl Lung Cancer Res* 2(3):172–179, 2013.

97. Takeda K, Mizushima T, Yokoyama Y, Hirose H, Wu X, Qian Y, Ikehata K, Miyoshi N, Takahashi H, Haraguchi N, Hata T, Matsuda C, Doki Y, Mori M, Yamamoto H. Sox2 is associated with cancer stem-like properties in colorectal cancer. *Sci Rep* 8(1):17639, 2018.

98. Bai J, Duan J, Liu R, Du Y, Luo Q, Cui Y, Su Z, Xu J, Xie Y, Lu W. Engineered targeting tLyp-1 exosomes as gene therapy vectors for efficient delivery of siRNA into lung cancer cells. *Asian J Pharm Sci* 15(4):461–471, 2020.

99. Zhou W, Xu M, Wang Z, Yang M. Engineered exosomes loaded with miR-449a selectively inhibit the growth of homologous non-small cell lung cancer. *Cancer Cell Int* 21(1):485, 2021.

100. Li Z, Yang L, Wang H, Binzel DW, Williams TM, Guo P. Non-small-cell lung cancer regression by siRNA delivered through exosomes that display EGFR RNA aptamer. *Nucleic Acid Ther* 31(5):364–374, 2021.

101. Zhou C, Zhu Y, Lu B, Zhao W, Zhao X. Survivin expression modulates the sensitivity of A549 lung cancer cells resistance to vincristine. *Oncol Lett* 16(4):5466–5472, 2018.

102. Kelly RJ, Lopez-Chavez A, Citrin D, Janik JE, Morris JC. Impacting tumor cell-fate by targeting the inhibitor of apoptosis protein survivin. *Mol Cancer* 10:35, 2011.

103. Lee JH, Choi JW. Application of plasmonic gold nanoparticle for drug delivery system. *Curr Drug Targets* 19(3):271–278, 2018.

104. Daraee H, Eatemadi A, Abbasi E, Fekri Aval S, Kouhi M, Akbarzadeh A. Application of gold nanoparticles in biomedical and drug delivery. *Artif Cells Nanomed Biotechnol* 44(1):410–422, 2016.

105. Li X, Corbett AL, Taatizadeh E, Tasnim N, Little JP, Garnis C, Daugaard M, Guns E, Hoorfar M, Li ITS. Challenges and opportunities in exosome research-perspectives from biology, engineering, and cancer therapy. *APL Bioeng* 3(1):011503, 2019.

106. Hidalgo M, Amant F, Biankin AV, Budinská E, Byrne AT, Caldas C, Clarke RB, de Jong S, Jonkers J, Mælandsmo GM, Roman-Roman S, Seoane J, Trusolino L, Villanueva A. Patient-derived xenograft models: An emerging platform for translational cancer research. *Cancer Discov* 4(9):998–1013, 2014.

107. Lin MT, Tseng LH, Kamiyama H, Kamiyama M, Lim P, Hidalgo M, Wheelan S, Eshleman J. Quantifying the relative amount of mouse and human DNA in cancer xenografts using species-specific variation in gene length. *BioTechniques* 48(3):211–218, 2010.

Index

A

A549 cells, 70, 97, 325, 326, 330, 331, 334, 362
AAT, *see* Alpha(1)-antitrypsin
ABB, *see* Airway-to-blood barrier
ABC, *see* ATP-binding cassette superfamily
ABPA, *see* Allergic bronchopulmonary
        aspergillosis
Absorption mechanism, 68
Absorption number, 33
ACI, *see* Anderson Cascade Impactor
Active pharmaceutical ingredients (APIs), 63, 152,
        206, 214, 372, 384
Adenocarcinoma, 240
Adenosine Triphosphate (ATP), 66
Advair® Diskus® (GlaxoSmithKline), 171
Aerodynamic diameter, 192, 208
Aerodynamic particle size distributions (APSD), 65
Aerodynamic size, 192
Aerolizer, 225
Aerosol-based delivery systems, 153–154
Aerosol deposition mechanisms
        diffusion, 460–461
        electrostatic precipitation, 461–462
        impaction (inertial deposition), 459
        interception, 461
        sedimentation (gravitational deposition),
                459–460
Aerosol drug delivery devices, 243–244
Aerosolized pulmonary delivery, 152
Aerosols, 20, 206
AFM, *see* Atomic force microscopy
AFM-based techniques, 223–224
AFM-infrared spectroscopy (AFM-IR), 224
Afrezza®, 53, 202
AgNPs, *see* Silver nanoparticles
Air jet milling, 164
Air-liquid-interface (ALI) model, 60, 69, 70, 86–87
AIR® technology, 210, 211
Airway
        conducting zones, 407–408
        inhaled particle transport, experimental
                models, 468–470
        respiratory zones, 407–408
        segments, 349
Airway epithelium, 456–457
Airway geometry, 9–10, 58

idealized extrathoracic geometries, 12–13
realistic extrathoracic geometries, 10–12
semi-realistic extrathoracic geometries, 10–12
in vitro measures of thoracic deposition, 13–14
Airway inflammatory diseases, 95
Airway surface liquid (ASL), 29, 31, 32, 34
Airway-to-blood barrier (ABB), 67, 68
Akita® Jet nebulizer, 442
Alberta Idealized Nasal Inlet, 13
Alberta Idealized Throat, 12, 22, 23
Albumin nanoparticles, 246, 360
ALI, *see* Air-liquid-interface
Alidornase alfa (PRX-110), 474
Allergic bronchopulmonary aspergillosis
        (ABPA), 285
Alpha(1)-antitrypsin (AAT), 474
Alveolar clearance mechanism, 51
Alveolar epithelium, 457–458
Alveolar interstitium, 111–112
Alveolar macrophages (AM), 457, 458
ALX-009, 474
ALX-0171, 473
AM, *see* Alveolar macrophages
Amino acid-based surface engineering, 360–362
Ammonium bicarbonate (ABC), 193
Amorphous solid dispersions (ASDs), 274, 291
Anderson Cascade Impactor (ACI), 22, 59, 363
Angiotensin converting enzyme receptor 2
        (ACE-2), 103
Antisolvent precipitation technique, 171
APIs, *see* Active pharmaceutical ingredients
Apparent permeation coefficient (P_a), 68
Apparent permeation flux (J_a), 68
APSD, *see* Aerodynamic particle size distributions
Area under the curve (AUC), 197
Aridol/Osmohale, 395
ASDs, *see* Amorphous solid dispersions
ASL, *see* Airway surface liquid
Aspartame particles, 192
Asprihale®, 413
Atomic force microscopy (AFM), 129–130,
        154, 220
ATP-binding cassette (ABC) superfamily, 66
AUC, *see* Area under the curve
AuNPs, *see* Gold nanoparticles
Autoradiographic visualization, 53
Azmacort®, 48

507

For Product Safety Concerns and Information please contact our EU
representative GPSR@taylorandfrancis.com
Taylor & Francis Verlag GmbH, Kaufingerstraße 24, 80331 München, Germany